D1331742

A full understanding of the developmental processes in individuals requires contributions from disciplines including developmental biology and psychology, physiology, neuropsychology, social psychology, sociology and anthropology. This ambitious and wide-ranging book is an attempt to present the findings from these and related areas to motivate a holistic view of human development from conception to death.

Distinguished scientists have combined their expertise in a synthesis of biological and social science that will demand the attention of all researchers and practitioners concerned with human development across the lifespan. Based on a Nobel symposium, the topics discussed range from the function and development of single cells to the whole organism interacting with its environment.

Drawing upon new theories and models, including the study of non-linear dynamic systems and chaos theory, this book represents a major step in the move towards an integrated science of human development.

The lifespan development of individuals: behavioral, neurobiological, and psychosocial perspectives

The lifespan development of individuals: behavioral, neurobiological, and psychosocial perspectives

A Synthesis

Edited by

DAVID MAGNUSSON
Stockholm University

in collaboration with

TORGNY GREITZ
Karolinska Hospital, Stockholm

TOMAS HÖKFELT
Karolinska Institute, Stockholm

LARS-GÖRAN NILSSON
Stockholm University

LARS TERENIUS
Karolinska Institute, Stockholm

BENGT WINBLAD
Karolinska Institute, Huddinge

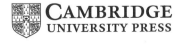

CAMBRIDGE
UNIVERSITY PRESS

Published by the Press Syndicate of the University of Cambridge
The Pitt Building, Trumpington Street, Cambridge CB2 1RP
40 West 20th Street, New York, NY 10011–4211, USA
10 Stamford Road, Oakleigh, Melbourne 3166, Australia

© Cambridge University Press 1996

First published 1996
Reprinted 1997
First paperback edition 1997

Printed in the United States of America

Library of Congress cataloging in publication data

The lifespan development of individuals: behavioral, neurobiological,
  and psychosocial perspectives: a synthesis / edited by David
  Magnusson, in collaboration with Torgny Greitz . . . [et al.].
      p. cm.
    Papers presented at a symposium, held at Södergarn Conference
  Center, Stockholm, June 1994.
    ISBN 0-521-47023-4 (hc)
      1. Developmental psychology — Congresses.   2. Developmental
  biology — Congresses.   3. Developmental neurophysiology — Congresses.
  I. Magnusson, David.
  BF713.5.L524   1996
  155 — dc20   95-13924
                                                                   CIP

A catalog record for this book is available from the British Library

ISBN 0-521-47023-4 Hardback
ISBN 0-521-62896-2 Paperback

Contents

Contributors to this volume

Tim Andrews
Department of Neurobiology, Duke University Medical Center, Durham, North Carolina, USA

Paul B. Baltes
Max-Planck-Institut for Human Development and Education, Berlin, Germany

Patrick Bateson
Sub-Department of Animal Behaviour, University of Cambridge, Cambridge, UK

Ursula Bellugi
Laboratory for Language Studies, The Salk Institute, La Jolla, California, USA

Robert B. Cairns
Center for Developmental Science, University of North Carolina, Chapel Hill, North Carolina, USA

Jean-Pierre Changeux
Institut Pasteur, Molecular Neurobiology Laboratory, Department of Biotechnology, Paris, France

Antonio R. Damasio
Department of Neurology, Division of Behavioral Neurology and Cognitive Neuroscience, University of Iowa College of Medicine, Iowa City, Iowa, USA

Hanna Damasio
Department of Neurology, Division of Behavioral Neurology and Cognitive Neuroscience, University of Iowa College of Medicine, Iowa City, Iowa, USA

Gerald M. Edelman
The Neurosciences Institute, La Jolla, California, USA

Caleb E. Finch
Neurogerontology Division, Andrus Gerontology Center and Department of Biological Sciences, University of Southern California, Los Angeles, California, USA

Marcia N. Gordon
Department of Pharmacology, Aging Studies Program, University of South Florida, Tampa, Florida, USA

Roger A. Gorski
*Department of Anatomy and Cell Biology and the Laboratory of Neuroendocrinology of the
Brain Research Institute, UCLA School of Medicine, Los Angeles, California, USA*

Gilbert Gottlieb
*Center for Developmental Science, University of North Carolina at Greensboro, Greensboro,
NC, USA*

Robert W. Goy
*Professor Emeritus of Psychology, Wisconsin Regional Primate Research Center, Madison,
Wisconsin, USA*

Peter Graf
University of British Columbia, Vancouver, Canada

David A. Hamburg
President, Carnegie Corporation of New York, New York, NY, USA

John Hardy
*Suncoast Alzheimer's Disease Laboratory, Departments of Psychiatry, Pharmacology,
Neurology and Biochemistry, University of South Florida, Tampa, Florida, USA*

Robert A. Hinde
The Master's Lodge, St. John's College, Cambridge, UK

Jerome Kagan
Department of Psychology, Harvard University, Cambridge, USA

Pierre Karli
*European Center for the History of Medicine, Faculty of Medicine, University Louis Pasteur,
Strasbourg, France*

Wolfgang Klein
Max-Planck-Institut für Psycholinguistik, Nijmegen, The Netherlands

Edward S. Klima
The Salk Institute for Biological Studies, La Jolla, California, USA

John C. Loehlin
Department of Psychology, University of Texas, Austin, USA

David Magnusson
Department of Psychology, Stockholm University, Stockholm, Sweden

David G. Morgan
*Department of Pharmacology, Aging Studies Program, University of South Florida,
Tampa, Florida, USA*

Richard G. M. Morris
*Centre for Neuroscience and Department of Pharmacology, University of Edinburgh
Medical School, Edinburgh, Scotland*

Dennis D. M. O'Leary
*Molecular Neurobiology Laboratory, The Salk Institute for Biological Studies, La Jolla,
California, USA*

Josef Perner
Laboratory of Experimental Psychology, University of Sussex, Brighton, UK

Dale Purves
Department of Neurobiology, Duke University Medical Center, Durham, North Carolina, USA

Osmund Reynolds
Department of Paediatrics, University College London Medical School, Rayne Institute, London, UK

David Riddle
Department of Neurobiology, Duke University Medical Center, Durham, North Carolina, USA

Sir Michael Rutter
MRC Child Psychiatry Unit, Institute of Psychiatry, London, UK

G. Tononi
The Neuroscience Institute, La Jolla, California, USA

Paul P. Wang
The Salk Institute for Biological Studies, La Jolla, California, USA

Franz E. Weinert
Max-Planck-Institut für Psychologische Forschung, München, Germany

Leonard White
Department of Neurobiology, Duke University Medical Center, Durham, North Carolina, USA

Dake Zheng
Department of Neurobiology, Duke University Medical Center, Durham, North Carolina, USA

Foreword: Towards a developmental science

A scientific study of the development of individuals, of the operative factors and the mechanisms by which they operate, is motivated for several reasons. The study of life processes is a scientific challenge per se, and knowledge about these processes is essential as a basis for prevention and prophylactic measures as well as for treatment of mental and somatic illnesses. Knowledge about the conditions which influence individual development is required for individuals and societies in their efforts to attain adequate standards of life during the various periods of the life cycle.

Individual development is a complex, multidetermined, and integrated process, which takes place progressively from conception to death. In this process, biological, mental, and behavioral factors are involved on the individual side and social and physical factors operate in the environments, which the individual encounters and has to deal with. The course and character of the development process depends on how the different operating factors, from the cellular level in the biological system to the specific elements of the culture, function throughout life.

New theories and models for complex, multidetermined processes have been launched in recent decades, successfully influencing the disciplines concerned. The study of nonlinear dynamic systems and chaos theory provides a case in point. A fundamental principle of such models is that complex, multidetermined processes cannot be understood or explained by the study of single variables, considered separately and taken out of context with other factors which operate simultaneously. For the topic that is the focus of this volume – individual development – this basic principle suggests that although research may have been successful within disciplines, concerned with specific aspects of the functioning and development of individuals, the exchange and integration of results and knowledge from different fields need to be encouraged.

The chapters of this volume cover a wide range of scientific disciplines, from those concerned with specific aspects of the functioning and development of single cells to those which focus on the functioning and development of the total organism in its continuous interaction with societies and cultures. Each of the contributions presents knowledge from a specific discipline, which it is necessary to consider when the goal is to understand and explain the process of individual development from conception to death. Knowledge from a single one of these sources is not enough.

As illustrated by the various chapters, for a full understanding and explanation of the developmental process of individuals, we need contributions from the *interface* of a number of traditional scientific disciplines: developmental biology, developmental psychology, physiology, neuropsychology, social psychology, sociology, anthropology and neighbouring disciplines.

The total space of phenomena involved in the process of lifelong individual development forms a clearly defined and delimited domain for scientific discovery which has to involve all these and other disciplines for effective investigation. This domain constitutes a scientific discipline of its own, *developmental science* (Magnusson & Cairns, in press).

SCIENTIFIC PROGRESS

A characteristic feature of progress in empirical sciences is increasing specialization. In natural sciences, when specialization has reached a certain stage new fields of discovery open up in the interface between traditionally well-defined subdisciplines. Specialization followed by integration has happened, for example, in the interface of physics and chemistry, and later in the interface of biology, chemistry and physics. The iterative process of specialization and integration is dependent on the existence of a general model of nature which serves as a common theoretical framework for the planning, implementation and interpretation of single studies in the natural sciences.

Most of the contributions to this volume reflect a high degree of specialization in a number of areas, all of which are relevant for understanding and explaining individual development. For a long time, specialists in medicine and psychology and other relevant disciplines have provided knowledge that is important for understanding and explaining how the individual develops and functions. For further real progress to be made in the emerging field of developmental science, the time has come to integrate the findings from the specialized areas, presented in this volume and elsewhere, in order to form a holistic perspective. What is needed is *a general model of homo and society* (Magnusson, in press). This model could serve as a common general theoretical framework for planning, implementation and interpretation of studies on the specific issues that are related to the various aspects and different levels of the individual developmental process across the lifespan. Such a framework would make it possible for endocrinologists to communicate with anthropologists, in the same way as the common theoretical model of nature enables nuclear physicists to communicate with astronomers. This is a challenging task and we have a long way to go. It is my hope and that of my colleagues in the organizing committee that the Nobel Symposium and this volume which emanates from it is a step in the right direction.

David Magnusson

REFERENCES

Magnusson, D. (1995) Individual development: a holistic integrated model. In Moen, Ph., Elder, Jr., G. H. & Luscher, Kurt (eds.) *Examining Lives in Context: Perspective on the Ecology of Human Development.* Washington, DC: American Psychological Association.

Magnusson, D. & Cairns, R. B. (in press) Developmental science: an integrated framework. In Cairns, R. B., Elder, Jr., G. H. & Costello, E. J. (eds.) *Developmental Science.* New York: Cambridge University Press.

Preface

Each year the Swedish Nobel Foundation selects, among a number of applications, two or three symposia to be organized as Nobel symposia. With reference to an application, supported by the Swedish Royal Academy of Sciences, a symposium with the title 'The lifespan development of individuals: a synthesis of biological and psychosocial perspectives' was funded for 1994. The chapters of this volume emanates from the symposium, which was held at Södergarn Conference Center, Stockholm, June 1994.

The aim of the symposium was to stimulate efforts to create more cross-disciplinary research on individual development in a holistic perspective, integrating knowledge from disciplines concerned with different aspects of the individual development processes. In order to meet this purpose, eminent researchers were invited to present their views on how their specific discipline can contribute to an understanding of the developmental processes of individuals. These presentations formed the basis for discussions, aimed at developing a holistic model of individual development.

The manuscripts for the symposium were distributed to participants beforehand and so could be used for discussion. After the symposium the authors revised their manuscripts, taking into consideration the comments made during the discussions.

Following an introductory chapter, which puts the rest of the book into an evolutionary perspective, the contributions are organized in six parts:

Part I early development
Part II the changing brain
Part III cognition and behavior
Part IV biology and socialization
Part V social competence
Part VI aging.

Each part is introduced by a brief summary and contains three chapters and a commentary.

The organizing committee for the symposium had the following composition: Professor Torgny Greitz, Karolinska Institute, Professor Tomas Hökfelt, Karolinska Institute, Professor David Magnusson, Stockholm

University (chairman), Professor Lars-Göran Nilsson, Stockholm University, Professor Lars Terenius, Karolinska Institute, and Professor Bengt Winblad, Karolinska Institute.

The organizing committee would like to express its gratitude to the Nobel Foundation for making the symposium possible by generous funding. Special thanks are given to Mrs Luki Hagen-Norberg for the skilful way in which she contributed to the organization of the symposium.

For the organizing committee
David Magnusson

1   Design for a life

PATRICK BATESON

INTRODUCTION

How does development work? In the past, when I have tried answers in terms of dynamic systems, some of my brightest students would react almost with outrage. They would listen with mounting irritation as I attempted to get them to understand how the various things that combine together give rise to behavioural development. Then one or other of them might say something like this: 'I don't understand all this stuff about systems. What gets it started in the first place?' Every so often I would get a similar response from some of my colleagues who were accustomed to the idea that research programmes hunted down the crucial factor that produced a qualitatively distinct effect. The talk of systems sounded to them like so much waffle. 'Science is about uncovering causes', they would tell me in a tone of voice usually reserved for a small child.

In recent years the mood has started to change. Experimentalists are now less likely to hold all but one variable constant. When a single independent variable is found to produce an effect, it is not immediately taken to be *the* cause, nor is everything else deemed unimportant. The nature of the feedback in free-running systems is such that the experimentalist's sharp distinction between independence and dependence evaporates. The dependent variable of a moment ago becomes the independent variable of the present.

Maybe these changes in thinking have come about because computer literacy has made it possible to think about the interplay between many different things with comparative ease. It is not difficult to construct simple working models on our personal computers. When the rules of operation are nonlinear, the behaviour of these models can change in complicated ways that are difficult to predict when the parameters are altered. Without basing them rigorously on what is known about behaviour and underlying mechanisms, such models merely serve to teach us a simple lesson about causality. But the more general point is that the development of individuals is readily perceived as an interplay between them and their environment. The current state influences which genes are expressed, and also the social and physical world.

Individuals are then seen as choosing and changing the conditions to which they are exposed.

As a result of the growing consensus about the systems view of behavioural development, I had intended to write optimistically about where the subject was going. It seemed as though the notion of the learnt/instinctive dichotomy of behaviour had fallen into disuse in most scientific discussions of the subject. Then I read a beautifully written book by Steven Pinker on human language called *The Language Instinct*. He writes:

> Language is a complex, specialised skill, which develops in the child spontaneously, without conscious effort or formal instruction, is deployed without awareness of its underlying logic, is qualitatively the same in every individual, and is distinct from more general abilities to process information or behave intelligently. For these reasons some cognitive scientists have described language as a psychological faculty, a mental organ, a neural system, and a computational module. But I prefer the admittedly quaint term 'instinct'. It conveys the idea that people know how to talk in more or less the sense that spiders know how to spin webs.
>
> (Pinker, 1994: 18)

Pinker knows that he teases and, in a great many ways, the book is wonderfully articulate, informative and sympathetic to modern thinking about behavioural development. Nevertheless, it seems to me that, on this particular developmental issue, he is fighting one of yesterday's battles. The modern debates about instinct are rarely about whether behavioural systems exist in the form that he uses to characterise language. If the debates occur at all they are about the sorts of confusion that arise when a great many different dimensions are collapsed into one. The word 'innate' has at least six separate meanings attached to it: present at birth; a behavioural difference caused by a genetic difference; adapted over the course of evolution; unchanging throughout development; shared by all members of a species; and not learned. 'Instinct' does indeed seem a little quaint now, but when it is used, is deployed in similar ways to innate. A further and special meaning is also attached to instinct, namely a distinctly organised system of behaviour driven from within. Does it follow that one of the meanings of innate or instinctive necessarily applies to a given activity when the justification for using another meaning has been demonstrated? Consider the following questions which might be applied to any pattern of behaviour:

(1) Does the activity appear at a particular stage in development?
(2) Are individual differences in the activity due to genetic differences?
(3) Was the activity adapted to its present function by the Darwinian process of evolution?
(4) Is the activity shared by all members of the species?
(5) Once present, is the frequency and form of the activity unchanged by experience?
(6) Does the activity develop without previous opportunities for learning?

(7) Does the activity have the characteristics of an organised behavioural system?

An unqualified 'Yes' or 'No' to any one of the above questions is liable to trigger an academic dispute. The practical difficulties in demonstrating, for instance, that a piece of behaviour is not learned are immense. Evidence that genetic relatives resemble each other behaviourally is open to the non-trivial objection that they are liable to share common experiences.

Leaving practical matters on one side, what would be implied if one of the answers to those questions was unequivocally 'Yes'? Would we be compelled to suppose that the answers to all the others could not possibly be 'No'? It does not take much thought to realise that we would not. For instance, if a behaviour pattern develops without obvious practice or example, the activity may subsequently be modified by learning. A blind baby may start to smile in the same way as a normal baby. But that does not mean that later on in their lives, sighted people will not modify their smiles to expressions that are characteristic of their own culture.

The major conclusion to draw from the debate about the use of the i-words is that clarity is never a fault. Say what you mean (even if it uses a bit more space) rather than unintentionally confuse your reader by employing a word that means so many different things to so many different people.

Reference to this debate, such as it has been, draws attention to some other respects in which we are genuinely better informed than we used to be. In his chapter in this book, Gottlieb deals with the history of these changes and I simply want to reiterate that many people have been involved (e.g. Magnusson, 1993; Rutter & Rutter, 1993; and articles in Gunnar & Thelen, 1989; Bateson, 1991; Smith & Thelen, 1993). Numerous factors affect the outcome of developmental processes. Dispositions to respond strongly to some features of the environment often develop without direct experience of those features and stereotyped motor patterns often develop without obvious opportunities for practice. But these aspects of a behavioural repertoire, once developed, may be modified by experience. Similarly, learning processes are also rule-governed and have an organisation that may develop without obvious practice but may also change with experience. The plain fact is that several different developmental processes may lead to the adaptive complexity of behaviour, but any given behaviour pattern may be affected by all or several of them.

The chances are that the various influences do not add together and, if that is the case, small changes in certain factors may sometimes make big differences to the outcome and large changes in others will have no effect whatsoever. Even when expressed like this, it is obvious why the old either/or oppositions applied to behaviour evaporated as knowledge advanced. The issues become obvious if the luxuriance of influences and outcomes shown in Figure 1.1 are considered.

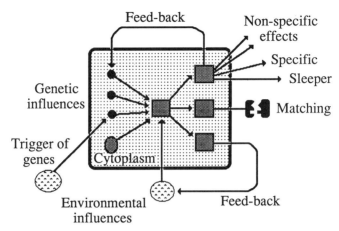

Figure 1.1. A schematic flow diagram of some of the events occurring during development. The neural structures required for the expression of behaviour depend on genes, cytoplasmic factors and environmental conditions, some of which trigger the expression of particular genes. Feedback onto genes to stop their expression may occur internally or be mediated through the environment. Some consequences of developmental processes are specific, some are general and some feed-forward to later stages in development and, in that sense, are 'sleepers'. Finally, some processes actively match the environment to the individual's characteristics.

The influences on behaviour may operate in a variety of different ways (enabling, initiating, facilitating, maintaining); they may also have radically different outcomes, some specific and some general. Developmental processes may be remarkably well buffered against fluctuations in the environment. Moreover, if an individual is prevented from developing in one way, the same behaviour pattern may sometimes develop in another way. Given their predispositions and proclivities, individuals may choose environments to which their characteristics are well adapted – 'niche-picking' as Scarr & McCartney (1983) called it. Even so, individuals are also equipped with conditional rules so that their behavioural development is directed down one of several different routes, depending on the prevailing conditions.

The trouble with the schematic flow diagram shown in Figure 1.1 is that it is not enormously rich in theory. Without a strong set of binding ideas, it is not easy to think about all aspects of the various strands of evidence, which often seem to point in opposite directions. Many mathematical techniques, such as catastrophe theory and 'chaos', have been developed to deal analytically with the complexities of dynamical systems. For all that, it is questionable whether the descriptive use of mathematics brings with it any explanatory power. Much more promising are those approaches that bind evidence across different levels of analysis. A remarkable attempt has been made by Edelman in his trilogy (Edelman, 1987, 1988, 1989).

Edelman sets his sights on an explanation for consciousness rather than development across the whole human lifespan, but the attempt to create a theory at different levels of organisation is attractive. Furthermore, central to his thinking is the notion of selection of the most appropriate subset from an array of alternative processes. This is a reworking of the three main stages of the Darwinian evolutionary argument, applied first to the workings of the immune system and then re-applied to behavioural development.

In my own work with Gabriel Horn, we have taken from behavioural development the specific example of imprinting (Bateson & Horn, 1994). Our model builds on a proposal that the behaviour of experienced animals relies on three subprocesses that analyse sequentially the features of stimuli, recognise those feature combinations that are familiar and organise appropriate responses (Figure 1.2). Like Edelman we tried to ensure that most of the subprocesses are as plausible in neural terms as current knowledge allows and that the whole system has the behavioural structure of an intact animal. The model exhibits a well-known feature of behavioural development seen in animals, tending to settle into familiar habits, while also able to build with increasing elaboration on the basis of previous perceptual experience. The pre-emptive effect of experience on control of the Executive module is shown in Figure 1.3. This feature means that other stimuli are less able to gain access to this module, even through the bypass, unless exposure to those novel stimuli is forced and prolonged. This aspect of the model simulates the closure of the sensitive period in development, which is known to be dependent on experience, at least in part. The greater the activating value of the features in the experienced stimuli, the more quickly the sensitive period comes to an end.

The case for some theory of mechanism is that it spawns explicit working models which bring with them mental discipline and expose weaknesses in a verbal argument that are all too easily missed. They can show how we are easily misled by the dynamics of development into supposing that the processes are so complicated that they are beyond comprehension. From the point of future empirical research, they can suggest profitable new lines of enquiry. They bring understanding of how real systems generate the seemingly elaborate things that we observe. Their predictions may be false, but they are worth testing just because the assumptions are rooted in psychological and biological reality.

I shall not go into these approaches any further because the general theme of this book has a broader scope. In separating out the great range of phenomena with which we deal, one approach is to consider the changing character of behaviour through the life cycle in terms of its utility. Instead of asking how individuals travel from conception to death, we can ask *why* they travel in just the way they do. What are the design principles on which their lives are constructed?

(a)

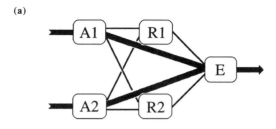

(b)

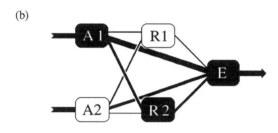

(c)

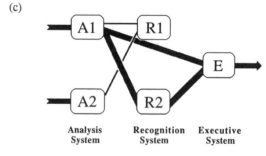

Analysis   Recognition   Executive
System   System   System

Figure 1.2. Simplified architecture of Bateson & Horn's (1994) model for imprinting. All modules in the Analysis System are initially linked to all modules in the Recognition System which, in their turn, are linked to all modules in the Executive System, only one of which is shown here. Initial strengths of links are indicated by the thickness of the lines. All modules in the Analysis System are also linked at maximum strength directly through a bypass to the module in the Executive System that controls filial behaviour (such as approach and following). The starting condition is shown in panel (a). Panel (b) shows the strengths of linkages between modules after the model has been exposed to a stimulus that activated Analysis module, A1. The spontaneous excitability in the Recognition module, R2, happened to be higher than that in R1 at the time that the input from A1 arrived; activity in R1 was inhibited. The strengthening rule is that modules are conjointly active. The weakening rule is that the upstream module is inactive when the downstream module is active. The completed process is shown in panel (c).

(a)

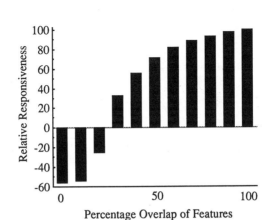

(b)

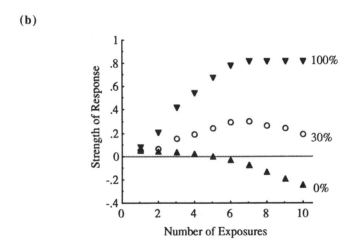

Figure 1.3. (a) The relative strength of response of the Bateson & Horn model after 10 exposures to a 10-feature stimulus and testing with stimuli that overlap in features with the familiar stimulus from 0% to 100%. The relative strength is the responsiveness to a stimulus divided by the responsiveness to the familiar stimulus and expressed as a percentage. (b) Changes in absolute responsiveness to stimuli that share all their features in common with the exposure stimulus (100%), some of their features (30%) or have no features in common (0%). The behavioural equivalent of a positive sign on the response is approach and of a negative sign withdrawal.

DARWINIAN DEVELOPMENT

A striking aspect of human development, when viewed in broad perspective, is how differently we behave at various points in our lives. Shakespeare put this idea into the mouth of Jacques in *As You Like It;*

All the world's a stage,
And all the men and women merely players.
They have their exits and their entrances,
And one man in his time plays many parts,
His acts being seven ages.

How do we make sense of these seven scenes? Why is the infant, mewling and puking in the nurse's arms, so different from the whining schoolboy, with his satchel and shining morning face, creeping like a snail unwillingly to school? Why is the lover, sighing like a furnace, with a woeful ballad made to his mistress' eyebrow, so unlike the middle-aged gentleman, with eyes severe and beard of formal cut, full of wise saws and modern instances? Shakespeare's flippant approach to lifespan studies would probably not have been sufficient to get his funding renewed: not familiar with the modern literature; not politically correct. And who would have ever suggested that a human butterfly could have reached its adult stage without first being a human caterpillar? Nevertheless, astute as ever about human nature, he spotted the marked discontinuities as we grow up and age. His seven ages do suggest that the changes in an individual's lifespan represent responses to different requirements in each scene in which he or she has to act.

I have argued in the past that it helps to think about such developmental problems from a functional and evolutionary standpoint (Bateson, 1981, 1987). It comes very naturally for biologists to think this way, although they have to remind themselves of an important qualification. Contemporary humans surely live in a dramatically changed environment from the one in which our ancestors evolved. Behaviour such as seeking out and being massively rewarded by sugar was doubtless of great importance to our ancestors in the world of our evolutionary adaptedness, to use John Bowlby's (1969) phrase. Nowadays, of course, our craving for sugar, fats and much else brings with it a host of the diseases of affluence.

Recognising that the adaptations of the past are not necessarily adaptations to the present may be useful when thinking about the problems of human lifespan. Even so, I must confess that I have felt a little diffident raising the matter again with colleagues many of whom have been trained as psychologists and may not much like what they regard as the biologists' messier habits. But I am emboldened to do so once again by the recent impact of Darwinian ideas on medicine.

In what is now regarded as a famous rallying point of Darwinian medicine, Williams & Nesse (1991) stressed the various ways in which a functional and evolutionary approach to medicine might open our eyes to problems that a purely mechanistic approach neglects. Fevers are uncomfortable and distressing to watch in someone you love and especially your own child. The traditional medical approach has been to try to reduce the temperature. However, if you ask why we should have a fever and when you know that experimental evidence suggests that raising the body temperature kills off invading bacteria, you are led to a very different response. You let the fever take its course as part of the natural attack on infection. I do not think that many would suggest that a completely non-interventionist approach to ill health is justified, but asking the question about utility does at least make you think in a different way.

Similarly, we are led to a different view of aging. To quote Shakespeare again, this time on the seventh age of man, 'Last scene of all, that ends this strange, eventful history, is second childishness and mere oblivion, sans teeth, sans eyes, sans taste, sans everything'. Why should this be? Here again medicine has avoided the question and looked for a cure for old age, even *the* cure – as though immortality were an option. The Darwinian response is couched very much in terms of life-history strategies. How many offspring should be conceived? How much investment should be put into each one? Answers to these questions relate to the resources available to members of a species and to finding trade-offs between quantity and quality of offspring. These trade-offs depend on the probabilities that adults will survive to breed again. It is a remarkable fact that, after the initial high mortality of early life, the probability of surviving from one year to the next is constant, in most wild-living birds and mammals at least, because accidents and disease affect all ages to the same extent. As a consequence, no surge in mortality occurs after a given period. Aging is not observed under natural conditions. So it was for humans. Everybody died before they were senile. Peter Medewar (1952) argued many years ago that, as a result, late-acting lethal genes were not removed by Darwinian evolution. Similarly, genes that had early benefits and late costs would not be removed. Jared Diamond (1991) drew an analogy with planned obsolescence in a car in which, if the manufacturer gets it right, everything wears out at the same time. Aging is *unplanned* synchronised obsolescence. It does not matter if repair mechanisms stop functioning because, in the environment of evolutionary adaptedness, nobody would have lived long enough to benefit from mutations that would have given them a longer life and another opportunity to reproduce. As Diamond points out, on this bleak view of aging we should not expect a cure for old age. No single immortality drug will ever be found that will remove the prospect of all those miseries of decaying senses, skeleton, musculature and mind that most of us have to expect. That is not to say that we cannot inhibit those harmful genes that are expressed late in life, but even such an orthodox programme of mechanistic medicine would be stimulated by the Darwinian approach.

Anyhow, as we think about the various stages of human development, asking what behaviour is for suggests at once that, in the environment of evolutionary adaptedness, some of our stage-specific patterns of behaviour were concerned with the peculiar problems associated with that stage. The process of assembly is long relative to the total lifespan and, as preparation for a reproductive life proceeds, the child has to survive. As a result, many aspects of his or her body, physiology and behaviour meet needs that are peculiar to the age. The adaptations of larval forms, such as tadpoles or caterpillars, with totally different bodies and behaviour from those of adults, provide the most striking examples of early specialisation in the animal kingdom. However, mammals also have their juvenile adaptations – the method of suckling being the most obvious. A different type of functional issue is to do with behaviour that is used in the assembly process. Some types of behaviour seem to function in this way, falling away like scaffolding round a building when the individual has matured. The biological utility of some behavioural mechanisms found in many developing animals seems to be the gathering of information or the guiding of their play with the environment.

When using a Darwinian approach to reinterpret developmental stages, we should not suppose that early experience has no long-term effects (Hinde & Bateson, 1984). Even metamorphosis does not necessarily erase previous memories. In certain moth species whose larvae can feed on more than one foodstuff, adult females are prone to lay eggs on the substrate on which they were reared. In amphibians, training during the larval phase can affect behaviour in adulthood. None of the explanations for a reorganisation of psychological structure requires that when one aspect of the structure changes, it all changes. Some behavioural systems may be adapted to both

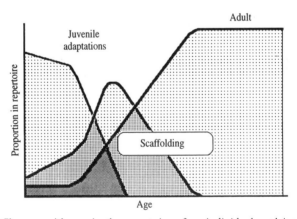

Figure 1.4. Changes with age in the repertoire of an individual explained in terms of the utility of the behaviour patterns. Early in life many forms of behaviour are specialized to meet needs that are peculiar to that stage. Later, some activities, like scaffolding on a building, are required for the assembly of adult behaviour. By degrees, the full repertoire of adult behaviour is established.

juvenile and adult life while others are not. Some may develop in fits and starts whereas others develop smoothly. The general point, depicted in Figure 1.4, is that changes in the repertoire of an individual as it grows older may reflect the immediate requirements at that stage or may anticipate needs that will arise in the future.

THE DEVELOPMENTAL JUKE-BOX

Another example of where the Darwinian approach may bring a refreshing new perspective on development is the induction of individual variation. Members of the same species, the same sex and the same age sometimes differ dramatically from each other. The variation commonly arises because an individual has the capacity to respond in more than one way according to the state of the local environment or its own body (Caro & Bateson, 1986). Individuals have many latent capacities that are only expressed under certain conditions. The developmental processes that are triggered provide useful adaptations to the environment. Such conditional responses during development are well known in the social insects, in which one sister might be adapted for producing thousands of eggs, another has massive jaws used in defence of the nest and yet another is equipped with foraging skills never expressed by the other two. Similar environmentally induced differences occur more frequently in mammals than had been realised (Lott, 1991). Young mammals may pick up crucial information from their mothers about when to wean themselves and how to develop afterwards on the basis of cues that they pick up from their nursing mothers. For instance, in an experiment on domestic cats, kittens of rationed mothers developed quite differently from those of mothers given *ad libitum* food. Play almost certainly has benefits for these animals. After weaning, they played more, compensating for loss of experience resulting from the relatively early break-up of the family group that would occur in a poor natural environment (Bateson, Mendl & Feaver, 1990). The individual is a juke-box, capable of playing many tunes but, in the course of its life, possibly playing only one of a set. The particular suite of adaptations that it does express is selected by the conditions in which it grows up.

Many of the animal examples of individuals developing in different modes were assumed to be different species living in the same place. Even when they were believed to belong to the same species, the different types were taken to have different genotypes responding to the environment that particularly favoured them. The mistake was easily made because, in addition to different bodies, the alternatives had different enzymes, presumably reflecting the expression of different genes.

When reflecting upon the design for a human life, the selection of appropriate modes of response gives us a novel way of thinking about individual differences. To underscore the point, the extreme alternative view is that every one of us has a single ideal state on which we should all converge, given perfect nourishment, stimulation and so forth. Anybody who failed to achieve that state had made the best of a bad job and, at the margins of existence, expressed pathological stunting of body and behaviour. One version of the general case that I wish to make is an idea developed by Waterlow (1990) about malnourishment. He and others have suggested that, far from expressing the devastating effects of bad diet, small size, reduced metabolic rate and reduced behavioural activity are all part of a suite of responses by humans to a world that does not have much food in it (see also Dasgupta, 1993, who brilliantly sets these ideas in a broad context). A political objection to this conjecture is that it encourages the rich of the world to look complacently at their fellow human beings and argue that, not only will the poor always be with us, but all is for the best; everybody expresses the morphology, physiology, biochemistry and behaviour that is best suited to their station. Given the real danger that such arguments may be mounted, let me scotch them immediately. The point is not that the qualities of life are identical for the rich and the poor. Rather, it may be that, if conditions are bad, the developmental response to those conditions is highly appropriate.

To show where it can take us, I shall apply this Darwinian thinking to a striking illustration of how adult characteristics may be predicted at a very early age. Among a large group of males, who were all breast-fed as babies, those who had the lowest weights at birth had the highest death rate from cardiovascular disease (Barker, 1991). Since poor maternal physique and health is associated with poor foetal growth, the argument based on utility is that, in bad conditions, mothers signal to their unborn child that the environment outside is harsh. As a result the babies are born with the suite of adaptations that would have adapted them well to poor, low-fat diets. However, they were inadequately adapted to the affluent environment in which they subsequently grew up. This is frank speculation, of course, but it is not a vacuous just-so story because it provides us with a set of questions that may be used to address data already available to us. It suggests, for instance, that people who were well adapted to good environments might be at greater risk in conditions of famine.

The selection of suites of responses appropriate for the environment in which the child grows up raises questions about why such systems once established are so difficult to reverse. The morphological cases are easier to understand because bodies, once formed, are not easily reshaped. Similarly, intricately interlocking metabolic pathways, once established, may have a stability that cannot be changed without threatening survival. The induced forms of behaviour may retain their stability because rejigging behavioural tactics, while beneficial in the long run, may mean that, during the new process of change, the individual requires a dependency on other members of his or her social group. Such help may not have been available to adults in the environment of evolutionary adaptedness.

If this argument is correct, it means that periods will be found in the life cycle when individual variation is particularly easily generated by differences in the environments in which they live. Parenthetically, two individuals may live in the same place at the same time and yet have different social environments from each other, since, as with siblings, one reacts to the personality and tastes of the other, thereby creating a separate space for itself (Plomin, DeFries & Fulker, 1988). The individual's environment, whether it be physical or social, will select an appropriate response. Once selected, a branching series of developmental events may be set in train. This process cannot be unscrambled and started again. It follows that periods in the life cycle will be found when individual variation in a particular domain is particularly easily generated by environmental differences. Conversely, at other stages, that domain of variation will be buffered from change.

These ideas lead naturally into the enormous developmental literature on sensitive periods (Bornstein, 1987). Sensitive periods are simply descriptions. Variation that is more easily generated at one stage of the life cycle than at others is not explained by saying that development took a particular course because the experience occurred within a sensitive period. At least, it is not explained without a very specific model of what controls the sensitivity, and such models grow out of considering particular cases. I shall turn to one that has attracted a great deal of attention, the development of preferences for particular sexual partners.

PARTNER CHOICE

The Darwinian evolutionary mechanism consists of three stages, namely (1) generation of variation among individuals, (2) differential reproductive success and (3) inheritance of the factors that gave rise to the variation. Design for a life can hardly miss out on the crucial middle stage involving mating and parenting where the interest of the evolutionary biologists has been especially intense (Betzig, 1988) and where developmental considerations are especially important (Rutter & Rutter, 1993). In as much as choice is possible, a sexual partner is preferred over others for many different reasons, particularly when a long-term relationship is contemplated. In ways that are obvious and others that are more subtle, the sexes differ in the characteristics which they consider desirable in a partner (Buss, 1985). Good partner choice in one set of conditions may not be equally satisfactory under different environmental conditions. Indeed, the evidence suggests that the combination of characteristics used in partner choice depends a great deal on the local environmental conditions, for very similar reasons advanced for body type (Alexander et al., 1979).

Sometimes a view is expressed that all the critical cues required for partner choice are carried in the face. Even a limited amount of self-reflection suggests that the claim is overstated. Nevertheless, one aspect of partner choice almost certainly involves the face because it depends on subtle recognition of individuals. I have argued by analogy with what we know about imprinting in birds that learning the features of closely related individuals is important in choice of a sexual partner (Bateson, 1983). This is because a balance must be struck between avoiding the costs of inbreeding too much and outbreeding too much. At least five reasons for avoiding inbreeding have been suggested. The most famous one is that deleterious genes are more likely to be fully expressed as a consequence of inbreeding. Another, probably more fundamental explanation is that fast-reproducing parasites are much better able to track their hosts' cell characteristics and thereby escape detection by immune systems; sexual reproduction with an unrelated individual makes that much more difficult.

At least eight costs of outbreeding too much have been suggested. One is that looking for mates that deviate substantially from close kin takes time and may result in a missed breeding season; travelling into another population in search of a mate, if that is what is required, may also be dangerous. Another is that systems can be independently inherited. George Bernard Shaw had the right idea when he was approached by a famous actress who wished to have a child by him. 'Imagine', she had gushed, 'what our child would be like with your brains and my beauty.' GBS was not tempted. His reply on one of his famous postcards was: 'What if the child had your brains and my beauty?' Independently segregating systems may, nevertheless, be well adapted to each other. But their independence may mean that those that work well together can easily become separated by outbreeding too much. One instance may be provided by teeth and jaws. Teeth size and shape are strongly inherited (see Hilson, 1986). So also is jaw size and shape, judging from famous paintings of the Habsburg family scattered round the museums of Europe. (Compare, for instance, the Dürer of the Holy Roman Emperor Maximilian I with the Velasquez of his great-great-great-grandson, Philip IV of Spain.) Despite developmental buffering mechanisms that harmonise disparities between the outcomes of different systems that are independently inherited, people with small jaws and teeth whose partners had big jaws and big teeth would probably have been laying down a lot of trouble for their descendants. In a world without dentists, ill-fitting teeth were probably a serious cause of mortality.

The pressures against inbreeding, on the one hand, and outbreeding, on the other, push in opposite directions (see Figure 1.5). Their resolution provides a nice justification for the discrepancy mechanism known from the psychological study of aesthetics, namely a preference for something a bit different from what you know, but not too different. If you learn about your close kin and prefer a sexual partner who looks a bit different, you may have chosen a first or second cousin and, in biological terms, you will be doing well (for further discussion see Thornhill, 1993).

An entrancing new technology enables the rank amateur to play Francis

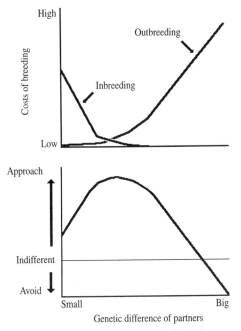

Figure 1.5. The genetic difference between partners affects how much their descendants suffer from the costs of inbreeding on the one hand and outbreeding on the other. The trade-off that minimised the combined costs of inbreeding and outbreeding affected the evolution of partner choice so that individuals now prefer partners who are somewhat related, but not too closely related, to themselves.

Galton's game with images of human faces, mixing them together to produce composite images that are astonishingly sharp. Even the composite of 20 faces looks good. Depending on how representative of the population is the range variation of photographs, it is possible to end up with an average 20-year-old, 30-year-old, 40-year-old, and so on. Similarly, an average Englishman, an average Greek woman, an average Japanese child might be produced. The faces are surprisingly beautiful and have prompted the speculation that similar averaging processes happen in the course of everyday human experience, setting our aesthetic standards. While the faces are beautiful, common experience suggests that they are not tremendously sexy. Recently, Perrett, May & Yoshikawa (1994) have found that they can be made more interesting by using a caricaturing algorithm that distorts the image away from a composite. This work encourages the thought that knowledge of several siblings' faces along with knowledge of the parents' faces would give a better sense of what an unknown cousin is like. The expectation would be that the composite face of close kin would lead to better cousin recognition than would any one face.

More than a hundred years ago Westermarck (1891) suggested that satisfying sexual relationships are not formed between people who have spent their childhood together. This view is supported by the behaviour of members of Israeli kibbutzim who rarely marry the people they have grown up with (Shepher, 1971; Talmon, 1964). Shepher had noted that a few individuals who married within their peer group in the kibbutz had entered the kibbutz usually after the age of six. He suggested, therefore, that development of sexual preferences is *complete* by the age of six in humans. To demonstrate a sensitive period of the type he was proposing, it would be necessary to show that adults who had left a kibbutz at the age of six were not sexually attracted by members of the opposite sex with whom they had been reared while still in the kibbutz. In any event, the kibbutz data have been fiercely attacked on methodological grounds (Leavitt, 1990).

Fortunately, data from another natural experiment allow a more careful analysis. Wolf & Huang (1980) investigated a form of arranged marriage that was practised in Taiwan. The wife-to-be was adopted into the family of the husband-to-be when she was a young girl. The marriage was formalised and consummated when the partners were adolescent. This form of arranged marriage, the 'minor marriage', could be compared with a more common form of arranged marriage, the 'major marriage', in which the partners met each other for the first time when they were adolescents. In a great many respects the minor marriages were less successful than the major marriages. They generated fewer children, the rates of infidelity were higher, and so forth. For instance, 15% of the minor marriages ended in divorce whereas only 6% of the major marriages did so. In a recent book Wolf (1995) has responded carefully to earlier criticisms of his work, showing by subtle analysis that the Westermarck hypothesis is strongly supported by the data. Moreover, he was able to show convincingly that girls adopted into families before the age of three have a lower fertility than girls adopted later. Other factors are also involved but the age-dependent phenomenon is highly robust.

Wolf quite properly concedes that his own data are mute on whether the process of generating indifference is complete by three years. Indeed, it seems highly unlikely that the process is complete by then, given the great changes in physical characteristics between the age of three and adolescence. A lot hinges on the type of relationship the couple have when they are young. If they play together and, as a result, see a lot of each other, the indifference is likely to be greater. By the time they are three, children are highly conscious of their gender and are much less likely to play with a member of the opposite sex, particularly a strange member (Maccoby, 1990; Howes & Phillipsen, 1992; Turner, Gervai & Hinde, 1993). It seems plausible then that a girl adopted when over three will be seen as a stranger by the boy and treated very differently from girls who are adopted when younger. What started as a functional argument leads into developmental questions about how preferences develop and how they are maintained.

DEVELOPMENT AFFECTS EVOLUTION

The benefits of bringing together how developmental processes work with why they work in the way they do flow both ways. It is not just that the study of the human lifespan can be helped by evolutionary biology. The study of evolution can benefit greatly from a thorough understanding of development – especially behavioural development (see Gottlieb, 1992).

Sudden changes in the environment may not lead to extinction because of the adaptability of organisms. Behavioural adaptability, mediated by learning processes, plays a particularly important role here. The adaptability allows time for efficient solutions to the environmental challenges to evolve. Sudden changes in the environment may also lead to the expression of characteristics that were not visible hitherto and provide the basis for further evolution. More importantly, the capacity to choose environments and companions, particularly sexual partners, can have dramatic effects on the course of evolution. Finally, the active control of the environment and particularly the social environment can lead to explosively rapid evolutionary change. These behavioural factors are likely to lie behind that most extraordinary aspect of human biology, namely the doubling of the brain size in two million years (see Bateson, 1988, 1990).

WHAT IS THE BIG IDEA?

The title of the talk, from which this chapter was derived, might have encouraged the thought that my theme was especially appropriate for a Sunday evening (when the talk was given), providing an answer to the question 'What is the meaning of it all?' The word 'design', after all, is heavily loaded with teleology. So let me emphasise that I wish to imply neither a designer nor conscious intention on the part of the person whose life is well designed from a biological standpoint. The astonishing consequence of Darwin's proposal is that exquisite adaptation arises as the result of a blind process. That was his Big Idea and it is one that can serve the study of behavioural development well in the sense that it makes us think about evolution and about utility. I have only touched on a few examples, namely adaptations for different stages of life and the triggering of appropriate repertoires for the conditions in which the individual grows up. A great deal more can be done in a similar vein.

The general point I have sought to establish is that the functional approach can helpfully reorder the material with which we have to deal in lifespan approaches to human development. The approach sets what we already know in ecological perspective and leads to interesting questions that would not otherwise have been asked. However, I should reiterate that what was good for the past is not necessarily good for the present where conditions are so different and changing with alarming speed as human population size surges upwards. Also, by planning and conscious actions each of us is able to affect the course of our lives. That aspect of design clearly lies outside the scope of this essay.

I dealt with another topic, namely the biological benefits during partner choice of self-centred knowledge and the pre-emptive effects of early experience. This discussion emphasised a different point. Arguments about utility may raise useful questions about developmental process. In the particular case I considered, the issues were to do with how partner preferences develop and how they are maintained. The return to mechanism brings me back to my starting point about systems.

We need ways of dealing with the complexity, even today when computer literacy is so much more widespread. The 'Why' questions help us to return to the 'How'. They clear the air for understanding the way in which developmental processes work. When the clarity is achieved, we have to shift mode. At that point, explanations for how things work gain their greatest power, I believe, when they take into account different levels of organisation. Whether one or more of those explanations will be a Big Idea remains to be seen. Even so, an enormous improvement in the quality of thought has already been achieved by abandoning the view that development is a linear chain of events. The treatment of the processes as systems, influenced by many things, with feedback and feed-forward and with numerous consequences, will be seen in the future as a major step in the direction of understanding what happens throughout the lifespan.

ACKNOWLEDGEMENTS

I am grateful to the following for their comments on a draft of this chapter: Dusha Bateson, Susan Oyama, Joan Stevenson-Hinde and Nick Thompson.

REFERENCES

Alexander, R. D., Hoogland, J. L., Howard, R. D., Noonan, K. M. & Sherman, P. W. (1979) Sexual dimorphisms and breeding systems in pinnipeds, ungulates, primates and humans. In Chagnon, N. A. & Irons, W. (eds.) *Evolutionary Biology and Human Social Behavior*. North Scituate, Mass.: Duxbury Press, pp. 402–35.

Barker, D. J. P. (1991) The intrauterine environment and adult cardiovascular disease. In Bock, G. R. & Whelan, J. (eds.) *The Childhood Environment and Adult Disease. CIBA Foundation Symposium 156*. Chichester: John Wiley, pp. 3–10.

Bateson, P. (1981) Ontogeny of behaviour. *British Medical Bulletin,* **37**, 159–64.

Bateson, P. (1983) Optimal outbreeding. In Bateson, P. (ed.) *Mate Choice*. Cambridge: Cambridge University Press, pp. 257–77.

Bateson, P. (1987) Biological approaches to the study of behavioural development. *International Journal of Behavioral Development,* **10**, 1–22.

Bateson, P. (1988) The active role of behaviour in evolution. In Ho, M.-W. & Fox, S. (eds.) *Process and Metaphors in Evolution*. Chichester: John Wiley, pp. 191–207.

Bateson, P. (1990) Animal communication. In Mellor, D. H. (ed.) *Ways of Communicating*. Cambridge: Cambridge University Press, pp. 35–55.

Bateson, P. (ed.) (1991) *The Development and Integration of Behaviour*. Cambridge: Cambridge University Press.

Bateson, P. & Horn, G. (1994) Imprinting and recognition memory: a neural net model. *Animal Behaviour*, **48**, 695–715.

Bateson, P., Mendl, M. & Feaver, J. (1990) Play in the domestic cat is enhanced by rationing the mother during lactation. *Animal Behaviour*, **40**, 514–25.

Betzig, L. (1988) Mating and parenting in Darwinian perspective. In Betzig, L., Borgerhoff Mulder, M. & Turke, P. (eds.) *Human Reproductive Behaviour*. Cambridge: Cambridge University Press, pp. 3–20.

Bornstein, M. H. (ed.) (1987) *Sensitive Periods in Development*. Hillsdale, NJ: Erlbaum.

Bowlby, J. (1969) *Attachment and Loss, Vol. 1. Attachment*. London: Hogarth Press.

Buss, D. M. (1985) Human mate selection. *American Scientist*, **73**, 47–51.

Caro, T. M. & Bateson, P. (1986) Organisation and ontogeny of alternative tactics. *Animal Behaviour*, **34**, 1483–99.

Dasgupta, P. (1993) *An Inquiry into Well-being and Destination*. Oxford: Oxford University Press.

Diamond, J. (1991) *The Rise and Fall of the Third Chimpanzee*. London: Hutchinson Radius.

Edelman, G. M. (1987) *Neural Darwinism*. New York: Basic Books.

Edelman, G. M. (1988) *Topobiology*. New York: Basic Books.

Edelman, G. M. (1989) *The Remembered Present*. New York: Basic Books.

Gottlieb, G. (1992) *Individual Development and Evolution*. Oxford: Oxford University Press.

Gunnar, M. R. & Thelan, E. (1989) *Systems and Development. The Minnesota Symposia on Child Psychology, Vol. 22*. Hillsdale, NJ: Erlbaum.

Hilson, S. (1986) *Teeth*. Cambridge: Cambridge University Press.

Hinde, R. A. & Bateson, P. (1984) Discontinuities versus continuities in behavioural development and the neglect of process. *International Journal of Behavioural Development*, **7**, 129–43.

Howes, C. & Phillipsen, L. (1992) Gender and friendship: relationships within peer groups of young children. *Social Development*, **1**, 230–42.

Leavitt, G. C. (1990) Sociobiological explanations of incest avoidance: a critical review of evidential claims. *American Anthropologist*, **92**, 971–93.

Lott, D. F. (1991) *Intraspecific Variation in the Social Systems of Wild Vertebrates*. Cambridge: Cambridge University Press.

Maccoby, E. E. (1990) Gender and relationships. *American Psychologist*, **45**, 513–20.

Magnusson, D. (1993) Human ontogeny. In Magnusson, D. & Casaer, P. (eds.) *Longitudinal Research on Individual Development: Present Status and Future Perspectives*. Cambridge: Cambridge University Press, pp. 1–25.

Medewar, P. B. (1952) *An Unsolved Problem in Biology*. London: H. K. Lewis.

Perrett, D. I., May, K. A. & Yoshikawa, S. (1994) Facial shape and judgements of female attractiveness. *Nature*, **368**, 239–42.

Pinker, S. (1994) *The Language Instinct*. London: Penguin.

Plomin, R., DeFries, J. C. & Fulker, D. W. (1988) *Nature and Nurture during Infancy and Early Childhood*. Cambridge: Cambridge University Press.

Rutter, M. & Rutter, M. (1993) *Developing Minds: Challenge and Continuity across the Lifespan*. New York: Basic Books.

Scarr, S. & McCartney, K. (1983) How people make their own environments: a theory of genotype → environment effects. *Child Development*, **54**, 424–35.

Shepher, J. (1971) Mate selection among second generation kibbutz adolescents and adults: incest avoidance and negative imprinting. *Archives of Sexual Behavior*, **1**, 293–307.

Smith, L. & Thelen, E. (1993) *A Dynamic Systems Approach to Development*. Cambridge, Mass.: MIT Press.

Talmon, Y. (1964) Mate selection in collective settlements. *American Sociological Review*, **29**, 491–508.

Thornhill, N. W. (ed.) (1993) *The Natural History of Inbreeding and Outbreeding*. Chicago, Ill.: University of Chicago Press.

Turner, P. J., Gervai, J. & Hinde, R. A. (1993) Gender-typing in young children: preferences, behaviour and cultural differences. *British Journal of Developmental Psychology*, **11**, 323–42.

Waterlow, J. C. (1990) Mechanisms of adaptation to low energy intakes. In Harrison, G. A. & Waterlow, J. C. (eds.) *Diet and Disease in Traditional and Developing Countries*. Cambridge: Cambridge University Press, pp. 5–23.

Westermarck, E. (1891) *The History of Human Marriage*. London: Macmillan.

Williams, G. C. & Nesse, R. M. (1991) The dawn of Darwinian medicine. *Quarterly Review of Biology*, **66**, 1–22.

Wolf, A. P. (1995) *Sexual Attraction and Childhood Association*. Stanford, Calif.: Stanford University Press.

Wolf, A. P. & Huang, C. (1980) *Marriage and Adoption in China, 1845–1945*. Stanford, Calif.: Stanford University Press.

PART I

EARLY DEVELOPMENT

This part concerns the early term of ontogenesis and deals mainly with the prenatal and perinatal periods. The main issue discussed by the four authors may be traced back to the relative influence of genes and environment and their interactions, including the impact of physiologic stimuli on gene expression. Also individual variations caused by damage to the developing brain have been considered. It is shown that to the outgrowth of the neurons exhibit a considerable degree of activity-dependent, developmental plasticity and this may also be true of cells in our sense organs.

The four authors addressed these issues from different aspects, each of them giving an account of the present knowledge in his field, viewed against the background of his own scientific experiences.

O'Leary (Chapter 2) shows, that in experiments on rats and rodents, cells of the different neocortical areas have equivalent functional capabilities, an observation that to a certain degree challenges the concept of the genetic specification of the cortex as it seems to indicate that its differentiation is not genetically determined, its neurons being from the beginning more or less equivalent. In O'Learys 'protocortex model' the neocortex differentiation requires instructions via afferent fibers, implying an influence of sensory stimulation on gene expression.

In Chapter 3 Loehlin attempts to investigate the relative influence of genes and the environment, by referring to quantitative statistical studies of lifespan development of human behavior characteristics such as intelligence, temperament and social attitudes, comparing groups of individuals that includes, for example, monozygotic and dizygotic twins as well as adopted children. His conclusions are that the relative influence of the genetic contribution increases over the lifespan and particularly so with regard to intelligence.

Reynolds (Chapter 4) has chosen to consider the influence of perinatal brain injury on individual development, since this cause of malfunctioning, although less common than congenital abnormalities and inherited diseases, can be eliminated in many instances by being adequately identified at an early stage – and thereby prevented – using modern imaging techniques such as *CT*, *MRI* and *PET* as well as physiologic measurements such as *MR*-spectroscopy. As an example, steroid treatment of mothers who will deliver before term prevents hyaline membrane disease and periventricular hemmorrhage, thus decreasing the number of disabling neuromotor impairments or impairments of cognitive functions.

In his discussion of the contributions to this section, Gottlieb in Chapter

5 focuses on the fact that O'Leary's discussion reduces the earlier 'uni-directional imbalance of the genetic predetermination' in the differentiation of neural structures and functions. He emphasizes the 'equipotentiality' of nerve cells and indicates that the functional anatomy of the nervous system is not entirely genetically predetermined.

Gottlieb, when discussing Loehlin's chapter, frequently refers to the multidirectional 'system model' used in developmental analysis in contrast to the purely statistical and unidirectional model used in qualitative behavior genetics. The latter model was applied in the investigations referred to by Loehlin and assumes, according to Gottlieb, the genetic and environmental contributions to be additive and not interactive. Gottlieb recognizes four levels of bidirectional influences in the 'systems model', genetic activity, neural activity, behavior and environment. He ends his discussion by questioning Loehlin's conclusions, claiming that 'heritability estimates apply only to populations and not to individuals'.

With regards to Reynolds's review, Gottlieb underlines the fact that premature children are at risk of perinatal brain damage, which in certain instances may be beneficially affected by nutritional supplementation, as is the case with lack of myelination in the corpus callosum of preterm infants. This he takes as an example of 'bidirectional' influences between the neural level and the environmental level in terms of the developmental 'systems model'.

2   Areal specialization of the developing neocortex: differentiation, developmental plasticity and genetic specification

DENNIS D. M. O'LEARY

The mammalian neocortex is responsible for diverse functions, ranging from the processing of visual, auditory and somatic sensations, the integration of this information into multimodal perceptions, and to even more complex phenomena such as learning, memory and behavior. These tasks are carried out by the functionally specialized areas of the neocortex, which are defined by differences in architecture and connections (Brodmann, 1909; Krieg, 1946). The developing neocortex, though, lacks many of these area-specific distinctions, and is more uniform across its extent. The immature neocortex undergoes considerable modification after neurogenesis which results in the emergence of the highly differentiated neocortical areas of the adult. The question considered in this chapter is how do areas of the neocortex acquire their unique characteristics? As discussed, increasing evidence suggests that many of the prominent features that distinguish areas of the neocortex are not determined at the time of neurogenesis, but instead are established through subsequent epigenetic interactions.

DISTINCT CORTICAL AREAS IN THE ADULT HAVE SIMILARITIES

Neocortical areas have prominent differences in connections, both efferent (i.e. outputs) and afferent (i.e. inputs), as well as in architecture, ranging from substantial variations in cell sizes and densities to differences in the distributions of extracellular matrix molecules and receptors for neurotransmitters. These area-specific characteristics contribute to the unique functional properties of the diverse neocortical areas. However, neocortical areas also have features in common. The most obvious one is that all areas have six main layers, a defining feature of the neocortex. Although laminar appearance differs from area to area, the principal characteristics of each layer, for example, the laminar arrangement of cortical projection neurons and terminations of afferent inputs, are constant: layer 6 neurons project to the thalamus and claustrum, layer 5 neurons project to the midbrain, hindbrain and spinal cord, neurons in layers 2 and 3 are the principal source of projections to other neo-cortical areas, while layer 4 receives the densest innervation from the thalamus (Gilbert, 1983; Jones, 1984). Other features are also surprisingly similar across areas. For example, the number of neurons found in a 'radial traverse' through the six layers is constant between diverse neocortical areas (with the exception of a greater number in primary visual cortex), even though cortical thickness varies considerably (Rockel, Hiorns & Powell, 1980; Hendry et al., 1987). The proportion of cells classified by shape as pyramidal or non-pyramidal, or as gabaergic – the predominant cortical inhibitory cell, is also similar (Winfield, Gatter & Powell, 1980; Hendry et al., 1987). Cortical neurons of other neurotransmitter or peptide phenotypes (see, for example, Fluxe et al., 1977; Peters, Miller & Kimerer, 1983; Morrison et al., 1983; Hendry, Jones & Emson, 1984), and even neurons of very rare biochemical phenotypes (Stephenson and Kushner, 1988), are also present in all neocortical areas. In brief, neurons representative of all the basic morphological and chemically defined phenotypes are widely distributed within the adult neocortex.

The structural and physiological similarities between areas of the adult neocortex have prompted many to propose that the different primary cortical areas share a common organizational scheme (Lorente de No, 1949; Creutzfeldt, 1977; Mountcastle, 1978; Powell, 1981; Eccles, 1984). This suggestion has been validated experimentally in animals by an analysis of the way in which somatosensory or auditory cortex processes visual input, an unusual circumstance achieved by misrouting retinal axons to somatosensory thalamic nuclei (Metin & Frost, 1989) or to auditory thalamic nuclei (Sur, Garraghty & Roe, 1988) deprived of their normal sensory input. In these animals, the receptive field and response properties of cells in somatosensory or auditory cortex to visual stimuli resemble those normally seen in visual cortex. Some cells in the somatosensory cortex to which visual input is directed were even found to have modality appropriate responses to both visual and somatosensory stimuli (Metin & Frost, 1989). The most straightforward explanation for these findings is that the primary sensory areas of the neocortex normally process in a fundamentally similar way sensory information relayed through the thalamus. In turn, this implies that the basic organization of cells and connections that underlie functional properties is also similar. In summary, the diverse areas of the adult neocortex seem to be constructed with the same basic types of cells organized in a similar way, yet each area has a unique functional identity which reflects the often dramatic differences between areas in architecture and connectivity.

UNIFORMITY IN THE DEVELOPING NEOCORTEX

Cortical neurons are generated in the dorsal telencephalic neuroepithelium of the lateral ventricle. The first neurons to be generated leave the neuroepithelium and accumulate beneath the pial surface, forming a transient layer termed the preplate (Marin-Padilla, 1971, 1972; Luskin & Shatz, 1985; Stewart & Pearlman, 1987; Chun & Shatz, 1989). Next, the neurons that populate layers 2 through 6 of the adult cortex are generated. These cells migrate superficially from the neuroepithelium along radial glia (Rakic, 1978, 1981), aggregate within the preplate, and form an undifferentiated layer called the cortical plate. As more cells are added to the cortical plate, it splits the preplate into a superficial, neuron-sparse marginal zone (future layer 1) located just beneath the pia, and a deep subplate layer located just beneath future layer 6 (Luskin & Shatz, 1985). The cortical plate subsequently matures in a deep to superficial pattern, with layer 6 being the first to differentiate and layer 2 the last (Rakic, 1974).

The developing neocortex lacks the area-specific features characteristic of the adult. For instance, cytoarchitecture is uniform across the developing neocortex. A striking feature of the primary sensory areas of the adult neocortex is the dense accumulation in layer 4 of small neurons with a 'stellate' morphology, resulting in a 'granular' appearance (Brodmann, 1909). The high density of stellate neurons is coincident with the dense layer 4 terminations of thalamocortical afferents from the principal sensory thalamic nuclei. The appearance of primary sensory areas is in sharp contrast to the appearance of 'agranular' areas of the neocortex, such as the primary motor cortex, which have a poorly defined, less dense layer 4. However, earlier in development, layer 4 of monkey primary motor cortex does have a granular appearance due to a high density of small neurons, and resembles that in somatosensory cortex (Huntley & Jones, 1991). Even the abrupt and dramatic cytoarchitectural border between visual areas 17 and 18 in the adult macaque monkey is not detectable early on and becomes apparent only after the cortex is invaded by thalamocortical afferents (Kostovic & Rakic, 1984). Another example of uniformity in the developing neocortex is the distribution of projection neurons. In the adult neocortex, the unique outputs of areas are reflected by the limited distributions of types of cortical projection neurons. However, during development all types of projection neurons are widely distributed across the neocortex (O'Leary et al., 1990; O'Leary & Koester, 1993).

Taken together, these comparisons between developing and adult neocortex suggest that the entire extent of the neocortical neuroepithelium is competent to generate the basic types of cortical neurons. Although the basic laminar organization of the neocortex appears to be determined in the neuroepithelium (McConnell, 1989; McConnell & Kaznowski, 1991; Katz & Callaway, 1992; O'Leary & Koester, 1993), considerable evidence indicates that many, if not all, of the 'area-specific' features are not committed properties and require extrinsic influences, for example thalamocortical input, that act later in development to shape them (O'Leary, 1989; Killackey, 1990; O'Leary, Schlaggar and Tuttle, 1994).

MECHANISMS INVOLVED IN THE DIFFERENTIATION OF AREA-SPECIFIC ARCHITECTURE AND EFFERENT PROJECTIONS

Two mechanisms, differential neuronal death and changes in neuronal morphology, each influenced by thalamocortical input, can account for much of the cytoarchitectural differences between areas. In rodents, about 30% of cortical neurons die, with most of the loss occurring in the superficial layers and to a lesser extent in layer 4 (Finlay & Slattery, 1983; Huemann et al., 1978; Windrem & Finlay, 1991). The number of surviving cells in layer 4 is governed in large part by the density of thalamic input. For example, removal of thalamocortical input to visual cortex produces large-scale neuronal degeneration in layer 4 and a loss of its granular appearance (Windrem & Finlay, 1991). Thalamocortical input also has dramatic influences on the dendritic development of cortical neurons (Harris & Woolsey, 1981; Peinado & Katz, 1990). For example, layer 4 stellate neurons in rat somatosensory cortex initially develop a small pyramidal morphology characteristic of layer 3 neurons and only later lose their apical dendrite and develop a stellate appearance (Peinado & Katz, 1990). This morphological change can be prevented by blocking the sensory information relayed by thalamocortical afferents from the periphery to somatosensory cortex in neonatal rodents. Thus, thalamocortical afferents can influence cytoarchitecture by regulating both cell death and dendritic elaboration and remodeling.

The set of output projections of a given neocortical area in the adult is only a subset of the projections that it originally elaborates. Selective axon or collateral elimination plays a major role in generating the characteristic patterning of the three major categories of cortical projections: callosal, intracortical, and subcortical projections. For example, the limited, discontinuous distributions of callosal neurons in adult cortex have been found to emerge from early widespread, continuous distributions of callosal neurons in all species examined, including primates (Killackey & Chalupa, 1986; Dehay et al., 1988), and in every cortical area studied (with the possible exception of the primary visual cortex of macaques; Dehay et al., 1988), by the selective elimination of a subset of the initially extended callosal axons (Innocenti, 1981; O'Leary, Stanfield & Cowan 1981; Ivy & Killackey, 1982; Chalupa and Killackey, 1989). Collateral elimination has also been implicated in the development of the mature connectional relationships between cortical areas in the same hemisphere (Price & Blackmore, 1985; Innocenti, Clarke & Kraftsik, 1986; Kennedy, Bullier & Dehay, 1989; Meissirel et al., 1990) as well as being instrumental in the refinement of horizontal connections within an area (Callaway & Katz, 1990), leading to the establishment of specific connections between groups of cells with like functional properties.

Collateral elimination is also prominent in the generation of area-specific efferent projections. The organization of the adult neocortex into functionally specialized areas requires that each area has efferent projections to specific structures in the brainstem and spinal cord. Layer 5 is the only source of cortical projections to the midbrain, hindbrain and spinal cord. In the adult, layer 5 neurons that project to these targets are limited to specific areas of the cortex that differs from target to target. However, as a population, developing layer 5 neurons in all areas of the developing neocortex initially extend a spinally directed primary axon and form collateral projections to the full set of brainstem targets (O'Leary et al., 1990). Area-specific, layer 5 projections emerge through the selective loss of different subsets of the initial set of collateral projections. For example, layer 5 neurons in motor cortex lose their axon collateral to the superior colliculus, while those in visual cortex lose their collateral projections to the inferior olive and dorsal column nuclei, as well as the segment of their primary axon caudal to the basilar pons (Stanfield et al., 1982; O'Leary & Stanfield, 1985; Stanfield & O'Leary, 1985a; Thong & Dreher, 1986; O'Leary & Terashima, 1988; O'Leary et al., 1990). Thus, the functionally appropriate efferent projections characteristic of the adult do not develop from the outset; instead, they are selected from a common projection pattern initially developed by layer 5 neurons across the entire neocortex.

The mechanisms that control the final pattern of cortical projections are poorly understood, but the evidence indicates that sensory input has a modulatory role. The elimination of callosal axons is altered by peripheral manipulations of either visual (Innocenti, 1986; Dehay et al., 1989; Dehay et al., 1991; Frost, May & Smith, 1990) or somatosensory (Koralex & Killackey, 1990) input, which alters either patterns of activity (e.g., strabismus) or absolute levels of activity (e.g., eyelid suture or pharmacological silencing of retinal activity). In these instances, callosal connections are retained between cortical areas that would normally lose them. Similarly, binocular eyelid suture disrupts the refinement of horizontal connections within visual cortex (Callaway & Katz, 1991). Thus sensory input plays an important role in the mature patterning of callosal and intracortical connections by influencing the pattern of axon elimination.

The evidence for sensory influences on the elimination of layer 5 axons is less direct than in the callosal projection, but is nevertheless intriguing. In rodents in which somatosensory information was misrouted to visual cortex during development, layer 5 neurons in visual cortex permanently retained their normally transient spinal axons – a projection characteristic of somatosensory cortex (O'Leary, 1992). A similar correlation can be derived from heterotopic cortical transplant experiments: transplants both receive sensory afferent input (Chang, Steedman & Lurd, 1986; Schlaggar & O'Leary, 1991; O'Leary, Schlagger & Stanfield, 1992) and permanently retain layer 5 collateral projections to subcortical targets (Stanfield & O'Leary, 1985b; O'Leary & Stanfield, 1989) appropriate for their new location. These observations are consistent with the idea that thalamocortical input or the sensory information relayed by this input may contribute to the development of area-specific patterns of layer 5 subcortical projections by influencing selective axon stabilization (or elimination).

PLASTICITY IN THE DEVELOPMENT OF AREA-SPECIFIC ARCHITECTURE AND CONNECTIONS

If the developing neocortex is truly similar across its extent and the differentiation of area-specific features is not rigidly specified, one would expect that the immature neocortex would be capable of considerable plasticity in its expression of area-specific features. This notion has been tested by heterotopic transplantation experiments. One set of experiments made use of 'barrels', which are unique functional and architectural groupings characteristic of the primary somatosensory cortex of adult rodents. Barrels, which process sensory information from large whiskers on the animal's face, are aggregations of layer 4 neurons surrounding a cluster of thalamic afferents and are distributed in a pattern that mirrors that of facial whiskers (Woolsey & Van Der Loos, 1970). Barrels are not apparent as the cortex is assembled, but emerge later from an initially uniform layer 4 through an interaction with thalamic afferents that relay sensory information from the whiskers (Woolsey, 1990). In one set of experiments, late embryonic visual cortex was transplanted into somatosensory cortex in newborn rats (Schlaggar & O'Leary, 1991) to challenge two hypotheses: first, that information intrinsic to somatosensory cortex is necessary to differentiate barrels; and second, that other neocortical areas are restricted in their fate such that they cannot differentiate the area-specific properties unique to somatosensory cortex. Inconsistent with these hypotheses, it was found that transplanted visual cortex developed the distinct features of normal barrels (Schlaggar & O'Leary, 1991). Since late embryonic visual cortex has the capacity to develop the functional and architectural groupings normally unique to somatosensory cortex, it must not be committed to develop the area-specific architecture and thalamocortical afferent characteristic of mature visual cortex, but instead is competent to form features characteristic of other neocortical areas. These findings also indicate that barrel architecture is not a specified feature of somatosensory cortex.

Other heterotopic transplantation experiments indicate that the areal location of a piece of developing neocortex has a decisive influence on the development of area-specific connections. For example, the layer 5 efferent projections permanently established by late fetal neocortex heterotopically transplanted to the neocortex of newborn rodents are appropriate for the transplant's new location. Visual cortical neurons transplanted to the sensorimotor cortex extend and permanently retain axons to the spinal cord, a subcortical target of sensorimotor cortex (Stanfield & O'Leary, 1985b;

O'Leary & Stanfield, 1989). Conversely, sensorimotor cortical neurons transplanted to visual cortex extend and then lose spinal axons, but retain a projection to the superior colliculus, a subcortical target of visual cortex (O'Leary & Stanfield, 1989). Heterotopic transplants also establish callosal and thalamic connections, both efferent and afferent, appropriate for their new location (Chang, Steedman & Lund, 1986; O'Leary & Stanfield, 1989; O'Leary et al., 1992). These experiments indicate that different areas of the developing neocortex are sufficiently alike that when heterotopically placed in the developing neocortex they will develop many of the area-specific features normally associated with their new location.

Similar conclusions can be drawn from studies in macaque monkeys which show that the border between primary visual cortex (area 17) and a secondary visual area (area 18) is capable of a large shift with dramatic consequences on the subsequent differentiation of the affected piece of cortex (Rakic, 1988; Dehay et al., 1989; Dehay et al., 1991). Such a border shift occurs in macaques in which both eyes were removed at mid-fetal stages. This manipulation results in a 50% or greater loss in the number of lateral geniculate neurons, the primary source of thalamic input to area 17, as well as a corresponding reduction in the total number of neurons in area 17 and its overall size. Features characteristic of area 17, indicating laminar thickness and appearance, laminar distributions of receptors for neurotransmitters and the presence of functional groupings specific to area 17 (i.e. blobs), are retained within the reduced area identified as area 17 based on cytoarchitectural appearance (Rakic, 1988; Rakic, Suner & Williams, 1991). However, in these monkeys a part of cortex normally contained within the borders of area 17 takes on the architectural characteristics of area 18. In addition, the callosal projections of area 17 are altered and resemble those of area 18 (Dehay et al., 1989). These findings provide further evidence that the architectural and connectional differentiation of a neocortical area can be developmentally controlled by epigenetic factors. Again, thalamocortical input has been suggested to have a critical, regulatory role in this phenomenon (Rakic, 1988).

These experimental findings indicate that diverse areas of the developing neocortex have similar potentials to differentiate the range of connectional and architectural features seen in the adult neocortex. The area-specific features that a part of the neocortex ultimately differentiates depends on where within the neocortex it develops, not on where it was generated. In other words, cortical plate neurons are not committed to a particular area fate when they leave the neuroepithelium. Studies which have investigated the spatial relationship between the neocortical neuroepithelium and the overlying cortical plate suggest a similar conclusion. Walsh & Cepko (1992, 1993) have used a battery of recombinant retroviruses with unique cDNA tags to show that clonally related cortical plate neurons commonly disperse widely in the neocortex, often scattering over many cortical areas. Given the small size of the neuroepithelium relative to the large size of overlying cortical plate, small dispersions of clonally related cells in the neuroepithelium could result in large displacements by the time the cells reach the cortical plate, especially since the radial glial scaffolding becomes progressively distorted (Misson et al., 1991). Indeed, cells in the neocortical neuroepithelium do move about randomly which results in the dispersion of once neighboring cells within the neuroepithelium (Fishell, Mason & Hatten, 1993). Other mechanisms also contribute to dispersion, such as the tangential migration of cells in the intermediate zone orthogonal to radial glia (O'Rourke et al., 1992) and the shifting of migrating cells from one radial glial fascicle to another (Austin & Cepko, 1990; Misson et al., 1991). The magnitude of dispersion of clonally related, cortical plate cells has led Walsh & Cepko (1992) to conclude that the specification of neocortical areas must occur after neurogenesis.

DEVELOPMENT OF AREA-SPECIFIC THALAMOCORTICAL PROJECTIONS

Thalamocortical input plays a fundamental role in defining neocortical areas, not only in the adult but also during development. In the adult, the modality of thalamic input dictates an area's functional identity. During development, thalamocortical afferents control the differentiation of neocortical areas from an initially 'uniform' cortical plane. A crucial issue in both cortical function and differentiation is defining the mechanisms that control the development of area-specific thalamocortical projections, and in turn the differentiation of cortical areas.

In the adult, thalamocortical projections are organized in an area-specific manner, that is specific thalamic nuclei project to specific neocortical areas; for example the lateral geniculate nucleus projects to primary visual cortex and the ventroposterior nucleus projects to primary somatosensory cortex (Hohl-Abrahao & Creutzfeldt, 1991). During development, thalamocortical axons target their appropriate cortical area with remarkable precision; thalamocortical axons rarely extend beyond their correct area or make gross directional errors (De Carlos, Schlagger & O'Leary, 1992), nor do they invade the cortical plate of inappropriate areas (Crandall & Caviness, 1984, De Carlos, et al., 1992). The establishment of area-specific thalamocortical projections argues for some form of specification in the developing cortex that generates position-dependent information.

Several lines of evidence suggest that thalamocortical axons use information available in the subplate layer to target their appropriate cortical areas. First, since the intracortical pathway of thalamocortical axons is centered on the subplate, they are in a position to be influenced by potential targeting cues associated with it (Miller, Chou & Finlay, 1993; Bicknese et al., 1994). Secondly, their 'decision' to invade an area of cortex is made within the subplate (Reinoso & O'Leary, 1990; Ghosh & Shatz, 1992). Third, thalamo-cortical axons grow past, rather than invading, the cortical plate overlying regions of the subplate pharmacologically depleted of neurons (Ghosh et al., 1990). Thus, the cues which set up specific thalamocortical relationships are likely to operate within the subplate. One way to lay down these cues would be for progenitor cells in the neuroepithelium to impart positional information to their progeny. Such a mechanism would require that gene expression be regulated in a position-dependent manner.

Evidence for position-dependent gene expression in the developing neo-cortex comes from the description of the expression patterns of mammalian homologues of the *Drosophila* gene, *empty spiracles* (Simeone et al., 1992). These genes, termed *Emx-1* and *Emx-2*, encode putative homeodomain transcription factors and have overlapping expression patterns in the de-veloping telencephalon. Within the embryonic mouse neocortex, *Emx-1* is expressed uniformly whereas *Emx-2* has a caudal to rostral graded pattern of expression, which strongly suggests that the graded expression of *Emx-2* is indeed position-dependent. Although the expression of *Emx-2* neither de-lineates nor predicts neocortical areas, *Emx-2* could direct a genetic cascade that regulates the position-dependent expression of genes encoding molecules that directly control the area-specific targeting of thalamocortical axons. This mechanism requires that the progeny of neighboring proliferative cells in the neocortical neuroepithelium maintain neighbor relationships in the subplate. If dispersion is substantial, targeting information very likely has a source other than subplate cells or is specified by interactions that occur after the preplate is established.

As described in a preceding section, the use of recombinant retroviruses to mark clonally related cells shows that neurons generated at later stages of corticogenesis, when the cortical plate is being assembled, disperse widely across diverse areas of the neocortex (Walsh & Cepko, 1992). For technical reasons, the recombinant retroviral method has not been successfully applied to study neuronal dispersion at earlier stages of corticogenesis, during the generation of the subplate. However, time-lapse videomicroscopy of fluores-cently labeled neuroepithelial cells and their progeny in fetal rat cortex maintained *in vitro*, indicates that subplate neurons and their progenitors maintain spatial relationships (O'Leary & Borngasser, 1992). Therefore, positional information imparted to subplate cells around the time they are generated could regulate the later deployment of guidance molecules to con-trol the area-specific targeting of thalamocortical axons. In this way, molecular information laid down in the subplate could influence the subsequent differentiation of area-specific features within the overlying cortical plate.

CONCLUSIONS

Evidence provided by a variety of experimental studies suggests that individual areas of the developing neocortex have the capacity to differentiate the range of architectural and connectional features characteristic of other neocortical areas. These findings do not rule out that neocortical neurons carry area-specific information, but they restrict the role required for this information in bringing about areal differentiation. Many studies indicate a pivotal role for thalamocortical afferents in the differentiation of the area-specific features that distinguish neocortical areas. Several lines of evidence are consistent with the idea that positional information is established in the cortical subplate and that this information controls the precise targeting of developing thalamocortical axons. In such a way, appropriate thalamocortical relationships can be established, which would allow these afferents to promote the differentiation of the functionally specialized and anatomically distinct areas of the adult neocortex.

ACKNOWLEDGMENT

Work on this topic in the author's laboratory is supported by NIH grant NS31558.

REFERENCES

Austin, C. P. & Cepko, C. L. (1990) Migration patterns in the developing mouse cortex. *Development*, **110**, 713–32.

Bicknese, A. R., Sheppard, A. M., O'Leary, D. D. M. & Pearlman, A. L. (1994) Thalamocortical axons extend along a chondroitin sulfate proteoglycan-enriched pathway coincident with the neocortical subplate and distinct from the efferent path. *Journal of Neuroscience*, **14**, 3500–10.

Brodmann, K. (1909) Lokalisationslehre der Groshirnrinde in ihren Principen dargestellt aug Grund des Zellen baue. Barth: Lepzig.

Callaway, E. M. & Katz, L. C. (1990) Emergence and refinement of clustered horizontal connections in cat striate cortex. *Journal of Neuroscience*, **10**, 1134–53.

Callaway, E. M. & Katz, L. C. (1991) Effects of binocular deprivation on the development of clustered horizontal connections in cat striate cortex. *Proceedings of the National Academy of Science of the USA*, **88**, 745–9.

Chalupa, L. M. & Killackey, H. P. (1989) Process elimination underlies ontogenetic change in the distribution of callosal projection neurons in the postcentral gyrus of the fetal rhesus monkey. *Proceedings of the National Academy of Science of the USA*, **86**, 1076–9.

Chang, F.-L. F., Steedman, J. G. & Lund, R. D. (1986) The lamination and connectivity of embryonic cerebral cortex transplanted into newborn rat cortex. *Journal of Comparative Neurology*, **244**, 401–11.

Chun, J. J. M. & Shatz, C. J. (1989) The earliest-generated neurons of the cat cerebral cortex: characterization by MAP-2 and neurotransmitter immunohistochemistry during fetal life. *Journal of Neuroscience*, **9**, 1648–67.

Crandall, J. E. & Caviness, V. S. (1984) Thalamocortical connections in newborn mice. *Journal of Comparative Neurology*, **228**, 542–6.

Creutzfeldt, O. D. (1977) Generality of the functional structure of the neocortex. *Naturwissen*, **64**, 507–17.

De Carlos, J. A., Schlaggar, B. L. & O'Leary, D. D. M. (1992) Targeting specificity of primary sensory thalamocortical axons in developing rat neocortex. *Society of Neuroscience Abstracts,* **18**, 57.

Dehay, C., Horsburgh, G., Berland, M., Killackey, H. & Kennedy, H. (1989) Maturation and connectivity of the visual cortex in monkeys altered by prenatal removal of spinal input. *Nature,* **337**, 265–7.

Dehay, C., Horsburgh, G., Berland, M., Killackey, H. & Kennedy, H. (1991) The effects of bilateral enucleation in the primate fetus on the parcellation of visual cortex. *Developmental Brain Research* **62**, 137–41.

Dehay, C., Kennedy, H., Bullier, J. & Berland, M. (1988) Absence of inter-hemispheric connections of area 17 during development in the monkey. *Nature,* **331**, 348–59.

Eccles, J. C. (1984) The cerebral neocortex. A theory of its operation. In Jones, E. G. & Peters, A. (eds.) *Cerebral Cortex. Vol. 2, Functional Properties of Cortical Cells.* New York: Plenum Press, pp. 1–36.

Fishell, G., Mason, C. A. & Hatten, M. E. (1993) Dispersion of neural progenitors within the germinal zones of the forebrain. *Nature,* **362**, 636–8.

Finlay, B. L. & Slattery, M. (1983) Local differences in the amount of early cell death in neocortex predict adult local specializations. *Science,* **219**, 1349–51.

Frost, D. O., Moy, Y. P. & Smith, D. C. (1990) Effects of alternating monocular occulsion on the development of visual callosal connections. *Experimental Brain Research,* **83**, 200–9.

Fuxe, K., Hokfelt, T., Said, S. I. & Mutt, V. (1977) Vasoactive intestinal polypeptide and the nervous system: immunohistochemical evidence for localization in central and peripheral neurons, particularly intracortical neurons of the cerebral cortex. *Neuroscience Letters,* **5**, 241–6.

Ghosh, A., Antonini, A., McConnell, S. K. & Shatz, C. J. (1990) Requirement for subplate neurons in the formation of thalamocortical connections. *Nature,* **347**, 179–81.

Ghosh, A. & Shatz, C. (1992) Pathfinding and target selection by developing geniculocortical axons. *Journal of Neuroscience,* **12**, 39–55.

Gilbert, C. D. (1983) Microcircuitry of the visual cortex. *Annual Review of Neuroscience,* **6**, 217–48.

Harris, R. M. & Woolsey, T. A. (1981) Dendritic plasticity in mouse barrel cortex following postnatal vibrassa follicle damage. *Journal of Comparative Neurology,* **196**, 357–76.

Hendry, S. H. C., Jones, E. G. & Emson, P. C. (1984) Morphology, distribution, and synaptic relations of somatostatin- and neuropeptide Y-immunoreactive neurons in rat and monkey neocortex. *Journal of Neuroscience,* **4**, 2497–517.

Hendry, S. H. C., Schwark, H. D., Jones, E. G. & Yan, J. (1987) Numbers and proportions of Gaba-immunoreactive neurons in different areas of monkey cerebral cortex. *Journal of Neuroscience,* **7**, 1503–19.

Hohl-Abrahao, J. C. & Creutzfeldt, O. D. (1991) Topographic mapping of the thalamocortical projections in rodents and comparison with that in primates. *Experimental Brain Research,* **87**, 283–94.

Huemann, D., Lueba, G. & Rabinowicz, G. (1978) Postnatal development of the mouse cerebral cortex. IV. Evolution of the total cortical volume, of the population of neurons and glial cells. *Journal für Hirnforschung,* **19**, 385–93.

Huntley, G. W. & Jones, E. G. (1991) The emergence of architectonic field structure and areal borders in developing monkey somatosensory cortex. *Neuroscience*, **44**, 287–310.

Innocenti, G. M. (1981) Growth and reshaping of axons in the establishment of visual callosal connections. *Science*, **212**, 824–7.

Innocenti, G. M. (1986) General organization of callosal connections in the cerebral cortex. In Jones, E. G. & Peters, A. (eds.) *Cerebral Cortex, Vol. 5*, Sensory motor areas and aspects of cortical connectivity. New York: Plenum, pp. 291–353.

Innocenti, G. M., Clarke, S. & Kraftsik, R. (1986) Interchange of callosal and association projections in the developing visual cortex. *Journal of Neuroscience*, **6**, 1384–409.

Ivy, G. O. & Killackey, H. P. (1982) Ontogenetic changes in the projections of neurocortical neurons. *Journal of Neuroscience*, **6**, 735–43.

Jones, E. G. (1984) Laminar distribution of cortical efferent cells. In E. G. Jones & A. Peters (eds.) *Cerebral Cortex. Vol. 1. Cellular Components of the Cerebral Cortex*. New York: Plenum, pp. 521–53.

Katz, L. C. & Callaway, E. M. (1992) Development of local circuits in mammalian visual cortex. *Annual Review of Neuroscience*, **15**, 31–56.

Kennedy, H., Bullier, J. & Dehay, C. (1989) Transient projection from the superior temporal sulcus to area 17 in the newborn macaque monkey. *Proceedings of the National Academy of Science of the USA*, **86**, 8093–7.

Killackey, H. P. (1990) Neocortical expansion: an attempt toward relating phylogeny and ontogeny. *Journal of Cognitive Neuroscience* **2**, 1–17.

Killackey, H. P. & Chalupa, L. M. (1986) Ontogenetic changes in the distribution of callosal projection neurons in the postcentral gyrus of the fetal rhesus monkey. *Journal of Comparative Neurology*, **244**, 33–48.

Koralek, K. A. & Killackey, H. P. (1990) Callosal projections in rat somatosensory cortex are altered by early removal of afferent input. *Proceedings of the National Academy of Science of the USA*, **87**, 1396–400.

Kostovic, I. & Rakic, P. (1984) Development of prestriate visual projections in the monkey and human fetal cerebrum revealed by transient cholinesterase staining. *Journal of Neuroscience*, **4**, 25–42.

Krieg, W. J. S. (1946) Connections of the cerebral cortex. I. The albino rat. A. Topography of the cortical areas. *Journal of Comparative Neurology*, **84**, 221–75.

Lorente de No, R. (1949) Cerebral cortex: Architecture, intracortical connections, motor projections. In Fulton, J. F., (ed.) *Physiology of the Nervous System*. Oxford: Oxford University Press, pp. 288–315.

Luskin, M. B. & Shatz, C. J. (1985) Studies of the earliest generated cells of the cat's visual cortex: cogeneration of subplate and marginal zones. *Journal of Neuroscience*, **5**, 1062–75.

Marin-Padilla, M. (1971) Early prenatal ontogenesis of the cerebral cortex (neocortex) of the cat (Felis domestica). A. Gogli study. I. The primoidal neocortical organization. *Zeittung für Anatomie und Ertwicklungseschichte*, **134**, 117–45.

Marin-Padilla, M. (1972) Prenatal ontogenetic story of the principal neurons of the neocortex of the cat (Felis domestica). A Golgi study. II. Developmental differences and their significances. *Zeittung für Anatomie und Ertwicklungseschichte*, **136**, 125–42.

McConnell, S. K. (1989) The determination of neuronal fate in the cerebral cortex. *Trends in Neuroscience*, **12**, 342–9.

McConnell, S. K. & Kaznowski, C. E. (1991) Cell cycle dependence of laminar determination in developing neocortex. *Science,* **254**, 282–5.

Meissirel, C., Dehay, C., Berland, M. and Kennedy, H. (1990) Incidence of visual cortical neurons which have axon collaterals projecting to both cerebral hemispheres during prenatal primate development. *Developments in Brain Research,* **56**, 123–6.

Metin, C. & Frost, D. O. (1989) Visual responses of neurons in somatosensory cortex of hamsters with experimentally induced retinal projections to somatosensory thalamus. *Proceedings of the National Academy of Science of the USA,* **86**, 357–61.

Miller, B., Chou, L. & Finlay, B. L. (1993) The early development of thalamocortical and corticothalamic projections. *Journal of Comparative Neurology,* **335**, 16–41.

Misson, J.-P., Austin, C. P., Takahashi, T., Cepko, C. L. & Caviness, V. S. Jr. (1991) The alignment of migrating neural cells in relation to the murine neopallial radial glial fiber system. *Cerebral Cortex,* **1**, 221–9.

Morrison, J. H., Benoit, P. J., Magistretti, P. J. & Bloom, F. E. (1983) Immunohisto-chemical distribution of pro-somatostatin-related peptides in cerebral cortex. *Brain Research,* **262**, 344–51.

Mountcastle, V. B. (1978) In Mountcastle V. B. & Edelman, G. M. (eds.) *The Mindful Brain.* Cambridge: MIT Press, pp. 7–50.

O'Leary, D. D. M. (1989) Do cortical areas emerge from a proto-cortex? *Trends in Neuroscience,* **12**, 400–6.

O'Leary, D. D. M., Bicknese, A. R., De Carlos, J. A., Heffer, C. D., Koester, S. E., Kutka, L. J. & Terashima, T. (1990) Target selection by cortical axons: alternative mechanisms to establish axonal connections in the developing brain. *Cold Spring Harbor Symposium on Quantitative Biology,* **55**, 543–68.

O'Leary, D. D. M. (1992) Development of connectional deversity and specificity in the mammalian brain by the pruning of collateral projections. *Current Opinion in Neurobiology,* **2**, 70–77.

O'Leary, D. D. M. & Borngasser, D. (1992) Minimal dispersion of neuroepithelial cells and their progeny during generation of the cortical preplate. *Society for Neuroscience Abstracts,* **18**, 925.

O'Leary, D. D. M. & Koester, S. E. (1993) Development of projection neuron types, axonal pathways and patterned connections of the mammalian cortex. *Neuron,* **10**, 991–1006.

O'Leary, D. D. M., Schlaggar, B. L. & Stanfield, B. B. (1992) The specification of sensory cortex: lessons from cortical transplantation. *Experimental Neurology,* **115**, 121–6.

O'Leary, D. D. M., Schlaggar, B. L. & Tuttle, R. (1994) Specification of neocortical areas and thalamocortical connections. *Annual Review of Neuroscience,* **17**, 419–39.

O'Leary, D. D. M. & Stanfield, B. B. (1985) Occipital cortical neurons with transient pyramidal tract axons extend and maintain collaterals to subcortical but not intracortical targets. *Brain Research,* **336**, 326–33.

O'Leary, D. D. M. & Stanfield, B. B. (1989) Selective elimination of axons extended by developing cortical neurons is dependent on regional locale: experiments utilizing fetal cortical transplants. *Journal Neuroscience,* **9**, 2230–46.

O'Leary, D. D. M., Stanfield, B. B. & Cowan, M. W. (1981) Evidence that the early postnatal restriction of the cells of origin of the callosal projection is due to the elimination of axon collaterals rather than to death of neurons. *Brain Research,* **1**, 607–17.

O'Leary, D. D. M. & Terashima, T. (1988) Cortical axons branch to multiple subcortical targets by interstitial axon budding: implications for target recognition and 'waiting periods'. *Neuron,* **1,** 901–10.

O'Rourke, N. A., Dailey, M. E., Smith, S. J. & McConnell, S. K. (1992) Diverse migratory pathways in the developing cerebral cortex. *Science,* **258,** 299–302.

Peinado, A. & Katz, L. C. (1990) Development of cortical spiny stellate cells: retraction of a transient apical dendrite. *Society for Neuroscience Abstracts,* **16,** 1127.

Peters, A., Miller, M. & Kimerer, L. M. (1983) Cholecystokinin-like immunoreactive neurons in rat cerebral cortex. *Neuroscience,* **8,** 431–48.

Powell, T. P. S. (1981) Certain aspects of the intrinsic organization of the cerebral cortex. In Pompeiana, O. & Ajmone Marsan, C. (eds.) *Brain Mechanisms and Perceptual Awareness.* New York: Raven Press, pp. 1–19.

Price, D. J. & Blakemore, C. (1985) Regressive events in the postnatal development of association projections in the visual cortex. *Nature,* **316,** 721–4.

Rakic, P. (1974) Neurons in the rhesus monkey visual cortex: systematic relation between time of origin and eventual disposition. *Science,* **183,** 425–7.

Rakic, P. (1978) Neuronal migration and contact guidance in primate telencephalon. *Postgraduate Medical Journal,* **54,** 25–40.

Rakic, P. (1981) Developmental events leading to laminar and areal organization of the neocortex. In Schmitt, F. O., Worden, F. G., Adelman, F. G. & Dennis, S. G. (eds.) *The Organization of the Cerebral Cortex.* MIT Press: Cambridge, Mass., pp. 74–8.

Rakic, P. (1988) Specification of cerebral cortical areas. *Science,* **241,** 170–6.

Rakic, P., Suner, I. & Williams, R. W. (1991) A novel cytoarchitectonic area induced experimentally within the primate visual cortex. *Proceedings of the National Academy of Science of the USA,* **88,** 2083–7.

Reinoso, B. S. & O'Leary, D. D. M. (1990) Correlation of geniculocortical growth into the cortical plate with the migration of their layer 4 and 6 target cells. *Society for Neuroscience Abstracts,* **16,** 439.

Rockel, A. J., Hiorns, R. W. & Powell, T. P. S. (1980) The basic uniformity in structure of the neocortex. *Brain,* 103, 221–44.

Schlaggar, B. L. & O'Leary, D. D. M. (1991) Potential of visual cortex to develop arrays of functional units unique to somatosensory cortex. *Science,* **252,** 1556–60.

Simeone, A., Guilsano, M., Acampora, D., Stornaiuolo, A., Rambaldi, M. & Boncinelli, E. (1992) Two vertebrate homeobox genes related to the Drosophila empty spiracles gene are expressed in the embryonic cerebral cortex. *European Molecular Biology Organization Journal,* **11,** 2541–50.

Stanfield, B. B. & O'Leary, D. D. M. (1985a) The transient corticospinal projection from the visual cortex during the postnatal development of the rat. *Journal of Comparative Neurology,* **238,** 236–48.

Stanfield, B. B. & O'Leary, D. D. M. (1985b) Fetal occipital cortical neurons transplanted to the rostral cortex can extend and maintain a pyramidal tract axon. *Nature,* **313,** 135–7.

Stanfield, B. B., O'Leary, D. D. M. & Fricks, C. (1982) Selective collateral elimination in early postnatal development restricts cortical distribution of rat pyramidal tract neurones. *Nature,* **298,** 371–3.

Stephenson, D. T. & Kushner, P. D. (1988) An atlas of a rare neuronal surface antigen in the rat central nervous system. *Journal of Neuroscience,* **8,** 3035–56.

Stewart, G. R. & Pearlman, A. L. (1987) Fibronectin-like immunoreactivity in the developing cerebral cortex. *Journal of Neuroscience,* **7,** 3325–33.

Sur, M., Garraghty, P. E. & Roe, A. W. (1988) Experimentally induced visual projections into auditory thalamus and cortex. *Science,* **242,** 1437–41.

Thong, I. G. & Dreher, B. (1986) The development of the corticotectal pathway in the albino rat. *Developmental Brain Research,* **25,** 227–38.

Walsh, C. & Cepko, C. L. (1992) Widespread dispersion of neuronal clones across functional regions of the cerebral cortex. *Science,* **255,** 434–40.

Walsh, C. & Cepko, C. L. (1993) Clonal dispersion in proliferative layers of developing cerebral cortex. *Nature,* **362,** 632–5.

Windrem, M. S. & Finlay, B. L. (1991) Thalamic ablations and neocortical development: effects on cortical cytoarchitecture and cell number. *Cereb Cortex,* **1,** 220–40.

Winfield, D. A., Gatter, K. C. & Powell, T. P. S. (1980) An electron microscopic study of the types and proportions of neurons in the cortex of the motor and visual areas of the cat and rat. *Brain,* **103,** 245–58.

Woolsey, T. A. (1990) Peripheral alteration and somatosensory development, In Coleman, J. R. (ed.) *Development of Sensory Systems in Mammals.* New York: John Wiley, pp. 416–516.

Woolsey, T. A. & Van Der Loos, H. (1970) The structural organization of layer IV in the somatosensory regions (SI) of mouse cerebral cortex: the description of a cortical field composed of discrete cytoarchitectonic units. *Brain Research,* **17,** 205–42.

3 Genes and environment

JOHN C. LOEHLIN

Genes and environments both play essential roles in human development. This is a point upon which all serious investigators nowadays agree. Certainly it is a point agreed on by behavior geneticists, the group with which I identify.

Some aspects of genes and of environments are uniform, or nearly so, for all members of a species. Other aspects show variation from individual to individual within a species. Both the species-constant and the individually distinctive characteristics may change through the lifespan. A full understanding of individual development must include both kinds of characteristics, but in practice we find the usual division of labor, with various scientific subspecialties focusing on one or another aspect of the overall developmental process. A central theme of the present volume is bringing together such differing perspectives.

Behavior geneticists concentrate chiefly, although not exclusively, on individual differences, the characteristics that vary from individual to individual within a species, and they seek to understand the extent to which these result from genetic or environmental variation. The observed differences reflect the same events and processes underlying all development, but are most directly informative concerning differences in them, that is, genetic or environmental characteristics or events that affect one individual but not another, or that affect different individuals to different degrees.

There are at least three good reasons for studying individual differences. First, a proper theory of development should account for how individuals differ as well as for how they are the same. Secondly, individual variation is basic to the Darwinian theory of evolution; genetic variation is a *sine qua non* of evolutionary change. Thirdly, in our own species, individual differences in cognitive skills, personality traits, and social attitudes are of immense social, political and educational concern. Many psychologists and others interested in understanding human development have had a great deal to say about them, and have spent a good deal of time discussing how they arise and whether and how much they can be changed. Understanding their origins does not automatically answer questions about how to change them, but it should help.

The traditional methods of human behavior genetics – twin, adoption, and family studies – are primarily directed toward partitioning the observed variation of a trait in some population into components associated with various categories of genetic and environmental causes. These are quantitative, 'how much', questions: how much of the variation in (say) academic achievement in some particular population is associated with genetic differences among the individuals in that population, and how much with differences in the environments to which they have been exposed? Of the latter, how much is due to the environment shared by family members, and how much to individually distinctive experience?

Various natural experiments, such as the comparison of monozygotic and dizygotic twins, or of ordinary and adoptive families, can be used to arrive at estimates of these proportions in human populations. Much of the early work in this area tended to use samples which were too small to do more than demonstrate *some* degree of genetic (or environmental) influence upon the trait being studied. During recent decades, however, there have been a number of large-scale studies carried out in the United States, Europe and Australia, and at least rough quantitative estimates can now reasonably be made for a number of human behavioral traits in these populations.

It should be kept in mind that such a 'how much' answer is a descriptive statement about the present characteristics of a population. It need carry no strong implications about modifiability. If genes or environments change, trait levels and trait variation can change, and the relative contributions of genes and environment to these can change as well. Some have seemed to find this an argument against ever assessing 'how much'. I have never understood this argument. For one thing, if you do not measure something, how will you ever know that it has changed? For another, the fact that something theoretically *can* change does not mean that it necessarily will change, or that it is likely to change very much in practice. Those are distinct questions, which can be empirically addressed, but only if one is willing to take the first step of assessing 'how much' for particular populations at particular times.

One may also need to assess 'how much' for particular ages. The changes in the proportion of trait variation attributable to various genetic and environmental causes may differ at different stages in life. In formulating a comprehensive lifespan theory of development, this fact should be of special interest, and I will emphasize age changes in this discussion.

AN EXAMPLE – INTELLIGENCE

One of the human characteristics for which we have the most evidence relevant to our topic – the contribution of genes and environment to individual differences in development – is intelligence. I will mostly use the term 'IQ' (intelligence quotient) rather than 'intelligence', both for brevity and as a reminder that the intelligence being measured is typically *relative* intelligence, that is, intellectual performance assessed relative to other individuals of the same age in the population, rather than ability in absolute terms.

The Louisville Twin Study

What do we know about how much the genes and environment contribute to IQ variation at different ages? Let us look at one important study. Figure 3.1 summarizes data from the Louisville Twin Study (Wilson, 1983). In this research, samples of monozygotic (MZ) and dizygotic (DZ) twins were followed longitudinally from birth until age 15, being tested every 3 months beginning at 3 months of age during the first year, every 6 months during the second and third years, annually thereafter until age 9, and once again at age 15. The IQ tests used varied with age. The two members of a twin pair were tested by different examiners. For various reasons, not every twin was tested at every age, and not all of the twins had reached the older ages at the time of the report. The actual numbers of twin pairs on which each point on the graph is based ranged from 72 to 146 for the MZs and 64 to 141 for the DZs.

The two curves at the top of the graph represent the intraclass correlations at various ages for the MZ pairs (empty squares) and the DZ pairs (filled

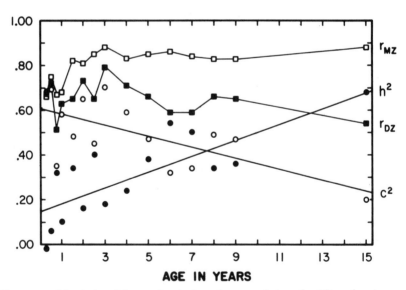

Figure 3.1. Identical and fraternal twin intraclass correlations for IQ, and estimates of genetic and shared environmental variation, in the Louisville Twin Study (data from Wilson, 1983). r_{MZ}, r_{DZ} = intraclass correlations for monozygotic and dizygotic twins; h^2, c^2 = proportions of variance attributable to genes and to shared environment.

squares). At 3 and 6 months, the correlations are virtually the same for both groups; thereafter the MZs are consistently higher, although only slightly so during the first 3 years, when both curves tend to rise. Thereafter, the MZ resemblance remains high, whereas the DZ resemblance begins to decline, dropping to a correlation of 0.54 at age 15.

What does this imply concerning the genetic and environmental contributions to individual differences in this population? In the lower part of the figure are shown, for each age, estimates of h^2, the proportion of population variance attributable to the genes (filled circles), and c^2, the proportion attributable to environmental factors shared by the twin pairs (empty circles). These estimates are obtained via formulas widely used in twin studies, h^2 as $2(r_{MZ} - r_{DZ})$, that is, twice the difference between the MZ and DZ correlations, and c^2 as $(r_{MZ} - h^2)$. I should emphasize that these are rough estimates, involving several assumptions that are unlikely to hold exactly for IQ, but they will serve our immediate purpose. Being based on differences between correlations, the estimates are also subject to a good deal of sampling fluctuation. To give a sense of their general trend over time I have fitted simple linear regression lines to the two sets of points; they are the straight lines shown on the figure.

As one can see, the heritabilities, the h^2s, start quite low, at around 15% by the regression line (the actual estimates at 3 and 6 months are closer to zero) and rise by age 15 to near 70%. The estimates of shared environmental effects, the c^2s, begin at above 60% and drop to about 25% by age 15. The residual portion of the variation, which would include measurement error and the effects of any environmental factors that are unique to an individual twin, is not shown explicitly on the graph, but by the subtraction $(1 - r_{MZ})$ can be estimated at about 34% at 3 months, declining to about 12% at 3 years, and fluctuating in the 12–17% range thereafter.

This is a single study based on twins. What about other twin studies? What about other behavior genetic designs, such as studies of adoptive families?

A meta-analysis of twin studies

The age trends in the Louisville study are generally consistent with the results of other twin studies. A meta-analysis of published twin studies between 1967 and 1985 was conducted by McCartney and her colleagues (McCartney, Harris & Bernieri, 1990). They reviewed 15 twin studies in which MZ and DZ intraclass correlations were reported, along with the ages of the twins. Although the ages ranged from 1 to 59 years, the bulk of the studies were done with children – the median age overall was 7.8 years. On the average, across studies, MZ correlations rose slightly with increasing age, and DZ correlations declined. The authors summarize the effects on the components of variance as follows: 'For intelligence, h^2 increased over time, more so when the less reliable preschool data were excluded. Conversely, es^2 [c^2], and to a lesser extent ens^2 [the residual variance], decreased over time' (McCartney et al., 1990, p. 232).

Adoption studies confirm these trends. Such studies yield a direct estimate of the effects of shared family environment, c^2. This is obtained simply from the correlation of genetically unrelated individuals reared together. The results are clear. In childhood, c^2 is appreciable – in two studies various correlations ranging from 0.11 to 0.49 were reported for genetically unrelated children reared together via adoption (Scarr & Weinberg, 1977; Loehlin, Horn & Willerman, 1989). By late adolescence or early adulthood, however, such correlations were essentially zero (Scarr & Weinberg, 1978; Loehlin et al., 1989). The Scarr and Weinberg results are based on two separate Minnesota samples studied at different ages; in our own study in Texas, the results are for the same individuals tested twice. In brief, in the populations studied, shared family environment had an effect in childhood in creating IQ resemblance among siblings, but the effect was only temporary.

Adoption studies also permit estimates of h^2 from the difference between genetically related and unrelated individuals growing up together in the same families. In both the Texas and Minnesota adoption studies estimates of h^2 were low at the early age, and substantial by the later one, again consistent with the twin studies.

As usual, however, not all the data are consistent. A recent combined analysis of twin and adoption data (Cardon et al., 1992) yielded rather stable estimates over the ages of 1–7 years for h^2 (≈ 0.57), c^2 (≈ 0.10) and the residual variance (≈ 0.33). It is not yet clear whether the rather complex analytic method used or the fact that the twin data were mostly confined to the first two years might have contributed to this outcome. Because these studies are ongoing, we may expect such matters to be clarified in due course. Another qualification should be made to these results (and to the personality data to follow). Measurement of human psychological traits at very early ages is an uncertain matter – it is always open to question whether intelligence as assessed at age 1 is really continuous with intelligence as assessed at age 7, or 27. Trends involving very early ages may, therefore, reflect changes in what is measured as well as changes in the presumed trait.

Summary: IQ

Granting some exceptions and qualifications, on the whole the twin and adoption studies agree in suggesting an interesting view of how individual differences in intellectual performance develop. At the start, the genes appear to carry little weight in accounting for individual differences in IQ, whereas shared family environment seems to play a substantial role. But as the individual is exposed to more varying environments, his genotype increasingly shapes his acquisition of intellectual skills and, by time adulthood is reached, the majority of the differences we observe reflect genetic differences, and few if any trace back to differences in family environments. Of the remaining variation, part reflects essentially random events – developmental accidents, errors of measurement – and part depends on potentially analyzable factors, such as genotype-environment interactions (in the statistical sense) and systematic environmental effects independent of genotype and family environment. These residual effects seem to be fairly modest for IQ – a bit larger very early; at a reasonably stable low level later on.

PERSONALITY

It is more difficult to summarize the data on how much the genes and environment contribute to variation on personality traits, if only because personality varies over a number of dimensions whose measurement is far from standardized, and therefore equivalences from study to study – and even from age to age within a study – are hard to establish with confidence. Nevertheless, at least in rough outline, certain similarities to the results for IQ emerge.

The Louisville Twin Study

The Louisville Twin Study assessed temperamental characteristics in its twins in several different ways – interviews with parents, ratings in laboratory situations, and so forth. A subgroup of the twins were studied right at the beginning. An observer rated the twins in the hospital, either within their first few days of life or (in the case of twins with medical problems) when their condition had stabilized prior to their release (Riese, 1990). The twins were rated in a standard way on six behavioral characteristics, such as activity, soothability, responsiveness, and so on. The average twin intraclass correlation across the six characteristics was 0.18 for MZ twins, 0.32 for same-sex DZs, and 0.23 for opposite-sex DZs. The numbers of pairs on which these correlations were based ranged from 38 to 72, so the differences among them should probably not be taken seriously. Nevertheless, on the face of it, there is no evidence for a genetic contribution to individual differences here at all, just a modest correlation of pair members, as high for DZ as for MZ twins. One would hardly describe this resemblance as due to shared family environment, to which the twins have not yet been exposed. It may well, however, reflect shared factors such as degree of prematurity, conditions of birth, common prenatal environment, and the like. (One might want to invoke such factors in the case of the very earliest IQ measures as well; it will be recalled that at 3 and 6 months there were strikingly similar IQ correlations for MZ and DZ pairs.)

On temperament ratings by laboratory personnel during the first year of life (at 9 and 12 months of age) there was still little if any greater resemblance for MZ than for DZ twins – the average correlations across four ratings were

0.54 for MZs and 0.47 for DZs at 9 months, and 0.40 and 0.52, respectively, at 12 months. But by the second year, the MZs were being rated as more and the DZs as less alike on the four traits – average ratings of 0.66 and 0.37 for MZs and DZs at 18 months, and 0.62 and 0.42 at 24 months (Wilson & Matheny, 1986). By middle childhood (ages 7–10) the differences between MZ and DZ correlations appear to be substantially larger (Matheny & Dolan, 1980), although shifts in the traits measured and in the method of measurement (to parent ratings) make detailed quantitative comparisons difficult.

Other twin studies

The meta-analysis mentioned earlier reviewed personality traits as well as IQ (McCartney et al., 1990). Correlations averaged across eight personality traits (activity-impulsivity, aggression, anxiety, dominance, emotionality, masculinity-femininity, sociability, and task orientation) declined with age for both MZ and DZ twins, about equally so. (For IQ, it will be recalled, there was a slight increase for MZs and a decrease for DZs.) This implies a more or less stable heritability over time for personality and a decline in the effect of shared family environment. In general, both MZ and DZ personality correlations were lower (by 20 points or so) than IQ correlations, leaving more scope for residual factors. A good part of this difference doubtless reflects the greater magnitude of measurement error typical in the personality domain. In comparing the IQ and personality results, it should also be noted that the personality studies reviewed tended to be based on older twins than the IQ studies. The median age for the IQ samples was in the neighborhood of 8 years; that for the personality trait samples was in the neighborhood of 16 years.

Adoptions

Adoption studies confirm a moderate effect of the genes and little enduring effect of shared environment on personality traits, as measured in late adolescence by personality questionnaires. In the Minnesota study, average correlations among several personality traits measured were 0.20 for biological siblings and 0.07 for adoptive siblings (Scarr et al., 1981). In one Texas adoptive sample, the average biological sibling correlation was 0.22 and the average adoptive sibling correlation was 0.01 (Loehlin, Willerman & Horn, 1985); in another sample using different questionnaires the corresponding figures were 0.10 and 0.05 (Loehlin, Willerman & Horn, 1987). In the latter sample, changes in means over a 10-year interval suggested that the adopted children as a group were tending to shift in the direction of their birth parents (Loehlin, Horn & Willerman, 1990), as one would expect if personality is increasingly reflecting the genes.

Configurational effects of genes?

There are other results that have been fairly common in behavior genetic studies in the personality domain. One is evidence for configurational effects of the genes, known to geneticists as genetic dominance and epistasis. A manifestation of this is DZ correlations that are less than half the size of corresponding MZ correlations. MZ twins have identical genotypes, so that they share all their individual genes and all configurational effects depending on multiple genes as well. Each DZ twin inherits a random half of his parents' genes. Two DZ twins will, on the average, therefore share half their individual genes, and thus half of any resemblance resulting from the average effects of individual genes. If there is a configurational effect that depends on a pair of genes, as would be the case in genetic dominance, there is a probability of one-quarter that both twins would have it, but as the number of genes involved in a configuration increases, the probability that both DZ twins will inherit all the genes in the pattern decreases rapidly towards zero. Thus a mixture of individual and configurational effects of genes will lead to DZ correlations less than half MZ correlations.

Table 3.1 shows some results for two traits measured in a large study of Swedish twins (Floderus-Myrhed, Pedersen & Rasmuson, 1980), comprising altogether over 12,000 pairs of twins, mostly adult. Several facts emerge from this table. First, the typical intraclass correlation for the MZ pairs is about 0.50; that for the DZ pairs about 0.20. That is, the DZ correlations tend overall to be less than one-half the MZ correlations, which could be evidence for configurational effects of the genes involved in personality. This is illustrated more explicitly in the far right-hand columns of the table, which show the extent to which the MZ correlation is more than twice the DZ correlation. All but one of these differences are positive, consistent with such an effect. Extraversion shows several relatively large differences, but also some small ones. Instability shows more uniformity. There does not seem to be any clear trend across the sexes or across ages in the tendency toward configurational effects.

Although differences such as these are consistent with configurational genetic effects on personality, environmental explanations have also been suggested, such as a systematic attempt by DZ twins to differentiate themselves from each other, or special similarities in treatment accorded to MZ twin pairs because of their striking resemblance. In principle, decisive evidence on these points could be provided by studies of MZ and DZ twins who have been reared apart in separate homes, and who would consequently not have been subjected to such special environmental effects. Recent studies have multiplied the amount of available data on the personalities of separated twins (Langinvainio et al., 1984; Pedersen et al., 1988; Tellegen et al., 1988). However, no clear picture has yet emerged (Loehlin, 1992).

Table 3.1. *Twin correlations for two personality traits in Sweden*

Trait and age group	MZ pairs		DZ pairs		MZ-2DZ	
	Males	Females	Males	Females	Males	Females
Instability						
16–28	0.53	0.62	0.24	0.29	0.05	0.04
29–38	0.39	0.51	0.19	0.24	0.01	0.03
39–48	0.40	0.42	0.16	0.18	0.08	0.06
Extraversion						
16–28	0.51	0.58	0.18	0.27	0.15	0.04
29–38	0.37	0.50	0.19	0.16	−0.01	0.18
39–48	0.46	0.51	0.21	0.14	0.04	0.23

Note: Numbers of pairs on which each correlation is based: 507–1240 for MZ groups, 814–1798 for DZ groups.
(Data from Floderus-Myrhed, Pedersen & Rasmuson, 1980.)

Sex and age differences in adulthood

There are some modest but probably real sex and age trends in Table 3.1 in the twin correlations themselves. For MZs on both traits and for DZs on instability the female pairs tend to have slightly higher intraclass correlations. (For the DZs on extraversion there is no consistent trend.) Except for the DZ males, the youngest group has slightly higher correlations than the rest. For the trait of instability in both sexes, and for extraversion in males, the changes in correlations are consistent with a modest drop in heritability after the youngest age group. A recent analysis of similar twin data from Finland found such a change for both traits in both sexes; in that study the youngest age group was 16–23 years, and longitudinal data confirmed the change to be an age rather than a cohort effect (Viken et al., 1994).

The same questionnaires were used with a somewhat older group of Swedish twins, averaging about 59 years of age, in the Swedish Adoption/ Twin Study of Aging (Pedersen et al., 1988). There were about 150 pairs of MZ twins and 204 pairs of DZ twins for whom scores were available for both twins. The correlations for MZ pairs were generally similar to those in Table 3.1 – 0.41 for instability and 0.54 for extraversion. The DZ correlations differed more – that for instability was a little higher, at 0.24, and that for extraversion was appreciably lower, at 0.06. Whether this difference is to be interpreted as a genuine age trend or as some artifact of sampling should probably be deferred pending replication in other studies.

Summary: personality

As things stand, the personality data are reasonably consistent with the following picture: (1) a moderate genetic influence on individual differences that emerges in childhood, peaks in young adulthood, and after a slight drop continues stable until fairly late in life; (2) an influence of shared family environment that decreases over time at least until late adolescence; (3) something else – perhaps nonadditive genetic effects or some special twin environmental factor – that tends to decrease DZ relative to MZ resemblance; and, lastly, (4) a remainder, partly measurement error, but partly, presumably, nonshared environmental effects, gene–environment interactions, and random developmental variation.

SOCIAL ATTITUDES

So far as I know, the heritability of social attitudes has only been studied among late-adolescents and adults, so that its direct empirical relevance to development is marginal. Nevertheless, it does raise some points of interest.

Initially, because attitudes on such matters as the appropriate treatment of criminals, the existence and nature of God, racial superiority, sexual liberty, political freedom, and the like, are so obviously learned from one's culture, and so obviously different from time to time and from place to place, it was assumed by behavior geneticists that their variation from person to person within a society would be almost entirely environmental. Moreover, since many attitudes are acquired in a familial context, much of that environment would be shared environment. As usual, things turned out to be not that simple.

An adoption study

Scarr and Weinberg's adoption study provides an instructive example (Scarr & Weinberg, 1981). As part of their study, the investigators thought it would be a nice idea to include a control variable *not* expected to be heritable. They picked the California F-Scale, a 20-item questionnaire in which the subject is invited to indicate the extent of his or her agreement with a number of statements about social and moral issues, a scale originally developed by its authors to measure tendencies toward authoritarianism (Adorno et al., 1950).

What happened was that the scale came out with correlations like those of a typical personality measure: biological parent–child correlations of 0.37 and 0.41 for fathers and mothers, adoptive parent–child correlations of 0.14 and 0.00, biological sibling correlations of 0.36, adoptive sibling correlations of 0.14 – all suggesting quite substantial heritability for whatever it was that the scale was measuring.

Twin studies

Such results are not unique to adoption studies. Martin and his colleagues reported data on social attitudes from adult twin samples in Australia and Great Britain (Martin et al., 1986). The Australia study used a conservatism scale in which respondents were asked to indicate their attitudes toward some 50 different topics ranging from jazz to the death penalty. The British study used a questionnaire in which the subject indicated degree of agreement with forty statements on such topics. The British questionnaire was scored for radicalism–conservatism and tough vs tendermindedness. In the larger Australian study, the correlations for conservatism for MZ twins were 0.60 and 0.64 for males and females, and 0.47, 0.46, and 0.41 for three DZ groups (male, female, and opposite-sex pairs). In the British study, the correlations ranged from 0.49 to 0.75 for MZ groups, and from 0.18 to 0.52 for DZs. The simple twin formulas discussed earlier would infer from these data the presence of both genetic and shared environmental contributions to variance. However, attitude scales such as these typically show quite high correlations between spouses, and different assumptions as to how these come about can have a marked effect on the amount of influence attributed to shared environment (Eaves, Eysenck & Martin, 1989). Multivariate analyses of the Australian twin data (Truett et al., 1992; Loehlin, 1993) suggest that there are both genetic and environmental factors in conservatism, the former more closely associated with (low) education and the latter with religious affiliation.

Summary: social attitudes

We may view this as a kind of cafeteria model of the acquisition of social attitudes. The individual does not inherit his ideas about fluoridation, royalty, women judges and nudist camps; he learns them from his culture. But his genes may influence which ones he elects to put on his tray. Different cultural institutions – family, church, school, books, television – like different cafeterias, serve up somewhat different menus, and the choices a person makes will reflect those offered him as well as his own biases. As he gets older, his choice of cafeterias will become important, in addition to his choice of dishes within them. As Martin and his colleagues put it, this model sees humans as 'exploring organisms whose innate abilities and predispositions help them select what is relevant and adaptive from the range of opportunities and stimuli presented by the environment' (Martin et al., 1986: 4368). Learning thus serves to 'augment rather than eradicate the effects of the genotype on behavior'. If such a model is correct we might reasonably expect that the heritability of social attitudes would follow a temporal course somewhat like that of IQ or personality, with an increase over time of the genetic contribution to individual differences and a decrease of the shared environmental contribution. It would seem worthwhile to investigate this. There might even be some advantages in studying such processes in this domain. First, it may well be that the effects occur at somewhat later ages, spread out over a longer period of time; this could facilitate their measurement. Secondly, specific inputs may be easier to identify. For example, the emergence of entirely new attitudes (toward television in courtrooms; toward the nations of the former Soviet Union) that can be dated within a relatively short time period could be exploited in certain research designs.

CONCLUSION

The notion that the genetic contribution to behavioral differences expands during individual development reflects a growing consensus among behavior geneticists. Plomin (1986: 328) refers to the principle of genetic effects being amplified as development proceeds. Scarr & McCartney (1983) stress the role of the genotype as the driving force behind development, by virtue of its effect on which environments are actually experienced. Bouchard and his colleagues (Bouchard et al., 1990: 228) use the phrase *nature via nurture*, referring to the role of the genes in influencing the character, selection and impact of experiences.

The notion of the declining influence of *imposed* environments on individual variation is also widely shared among human behavior geneticists. A recent, forceful expression of this view is contained in Rowe's (1994) book *The Limits of Family Influence*.

One should not misinterpret this position. It does not hold that the environment is unimportant to development. On the contrary it regards it as essential. What it *does* hold is that during development the organism–environment transactions that lead to individual behavioral differences increasingly reflect the influence of the genes; and that they decreasingly reflect the influence of shared family environment. It should be kept in mind that the reference here is to a not-too-extreme range of ordinary environments, that is, to the bulk of the population variation as we observe it in Western countries. The effects of extreme environments are a topic for separate study – one should surely not blindly generalize the results of typical twin and adoption studies to such conditions. After all, we can easily think of simple environmental manipulations, such as the administration of a large dose of potassium cyanide, that will have a spectacular effect on intelligence, personality, and social attitudes, reducing all to zero, but we do not assume that such factors account for much of the variation we observe under ordinary circumstances.

The story is far from settled in all its details, but at least a general picture is emerging. It is hoped that this broad picture will help provide some orientation as to what one should look for, and where and when one should look for it, in studying the detailed mechanisms of behavioral development.

Of course, behavior geneticists need not stop with the broad picture. A current focus of research interest in the field is to go beyond the general genetic and environmental categories that I have so far discussed. On the genetic side, this includes searching for particular genetic loci that have detectable effects on the variation of the quantitative traits under study. On the environmental side, this includes examining the genetic causation of the environment – the role of the genotype in creating, evoking, or selecting environmental inputs to the organism. Business is currently brisk in both lines of investigation (Plomin, Owen & McGuffin, 1994).

REFERENCES

Adorno, T. W., Frenkel-Brunswik, E., Levinson, D. J. & Sanford, R. N. (1950) *The Authoritarian Personality*. New York: Harper.

Bouchard, T. J., Jr., Lykken, D. T., McGue, M., Segal, N. L. & Tellegen, A. (1990) Sources of human psychological differences: The Minnesota Study of Twins Reared Apart. *Science*, **250**, 223–8.

Cardon, L. R., Fulker, D. W., DeFries, J. C. & Plomin, R. (1992) Continuity and change in general cognitive ability from 1 to 7 years of age. *Developmental Psychology*, **28**, 64–73.

Eaves, L. J., Eysenck, H. J. & Martin, N. G. (1989) *Genes, Culture and Personality: An Empirical Approach*. London: Academic Press.

Floderus-Myrhed, B., Pedersen, N. & Rasmuson, I. (1980) Assessment of heritability for personality, based on a short-form of the Eysenck Personality Inventory: a study of 12,898 twin pairs. *Behavior Genetics, 10*, 153–62.

Langinvainio, H., Kaprio, J., Koskenvuo, M. & Lönnqvist, J. (1984) Finnish twins reared apart. III: Personality factors. *Acta Geneticae Medicae et Gemellologiae*, **33**, 259–64.

Loehlin, J. C. (1992) *Genes and Environment in Personality Development*. Newbury Park, Calif.: Sage.

Loehlin, J. C. (1993) Nature, nurture, and conservatism in the Australian twin study. *Behavior Genetics*, **23**, 287–90.

Loehlin, J. C., Horn, J. M. & Willerman, L. (1989) Modeling IQ change: evidence from the Texas Adoption Project. *Child Development*, **60**, 993–1004.

Loehlin, J. C., Horn, J. M. & Willerman, L. (1990) Heredity, environment, and personality change: Evidence from the Texas Adoption Project. *Journal of Personality*, **58**, 221–43.

Loehlin, J. C., Willerman, L. & Horn, J. M. (1985) Personality resemblances in adoptive families when the children are late-adolescent or adult. *Journal of Personality and Social Psychology*, **48**, 376–92.

Loehlin, J. C., Willerman, L & Horn, J. M. (1987) Personality resemblance in adoptive families: a 10-year follow-up. *Journal of Personality and Social Psychology*, **53**, 961–9.

Martin, N. G., Eaves, L. J., Heath, A. C., Jardine, R., Feingold, L. M. & Eysenck, H. J. (1986) Transmission of social attitudes. *Proceedings of the National Academy of Sciences of the USA*, **83**, 4364–8.

Matheny, A. P., Jr. & Dolan, A. B. (1980) A twin study of personality and temperament during middle childhood. *Journal of Research in Personality*, **14**, 224–34.

McCartney, K., Harris, M. J. & Bernieri, F. (1990) Growing up and growing apart: a developmental meta-analysis of twin studies. *Psychological Bulletin*, **107**, 226–37.

Pedersen, N. L., Plomin, R., McClearn, G. E. & Friberg, L. (1988) Neuroticism, extraversion, and related traits in adult twins reared apart and reared together. *Journal of Personality and Social Psychology*, **55**, 950–7.

Plomin, R. (1986) *Development, Genetics, and Psychology*. Hillsdale, NJ: Erlbaum.

Plomin, R., Owen, M. J. & McGuffin, P. (1994) The genetic basis of complex human behaviors. *Science*, **264**, 1733–9.

Riese, M. L. (1990) Neonatal temperament in monozygotic and dizygotic twin pairs. *Child Development*, **61**, 1230–7.

Rowe, D. C. (1994) *The Limits of Family Influence: Genes, Experience, and Behavior*. New York: Guilford.

Scarr, S. & McCartney, K. (1983) How people make their own environments: A theory of genotype → environment effects. *Child Development*, **54**, 424–35.

Scarr, S. & Weinberg, R. A. (1977) Intellectual similarities within families of both adopted and biological children. *Intelligence*, **1**, 170–91.

Scarr, S. & Weinberg, R. A. (1978) The influence of 'family background' on intellectual attainment. *American Sociological Review*, **43**, 674–92.

Scarr, S & Weinberg, R. A. (1981) The transmission of authoritarianism in families: Genetic resemblance in social-political attitudes? In Scarr, S. (ed.) *Race, Social Class, and Individual Differences in IQ*. Hillsdale, NJ: Erlbaum, pp. 399–427.

Scarr, S., Webber, P. L., Weinberg, R. A. & Wittig, M. A. (1981) Personality resemblance among adolescents and their families in biologically related and adoptive families. *Journal of Personality and Social Psychology*, **40**, 855–98.

Tellegen, A., Lykken, D. T., Bouchard, T. J., Jr., Wilcox, K. J., Segal, N. L. & Rich, S. (1988) Personality similarity in twins reared apart and together. *Journal of Personality and Social Psychology*, **54**, 1031–9.

Truett, K. R., Eaves, L. J., Meyer, J. M., Heath, A. C. & Martin, N. G. (1992) Religion and education as mediators of attitudes: a multivariate analysis. *Behavior Genetics*, **22**, 43–62.

Viken, R. J., Rose, R. J., Kaprio, J. & Koskenvuo, M. (1994) A developmental genetic analysis of adult personality: extraversion and neuroticism from 18 to 59 years of age. *Journal of Personality and Social Psychology*, **66**, 722–30.

Wilson, R. S. (1983) The Louisville Twin Study: developmental synchronies in behavior. *Child Development*, **54**, 298–316.

Wilson, R. S. & Matheny, A. P., Jr. (1986) Behavior-genetics research in infant temperament: the Louisville Twin Study. In Plomin, R. & Dunn, J. (eds.) *The Study of Temperament*. Hillsdale, NJ: Erlbaum, pp. 81–97.

4 Causes and outcome of perinatal brain injury

OSMUND REYNOLDS

The perinatal period runs from 24 weeks of gestation to one week after birth. Deaths of babies within this period are defined by the perinatal mortality rate. This rate has been falling steadily for many years in developed countries and it is now at a low level. For example, in England and Wales it fell from 42 deaths per 1000 births at the end of the Second World War in 1945 to under 8 per 1000 in 1993. The deaths are roughly equally apportioned between stillbirths and deaths of liveborn infants during the first week of life. Deaths of liveborn infants are generally due to congenital abnormalities, birth asphyxia, or problems associated with preterm birth (birth before 37 weeks of gestation). Mortality rates in all three categories have fallen sharply in developed countries, but they continue to take a heavy toll in underdeveloped ones. The same influences that cause death can cause long-term neurodevelopmental impairment. At school age congenital abnormalities and inherited illnesses account for the large majority of severely disabled children. Down's syndrome is the major contributor. In a significant minority of disabled children, birth asphyxia is responsible. There has been much debate about the contribution of birth asphyxia to neurodevelopmental disabilities, particularly cerebral palsy. Recent estimates suggest that in developed countries about 15–20% of cases of cerebral palsy are attributable to this cause with most of the others due to congenital defects. In total, birth asphyxia is thought to be responsible for about 5% of severely disabled children at school age and about another 5% of those with lesser disabilities (Alberman, 1982).

Preterm infants, particularly the smallest ones, are very prone to develop cerebral injury in the perinatal period, especially during the first days of life. This injury is usually due to cerebral haemorrhage or to hypoxia-ischaemia – which is also responsible for the damage which occurs during birth asphyxia in more mature infants.

The survival rates of very preterm (less than 33 weeks gestation) or very low birthweight (VLBW, less than 1500 g) infants have increased dramatically in recent years (Alberman & Botting, 1991). This development is largely due to the introduction of neonatal intensive care, which involves such procedures as mechanical ventilation and total parenteral nutrition. Over 50% of infants born at 24 and 25 weeks of gestation now survive if they are admitted to modern neonatal intensive care units, and survival is being reported as early as 22 and 23 weeks. The high incidence of perinatal cerebral injury in these smallest infants, together with the massive increase in the overall chances of survival has caused considerable concern that the total number of children surviving with serious disabilities would increase. However, follow-up studies are generally reassuring. They show that a large majority of infants surviving from neonatal intensive care units are normal children at school age, but among the very smallest ones (< 1000 g) the risk of disability is high – about 20% (Stewart, 1994). Because the numbers are so small, the contribution of disabled VLBW infants to the total number of seriously disabled children in general is also bound to be small. Alberman (1982) put it about 2%. Some studies have suggested a trend towards an increase (Hagberg et al., 1984; Pharoah et al., 1990), but more recently evidence for a decrease has been found (Krägeloh-Mann et al., 1994), suggesting the improved effectiveness of intensive care.

So although most vulnerable or ill newborn babies who are at high risk for perinatal brain injury survive as normal children, a much smaller number survive disabled. If this number, as well as perinatal deaths, are to be minimised, it is important to learn more about the pathogenesis, prevention and prognostic significance of the major causes of perinatal brain injury, namely cerebral haemorrhage in preterm infants, and hypoxic-ischaemic injury in both preterm and term ones. The recent introduction of non-invasive techniques for investigating the structure and function of the brain in ill babies has proved valuable for addressing these issues. The purpose of this chapter is to consider what has been learnt from the application of some of these techniques. Consideration will also be given to the possible role of minor degrees of perinatal damage in causing subtle learning difficulties in surviving preterm infants. Prevalent causes of brain injury in the past, such as hyperbilirubinaemia and hypoglycaemia, which are now easy to detect and treat, will not be considered; nor will the uncommon idiopathic cerebral infarctions (usually of the middle cerebral artery) occasionally seen in term infants, or the adverse cerebral consequences of rare inborn errors of metabolism, which sometimes become manifest in the first week of life.

CEREBRAL LESIONS IN PRETERM INFANTS

Periventricular haemorrhage

Pathogenesis

For many years it was well known that periventricular haemorrhage (PVH) was very common at autopsy in VLBW infants, affecting about 75% of them (Pape & Wigglesworth, 1979). This haemorrhage arises in the germinal layer and may spread to the lateral ventricles, sometimes leading to hydrocephalus, or damage to the brain parenchyma. Until the 1970s it was usually believed that survival with PVH was unlikely, but studies with computerized tomography then gave the rather surprising result that about one third of all VLBW survivors had PVH (Papile et al., 1978). This finding caused considerable anxiety at the time because many observers thought that the PVHs would inevitably lead to adverse sequelae. Computerized tomography has the disadvantage that it involves considerable ionizing radiation and also that the baby has to be taken to the machine, so the discovery in 1978 that the neonatal brain could be imaged with ultrasound, using portable equipment at the cotside, was a useful advance (Pape et al., 1979). Ultrasound imaging has subsequently been very extensively employed for the investigation of PVH, and much information has emerged (for review see Reynolds & Wyatt, 1992). For example, it is known that bleeding usually arises during the first two days of life and only very rarely after the fifth day (whatever the gestational age of the baby). About 30–50% of all VLBW or very preterm infants are affected and the incidence decreases sharply with increasing gestation from about 80% at 26 weeks to 15–20% at 32 weeks. The germinal layer largely involutes by 34 weeks, so PVH is almost exclusively a problem affecting very preterm infants. Some recent studies are tending to show a reduction in incidence, probably due to increased understanding and amelioration of the likely causal antecedents (Philip et al., 1987; Cooke, 1994).

Early pathological studies suggested that PVH arose from rupture of the terminal (thalamostriate) vein draining the germinal layer (Towbin, 1968; Cole et al., 1974). Abnormal haemostasis and the presence of hyaline membrane disease (surfactant-deficient respiratory distress syndrome) were also thought to be implicated (Gray et al., 1968; Harrison, Heese & Klein, 1968). In 1974, Cole et al. showed that abnormalities of haemostasis were unlikely to be importantly involved and postulated that haemodynamic factors were more relevant. Hambleton and Wigglesworth concluded in 1976 that the bleeding originated from capillaries in the germinal layer, most commonly over the head of the caudate nucleus opposite the foramen of Munro, a finding much amplified later by Pape & Wigglesworth (1979). The capillary network in the germinal layer is supplied largely by Heubner's artery, a branch of the anterior cerebral artery, and drained via a rich system of venules into the terminal vein. Animal modelling of PVH was first attempted by Reynolds et al. who in 1979 showed that bleeding from the capillaries and venules of the germinal layer of the exteriorized preterm sheep fetus could be provoked by a combination of impaired gas exchange with increased arterial or venous pressure (or both). In the same year, Lou, Lassen & Friis-Hansen (1979) demonstrated that autoregulation of cerebral blood flow was often defective in small preterm infants and that flow was pressure-passive. When ultrasound imaging became available, the scene was therefore set for testing the hypothesis that variables affecting cerebral haemodynamics were involved in the pathogenesis of PVH. Very many studies have been done. They give reasonably comparable results, and no attempt will be made to review them here. Important conclusions included that prenatal and intrapartum events are not the major causes of bleeding, though they may predispose to it, and that the presence and severity of respiratory illnesses, which are very common in preterm infants are major contributors (Reynolds & Wyatt, 1992). A reasonable consensus exists that bleeding into the germinal layer arises with increasing frequency as gestation decreases partly because of the increasing quantity of germinal layer, and also because of the parallel increase in the likelihood of respiratory problems. These problems cause perturbations in cerebral haemodynamic variables which lead to rupture of vulnerable vessels. For example, the smallest infants often show abnormalities of arterial oxygen (PaO_2) and carbon dioxide ($PaCO_2$) tensions, due to immature control of breathing, even if no frank pulmonary illness is present. $PaCO_2$ is a very major determinant of cerebral blood flow which increases with rising $PaCO_2$. Very low PaO_2 also increases blood flow and may be capable of directly damaging the germinal layer vessels. With increasing severity of respiratory problems, abnormalities of the blood gases are more likely, and any acute deterioration can provoke an increase in arterial blood pressure, which, since autoregulation is impaired, will cause an increased distending pressure in vulnerable capillaries. Such a distending pressure is much easier to achieve in the cerebral blood vessels of a preterm baby than in an adult because the head is compliant and not a 'closed box'. In the worst case, if a tension pneumothorax develops, venous pressure rises, in addition to the above sequence of events. Since there are no valves in the veins draining the brain, this pressure can also be transmitted to the capillaries in the germinal layer; pneumothorax, unless promptly treated is a very potent cause of PVH. If damage to the vessels has previously occurred due, for example, to hypotension, rupture is more likely and if haemostasis is defective, bleeding will be more severe. Much animal experimentation supports this line of reasoning (Goddard-Finegold, 1989).

Prevention

Although other factors are sure to be identified, the above summary of probable pathogenetic factors involved in PVH allows hypotheses for prevention to be set up and tested. Prevention of preterm birth would be the best approach, but this is proving very difficult. Amelioration of respiratory illnesses also has a sound basis. Current evidence is that antenatal steroid treatment of mothers who will deliver before term reduces the incidence of hyaline membrane disease and of PVH (Crowley, Chalmers & Kierse, 1990). Postnatal treatment by surfactant replacement has so far not been associated with a fall in the incidence of PVH, and care has to be taken with the mechanics of administration, for fear of provoking haemorrhage by seriously perturbing the blood gases or overdistending the lungs (Edwards et al., 1992). Treatment with the prostaglandin inhibitors indomethacin (Ment et al., 1994) and ethamsylate (Benson et al., 1986) has been shown in controlled trials to lower the incidence of PVH, but some concern exists that they might at the same time increase the incidence of hypoxic-ischaemic damage at the periventricular watershed zones and cause periventricular leukomalacia (see below). Muscle relaxation with pancuronicum has been found effective in babies selected for treatment because of fluctuating cerebral blood flow velocities (Perlman et al., 1985), and there is some evidence that stabilization of variables that control cerebral haemodynamics, such as the blood gases and blood pressure, at as close to normal levels as possible has a protective effect (Szymonowicz et al., 1986). Careful conduct of labour and delivery, with the aim, in particular, of avoiding hypotension, also has merit. It is probable that the reduction in the incidence of PVH being reported from some centres reflects the effects of the measures enumerated above.

Complications

Germinal layer haemorrhages and small intraventricular haemorrhages generally resolve within a week or two. When the germinal layer involutes there is then no residual anatomical evidence that a PVH has taken place. In a proportion of survivors, however, relatively serious complications can occur. Ventricular dilatation and frank hydrocephalus may develop due to a clot in the ventricular system or at the base of the brain. This complication is difficult to treat and may be fatal. Lumbar punctures are sometimes effective but ventriculo-peritoneal shunts are often required.

The other major complication is haemorrhagic parenchymal infarction. Particularly when unilateral, this lesion is often due to obstruction of flow through the terminal vein due to a large germinal layer and intraventricular haemorrhage (Figure 4.1). Infarction of brain tissue drained by this vein may involve the caudate nucleus and, particularly, the internal capsule. Bilateral infarctions may be due to the same cause or to bleeding spreading into tissue damaged by arterial hypoxia-ischaemia. In either case bilateral haemorrhagic parenchymal infarctions are often fatal. Prevention of the complications of PVH is most likely to be achieved by prevention of the initiating germinal layer bleed.

Periventricular leucomalacia

Periventricular leukomalacia (PVL) (Figure 4.2) mainly affects infants born before 35 weeks of gestation and has a prevalence of about 5–10% in survivors. It often coexists with PVH. The condition was first clearly recognised by Banker & Larroche in 1962, and its pathological findings and likely cause were amplified by de Reuek (1971), Armstrong & Norman (1974), Takashima & Tanaka (1978), and Pape & Wigglesworth (1979). These and many later studies show clearly that PVL principally affects the watershed

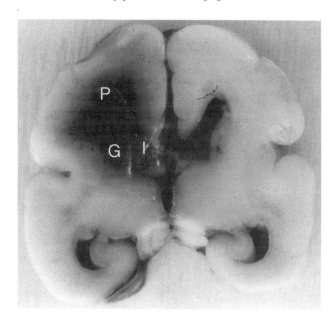

Figure 4.1. Coronal section of the brain of an infant born at 24 weeks of gestation who died aged four days. A large PVH is present which originated in the germinal layer (G), ruptured into the lateral ventricle to cause an intraventricular haemorrhage (I) and provoked a parenchymal haemorrhage (P) due to venous infarction. (From Gould et al., 1987.)

zones between the centrifugal and centripetal arterial supplies of the developing brain, especially near the dorsolateral angle of the lateral ventricles and at the trigone.

Typically, the internal capsule is involved, and since the long motor fibres leading to the contralateral legs are often symmetrically affected, spastic diplegia, and with more extensive lesions tetraplegia, are to be expected. There is little doubt that PVL is caused by hypoxaemia and hypotension, which leads to necrosis in the watershed zones. The sequelae include the development of cystic changes (Figure 4.2), or passive ventricular dilatation which may be difficult or impossible to distinguish by ultrasound imaging from that which follows intraventricular haemorrhage and partial obstruction to the flow of cerebrospinal fluid. The two situations may coexist. Obtaining accurate information about the timing and factors involved in the initiation of PVL is much more difficult than for PVH, because the early stages cannot be visualized with any confidence by ultrasound (Hope et al., 1988). In some instances persistently increased echodensities may indicate PVL, but for a certain diagnosis cyst formation, which may take a month or more, has to be awaited. Lesser degrees of PVL are often missed completely by ultrasound

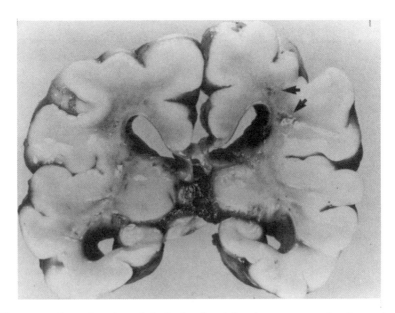

Figure 4.2. Coronal section of the brain of an infant born at 34 weeks of gestation who died aged 11 days. Multiple small cavities caused by PVL can be seen (arrows). (From Wigglesworth, 1984.)

imaging. Magnetic resonance spectroscopy (see below) has proved useful for separating infants with increased echodensities into those with a good, from those with a bad, prognosis. In a (probably small) proportion of cases, cysts are present in the first few days of life, indicating that the initiating insult was antenatal (Behar et al., 1988). Affected infants often have other evidence of fetal compromise, such as poor growth or sepsis. More often the cysts appear much later indicating that the initiating insult was intrapartum (in which case PVL can be regarded as a manifestation of birth asphyxia in the preterm infant) or in the first few days of life – at a time when these infants are very prone to hypotension and hypoxaemia.

Prognosis of PVH and PVL

Ultrasound-imaging is very useful for relating the presence or absence of PVH and PVL to neurodevelopmental outcome in childhood. Numerous studies have been done. They give broadly comparable results. For example, in one cohort study of 342 very preterm infants without congenital malformations whose brains were prospectively scanned and who were then examined in great detail at 1, 4 and 8 years of age, it was found that valuable prognostic information could be obtained as early as the first week of life

(Stewart et al., 1987). Also, by the time the infants were discharged from the neonatal unit, they could be assigned to one of three groups at low, intermediate and high risk of neurodevelopmental impairments detectable at one year of age. The largest group comprised 275 (80%) infants with normal scans or uncomplicated PVH (PVH not associated with haemorrhagic parenchymal infarction and not followed by ventricular dilatation with cerebrospinal fluid). These infants were at low risk, with only a 4% probability of a disabling impairment at one year. In contrast, a small group of 26 (8%) infants with posthaemorrhagic hydrocephalus or cerebral atrophy (any definite loss of brain tissue) were at high risk, with a probability of a disabling impairment of 58% (and of any impairment of 88%). Between the low risk and high risk groups lay the 41 (12%) infants with ventricular dilatation who were at intermediate risk, with a 27% probability of a disabling impairment. At 4 years, these findings were generally confirmed, although cognitive impairments (usually minor) that were not closely related to the ultrasound findings had by then begun to emerge (Costello et al., 1988). The oldest 206 children were reexamined at 8 years (Roth et al., 1993). Their median birthweight had been 1337 (range 600–2500) g and gestational age 30 (24–32) w. Some of the results are summarized in Figure 4.3.

The 112 infants discharged with normal scans had only a 4% (95% CI, 1–6%) probability of a major (disabling) impairment. Interestingly, the incidence of impairment was no different in the 55 children who had had uncomplicated PVH, confirming the findings in the children when they were younger. Proliferation of glia, particularly oligodendroglia, will have been under way in the germinal layer at the stage when the GLHs took place, and it had been thought that the disruption involved might lead to adverse sequelae due, for example, to defective myelination. The data shown in Figure 4.3 indicate no difference in outcome on a wide range of measures, compared with children with normal scans, and they apparently refute this possibility. The 39 infants with ventricular dilatation, hydrocephalus or cerebral atrophy, whether due to loss of brain tissue following haemorrhagic parenchymal infarction or to cystic PVL had a poor prognosis. For example, compared with infants with normal scans, those with atrophy had a 20-fold increase in the probability of a disabling neuromotor impairment, such as spastic tetraplegia, hemiplegia or athetosis; and they also had a 10-fold increase in the probability of a Weschler Intelligence Scale for Children (WISC-R) IQ below 70. In the cohort as a whole, lesions detected by ultrasound that led to an increased risk of disabling impairment were always seen to develop during the neonatal period, except in two infants, one presenting with generalised cerebral atrophy and another with ventricular dilatation within the first 12 hours after delivery. It follows that they were almost always initiated close to the time of delivery or during the first days of life.

Although the *proportion* of infants in this study with normal ultrasound scans who developed major disabling impairments was low the *number* (five)

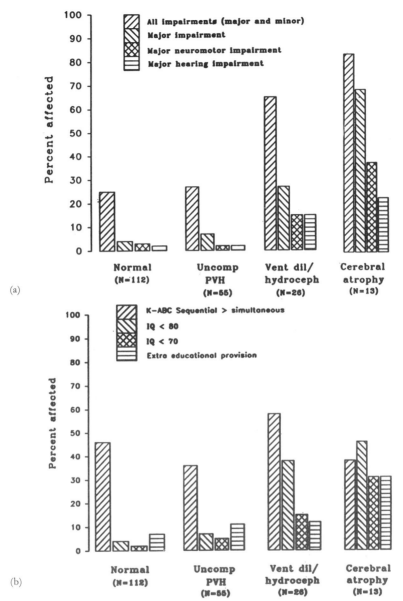

Figure 4.3. Relation between the ultrasound appearance of the brain of 206 very preterm
(< 33 w gestation) infants on discharge from the neonatal unit and neurodevelopmental status at eight years of age. Uncomplicated PVH = PVH not
associated with dilatation of the ventricles with cerebrospinal fluid or
haemorrhagic parenchymal infarction; hydrocephalus (n = 5) = width of a
lateral ventricle 5 mm or more above the 97th centile; cerebral atrophy = any
loss of brain tissue, including cysts and generalized atrophy. (a) *All impairments*. Major impairments = impairments causing disability. (b) *Cognitive
impairments*. K-ABC sequential > simultaneous = a significant difference in
processing scores (> 11 points). IQ = WISC IQ. (From Roth et al., 1993.)

represented 20% of those so impaired and the 23 with minor (mostly cognitive) impairments represented 50% so, especially for minor impairments, causes other than lesions visualised by ultrasound were operating. On cognitive testing, as many as 38% of the whole cohort had significantly higher verbal than performance IQs on the WISC-R subscales, although their full-scale IQs were usually normal (Figure 4.3b). An even higher proportion, 44%, showed a significant difference of sequential over simultaneous processing on testing with the Kaufman Assessment Battery for Children (K-ABC). These differences appeared consistent with impaired interhemispheric connection. More recently evidence for impairment of posterior (but not anterior) callosal function has been found in a sample of children from the cohort (Kirkbride et al., 1994), and very preliminary evidence obtained by magnetic resonance imaging among children who had reached 14 years of age suggests thinning in this area. The explanation for impaired callosal function could be that minor degrees of hypoxic-ischaemic injury, undetected by ultrasound imaging (Hope et al., 1988), could have affected the callosal fibres, which lie very close to the typical site for periventricular leukomalacia. Alternatively nutritional influences in the neonatal period may have been involved, and could possibly have adversely affected myelination, which does not begin in the corpus callosum until after term. Such an explanation is consistent with evidence that infants who grow poorly *in utero* do worse in terms of neurodevelopment than those who grow well and also that nutritional supplementation in preterm infants improves outcome (Lucas et al., 1990).

The data summarized above indicate that in very preterm infants without congenital malformations disabling neurodevelopmental impairments are usually, but not always, the result of obvious perinatal brain injury. This injury is initiated either by PVH, which can lead to haemorrhagic parenchymal infarction or to ventricular dilatation and frank hydrocephalus; or by hypoxia-ischaemia, which can be followed by cystic PVL, or by ventricular dilatation which is difficult or impossible to distinguish from that following PVH. Lesser degrees of hypoxia-ischaemia could be responsible for subtle cognitive difficulties capable of interfering with learning, but other explanations may well be involved.

BIRTH ASPHYXIA

Birth asphyxia may be defined as critically impaired intrapartum gas exchange, which can lead to hypoxic-ischaemic encephalopathy. Influences that adversely affect placental function, such as pre-eclamptic toxaemia and postmaturity, may predispose infants to birth asphyxia, and causal events during labour include separation of the placenta and prolapse of the umbilical cord. In very acutely asphyxiated infants, the basal ganglia are particularly prone to damage. More commonly, asphyxia is less acute and complicated by hypotension, leading to injury in the parasaggital areas at the boundary zones between the territories of the anterior, middle and posterior cerebral arteries. An inadequate oxygen supply to the bases of the cortical sulci causes subcortical leukomalacia with lesions similar in nature to those of PVL in preterm infants.

Birth asphyxia is much more readily recognized in term than in preterm infants. The physical signs depend on the severity of hypoxic-ischaemic encephalopathy. Grading systems based on these signs have been devised which give prognostic information (Sarnat & Sarnat, 1976; Levene, 1988). Infants with mild encephalopathy (minor disturbances of tone, hyperalertness, slight feeding difficulties lasting for a few days) generally recover completely. Those with moderate encephalopathy (lethargy, convulsions, poor feeding, signs of recovery by 1 week of age) have a variable prognosis; and those with severe encephalopathy (coma, profound hypotonia, inadequate breathing) usually die or survive with severe disabilities.

Prevention of birth asphyxia depends on identification of fetuses at risk and appropriate obstetric intervention. However, in many instances, it is unforeseen. Continuous electronic monitoring of the fetal heart-rate has been much used in an attempt to identify fetuses whose oxygen supply is impaired during labour, but convincing evidence of an important beneficial effect on outcome is lacking. Methods for the treatment of asphyxiated infants are unsatisfactory. Apart from rapid resuscitation, maintenance of oxygenation and cardiac output, and prevention of seizures, little can at present be done. In the future, cerebroprotective strategies may find a role (see below).

Cerebral oxidative metabolism and haemodynamics

Several methods have been used to investigate the progression of abnormal cerebral pathophysiology in birth-asphyxiated babies (and other babies with cerebral problems), for example, electrocencephalography, Dopper velocimetry of cerebral vessels, and imaging with computerized tomography, magnetic resonance and position emission tomography, as well as ultrasound. These methods provide useful information and can give a guide to prognosis.

Recently, two new methods, magnetic resonance spectroscopy and near infrared spectroscopy have been introduced for the investigation of cerebral oxidative metabolism and haemodynamics. These methods provide complimentary information about cerebral events in asphyxiated infants (and other infants with cerebral injury), for reasons illustrated in Figure 4.4, which is a simplified diagram representing oxidative phosphorylation. Electrons passing down the respiratory transport chain in the inner mitochondrial membrane initiate the synthesis of adenosine triphosphate (ATP) (the major fuel for all cellular activities), from adenosine diphosphate (ADP) and inorganic orthophosphate (Pi). The electrons then reduce cytochrome aa_3 (also known as cytochrome c oxidase) the terminal member of the chain. Cytochrome aa_3 is reoxidized by molecular oxygen, a reaction accounting for about 95% of the oxygen consumption of the body. Phosphorus (^{31}P) magnetic resonance

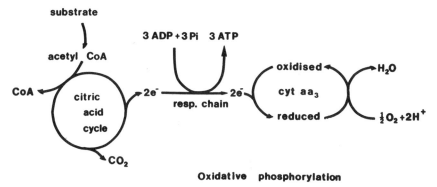

Figure 4.4. Simplified diagram of oxidative phosphorylation. (From Wyatt, Edwards, Azzopardi, et al., 1989.)

spectroscopy allows the non-invasive measurement of ATP and its 'buffer' phosphocreatine (PCr). Intracellular pH (pH_i) can be derived from the difference in resonance frequency between PCr and Pi, and proton ('H) spectroscopy can be used to measure lactate (and other proton-containing compounds). Near infrared spectroscopy allows observations to be made of a range of other important indices of cerebral oxygenation and haemo-dynamics.

Magnetic resonance spectroscopy (MRS)

If the oxygen supply to tissue is critically curtailed, or the mitochondrial mechanisms for consuming oxygen are damaged, [ATP] tends to fall. However, the buffering action of the creatine kinase reaction ensures that the fall is initially extremely small. This reaction causes a reduction in [PCr] in the tissue, counterbalanced by a reciprocal rise in [Pi]. Hence the ratio [PCr]/[Pi] falls. This ratio is directly related to the phosphorylation potential and is widely used as an index of the energy state or reserve of the tissue. Only when [PCr]/[Pi] decreases to a low level does [ATP] also fall.

Secondary energy failure

Studies by ^{31}P MRS of the brain in severely birth-asphyxiated babies have shown, rather surprisingly, little or no abnormality in the hours following delivery (Figure 4.5). Subsequently, however, [PCr]/[Pi] (recorded from the temporo-parietal cortex) gradually fell, with a nadir at 2–4 days of age, in spite of normal values for arterial oxygen saturation, blood pressure and blood glucose (Hope et al., 1984; Azzopardi et al., 1989). In the worst affected infants [ATP] then fell and death ensued (Figure 4.5a). In survivors, the spectra usually returned to normal within about two weeks, except that the total [31]P

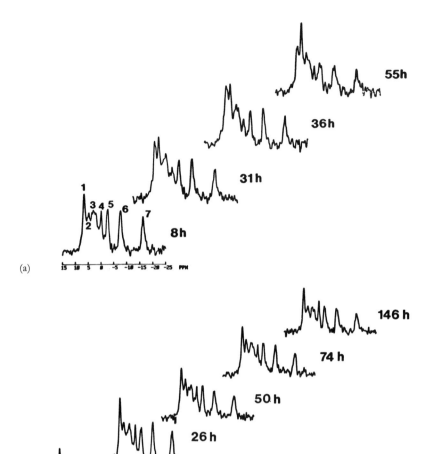

Figure 4.5. ^{31}P magnetic resonance spectra obtained from the temporo-parietal cortex of two severely birth-asphyxiated infants born at 37 and 36 weeks of gestation. Postnatal ages at the time of study are indicated. The peak-assignments are 1, phosphomonoesters; 2, Pi; 3, phosphodiesters; 4, PCr; 5, 6 and 7, the γ, α and β phosphates of ATP (with small contributions from other nucleotide triphosphates). (a) The spectrum at 8 h was normal: [PCr]/[Pi] then fell, to a minimum of 0.32 at 55 h and [ATP] also fell: pH$_i$ was normal, 7.06 at 8 h, and rose to a maximum of 7.28 at 36 h. The infant died at 60 h. (b) The spectrum at 4 h was normal: [PCr]/[Pi] fell to a minimum of 0.65 at 50 h but recovered to normal by 146 h: [ATP] never fell. pH$_i$ was 7.08 at 4 h and rose to a maximum of 7.23 at 26 h. The infant died aged 27 days with global cerebral atrophy. (From Axxopardi et al., 1989.)

signal was reduced, indicating loss of brain cells (Figure 4.5b). The explanation offered for this sequence of changes was that the brain had suffered an acute episode of hypoxia-ischaemia, causing 'primary' energy failure, during labour, but which had been reversed by resuscitation at delivery, so that the energy state of the brain had returned to normal. The subsequent changes in ^{31}P spectra were attributed to a 'secondary' phase of energy impairment or failure which had been set of by the 'primary' phase, or events associated with it.

Prognosis

MRS has proved useful for exploring the prognosis of secondary energy failure. Azzopardi et al. (1989) studied 61 infants recruited because of evidence or suspicion of hypoxic-ischaemic brain injury, many of whom had sustained birth asphyxia. Clear evidence emerged that the chances of survival and the severity of neurodevelopmental impairments at 1 year of age were directly related to the maximum detected extent of energy failure during the first days of life, as judged by minimum values for [PCr]/[Pi] (Figures 4.6 and 4.7). If [ATP]/[Ptot] (total phosphorus signal) fell, death was almost inevitable. More recently, Roth et al. (1992), as part of the same study, recruited a further group of birth-asphyxiated babies, so that data from a total of 52 babies, studied specifically because of birth asphyxia, were available for anlaysis. The babies had been in very poor condition at birth: their mean arterial base excess in cord blood or shortly after delivery was -20 mmol. l^{-1}, 38 had fits, and 26 required mechanical ventilation. The results extended those of Azzopardi et al. and confirmed the bad prognosis of secondary energy failure. The sensitivity, specificity and positive predictive value for death or multiple disabling impairments of [PCr]/[Pi] values lower than 2.5 standard deviations below the mean normal value were 72%, 92% and 91% respectively. Ten of the 14 multiply disabled infants were very severely affected, six had tetraplegia, five diplegia, and seven were cortically blind. Roth et al. (1992) also investigated the relation between minimum values for [PCr]/[Pi] and head growth. They found that although the infants had normal head circumferences at birth, head growth was slowest, leading to microcephaly in those whose values for [PCr]/[Pi] fell the most (Table 4.1). The results of these studies may be summed up as showing that secondary energy failure leads both to neurodevelopmental disabilities and to microcephaly. The worse the energy failure, the worse the outcome is likely to be.

Studies with MRS will probably provide increasing information over the next few years. Localization has so far been crude, but improvements in the capabilities of the technique now permit data to be acquired from small (4 ml) regions of the brain both for ^{31}P, and for ^{1}H spectra (Cady & Reynolds, 1995). Data are already emerging that lactate, indicating anaerobic glycolysis, is detectable in the brains of newborn infants, particularly if they are born

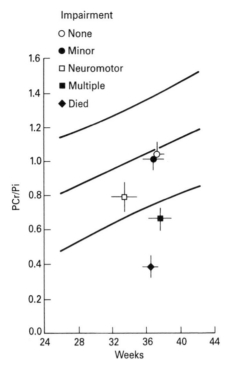

Figure 4.6. Relation between minimum recorded values for cerebral [PCr]/[Pi]
during the first 6 days of life, death, and neurodevelopmental impairments
at one year of age in 61 infants studied because of evidence or suspicion
of perinatal hypoxic-ischaemic brain injury. The regression and 95%
confidence limits for normal values versus gestational plus postnatal age
(weeks) are shown. Minor impairment = disorders of tone or reflexes not
causing disability; neuromotor impairment = major neuromotor impairment causing disability; multiple impairments = more than one disabling
impairment, including neuromotor, neurosensory (vision or hearing),
neurobehavioural and psychometric, often together with microephaly.
Mean values ± SEM are shown. (Constructed from the data of Azzopardi
et al., 1989.)

preterm or suffer intrauterine growth retardation. Increased lactate, following
birth asphyxia like low [PCr]/[Pi], indicates a bad prognosis (Groenendaal
et al., 1994; Penrice et al., 1994).

Progression from primary to secondary energy failure

Since the prognosis of secondary energy failure is so bad it becomes important
to understand the mechanisms involved, and to devise preventive strategies.
It was assumed above that an acute intrapartum episode of hypoxia-ischaemia

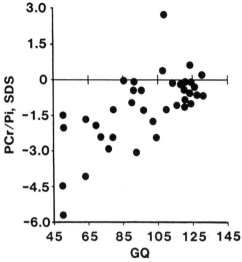

Figure 4.7. Relation between minimum values during the first six days of life for
[PCr]/[Pi], expressed as standard deviation scores (SDS) and Griffiths
General Quotient (GQ) at one year of age in 38 infants studied by MRS
because of evidence or suspicion of hypoxic-ischaemic brain injury. Values
for GQ < 50 were recorded as 50. (From Azzopardi et al., 1989.)

Table 4.1. *Head growth in 52 birth-asphyxiated infants*

PCr/Pi SDS	Discharge or death			Age one year			OFC growth velocity (cm/yr)
	n	OFC (cm)	OFC SDS	n*	OFC (cm)	OFC SDS	
> −1.99	25	34.9 (2.7)	−0.8 (1.5)	21	46.2 (2.0)	−0.9 (2.2)	10.4 (3.1)
−2.00 to −3.99	11	34.9 (2.5)	0.6 (1.5)	7	45.5 (2.0)	−1.5 (1.6)	9.5 (2.7)
< −4.00	16	35.7 (1.7)	0.0 (1.5)	5	41.2 (2.1)	−4.8 (2.0)	5.6 (2.1)

Notes: Occipto frontal head circumference (OFC) and OFC standard deviation score
(SDS) on discharge or death at a median age of 16 (range one to 94) days and at 12
(range 11 to 13) months, and OFC growth velocity, according to PCr/Pi SDS.
*15 infants died; values were missing for four. Mean values (SD) are given.
(From Roth et al., 1993).

was responsible for the initiating reactions. However, until very recently it had not been shown that an acute reversed cerebral hypoxic-ischaemic insult mimicking birth asphyxia and causing primary energy failure could lead, after a delay of many hours, to a secondary phase, as seen in the human infant. Lorek et al. (1994) carried out studies on newborn piglets to investigate whether this progression could be reproduced. The piglets were subjected to occlusion of the internal carotid arteries and hypoxaemia, which was reversed after an hour. Cerebral [PCr]/[Pi] fell to zero but it returned to baseline levels on reperfusion and reoxygenation of the brain. By 24–48 hours later exactly the same changes had developed as seen in birth-asphyxiated human infants. [PCr]/[Pi] and [ATP]/[Ptot] fell again, in spite of normal oxygen and substrate supply to the brain. The extent of the secondary fall in [PCr]/[Pi] was shown to be directly proportional to the severity of the primary insult, as judged by depletion of ATP. During primary energy failure, the lactate levels in the brain increased greatly, returning close to baseline before increasing again during the secondary phase. At the same time the spin-spin (transverse) relaxation time of proton containing metabolites varied in a manner consistent with the development of cytotoxic oedema – particularly, in the secondary phase, neuronal oedema (Cady et al., 1994). Neuropathological studies showed changes closely similar to those in birth-asphyxiated infants, and evidence of a relation between the extent of energy failure and the proportion of cells affected by programmed cell death (Mehmet et al., 1994). This animal model of the progression from primary to secondary energy failure is suitable for investigating further the biochemical and molecular mechanisms involved, and also for testing cerebroprotective methods for preventing the progression.

Prevention

The best way to prevent secondary energy failure with its very bad prognosis in the asphyxiated human infant would be to prevent, by suitable obstetric surveillance and intervention, the primary hypoxic-ischaemic insult which initiates the processes leading to it. If that is not feasible, it is possible that in the future methods for cerebroprotection that can be applied after the acute insult may become established. Very many mechanisms have been invoked to explain the progression from primary to secondary energy failure. For example, one much-canvassed possibility is that excitatory neurotransmitters, particularly glutamate, which are released at the synapses in response to acute hypoxia-ischaemia may, by stimulating N-methyl D-aspartate (NMDA) and other receptors, cause massive calcium entry to cells and damage to the mitochondrial electron transport chain. Other mechanisms that have been invoked include those involving prostanoids, nitric oxide, free radicals, immune mechanisms, phagocytes, growth factors and impaired protein synthesis. As more is learnt about these mechanisms and how to interrupt them, therapy immediately after delivery in severely asphyxiated infants may be justifiable, but only if it has been shown by animal experimentation to be sensible. For example, a mixture of oxygen-free radical scavengers and magnesium, which blocks both voltage-dependent and NMDA-receptor associated channels, has shown considerable promise in animals, when given after a cerebral hypoxic-ischaemic insult (Thordstein et al., 1993). Also, mild hypothermia, which would be relatively simple to apply to newborn infants, has recently been found markedly to ameliorate secondary energy failure following an acute reversed cerebral hypoxic-ischaemic insult in the newborn piglet (Thoresen et al., 1995). The prevention of secondary energy failure in newborn animals such as the piglet could prove to be a suitable initial end-point for the testing of cerebroprotective strategies, though long-term follow-on studies will also be needed.

Near infrared spectroscopy (NIRS)

NIRS has recently been applied to the investigation of perinatal brain injury and it shows considerable promise for the future. The technique depends on the transmission through the brain of light in the near infrared region of the spectrum (700–1000 nm). The light is absorbed in predictable ways by the chromophores oxyhaemoglobin, deoxyhaemoglobin and oxidized cytochrome aa$_3$ (or cytochrome c oxidase), the terminal member of the mitochondrial electron transport chain (Figure 4.4). Changes in the intracerebral concentrations of these compounds can be recorded continuously from newborn infants at the cot side (Wyatt et al., 1986) and methods have been described for the measurement of cerebral blood flow (Edwards et al., 1988), blood volume (Wyatt et al., 1990), venous saturation (Skov et al., 1993) and the carbon dioxide reactivity of the cerebral circulation (Wyatt et al., 1991). NIRS can also be used to make observations from the brain of the human infant during labour, including measurement of mean cerebral oxygen saturation (Peebles et al., 1992). Uterine contractions accompanied by reductions in fetal heart rate were associated with falls in saturation, whereas those without these reductions were not. Studies of a number of interventions that might influence perinatal cerebral haemodynamics and oxygenation are underway. So far, only normal labours have been investigated but, in the future, studies of compromised fetuses are likely to shed new light on the relation between intrapartum events and long-term outcome.

Studies of influences that might cause dangerous pertubations of cerebral haemodynamics in newborn infants include one of the indomethacin treatment of patent ductus arteriosus. Major reductions were found in cerebral blood flow, oxygen delivery and carbon dioxide reactivity, and also in the concentration of oxidized cytochrome aa$_3$, thus indicating a reduction in intracellular oxygen availability (Edwards et al., 1990; McCormick et al., 1993).

Of particular relevance to the possibility of preventing secondary energy failure is the finding that abnormalities are detectable by NIRS in the brains of newborn infants at a time when the ^{31}P spectra are still normal shortly after delivery. Current evidence is that cerebral blood flow, blood volume and venous saturation are all raised, and that the carbon dioxide reactivity of the circulation is almost abolished (McCormick et al., 1991; Skov et al., 1993). These observations need confirmation, but if substantiated they could eventually be used to identify infants destined to develop secondary energy failure, and who might then justifiably be enrolled into controlled trials of cerebro-protection. Other methods for identifying these infants could include electroencephalography (Murdoch-Eaton et al., 1992) and Doppler velocimetry (Levene, 1988).

SUMMARY AND CONCLUSIONS

The major causes of perinatal brain injury are cerebral periventricular haemorrhage in preterm infants, and hypoxia-ischaemia in both preterm and term ones.

These types of injury are responsible for permanent neurodevelopmental impairments in a significant minority of impaired children and adults. Much has been learnt about the causal antecedents of cerebral haemorrhage in preterm infants and methods of prevention are becoming reasonably soundly based. Birth asphyxia causes hypoxic-ischaemic injury to the brain, and this type of injury is also responsible for periventricular leukomalacia in preterm infants. Acute hypoxia-ischaemia, which is then reversed (as in birth asphyxia), can set off a chain of cerebral metabolic reactions culminating in severe delayed (or 'secondary') energy failure which is at its worst two to four days later, and which is detectable by phosphorus magnetic resonance spectroscopy. In the future it may be possible to interrupt these reactions, thus improving the prognosis of the infants. The new technique of near infrared spectroscopy gives information about cerebral oxidative metabolism and haemodynamics – before delivery as well as afterwards – that is relevant to the pathogenesis of perinatal brain injury.

Ultrasound imaging of the brain in the neonatal period provides very valuable information about the long-term sequelae of cerebral haemorrhage and periventricular leukomalacia in very preterm infants. The more extensive forms of these conditions account for most of the disabling neurodevelopmental impairments found in these infants when they reach school age. Some of the lesser cognitive impairments found may also be due to perinatal hypoxic-ischaemic injury though other influences could well be operating. In birth-asphyxiated infants, magnetic resonance spectroscopy has shown that the extent of permanent neurodevelopmental sequelae is directly related to the severity of cerebral energy failure in the first days of life. To what extent the various aspects of brain plasticity modulate outcome in brain-injured infants is virtually unknown; some infants with large localized lesions progress surprisingly well.

The ability to employ non-invasive methods including, among others, ultrasound imaging and magnetic resonance spectroscopy to examine the brain in the perinatal period allows the prevalence and mechanisms of brain-damaging influences to be explored, preventive measures and treatments to be tested, and the prognosis of small ill infants to be assigned with reasonable confidence. The ability to form a clear opinion about prognosis has important implications for the care of ill infants. The parents of those whose prognostic indicators are good can be reassured, early warning can be given if a serious impairment can be foreseen and, if the prognosis is extremely bad, informed decisions can be made about how far to pursue treatment.

Perinatal brain injury is clearly involved in the development over the lifespan of a small minority of individuals. Many questions remain unanswered. For example, the extent to which it contributes to neuropsychiatric illness in adult life is unresolved. Genetic factors clearly have the main influence, though environmental influences are also important. Clues exist that perinatal hypoxic-ischaemic brain injury, one such influence, may be more important than is currently recognized. In the future, it will be increasingly possible to relate the presence of objectively determined perinatal cerebral lesions to neuropsychiatric outcomes in later childhood and adult life.

ACKNOWLEDGEMENTS

The author gratefully acknowledges the help of numerous colleagues, including particularly E. B. Cady, D. T. Delpy, A. D. Edwards, Ann L. Stewart and J. S. Wyatt.

REFERENCES

Alberman, E. D. (1982) The epidemiology of congenital defects: a pragmatic approach. In M. Adinolfi & P. Benson, et al. (eds.) *Paediatric Research: A Genetic Approach* London, Heinemann, pp. 1–28.

Alberman, E. D. & Botting, B. (1991) Trends in prevalence and survival of very low birthweight infants, England and Wales. 1983–1987. *Archives of Disease in Childhood,* **66**, 1304–8.

Armstrong, D. & Norman, M. G. (1974) Periventricular leucomalacia in neonates: complications and sequelae. *Archives of Disease in Childhood,* **49**, 367–75.

Azzopardi, D., Wyatt, J. S., Cady, E. B., Delpy, D. T., Baudin, J., Stewart, A. L., Hope, P. L., Hamilton, P. A. & Reynolds, E. O. R. (1989) Prognosis of newborn infants with hypoxic-ischaemic brain injury assessed by phosphorus magnetic resonance spectroscopy. *Pediatric Research,* **25**, 445–51.

Banker, B. & Larroche, J. C. (1962) Periventricular leucomalacia of infancy. *Archives of Neurology,* **7**, 386–410.

Behar, R., Wozniak, P., Allard, A., Benirschke, K., Vaucher, Y., Coen, R., Berry, C., Schragg, P., Villegas, I. & Resnik, R. (1988) Antenatal origin of neurologic damage in newborn infants. *American Journal of Obstetric Gynecology*, **159**, 357–63.

Benson, J. W. T., Drayton, M. R., Hayward, C., Murphy, J. F., Osborne, J. P., Rennie, J. M., Schulte, J. F., Speidel, B. D. & Cooke, R. W. I. (1986) Multicentre trial of ethamsylate for prevention of periventricular haemorrhage in very low birthweight infants. *Lancet*, **ii**, 1297–9.

Cady, E. B., Lorek, A., Penrice, J., Wylezinska, M., Cooper, C. E., Brown, G. C., Owen-Reece, H., Kirkbride, V., Wyatt, J. S. & Reynolds, E. O. R. (1994) Brain-metabolite transverse relaxation times in magnetic resonance spectroscopy increase as adenosine triphosphate depletes during secondary energy failure following acute hypoxia-ischaemia in the newborn piglet. *Neuroscience Letters*, **182**, 201–4.

Cady, E. B. & Reynolds, E. O. R. (1995) Pediatric brain spectroscopy: clinical utility. In D. M. Grant & R. K. Harris (eds.) *Encyclopedia of Nuclear Magnetic Resonance.* Chichester: John Wiley, (not yet out).

Cole, V. A., Durbin, G. M., Olaffson, A., Reynolds, E. O. R., Rivers, R. P. A. & Smith, J. F. (1974) Pathogenesis of intraventricular haemorrhage in newborn infants. *Archives of Disease in Childhood*, **49**, 722–8.

Cooke, R. W. I. (1994) Survival and cerebral morbidity in preterm infants. *Lancet*, **343**, 1578.

Costello, A. M. de L., Hamilton, P. A., Baudin, J., Towsend, I., Bradford, B. C., Stewart, A. L. & Reynolds, E. O. R. (1988) Prediction of neurodevelopmental impairment at 4 years from brain ultrasound appearance in very preterm infants. *Developmental Medicine and Child Neurology*, **30**, 711–22.

Crowley, P., Chalmers, I. & Kierse, M. J. N. C. (1990) The effects of corticosteroid administration before preterm delivery: an overview of the evidence from controlled trials. *British Journal of Obstetric Gynaecology*, **97**, 11–25.

de Reuek, J. (1971) The human periventricular arterial supply and the anatomy of cerebral infarctions. *European Neurology*, **5**, 321–34.

Edwards, A. D., McCormick, D. C., Roth, S. R., Cope, M., Wyatt, J. S., Delpy, D. T. & Reynolds, E. O. R. (1992) Cerebral haemodynamic effects of surfactant administration investigated by near infrared spectroscopy. *Pediatric Research*, **32**, 532–6.

Edwards, A. D., Wyatt, J. S., Richardson, C., Potter, A., Cope, M., Delpy, D. T. & Reynolds, E. O. R. (1990) Effects of indomethacin on cerebral haemodynamics in very preterm infants. *Lancet*, **335**, 1491–5.

Edwards, A. D., Wyatt, J. S., Richardson, C., Delpy, D. T., Cope, M. & Reynolds, E. O. R. (1988) Cotside measurement of cerebral blood flow in ill newborn infants by near infrared spectroscopy. *Lancet*, **ii**, 770–1.

Goddard-Finegold, J. (1989) Experimental models of intraventricular hemorrhage. In K. E. Pape & J. S. Wigglesworth (eds.) *Perinatal Brain Lesions.* Oxford: Blackwell, pp. 115–34.

Gould, S. J., Howard, S., Hope, P. L. & Reynolds, E. O. R. (1987) Periventricular intraparenchymal cerebral haemorrhage in preterm infants: the role of venous infarction. *Journal of Pathology*, **151**, 197–202.

Gray, O. P., Ackerman, A. & Fraser, A. J. (1968) Intracranial haemorrhage and clotting defects in low birthweight infants. *Lancet*, **i**, 545–7.

Groenendaal, I., Veenhoven, R. H., van der Grond, J., Jansen, G. H., Witkamp, T. D. & de Vries, L. S. (1994) Cerebral lactate and n-acetyl-aspartate/choline ratios in asphyxiated full-term neonates demonstrated in vivo using proton magnetic resonance spectroscopy. *Pediatric Research*, **35**, 148–51.

Hagberg, B., Hagberg, G. & Olow, I. (1984) The changing panorama of cerebral palsy in Sweden. IV: Epidemiological trends 1959–78. *Paediatrica Scandinavica*, **73**, 433–40.

Hambleton, G. & Wigglesworth, J. S. (1976) Origin of intraventricular haemorrhage in the preterm infant. *Archives of Disease in Childhood*, **51**, 651–9.

Hamilton, P. A., Hope, P. L., Cady, E. B., Delpy, D. T., Wyatt, J. S. & Reynolds, E. O. R. (1986) Impaired energy metabolism in brains of newborn infants with increased cerebral echodensities. *Lancet*, **i**, 1242–6.

Harrison, V. C., Heese, H. V. & Klein, M. (1968) Intracranial haemorrhage associated with hyaline membrane disease. *Archives of Disease in Childhood*, **43**, 116–20.

Hope, P. L., Costello, A. M. de L., Cady, E. B., Delpy, D. T., Tofts, P. S., Chu, A., Hamilton, P. A., Reynolds, E. O. R. & Wilkie, D. R. (1984) Cerebral energy metabolism studied with phosphorus NMR spectroscopy in normal and birth-asphyxiated infants. *Lancet*, **ii**, 366–70.

Hope, P. L., Gould, S. J., Howard, S., Hamilton, P. A., Costello, A. M. de L. & Reynolds, E. O. R. (1988) Precision of ultrasound diagnosis of pathologically verified lesions in the brains of very preterm infants. *Developmental Medicine and Child Neurology*, **30**, 457–71.

Kirkbride, V., Baudin, J., Lorek, A., Meek, J., Penrice, J., Townsend, J., Roth, S., Edwards, A. D., McCormick, D., Reynolds, D. & Stewart, A. (1994) Motor tests of interhemispheric control and cognitive function in very preterm infants at eight years. *Pediatric Research*, **36**, 20A.

Krägeloh-Mann, I., Hagberg, G., Meisner, C., Schelp, B., Maas, G., Eeg-Olofson, K. E., Selbman, H. K., Hagberg, B. & Michaelis, R. (1994) Bilateral spastic cerebral palsy – a comparative study between south-west Germany and western Sweden. II: Epidemiology. *Developmental Medicine and Child Neurology*, **36**, 473–83.

Levene, M. I. (1988) Management and outcome of birth asphyxia (1988) In M. I. Levene, M. J. Bennett & J. Punt (eds.) *Fetal and Neonatal Neurology and Neurosurgery*. Edinburgh: Churchill Livingstone, pp. 383–92.

Lorek, A., Takei, Y., Cady, E. B., Wyatt, J. S., Penrice, J., Edwards, A. D., Peebles, D., Wylezinska, M., Owen-Reece, H., Kirkbride, V., Cooper, C. E., Aldridge, R. F., Rosh, S. C., Brown, G., Delpy, D. T. & Reynolds, E. O. R. (1994) Delayed ('secondary') energy failure following acute cerebral hypoxia-ischaemia in the newborn piglet: continuous 48-hour studies by phosphorus magnetic resonance spectroscopy. *Pediatric Research*, **36**, 699–706.

Lou, H. C., Lassen, N. A. & Friis-Hansen, B. (1979) Impaired autoregulation of cerebral blood flow in the distressed newborn infant. *Journal of Pediatrics*, **94**, 118–21.

Lucas, A., Morley, R., Cole, T. J., Gore, S. M., Lucas, P. J., Crowle, P., Pearse, R., Boon, A. J. & Powell, R. (1990) Early diet in preterm babies and neurodevelopmental status at 18 months. *Lancet*, **i**, 1477–81.

McCormick, D. C., Edwards, A. D., Brown, G. C., Wyatt, J. S., Potter, A., Delpy, D. T. & Reynolds, E. O. R. (1993) Effects of indomethacin on cerebral oxidised cytochrome oxidase in preterm infants. *Pediatric Research*, **33**, 603–8.

McCormick, D. C., Edwards, A. D., Roth, S. C., Wyatt, J. S., Elwell, C. E., Cope, M., Delpy, D. T. & Reynolds, E. O. R. (1991) Relation between cerebral haemodynamics and outcome in birth asphyxiated infants studied by near infrared spectroscopy. *Pediatric Research*, **37**, 637.

Mehmet, H., Yue, X., Squier, M. V., Lorek, A., Cady, E. B., Penrice, J., Sarraf, C., Peebles, D., Wylezinska, M., Kirkbride, V., Cooper, C., Brown, G., Wyatt, J. S., Delpy, D. T., Reynolds, E. O. R. & Edwards, A. D. (1994) Increased apoptosis in the cingulate sulcus of newborn piglets following transient hypoxia-ischaemia is related to the degree of high energy phosphate depletion during the insult. *Neuroscience Letters*, **181**, 121–5.

Ment, L. R., Oh, W., Ehrenkrantz, R. A., Philip, A. G. S., Vohr, B., Allan, W., Duncan, C. C., Scott, D. T., Taylor, K. J. W., Katz, K. H., Schneider, K. C. & Makuch, R. W. (1994) Low dose indomethacin and prevention of intraventricular hemorrhage: a multicenter randomized trial. *Pediatrics*, **93**, 543–50.

Murdoch-Eaton, D., Connell, J., Dubowitz, V. & Dubowitz, L. (1992) Monitoring of the electroencephalogram during intensive care. In Eyre, T. J. (ed.) *The Neurophysiological Examination of the Newborn Infant*. Lavenham: McKeith Press, pp. 48–65.

Pape, K. E., Blackwell, R. J., Cusick, G., Sherwood, A., Houang, M. T. W., Thorburn, R. J. & Reynolds, E. O. R. (1979) Ultrasound detection of brain damage in preterm infants. *Lancet*, **i**, 1261–4.

Pape, K. E. & Wigglesworth, J. S. (1979) *Haemorrhage, Ischaemia and the Perinatal Brain*. London, Heinemann.

Papile, L. A., Burstein, J., Burstein, R. & Koffler, H. (1978) Incidence and evolution of subependymal and intraventricular hemorrhage: a study of infants with birth weights less than 1500 gm. *Journal of Pediatrics*, **92**, 529–34.

Peebles, D. M., Edwards, A. D., Wyatt, J. S., Bishop, A. P., Cope, M., Delpy, D. T. & Reynolds, E. O. R. (1992) Changes in human fetal cerebral haemoglobin concentration and oxygenation during labour measured by near infrared spectroscopy. *American Journal of Obstetrics and Gynecology*, **166**, 1369–73.

Penrice, J., Cady, E. B., Lorek, A., Wylezinska, M., Wyatt, J. S. & Reynolds, E. O. R. (1994) Localised ^{1}H magnetic resonance spectroscopy of the brain in normal and perinatally asphyxiated infants. *Pediatric Research*, **34**, 33A.

Perlman, J. M., Goodman, S., Kreusser, K. L. & Volpe, J. J. (1985) Reduction in intraventricular hemorrhage by elimination of fluctuating cerebral blood flow in preterm infants with respiratory distress syndrome. *New England Journal of Medicine*, **312**, 1353–7.

Philip, A. G. S., Allan, W. C., Tito, A. M. & Wheeler, L. R. (1987) Intraventricular haemorrhage in preterm infants: declining incidence in the 1980s. *Pediatrics*, **84**, 797–801.

Pharoah, P. O. D., Cooke, T., Cooke, R. W. I. & Rosenbloom, L. (1990) Birthweight specific trends in cerebral palsy. *Archives of Disease in Childhood*, **65**, 602–6.

Reynolds, E. O. R. & Wyatt, J. S. (1992) Perinatal brain injury. In Asbury, A. K., McKhann, G. M. & McDonald, W. I. (eds.) *Diseases of the Nervous System*, 2nd edn. WB Sanders: Philadelphia, PA, pp. 584–97.

Reynolds, M. L., Evans, C. A. N., Reynolds, E. O. R., Saunders, N. R., Durbin, G. M. & Wigglesworth, J. S. (1979) Intracranial haemorrhage in the preterm sheep fetus. *Early Human Development*, **3**, 163–86.

Roth, S. C., Edwards, A. D., Cady, E. B., Delpy, D. T., Wyatt, J. S., Azzopardi, D., Baudin, J., Townsend, J., Stewart, A. L. & Reynolds, E. O. R. (1992) Relation between cerebral oxidative metabolism following birth asphyxia and neurodevelopmental outcome and brain growth at one year. *Developmental Medicine and Child Neurology*, **34**, 285–95.

Roth, S. C., Baudin, J., McCormick, D. C., Edwards, A. D., Townsend, J., Stewart, A. L. & Reynolds, E. O. R. (1993) Relation between ultrasound appearance of the brain in very preterm infants and neurodevelopmental impairment at eight years. *Developmental Medicine and Child Neurology*, **35**, 715–28.

Sarnat, H. B. & Sarnat, M. S. (1976) Neonatal encephalopathy following fetal distress. *Archives of Neurology*, **33**, 696–705.

Skov, L., Pryds, O., Greisen, G. & Lou, H. (1993) Estimation of cerebral venous saturation in newborn infants by near infrared spectroscopy. *Pediatric Research*, **33**, 52–5.

Stewart, A. L. (1994) Outcome. In Harvey, D., Cooke, R. W. I. & Levitt, G. (eds.) *The Baby Under 1000 g*, 2nd edn. Potters Bar: Wright.

Stewart, A. L., Reynolds, E. O. R., Hamilton, P. A., Baudin, J., Costello, A. M. de L., Bradford, B. C. & Wyatt, J. S. (1987) Probability of neurodevelopmental disorders estimated from ultrasound appearance of brain in very preterm infants. *Developmental Medicine and Child Neurology*, **29**, 3–11.

Szymonowicz, N., Yu, V. Y. H., Walker, A. & Wilson, F. (1986) Reduction in periventricular haemorrhages in preterm infants. *Archives of Disease in Childhood*, **61**, 661–5.

Takashima, J. & Tanaka, K. (1978) Development of cerebral architecture and its relationship to periventricular leukomalacia. *Archives of Neurology*, **35**, 11–16.

Thoresen, M., Penrice, J., Lorek, A., Cady, E. B., Wylezinska, M., Kirkbride, V., Cooper, C. E., Brown, G. C., Edwards, A. D., Wyatt, J. S. & Reynolds, E. O. R. (1994) Mild hypothermia following severe hypoxia-ischaemia ameliorates delayed cerebral energy failure in the newborn piglet. *Pediatric Research*, **37**, 667–70.

Thordstein, M., Bagenholm, R., Thiringer, K. & Kjellmer, I. (1993) Scavengers of free oxygen radicals in combination with magnesium ameliorate perinatal hypoxic-ischaemic damage in the rat. *Pediatric Research*, **34**, 23–6.

Towbin, A. (1968) Cerebral intraventricular hemorrhage and germinal matrix infarction in the fetus and premature newborn. *American Journal of Pathology*, **52**, 121–40.

Wigglesworth, J. S. (1984) *Perinatal Pathology*. Philadelphia, PA.: Saunders.

Wyatt, J. S., Cope, M., Delpy, D. T., Wray, S. & Reynolds, E. O. R. (1986) Quantitation of cerebral oxygenation and haemodynamics in sick newborn infants by near infrared spectrophotometry. *Lancet*, **ii**, 1063–6.

Wyatt, J. S., Cope, M., Delpy, D. T., Richardson, C. E., Edwards, A. D., Wray, S. & Reynolds, E. O. R. (1990) Quantitation of cerebral blood volume in human infants by near infrared spectroscopy. *Journal of Applied Physiology*, **68**, 1086–91.

Wyatt, J. S., Edwards, A. D., Azzopardi, D. & Reynolds, E. O. R. (1989) Magnetic resonance and near infrared spectroscopy for the investigation of perinatal hypoxic-ischaemic brain injury. *Archives of Disease in Childhood*, **64**, 953–63.

Wyatt, J. S., Edwards, A. D., Cope, M., Delpy, D. T., McCormick, D. C., Potter, A. & Reynolds, E. O. R. (1991) Response of cerebral blood volume to changes in arterial carbon dioxide tension in preterm and term infants. *Pediatric Research*, **29**, 553–7.

5 Commentary **A systems view of psychobiological development***

GILBERT GOTTLIEB

THE FIRST PERIOD (ROUGHLY 1800-90)

The triumph of epigenesis over the concept of preformation ushered in the era of truly developmental thinking. Namely, the notion that to understand the origin of any phenotype it is necessary to study its development in the individual. This insight has been with us since at least the beginning of the 1800s when Etienne Geoffroy Saint-Hilaire (1825) advanced his hypothesis that the originating event of evolutionary change was an anomaly of embryonic or fetal development. The origin or initiation of evolutionary change was thus seen as a change in the very early development of an atypical individual. Although not a believer in evolution (in the sense that a species could become so modified as to give rise to a new species), Karl Ernst von Baer (1828) used the description of individual development as a basis for classifying the relationships among species: those that shared the most developmental features were classified together, while those that shared the fewest features were given a remote classification. It was von Baer who noticed that vertebrate species are much more alike in their early developmental stages than in their later stages. This was such a ubiquitous observation that von Baer formulated a law to the effect that development in various vertebrate species could be universally characterized as progressing from the homogeneous to the heterogeneous. As individuals in each species reached the later stages of their development they began to differentiate more and more away from each other, so there was less and less resemblance as each species reached adulthood. Figure 5.1 is a reproduction of von Baer's classification of various classes of vertebrate species based on his developmental observations.

---

* The reader will note that the title of this chapter is 'A Systems View', not '*The* Systems View'. To partially illustrate the variety of developmental systems views in the behavioral sciences, the interested reader is referred to Ford & Lerner's (1992) description of their version of a systems view of human development and, at an even more abstract level, Oyama's (1985) depiction of her ideas about developmental systems and evolution. Figure 5.4 gives the essence of my notion of a developmental psychobiological systems approach as I have worked it out, beginning with the related notions of structure–function bidirectionality and probabilistic epigenesis in 1970.

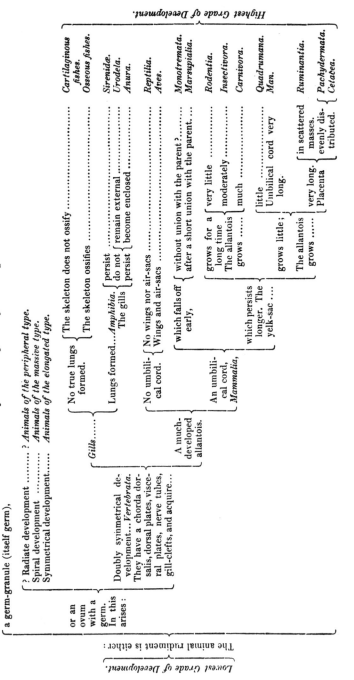

Figure 5.1. Von Baer's developmental classification of various classes of vertebrate animals (fish, amphibians, reptiles, birds, mammals – Monotremata through Cetacea – along right vertical axis. His three other 'types' of bodily organization are briefly designated in upper left of figure. Von Baer's scheme is not evolutionary in the conventional sense of ancestors giving rise to descendants. Rather he sees an increasing complexity of prenatal structural organization going from the top to the bottom of the figure. For von Baer, the most complex prenatal structural organizations reflect the highest grade of ontogenetic development. Grades of development proceed from lowest (beginning on left side of figure) to highest (right side of figure), whereas structural organizational complexity goes from lowest (top) to highest (bottom) on right vertical axis. (From von Baer, 1828, translated by Henfry & Huxley, 1853.)

THE SECOND PERIOD (ROUGHLY 1890–1935)

While von Baer's emphasis on the importance of developmental description represented a great leap forward in understanding the question of 'what', it did not come to grips with the problem of 'how'; namely, he and his predecessors evinced no interest in the mechanisms or means by which each developmental stage is brought about – it simply was not a question for them. It remained for the self-designated *experimental* embryologists of the late 1800s to ask that developmental question: Wilhelm His, Wilhelm Roux and Hans Driesch. As His wrote (1888, p. 295) in reference to von Baer's observations:

By comparison of [the development of] different organisms, and by finding their similarities, we throw light upon their probable genealogical relations, but we give no direct explanation of their growth and formation. A direct explanation can only come from the immediate study of the different phases of individual development. Every stage of development must be looked at as the physiological consequence of some preceding stage, and ultimately as the consequence of the acts of impregnation and segmentation of the egg . . .

It remained for Roux, in 1888, to plunge a hot needle into one of the two existing cells after the first cleavage in a frog's egg, thereby initiating a truly *experimental* study of embryology.

The arduously reached conclusion – the one we hold today – that individual development is most appropriately viewed as a hierarchically organized system began with Hans Driesch being dumbfounded by the results of his replication of Roux's experiment. While Roux found that killing one cell and allowing the second cleavage cell to survive resulted in a half-embryo in frogs, Driesch (reviewed in 1908) found that disattaching the first two cells in a sea urchin resulted in two fully formed sea urchins, albeit diminished in size. (When the disattachment procedure was later used in amphibians, two fully formed embryos resulted as in Driesch's experiment with sea urchins – Mangold & Seidel, 1927.) Driesch came to believe there is some nonmaterial vitalistic influence (an 'entelechy') at work in the formation of the embryo, one that will forever elude our best experimental efforts, so he eventually gave up embryology in favor of the presumably more manageable problems of psychology. Since Driesch found that a single cell could lead to the creation of a fully formed individual, he gathered, quite correctly, that each cell must have the same prospective potency, as he called it, and could in principle become any part of the body. He thought of these cells as *harmonious-equipotential systems*. For Driesch, the vitalistic feature of these harmonius-equipotential systems is their ability to reach the same outcome or end-point by different routes, a process which he labelled *equifinality*. Thus, in the usual case, there are two attached cleavage cells giving rise to an embryo, whereas in the unusual case, there are two separated cleavage cells, each giving rise to an embryo. While to Driesch these experimental observations provided the most elementary or 'easy' proofs of vitalism, for those still laboring in the field of embryology today they continue to provide a provocative challenge for experimental resolution and discovery. For the present purposes, it is important to note that, if each cell of the organism is a harmonious-equipotential system, then it follows that the organism itself must be such a system. Driesch's notion of equifinality – that developing organisms of the same species can reach the same endpoint via different developmental pathways – has become an axiom of developmental systems theory.* In a systems view of developmental psychology, equifinality means (a) that developing organisms which have different early or 'initial' conditions can reach the same endpoint and (b) that organisms that share the same initial condition can reach the same endpoint by different routes or pathways (cf. Ford & Lerner, 1992). Both of these points have been empirically demonstrated by the behavioral research of D. B. Miller (Miller, Hicinbothom & Blaich, 1990) and R. Lickliter (Banker & Lickliter, 1993) in birds, and by Nöel (1989) and Carlier et al. (1989), among others, in mammals. The uniquely important development principle of equifinality is rarely explicitly invoked in theoretical views of developmental psychology, so it may seem unfamiliar to many readers.

THE THIRD PERIOD (ROUGHLY 1935 TO THE PRESENT)

As we move from the late 1800s to the 1930s in our brief overview of the precursors to our present concept of the systems nature of development, we encounter the insights of the systems- or organismically-oriented embryologists, Paul Weiss and Ludwig von Bertalanffy, and the geneticist Sewall Wright.

In his wonderfully lucid and historically complete opus on the topic of development, *Modern Theories of Development: An Introduction to Theoretical Biology*, originally published in German in 1933, von Bertalanffy introduced the system theory, as he called it, as a way of avoiding the pitfalls of machine theory, on the one hand, and vitalism, on the other. The error of the machine theory of development, as von Bertalanffy saw it, was the attempt to analyze the various aspects of the developmental process into their individual component parts or mechanisms, conceived of as proceeding independently of one another. Von Bertalanffy believed that the fundamental error of the classical concept of mechanism, which was adopted wholesale from physics,

---

* To the best of my knowledge, Egon Brunswik (1952) was the first to call attention to equifinality as an important principle of psychological development in his infrequently cited monograph for the International Encyclopedia of Unified Science, *The Conceptual Framework of Psychology*.

lay in its application of an additive point of view to the interpretation of living organisms.

'Vitalism, on the other hand, while being at one with the machine theory in analyzing the vital processes into occurrences running along their separate lines, believed these to be co-ordinated by an immaterial, transcendent entelechy. Neither of these views is justified by the facts. We believe now that the solution of this antithesis in biology is to be sought in an *organismic* or *system theory* of the organism which, on the one hand, in opposition to machine theory, sees the essence of the organism in the harmony and co-ordination of the processes among one another, but, on the other hand, does not interpret this co-ordination as vitalism does, by means of a mystical entelechy, but through the forces immanent in the living system itself'.

(von Bertalanffy, 1933/1962: 177–8)

Nowadays, we make von Bertalanffy's point by distinguishing between theoretical and methodological reductionism. Theoretical reductionism seeks to explain the behavior of the whole organism by reference to its component parts – a derivative of the older additive, physical concept of mechanism – while methodological reductionism holds that not only is a description of the various hierarchically organized levels of analysis of the whole organism necessary but that a depiction of the bidirectional traffic between levels is crucial to a developmental understanding of the individual.* For purposes of recognizing historical precedent, it is appropriate here to present the diagrams of Paul Weiss and Sewall Wright as they exemplify the strictly methodological reductionism of the hierarchically organized systems view of development. (I use what I hope is not an annoying plural form of system because the various levels of organismic functioning constitute within themselves systems of analysis: the organism–environment ecological system, the nervous system, the genomic system, for example. Von Bertalanffy himself later (1950) came to use the plural form in his conception of General Systems Theory.)

In Paul Weiss's (1959) diagram of the hierarchy of reciprocal influences, as shown in Figure 5.2, there are seven levels of analysis. The *gene* (DNA) is the ultimately reduced unit in an ever-expanding analytic pathway that moves from gene to *chromosome* – where genes can influence each other – from cell *nucleus* to cell *cytoplasm*, from cell to tissue (organized arrangements of cells that form organ systems – the nervous system, circulatory system, musculo-skeletal system, etc.), all of which make up the organism that interacts with the external environment. The entire schema represents a hierarchically organized system of increasing size, differentiation and complexity, in which each component affects, and is affected by, all the other components, not only at its own level but at lower and higher levels as well. Thus, the

* When I first introduced the notion of structure-function bidirectionality in connection with the concept of probabilistic epigenesis in an essay on developmental psychobiology (Gottlieb, 1970), I was unaware of the compatibility with the physiological notions already expressed by Paul Weiss and Sewall Wright as described below.

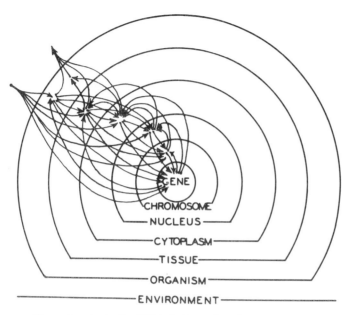

Figure 5.2. The embryologist Paul Weiss's hierarchy of reciprocal influences moving
back and forth from the lowest level of organization (gene) to the highest
level (external environment). (From Weiss, 1959.)

arrows in Figure 5.2 not only go upward from the gene, eventually
reaching all the way to the external environment through the activities of
the whole organism, but the arrows of influence return from the external
environment through the various levels of the organism back to the genes.
While the feed-forward or feed-upward nature of the genes has always
been appreciated, the feedbackward or feed-downward influences have
usually been thought to stop at the cell membrane. The newer conception
is one of a totally interrelated, fully coactional system in which the activity
of the genes themselves can be affected through the cytoplasm of the cell
by events originating at any other level in the system, including the
external environments. It is known, for example, that external environmental factors such as social interactions, changing day length, and so on
can cause hormones to be secreted (review by Cheng, 1979), which, in
turn, result in the activation of DNA transcription inside the nucleus of
the cell (i.e., 'turning genes on'). There are now many empirical examples
of external sensory and internal neural events that excite and inhibit gene
expression (e.g., Anokhin et al., 1991; Calamandrei & Keverne, 1994;
Mauro et al., 1994; Rustak et al., 1990) thereby supporting the *bidirectionality* of influences among the various levels of analysis from gene to
environment (discussed further below).

Since Weiss was an experimental embryologist it was probably merely by

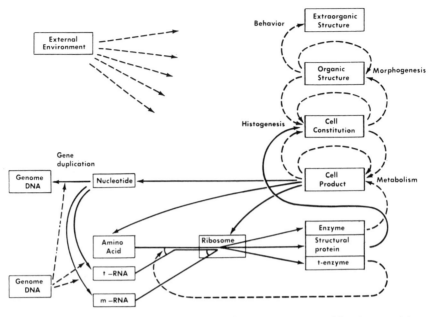

Figure 5.3. The fully coactive or interactional system, as presented by the geneticist
Sewall Wright (1968).

oversight that he did not explicitly include a developmental dimension in his
figure. Yet another not explicitly developmental schematic of a systems view
was put forward by Sewall Wright in 1968. As shown in Figure 5.3, once
again, the traffic between levels is bidirectional and the activity of the genes
is placed firmly inside a completely coactional system of influences. It is but
a small step to apply this way of thinking to the process of development (see
Figure 5.4 below).

As some behavioral scientists, including developmental psychologists, seem
to be unaware of the fact that the genes (DNA) themselves are subject to
influences from higher levels during the course of development, it is useful
to stress that contingency as a part of the *normal* process of development,
along with the better-known deleterious effects of environmentally induced
mutations of the genetic material. For example, there is a category of genetic
activity called 'immediate early gene expression', which is specifically responsive to sensory stimulation and results in a higher number of neurons in the
brains of developing animals that have been appropriately stimulated and a
deficiency in the number of cortical neurons in animals that have been
deprived of such normal sensory stimulation (e.g., Rosen et al., 1992, and
references therein). It was not so long ago that neuroscientists of very high
repute, including at least one eventual Nobel prize winner, were writing in
a vein that would seem to make sensory-stimulated immediate early gene

expression an impossibility, much less an important feature of normal neurobehavioral development. For example, Roger Sperry wrote in 1951 (p. 271): 'the bulk of the nervous system must be patterned without the aid of functional adjustment' or, 'Development in many instances. . . is remarkably independent of function, even in. . . [the] sense. . . [of]. . . function as a general condition necessary to healthy growth.' Twenty years later, Sperry (1971, p. 32) continued to observe: 'In general outline at least, one could now see how it could be entirely possible for behavioral nerve circuits of extreme intricacy and precision to be inherited and organized prefunctionally solely by the mechanisms of embryonic growth and differentiation.' Sperry was not alone in expressing a genetically predeterministic conception of neural and behavioral epigenesis. Viktor Hamburger, perhaps the foremost student of Nobel laureate Hans Spemann, echoed Sperry's beliefs on several occasions which, to his credit, he later ameliorated:

'The architecture of the nervous system, and the concomitant behavior patterns result from self-generating growth and maturation processes that are determined entirely by inherited, intrinsic factors, to the exclusion of functional adjustment, exercise, or anything else akin to learning [Hamburger, 1957, p. 56, reiterated *in toto* in 1964. 21]'.*

With noted authorities on the development of the nervous system making such statements in books and articles apt to be read by biologically-oriented psychologists, it is not surprising that a genetically predeterministic view entered into psychology, especially a psychology trying to recover its balance from accusations of (the other error) environmentalism. One of the values of a systems view of development is the explicit utilization of both genetic and experiential influences, not merely a nervous and often empty lip service averring that both are surely necessary.

THE PRESENT PERIOD (AROUND 1995)

In the past, I have presented on several occasions a simplified scheme of a systems view of psychobiological development that incorporates the major points of von Bertalanffy's, Weiss's, and Wright's thinking on the subject, and adds some detail on the organism–environment level that seems useful for a thoroughgoing behavioral and psychobiological analysis (Gottlieb, 1970, 1991, 1992). Whatever merit this way of thinking about development may have certainly must be traced to the pioneering efforts of psychobiological

---

* As a tribute to his long and productive career in neuroembryology, the *International Journal of Developmental Neuroscience* publishes a Viktor Hamburger Award Review. In 1993, the award went to Ira B. Black, who published a review on 'Environmental regulation of brain trophic interactions, which detailed the influence of neural activity on multiple trophic (growth) factors during development, further attesting to the feasibility of working out the bidirectional relations depicted here in Figure 5.4. The author himself raised that optimistic question at the conclusion of his review (p. 409): 'Are we now in a position to move from environmental stimulus to impulse activity, trophic regulation, mental function and behavior . . . ?'

BIDIRECTIONAL INFLUENCES

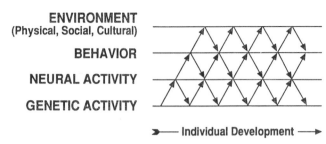

ENVIRONMENT
(Physical, Social, Cultural)
BEHAVIOR
NEURAL ACTIVITY
GENETIC ACTIVITY

➤— **Individual Development** —➤

Figure 5.4. The author's version of a systems view of psychobiological development. (From Gottlieb, 1991, 1992.)

theoreticians such as Z.-Y. Kuo (summarized in 1976), T. C. Schneirla (1960), and D. S. Lehrman (1970). At present, this way of thinking is being used both implicitly and explicitly by a number of more recent psychobiologically oriented theorists (e.g., Cairns, Gariépy & Hood, 1990; Edelman, 1988; Ford & Lerner, 1992; Griffiths & Gray, 1994; Hinde, 1990; Johnston & Hyatt, 1994; Magnusson & Törestad, 1993; Oyama, 1985).

As shown in Figure 5.4, I have reduced the levels of analysis to three functional organismic levels (genetic, neural, behavioral) and an environmetal level subdivided into three components (physical, social, cultural).* While those of us who work with nonhuman animal models stress the influence of the physical and social aspects of the environment, those who work with humans prominently include cultural aspects as well. The criticism that I hear most of this admittedly simple-minded scheme is not that it is overly simple but, rather, that it is too complex, not only with too many influences but too many influences running in too many directions: in short, a developmental systems approach is unmanageable and just not useful for analytic purposes. What I hope to show in the remainder of this chapter is that such a scheme is not only useful but that it represents individual development at a suitable level of complexity that does justice to the actualities of developmental influences.†

---

* Gariépy (1995) has correctly pointed out that psychological functioning as such is not included in the four levels of my systems diagram (Figure 5.4). The reason for that omission is that psychological functioning or mediation (perception, thinking, attitudes, love, hate, and so on) must be inferred from analysis at the overt level of behavior and the environment, as made clear by the notion of methodological behaviorism introduced by E. C. Tolman in 1932. In this sense, all psychologists are methodological (not theoretical) behaviorists (cf. Brunswik, 1952).

† At the conclusion of their review of genotype and maternal environment, Roubertoux, Nosten–Bertrand & Carlier (1990, p. 239) observe: 'The effects constitute a very complex network, which is probably discouraging for those who still hope to establish a simple relation between the different levels of biological organization, and particularly the molecular and the behavioral. The picture is indeed more complicated.'

Before turning to a review of several research programs that, among them, link all four levels of analysis in Figure 5.4, I want to offer a definition of the term *experience* that will allow me to discuss experiential events occurring at each level of analysis, not just at the organism–environment level. Experience is synonymous with function or activity, and is construed very broadly to include the activity of genes, the electrical activity of nerve cells, and their processes, impulse condition, neurochemical and hormonal secretion, the use and exercise of muscles and sense organs (whether interoceptive, proprioceptive, exteroceptive), and of course the behavior of the organism itself. Thus, the term experience, as used here, is not synonymous with 'environment', but rather stresses functional *activity* at all four levels of analysis. The contribution of such functions to development can take any of three forms. First, it can be of an *inductive* nature, channeling development in one direction rather than another. Secondly, it can be of a *facilitative* (temporal or quantitative) nature, influencing thresholds or the rate at which structural and physiological maturation, or behavioral development, occurs. Thirdly, it can be of a *maintenance* nature, serving to maintain the integrity of already formed neural or behavioral systems. The various courses these three experiential influences can take during development are shown in Figure 5.5. Patrick Bateson (Chapter 1) has added the notion that certain organism–environment encounters serve to trigger or stimulate the expression of previously organized behavior or responses.

A developmental psychobiological systems view

In summary, in its finished form, the developmental psychobiological systems approach that I have described involves a temporal description of activity at four levels of analysis (genetic, neural, behavioral, environmental) and the bidirectional effects of such activity among the four levels. When I first put forth the related notions of bidirectionality and probabilistic epigenesis in 1970, they were largely intuitive. They seem now to be established facts in many, if not all, quarters. Given the experimental–embryological heritage of all systems view, two further assumptions or propositions are warranted. Because of the early equipotentiality of cells and the fact that only a small part of the genome is expressed in any individual (Gottlieb, 1992), what is actually realized during the course of individual development represents only a fraction of many other possibilities. Finally, a developmental systems view entails the notion of equifinality, that is, the possibility of variation in pathways to common developmental endpoints.

I will now turn to an application of the present developmental systems concept to the foregoing empirical papers by Dennis O'Leary, Osmund Reynolds, and John C. Loehlin.

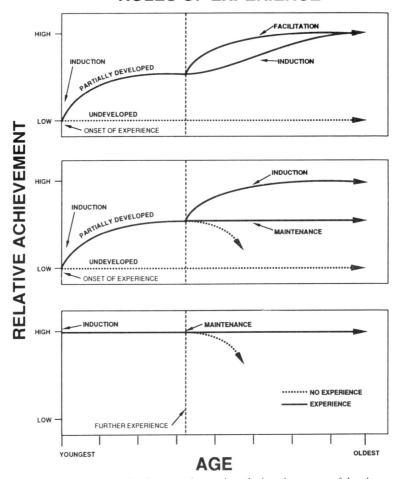

Figure 5.5. The various roles that experience plays during the course of development at the environmental, behavioral, neural, and genetic levels of analysis. (From Gottlieb, 1992.)

EQUIPOTENTIALITY AND THE INFLUENCE OF NEURAL ACTIVITY ON THE DIFFERENTIATION OF THE CEREBRAL CORTEX: DENNIS O'LEARY'S REVIEW

Although O'Leary's discussion includes factors in addition to equipotentiality and functional activity, it is those aspects of his review that I wish to emphasize here, in keeping with the aim of illustrating the utility of a systems view of psychobiological development.

As documented elsewhere (Gottlieb, 1992), the current definition of epigenesis holds that individual development is characterized by an increase in complexity of organization – that is, the emergence of new structural and functional properties and competencies – at all levels of analysis as a consequence of horizontal and vertical coactions among its parts, including organism–environment coactions. Nowhere is the epigenetic character of development better seen than in the differentiation of the brain, as Dennis O'Leary's review makes clear. Early on there is a uniformity of cyto-architecture across all cortical areas, such that the striking borders between cortical areas in the adult are indistinguishable at early stages. A second feature of adult development is the exquisitely precise patterns of synaptic connectivity both within the cortex itself and with noncortical structures. These gradually emerge from initially very widely distributed patterns of projections where axons go every which way in an early period of over exuberant projection. The precision of the adult pattern of synaptic connections emerges under the influence of activity-dependent processes, whereby nonfunctional connections are lost (pruned back by the absence of functional activity). Thus, selective axon elimination results in area-specific patterns of cortical efferent projections, a developmental process which is in stark contrast to older notions of a sheerly genetically determined blueprint for the brain areas and their interconnections. In fact, out of this work has come the felicitous phrase *activity-dependent gene expression* (review in Changeux & Konishi, 1987), which meshes well with the developmental systems view presented here. As Edelman's reviews (1988, and in Chapter 9) make clear, as research progresses the contribution of factors 'upstream' from the genes are now being widely recognized in developmental neuroscience, redressing the earlier unidirectional imbalance of the genetic predetermination of neural structures and functions. The activity-dependent outgrowth of neurons and 'overshoot' phenomena in developing neural networks have recently been reviewed and modeled by van Ooyen and van Pelt (1994).

With respect to the topic of equipotentiality, while we are familiar with the notion of the early equipotentiality of cells from the work of Driesch reviewed above, the findings reviewed by O'Leary having to do with the equivalent functional capabilities of the different sensory cortical areas in adult brains are remarkable. Namely, when visual input from the retinal axons from the eyes is rerouted to the somatosensory and auditory cortices instead of the visual cortex, the receptive field and response properties of the cells in the somatosensory and auditory cortices to visual stimulation resembled those normally seen in the visual cortex. This would imply that the early equipotentiality of these cells is maintained into adulthood, a fact that would be masked under normal conditions where each primary sensory cortex receives input only from its usual peripheral sources.

Thus, research in developmental neuroscience supports the developmental psychobiological notions of equipotentiality, bidirectionality, and the importance of neural activity for gene expression in the normal segregation of the cortical areas.

CAUSES AND OUTCOMES OF PERINATAL BRAIN
INJURY: OSMUND REYNOLD'S RESEARCH

While the human newborn is motorically highly immature ('altricial') at birth, all of its sensory systems become capable of functioning prior to birth, which makes the human (and other primate) infants unique among altricial mammals with respect to the precocity of their sensory development (Gottlieb, 1971). Thus, in the human fetus and infant, the early cerebral basis of perceptual and cognitive functioning begins in a substantial way in the prenatal period. Since normal blood flow and oxygenation are critically important to the health and sustenance of brain cells, and preterm (prematurely born) infants often have problems with cerebral hemorrhaging and respiration, it follows that premature infants are at risk for perinatal brain damage. While the usual period of gestation for the human fetus is around 265 days or about 38 weeks, over half of the premature infants born as early as 24 or 25 weeks of gestation survive if they are placed in neonatal intensive care units (*Reynolds, Chapter 4*). These survivors are most at risk for perinatal brain damage, and it is this population that the neonatal pediatrician Osmund Reynolds has been studying in a longitudinal fashion for the past decade or so. The general procedure has been to identify the type and extent of brain injury through various brain-imaging techniques and then to follow the course of neurocognitive development up through school age.

Perhaps the most striking and hopeful feature of Reynold's review, as shown in his Figure 4.3a, is that so many of these prematurely born infants did not evince major (disabling) cognitive impairments when they were examined at 8 years of age. It was primarily the infants who evinced gross brain damage during the neonatal period who showed major cognitive deficits upon reaching school age. These prematures had enlarged ventricles, hydrocephaly, and frank cerebral atrophy at birth, so it is not unexpected that they would be apt to manifest fairly serious cognitive deficits, as measured by IQ tests, in their school years. Concerning the large majority of children without major impairments, Reynolds raises the question of whether almost 50% of this population may suffer a subtle cognitive processing deficiency at school, as judged by their performance on the Kaufman Assessment Battery for Children (K-ABC in Reynolds' Figure 4.3b). Reynolds reports that 48% of these otherwise normal children show a significant difference between sequential over simultaneous processing on the K-ABC, a finding that would be consistent with an impairment in the functioning of the corpus callosum, the structure which unites the two hemispheres of the brain. This sort of microscopic callosal damage would not be detectable by the imaging techniques employed when these children were neonates. Another possibility raised by Reynolds is that nutritional problems in the neonatal period may have adversely affected the myelination of the corpus callosum, which does not begin until after term. Reynolds points out that nutritional supplementation in preterm infants improves outcome, so, in terms of our developmental systems model (Figure 5.4), this would involve bidirectional influences between the neural level and the environmental level, if we think of nutritional supplementation as a physical influence provided by the external environment of the preterm infant.

Since birth asphyxia is the other main perinatal insult that Reynolds describes in his chapter, I did want to bring in the possibility of another facilitating experience at the environmental level that could be utilized with carefully selected subgroups of preterm infants, a physical procedure that enhances the neonate's respiration and cardiac function when successfully applied: a neonatal waterbed. Since the somesthetic, vestibular, and proprioceptive sensory systems develop very early in fetal development (Gottlieb, 1971), Anneliese Korner decided that it would be a useful intervention with preterm infants to replace some of the uterine stimulation of which they are deprived when they are born long before term, so, over a period of 20 years, she worked out the details and developed a neonatal waterbed (review in Korner, in press). The bed provides very low amplitude (2.4 mm) head-to-foot oscillations that benefit the infants' respiratory efforts. Korner chose a temporal pattern within the range of maternal biological rhythms so as not to interfere with the developing organization of the infants' own biological rhythms; namely, slightly irregular rhythms in the lower range of maternal resting respirations (12–14 pulses per minute) that the infant would experience in the third trimester of pregnancy. Since prematures often evince apnea, and apnea can cause brain damage, one of the first payoffs of the waterbed stimulation was a reduction of apnea in polygraphically monitored prematures that were placed on oscillating waterbeds (see Figure 5.6). It was the most severe types of apnea that were significantly reduced, ones which are associated with slowing of the heart rate to less than 80 beats per minute. In further studies, it was determined that quiet sleep was significantly increased and crying significantly decreased when the infants were on the waterbeds.

Since the original aim of Korner's research with the preterm waterbed was to study its effect on neurobehavioral development, she undertook a longitudinal study of 56 premature infants whose gestational ages ranged from 22 to 32 weeks and followed them through 35 weeks of postconceptional age. In comparison to control infants, the waterbed group showed significantly more mature motor behavior, were significantly less irritable, were more than twice as often in the visually alert inactive state, and performed significantly better at attending and pursuing visual and auditory stimuli. Thus, it can be concluded that the compensatory movement stimulation provided by waterbeds is likely to enhance the neurobehavioral development of preterm infants. For very tiny, fragile babies or other infants in whom even the slightest passive movement might cause discomfort, the use of a nonoscillating waterbed is preferable to the oscillating waterbed. Moreover, while there is a

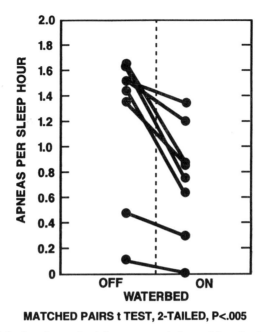

MATCHED PAIRS t TEST, 2-TAILED, P<.005

Figure 5.6. Episodes of apnea in eight premature infants while off and on an oscillating waterbed. (From Korner et al. 1978. Reproduced by permission of *Pediatrics*, Vol. 61, p. 528, copyright 1978.)

theoretical rationale for providing preterms with compensatory tactile-vestibular-proprioceptive stimulation because they are largely deprived of this developmentally important form of stimulation when growing to term in incubators, there is no such rationale for post-term infants, who experience ample movement stimulation in the course of ordinary maternal care (Korner, in press).

Before leaving the topic of sensory stimulation and its beneficial role in the neural and behavioral development of preterm infants, it is important to note that the preterm infant is also readily subject to overstimulation because of its neurobehavioral immaturity and the unusual opportunities for high levels of stimulation not normally encountered *in utero*. Work in my laboratory with 'preterm' animals indicates that combining waterbed stimulation with concurrent social (auditory) stimulation from the parent is disruptive in the preterms but not so in the post-term animals (Radell & Gottlieb, 1992). It is the concurrent nature of the stimulation which is disruptive because successive rather than simultaneous waterbed and auditory stimulation is not disruptive to the preterm animals. In human prematures, Eckerman et al. (1994) have found that when an adult concurrently talks to and lightly strokes a premature, the infant finds the experience noxious and evinces strong signs of withdrawal, indicating sensory overload or over arousal, as in the animal work. So, we need to be quite sensitive and alert to the possibility of noxious and, possibly, even damaging overstimulation when interventions are undertaken with prematurely born infants who would otherwise not experience certain kinds and combinations of sensory stimulation if they were safely stowed in utero. With this strong qualification, it would seem useful to consider that mild levels of compensatory tactile, vestibular, and proprioceptive stimulation such as that encountered in utero may well facilitate the neural and behavioral development of preterm infants, perhaps even those who have sustained subtle forms of perinatal brain injury.

While animal research indicates that the neonatal intensive care unit may be an overstimulating auditory environment (e.g., Philbin, Ballweg & Gray, 1994), the somesthetic, vestibular, and proprioceptive modalities represent a sensory deprivation condition from the standpoint of the fetus, as Korner's results would tend to suggest. Thus, it seems clear from the animal and human literature that neonatal pediatricians should consider taking steps to reduce the auditory and visual stimulation impinging on the premature, while mildly enhancing tactile, vestibular, and proprioceptive stimulation, as the latter facilitate respiration and cardiac function in the otherwise uncompromised preterm infant. These suggestions are further based on the fact that the somesthetic, vestibular, and proprioceptive systems develop very early in the fetus, whereas the auditory and visual systems are the last to develop. Since the auditory and visual systems are the most immature, they would be the most subject to overloading in the premature. Sensory overload occurs in premature animals when they are exposed to higher levels of stimulation than they would ordinarily experience in utero. To be specific, when enhanced auditory and visual stimulation are concurrent with each other, or separately combined with stimulation in other modalities, that results in 'developmental intersensory interference', a phenomenon well-documented in preterm animals and suspected but not well-documented in humans (Gottlieb, Tomlinson & Radell, 1989; Kenny & Turkewitz, 1986; Lickliter, 1993; Lickliter & Banker, 1994; Radell & Gottlieb, 1992). Developmental intersensory interference means that the usual learning, perceptual, or adaptive behavioral capacities of the premature are inhibited by certain *kinds* of stimulation (McBride & Lickliter, 1994), by precocious stimulation, or by exposure to concurrent stimulation in two sensory modalities, one of which is elevated above that encountered in the prenatal period.

GENES AND ENVIRONMENT: JOHN C. LOEHLIN'S REVIEW

Loehlin's review provides us with an opportunity to consider broader issues, particularly the question of whether the largely statistical approach of quantitative behavior genetics provides data of developmental significance. In order to answer that question, we need to agree on the content and procedure of developmental science. To put the matter in its simplest terms, it seems to me that there are two stages involved in developmental inquiry. In the first stage, a phenomenon would be identified that changes over some short or longer course of the lifetime. In the second stage experiments or other analytic procedures would be engaged in to specify the influences that cause the phenomenon in question to change as it does in the normal course of living. In short, the first stage identifies the 'what' for analysis and the second stage deals with the 'how' or the processes producing the change in the 'what'. In a systems view of development, these processes would be occurring at each of the four levels shown in Figure 5.4, not just at the genetic and environmental levels.

As Loehlin makes clear in his review, the procedures of quantitative behavior genetics deal with 'how much' and not how. So, the statements in his review are necessarily restricted to the size of the genetic and environmental influences on a given phenotypic outcome at various stages of the lifespan, not the developmental question of how genes and environment contribute to the outcome. A further problem with the heritability statistic employed by quantitative behavior geneticists is that it assumes that the genetic and environmental contributions are additive and not interactive, whereas developmental analysis is firmly rooted in interactionism.

Loehlin reviews lifespan trends in heritability in three important human functions: IQ, personality traits, and social attitudes. Although there are some exceptions noted by Loehlin, what he wishes quite reasonably to stress as a general trend is that heritability increases over the lifespan in all three areas. Technically interpreted, what this means is that as humans move through the lifespan, genes account for more of the variance than environment with respect to differences in intellectual functioning, personality, and social attitudes. Heritability estimates apply only to populations and not to individuals, so it would be inappropriate to generalize these results to individuals. But if this generalization can not be made, then I would hold that the results are without significance: the results do not suggest anything beyond themselves. No scientist would be satisfied with results that do not suggest anything beyond themselves, so it is understandable to find Loehlin and his colleagues making statements about the influence of genes on individual development. To quote Loehlin (this volume),

'The notion that the genetic contribution to behavioral differences expands during individual development reflects a growing consensus among behavior geneticists. Plomin . . . refers to the principle of genetic effects being amplified as development proceeds. Scarr and McCartney . . . stress the role of the genotype as the driving force behind development . . . Bouchard and his colleagues . . . use the phrase *nature via nurture*, referring to the role of the genes in influencing the character, selection, and impact of experiences. The notion of the declining influence of *imposed* environments on individual variation is also widely shared among human behavior geneticists'.

Loehlin goes on to say,

'One should not misinterpret this position. It does not hold that the environment is unimportant to development. On the contrary, it regards it as essential. What it *does* hold is that during development the organism–environment transactions that lead to individual behavioral differences increasingly reflect the influence of the genes; and that they decreasingly reflect the influence of shared family environment'.

Thus, in order for us not to mistakenly generalize the results to individual development, Loehlin is forced to reiterate the results themselves, thereby correctly restricting their generalizability to themselves.

As shown in prior Figure 5.4, a developmental analysis ultimately entails a description of genetic activity – which genes are turned on and by what influences – as well as the description of specific aspects of environmental influences, whether physical, social, or cultural. The purely statistical approach of quantitative behavior genetics does not allow any such specifications, but only the more general 'how much', as Loehin himself acknowledges.

Perhaps others will see bridges or implications that I have overlooked, but I do not see how an essentially contentless quantitative behavior genetics can help us understand individual development, if the understanding of individual development is our aim. As Thelen (1990) has shown, a developmental understanding of individual differences requires different assumptions than those of quantitative behavior genetics. One of these is the probabilistic character of development, and the other is the non-exclusive causality of genes and environment (reviewed in detail by Wahlsten & Gottlieb, in press). While, as shown in Figure 5.4, the role of genetic activity is an essential component of developmental analysis, to quote the well-known behavior geneticist Sandra Scarr (in press): 'Behavior genetics is not the study of species invariants or of gene action pathways that affect behaviors.' The implication that one needs to be interested in species invariants to be concerned with gene action pathways is dispelled by a quote from the developmental behavior geneticist J.-L. Gariépy (1995, p. 214): 'A major achievement of the modern systemic approach has been the formulation of a unified framework showing that the same processes that give rise to regularities in development also account for variability in individual development.'

CHARTING RECIPROCAL INFLUENCES AMONG ENVIRONMENT, BEHAVIOR, AND NEURAL ACTIVITY: DEVELOPMENT OF SPECIES IDENTIFICATION IN THE MALLARD DUCK EMBRYO AND HATCHLING

Since I would like to end on a more positive note, I would like to briefly review some of my own work as a further illustration of a systems view of psychobiological development.

A very interesting phenomenon for developmental analysis is presented by the fact that hatchlings in all precocial avian species tested to date are uniquely sensitive to the maternal assembly call of their own species in the absence of prior exposure to the hen. That is, when faced with a simultaneous auditory choice test between the maternal call of their own species and an alien maternal call, maternally naive hatchlings unerringly approach the maternal call of their own species (reviews in Gottlieb, 1981; Miller, 1988). Since this ability of mallard ducklings has all the hallmarks of innate behavior, I undertook a developmental analysis of the phenomenon. Since these birds were hatched in incubators the only prior vocal-auditory experience they had was hearing their own embryonic vocalizations and those of siblings. With the assistance of John Vandenbergh (Gottlieb & Vandenbergh, 1968), I developed a technique for muting embryos so they could not hear their own voices prior to hatching. When these devocalized birds were tested after hatching, their absolute preference for the maternal call of their own species was no longer present; they would respond as readily to a chicken maternal call as to a mallard maternal call in a simultaneous auditory choice test. By doing behavioral choice tests with artificially altered mallard maternal calls, I was able to learn that the acoustic basis of the vocal mallard duckling's selective perception of the mallard maternal call was based on two features of the call: its rhythmic organization around 3–5 notes/second and its low and high frequency components (400–2300 Hz). When the embryo was deprived of hearing its own vocalizations or those of siblings, two perceptual deficits occurred: they were not sensitive to the high-frequency components of the maternal call and their restricted range of sensitivity to the rhythmic aspect was enlarged to include 2 notes/second as well as 3–5 notes/second. The chicken call became as attractive as the mallard call to muted ducklings because the chicken call has the same low frequency components as the mallard call and the repetition rate of the chicken call is 2 notes/second. Because of a recent collaboration with avian neurophysiologists (the late Sergei Khayutin and Lubov Dmitrieva) in the Institute of Higher Nervous Activity and Neurophysiology, Russian Academy of Sciences, I have been able to take the experimental analysis to the level of neural activity. In particular, we have investigated the role of normally occurring embryonic auditory experience in the development of high–frequency sensitivity in vocal and muted mallard duck embryos and hatchlings.

Before describing the results of our auditory neurophysiological investigation, I need to tell you a bit more about our behavioral findings. After finding the high-frequency deficiency in the muted birds, we examined frequency analyses of the mallard duck embryo's vocalizations and found an almost perfect fit between the frequency components of the embryo's contact call (1500–2500 Hz) and the perceptual deficit in the muted hatchlings' response to the mallard maternal call (1600–2300 Hz). The match of high frequencies in the embryonic and maternal calls is shown in Figure 5.7.

In order to determine whether the high-frequency perceptual deficit in the muted ducklings was a consequence of the muted embryo not hearing

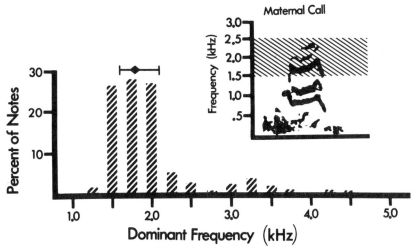

Figure 5.7. The frequency of most of the contact notes emitted by mallard duck embryos is between 1500 and 2500 Hz, which matches the upper frequency range of the mallard maternal call. (From Scoville, 1982.)

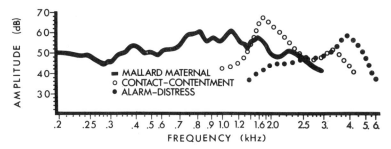

Figure 5.8. Peak frequency (Hz) bands of the mallard maternal call and the embryonic contact and alarm calls. (From Gottlieb, 1975b.)

the high frequencies in its contact call, I performed an experiment in which muted embryos were exposed to tape recordings of either a contact call (1500–2500 Hz) or an alarm-distress call (>3000 Hz) and then tested them after hatching with a normal mallard maternal call versus the same call with high frequencies above 1800 Hz deleted. The muted birds that were exposed to the contact call preferred the normal maternal call over the low-frequency maternal call, whereas the muted birds exposed to the alarm-distress call did not discriminate between the normal and low-frequency maternal calls. The peak frequency bands of the normal mallard maternal call and the embryonic contact and alarm calls are shown in Figure 5.8. (This research was published in Gottlieb, 1975a, b.)

The highly specific fit between the embryonic auditory experience of the frequencies in the contact call and the postnatal auditory perceptual performance of the muted ducklings indicates that the maturation of high-frequency sensitivity is not only endogenously driven, but there is an external experiential component that also contributes to the process. At the time this research was done, Patrick Bateson (1976) pointed out that theorists who concern themselves with innate behavior assume that the development of such behavior is not critically linked to any specific prior experience, but rather that it will exhibit itself provided only that rather general (nonspecific) life-sustaining conditions prevail during ontogeny. The assumption that innate behavior derives exclusively fron neural maturation without the benefit or necessity of specific experiences is not confined to classical ethological theory – it would seem to be a fairly widely held view in the psychological field as well. The present results called for a revision in that view and offered support for the contention that during the evolution of species-specific behavior, natural selection involved a selection of the entire developmental manifold, including not only the neuroembryological but also the normally occurring experiential features of ontogeny. This contention is in accord with recent advances in developmental neurobiology, which call for an appreciation of the experiential component in inducing, facilitating, and maintaining species-typical neural end-products, as exemplified in Dennis O'Leary's review. Thus, when Lubov Dmitrieva, of the former Soviet Union, offered to investigate the present behavioral phenomenon at the neurophysiological level by using the brain stem auditory evoked response (BAER) technique, I was delighted.

Dmitrieva and I (Dmitrieva & Gottlieb, 1993) examined the neuro-physiological development of the auditory system of the mallard duck embryo on day 24 of incubation (2–3 days before hatchling), in hatchlings, and in two-day-old ducklings. The day-24 embryos provide a benchmark in the sense that their responsiveness is based on the maturation of the auditory system prior to embryonic vocalization and vocal-auditory experience (the embryos begin vocalizing later on day 24). We examined the latency and threshold of the first wave of the BAER in two groups of birds: ones that had been muted on day 24 and kept in auditory isolation (auditory deprivation group) until tested and vocal embryos that had been exposed to tape recordings of the embryonic contact call (stimulation with contact calls). Since the latency and threshold findings were highly similar, I will present only the threshold findings.

As can be seen in Figure 5.9, auditory deprivation virtually arrested auditory development beyond day 24 of embryonic development. On day 24, prior to vocal-auditory experience, the embryos are most sensitive to 1000, 1500, and 2000 Hz, and, subsequent to day 24, their threshold drops only slightly in the absence of auditory experience. On the contrary, as can be seen in Figure 5.10, when the birds are exposed to the embryonic contact call (CT), their thresholds plunge to their most mature level in the two days prior to

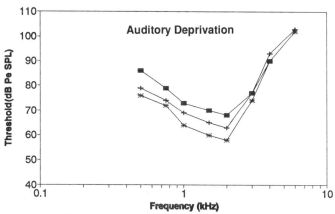

Figure 5.9. Threshold of the brain stem auditory evoked response in aurally deprived day-24 mallard duck embryos (■), hatchlings (+), and two-day-old ducklings (*). (From Dmitrieva & Gottlieb, 1993.)

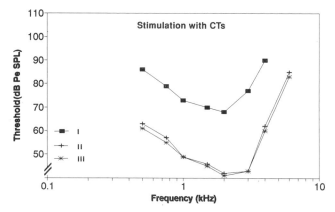

Figure 5.10. Threshold of the brain stem auditory evoked response in hatchlings (+) and two-day-old ducklings (*) that were exposed to embryonic contact calls from day 24 of embryonic development through two days after hatching. The top line (■) shows the threshold of the day-24 embryo prior to auditory experience. (From Dmitrieva & Gottlieb, 1993.)

hatching and show no further improvement in the two days after hatching despite continued exposure to the tape-recorded CTs, their own and sibling vocalizations. The most extraordinary finding is that exposure to the 1500–2500 Hz contact call markedly affected thresholds both below and above that frequency range. Thus, the auditory experience accelerated the development of the receptor epithelium of the entire cochlea, accelerating the developmental shift of responsive frequencies along the cochlea, and furthering the maturation of subsequent tonotopic areas in nuclei higher in the auditory pathway. Scanning electron microscope studies have shown that the auditory epithelium of avian embryos exposed to enhanced auditory stimulation is always larger than the auditory epithelium of control embryos (Golubeva & Tikhonov, 1985).

The present neurophysiological results mesh well with my behavioral studies in two ways. That the auditory experiential enhancement has its greatest effect during the embryonic period from days 24–26 (hatching) correlates precisely with the auditory perceptual malleable and critical periods found in my behavioral studies. Namely, this embryonic period is one in which mallard ducklings are most susceptible to exposure to an alien species maternal call (Gottlieb, 1987), and it is also the period during which exposure to the embryonic contact call establishes species-specific auditory responsiveness to the mallard maternal call itself (Gottlieb, 1975b, 1985). Thus, we have a very nice fit between the neural and behavioral levels of analysis, and we have identified the facilitating role of normally occurring embryonic auditory experience in furthering species-typical neural and behavioral development. So, we have traversed three of the four levels of analysis for a given phenomenon, and, given that developmental-genetic techniques are currently available to get at gene activity, it is possible to take the study to the genetic level of analysis.

In conclusion, a systems view of psychobiological development is an achievable goal, at least within the confines of animal experimentation. It is quite rewarding to note that Ford & Lerner (1992) explicitly advocate the utility of the systems concept for developmental psychologists who work with human beings. As I noted earlier, similar points of view have been put forward by psychobiologically-oriented developmentalists such as Cairns, Gariépy, & Hood (1990), Edelman (1988), Griffiths & Gray (1994), Hinde (1990), Johnston & Hyatt (1994), Magnusson & Törestad (1993), and Oyama (1985), and this represents a realization of the pioneering theoretical efforts of Z.-Y. Kuo, T. C. Schneirla, and D. S. Lehrman. Since the systems view dates to at least as early as Hans Driesch's theorizing about his embryological experiments in the 1890s, it can not be called a 'paradigm shift', but certainly it is something relatively new in the field of developmental psychology.

SUMMARY AND CONCLUSION

Developmental thinking began in the early 1800s coincident with the triumph of epigenesis over the concept of preformation. Though practiced only at the descriptive level in the First Period, it was realized that to understand the origin of any phenotype it is necessary to study its development in the individual. Late in the 1800s, in the Second Period, developmental description was superseded by an experimental approach in embryology. A field or systems view was born when the results of Hans Driesch's experiments made it necessary to conceptualize embryonic cells as harmonious-equipotential systems. Steering a careful path between mechanical-reductive and vitalistic-constructive viewpoints, in the Third Period, Ludwig von Bertalanffy formalized an organismic systems view for experimental embryology, which was later worked out in detail by the embryologist Paul Weiss and the geneticist Sewall Wright. In the Present Period, a systems view of development has begun to infiltrate into developmental psychology and developmental neurobiology. Although there are dissenters, a systems view seems workable and thus useful in thinking about human as well as nonhuman animal psychological development.

REFERENCES

Anokhin, K. V., Mileusnic, R., Shamakina, I. Y. & Rose, S. (1991) Effects of early experience on c-fos gene expression in the chick forebrain. *Brain Research,* **544,** 101–7.

von Baer, K. E. (1828) *Über Entwickelungsgeschichte der Thiere: Beobachtung und Reflexion.* Part one. Königsberg: Bornträger. (Reprinted 1966 by Johnson Reprint Corporation.)

Banker, H. & Lickliter, R. (1993) Effects of early and delayed visual experience on intersensory development in bobwhite quail chicks. *Developmental Psychobiology,* **26,** 155–70.

Bateson, P. P. G. (1976) Specificity and the origins of behavior. *Advances in the Study of Behavior,* **6,** 1–20.

von Bertalanffy, L. (1933/1962) *Modern Theories of Development: An Introduction to Theoretical Biology.* New York: Harper. (Originally published in German in 1933.)

von Bertalanffy, L. (1950). *A systems view of man.* Boulder, Colo.: Western Press.

Black, I. B. (1993) Environmental regulation of brain trophic interactions. *International Journal of Developmental Neuroscience,* **11,** 403–10.

Brunswik, E. (1952) *The Conceptual Framework of Psychology.* Chicago, Ill.: University of Chicago Press.

Cairns, R. B., Gariépy, J.-L. & Hood, K. E. (1990) Development, microevolution, and social behavior. *Psychological Review,* **97,** 49–65.

Calamandrei, G. & Keverne, E. B. (1994) Differential expression of Fos protein in the brain of female mice is dependent on pup sensory cues and maternal experience. *Behavioral Neuroscience,* **108,** 113–20.

Carlier, M., Roubertoux, P., Kottler, M. L. & Degrelle, H. (1989) Y chromosome and aggression in strains of laboratory mice. *Behavior Genetics,* **20,** 137–56.

Changeux, J.-P. & Konishi, M. (eds.) (1987) *The Neural and Molecular Bases of Learning.* Chichester: John Wiley.

Cheng, M.-F. (1979) Progress and prospects in ring dove: a personal view. *Advances in the Study of Behavior,* **9,** 97–129.

Dmitrieva, L. P. & Gottlieb, G. (1993) Influence of auditory experience on the development of brain stem auditory-evoked potentials in mallard duck embryos and hatchlings. *Behavioral and Neural Biology,* **61,** 19–28.

Driesch, H. (1908/1929) *The Science and Philosophy of the Organism,* 2nd edn. London: A. & C. Black.

Eckerman, C. O., Oehler, J. M., Medvin, M. B. & Hannan, T. E. (1994) Premature newborns as social partners before term age. *Infant Behavior and Development*, **17**, 55–70.

Edelman, G. (1988) *Topobiology*. New York: Basic Books.

Ford, D. H. & Lerner, R. M. (1992) *Developmental systems theory: an interactive approach*. Newbury Park, Calif.: Sage Publications.

Gariépy, J.-L. (1995) The evolution of a developmental science: Early determinism, modern interactionism, and a new systemic approach. *Annals of Child Development*, **11**, 167–222.

Golubeva, T. B. & Tikhonov, A. V. (1985) The voice and hearing of birds in ontogeny. *Acta XVIII International Ornithological Congress*. Moscow: Nauka, pp. 259–74.

Gottlieb, G. (1970) Conceptions of prenatal behavior. In Aronson, L. R., Tobach, E., Lehrman, D. S. & Rosenblatt, J. S. (eds.) *Development and Evolution of Behavior*. San Francisco, Calif.: W. H. Freeman, pp. 111–37.

Gottlieb, G. (1971) Ontogenesis of sensory function in birds and mammals. In Tobach, E., Aronson, L. R. & Shaw, E. (eds.) *The Biopsychology of Development*. New York: Academic Press, pp. 67–128.

Gottlieb, G. (1975a) Development of species identification in ducklings. I. Nature of perceptual deficit caused by embryonic auditory deprivation. *Journal of Comparative and Physiological Psychology*, **89**, 387–99.

Gottlieb, G. (1975b) Development of species identification in ducklings. II. Experiential prevention of perceptual deficit caused by embryonic auditory deprivation. *Journal of Comparative and Physiological Psychology*, **89**, 675–84.

Gottlieb, G. (1981) Roles of early experience in species-typical perceptual development. In Aslin, R. N., Alberts, J. R. & Petersen, M. R. (eds.) *Development of Perception, Vol. 1*, pp. 5–44. New York: Academic Press.

Gottlieb, G. (1985) Development of species identification in ducklings. XI. Embryonic critical period for species-typical perception in the hatchling. *Animal Behaviour*, **33**, 225–33.

Gottlieb, G. (1987) Development of species identification in ducklings. XIII. A comparison of malleable and critical periods of perceptual development. *Developmental Psychobiology*, **20**, 393–404.

Gottlieb, G. (1991) Experiential canalization of behavioral development: theory. *Developmental Psychology*, **27**, 4–13.

Gottlieb, G. (1992) *Individual Development and Evolution: The Genesis of Novel Behavior*. New York: Oxford University Press.

Gottlieb, G., Tomlinson, W. T. & Radell, P. L. (1989) Developmental intersensory interference: premature visual experience suppresses auditory learning in ducklings. *Infant Behavior and Development*, **12**, 1–12.

Gottlieb, G. & Vandenbergh, J. G. (1968) Ontogeny of vocalization in duck and chick embryos. *Journal of Experimental Zoology*, **168**, 307–25.

Griffiths, P. E. & Gray, R. D. (1994) Developmental systems and evolutionary explanation. *Journal of Philosophy*, **91**, 277–304.

Hamburger, V. (1957) The concept of 'development' in biology. In Harris, D. H. (ed.) *The Concept of Development*. Minneapolis, Minn.: University of Minnesota, pp. 49–58.

Hamburger, V. (1964) Ontogeny of behaviour and its structural basis. In Richter, D. (ed.), *Comparative Neurochemistry*. Oxford: Pergamon Press, pp. 21–34.

Henfry, A. & Huxley, T. H. (1853) *Scientific Memoirs, Selected from the Transactions of Foreign Academies of Science, and from Foreign Journals. Natural History.* London: Taylor and Francis.

Hinde, R. A. (1990) The interdependence of the behavioral sciences. *Philosophical Transactions of the Royal Society, London, B,* **329**, 217–27.

His, W. (1888) On the principles of animal morphology. *Proceedings of the Royal Society of Edinburgh,* **15**, 287–98.

Johnston, T. D. & Hyatt, L. E. (1994) Genes, interactions, and the development of behavior. Unpublished manuscript.

Kenny, P. A. & Turkewitz, G. (1986) Effects of unusually early visual stimulation on the development of homing behavior in the rat pup. *Developmental Psychobiology,* **19**, 57–66.

Korner, A., Guillenminault, C., van den Hoed, J. & Baldwin, R. B. (1978) Reduction in sleep apnea and bradycardia in preterm infants on oscillating water beds: A controlled polygraphic study. *Pediatrics,* **61**, 528–33.

Korner, A. in press. Vestibular stimulation as a neurodevelopmental intervention with preterm infants: Findings and new methods for evaluating intervention effects. In Goldson, E. (ed.) *Nurturing the Premature Infant: Developmental Interventions in the Neonatal Intensive Care Nursery.* New York: Oxford University Press.

Kuo, Z.-Y. (1976) *The Dynamics of Behavior Development.* New York: Plenum Press.

Lehrman, D. S. (1970) Semantic and conceptual issues in the nature-nurture problem. In Aronson, L. R., Lehrman, D. S., Tobach, E. & Rosenblatt, J. S. (eds.) *Development and Evolution of Behavior.* San Francisco, Calif.: W. H. Freeman, pp. 17–52.

Lickliter, R. (1993) Timing and the development of perinatal perceptual organization. In Turkewitz, G. & Devenny, D. A. (eds.) *Developmental Time and Timing.* Hillsdale, NY: Erlbaum, pp. 105–23.

Lickliter, R. & Banker, H. (1994) Prenatal components of intersensory development in precocial birds. In Lewkowicz, D. J. & Lickliter, R. (eds.) *Development of Intersensory Perception: Comparative Aspects.* Hillsdale, NJ: Erlbaum, pp. 59–80.

McBride, T. & Lickliter, R. (1994) Specific postnatal auditory stimulation interferes with species-typical visual responsiveness in bobwhite quail chicks. *Developmental Psychobiology,* **27**, 169–83.

Magnusson, D. & Törestad, B. (1993) A holistic view of personality: a model revisited. *Annual Review of Psychology,* **44**, 427–52.

Mangold, O. & Seidel, F. (1927) Homoplastische und heteroplastische Verschmelzung ganzer Tritonkeime. Roux's *Archiv für Entwicklungsmechanik der Organismen,* **111**, 593–665.

Mauro, V. P., Wood, I. C., Krushel, L., Crossin, K. L. & Edelman, G. M. (1994) Cell adhesion alters gene transcription in chicken embryo brain cells and mouse embryonal carcinoma cells. *Proceedings of the National Academy of Sciences USA,* **91**, 2868–72.

Miller, D. B. (1988) Development of instinctive behavior: an epigenetic and ecological approach. In Blass, E. M. (ed.), *Handbook of Behavioral Neurobiology, Vol. 9: Developmental Psychology and Behavioral Ecology.* New York: Plenum Press, pp. 415–44.

Miller, D. B., Hicinbothom, G. & Blaich, C. F. (1990) Alarm call responsivity of mallard ducklings: multiple pathways in behavioral development. *Animal Behaviour,* **39**, 1207–12.

Nöel, M. (1989) Early development in mice. V. Sensorimotor development of four coisogenic mutant strains. *Physiology and Behavior,* **45**, 21–6.

van Ooyen, A. & van Pelt, J. (1994) Activity-dependent outgrowth of neurons and overshoot phenomena in developing neural networks. *Journal of Theoretical Biology,* **167**, 27–43.

Oyama, S. (1985) *The Ontogeny of Information.* New York: Cambridge University Press.

Philbin, M. K., Ballweg, D. D. & Gray, L. (1994) The effect of an intensive care unit environment on the development of habituation in healthy avian neonates. *Developmental Psychobiology,* **27**, 11–22.

Radell, P. L. & Gottlieb, G. (1992) Developmental intersensory interference: augmented prenatal sensory experience interferes with auditory learning in duck embryos. *Developmental Psychology,* **28**, 795–803.

Rosen, K. M., McCormack, M. A., Villa-Komaroff, L. & Mower, G. D. (1992) Brief visual experience induces immediate early gene expression in the cat visual cortex. *Proceedings of the National Academy of Sciences, USA,* **89**, 5437–41.

Roubertoux, P. L., Nosten-Bertrand, M. & Carlier, M. (1990) Additive and interactive effects of genotype and maternal environment. *Advances in the Study of Behavior,* **19**, 205–47.

Roux, W. (1888/1974) Contributions to the developmental mechanics of the embryo. Translated from the German in 1974, in Willier, B. H. & Oppenheimer, J. M. (eds.) *Foundations of Experimental Embryology.* New York: Hafner, pp. 2–37.

Rustak, B., Robertson, H. A., Wisden, W. & Hunt, S. P. (1990) Light pulses that shift rhythms induce gene expression in the suprachiasmatic nucleus. *Science,* **248**, 1237–40.

Saint-Hilaire, E. G. (1825) Sur les déviations organiques provoquées et observées dans un établissement des incubations artificielles. *Mémoires. Museum National d'Histoire Naturelle (Paris),* **13**, 289–96.

Scarr, S. (1995) Behavior genetic and socialization theories of intelligence: truce and reconciliation. In Sternberg, R. J. & Grigorenko, E. L. (eds.) *Intelligence: Heredity and Environment.* New York: Cambridge University Press, in press.

Schneirla, T. C. (1960) Instinctive behavior, maturation – experience and development. In Kaplan, B. & Wapner, S. (eds.) *Perspectives in psychological theory – Essays in honor of Heinz Werner,* pp. 303–34. New York: International Universities Press.

Scoville, R. (1982) Embryonic development of vocalization in Peking ducklings. (*Anas platyrrhynchos*). Unpublished doctoral dissertation, University of North Carolina at Chapel Hill.

Sperry, R. W. (1951) Mechanisms of neural maturation. In Stevens, S. S. (ed.) *Handbook of Experimental Psychology.* New York: John Wiley, pp. 236–80.

Sperry, R. W. (1971) How a developing brain gets itself properly wired for adaptive function. In Tobach, E., Aronson, L. R. & Shaw, E. (eds.) *The Biopsychology of Development.* New York: Academic Press, pp. 28–34.

Thelen, E. (1990) Dynamical systems and the generation of individual differences. In Colombo, J. & Fagen, J. (eds.) *Individual Differences in Infancy: Reliability, Stability, Prediction.* Hillsdale, NJ: Erlbaum, pp. 19–43.

Tolman, E. C. (1932) *Purposive Behavior in Animals and Man.* New York: Century.

Wahlsten, D. & Gottlieb, G. (1995) The invalid separation of the effects of nature and nuture: lessons from animal experimentation. In Sternberg, R. J. & Grigorenko, E. L. (eds.) *Intelligence: Hereditary and Environment*. New York: Cambridge University Press, in press.

Weiss, P. (1959) Cellular dynamics. *Review of Modern Physics*, **31**, 11–20.

Wright, S. (1968) *Evolution and the Genetics of Populations, Vol. 1: Genetic and Biometric Foundations*. Chicago, Ill.: University of Chicago Press.

PART II
THE CHANGING BRAIN

This part on the changing brain deals with fundamental neural mechanisms ranging from structures underlying chemical signaling in the brain, the neurotransmitter receptors, through one of the most fascinating processes in neural function, the ability of brain to acquire and store information and through a thoughtful analysis of the eternal question of a possible relation between brain size and 'intelligence', to an in-depth discussion of a global theory of higher neuronal functions. These different aspects were intensely dealt with in the discussion section and expanded to questions of general nature bordering and interlocking with many other topics in other parts of the book.

Ever since the work of Ehrlich and Langley, the receptors for chemical messengers have represented a central but elusive theme, and only recently have we been able to understand their exact molecular structure. In Chapter 6, Changeux describes the structural and biochemical properties of the transmembrane macromolecule complex of the nicotinic receptor, which is present both in the brain and also is the critical 'sensor' at the neuromuscular junction. It has turned out that this receptor is just one of several members of a family which form ion channels and which share the feature of four or sometimes five membrane spanning domains. Changeux contrasts these receptors with the other major family characterized by seven membrane spanning elements which via heterotrimeric G proteins mediate a cascade of intracellular reactions. It is already known that altered receptor function in several cases can lead to a specific disorder, and the enormous diversity of some receptor subtypes has provided new possibilities for developing important drugs for treatment of various mental and neurological diseases. It will be a monumental task to study in detail the expression of receptors in the nervous system during the lifespan and to understand their role in the development of individuals. It is clear that complex changes, for example in composition of subunits, occur during development. Modifications of these changes may influence neuronal function, lead to disease states and alter sensitivity to drug treatment. In fact, using modern imaging techniques such as positron emission tomography it is possible to visualize receptor mechanisms in living human brains under normal and pathological conditions.

Synapses and chemical transmission are also central for the understanding of the brain functions dealt with by Morris (Chapter 7) who dissects possible mechanisms underlying synaptic plasticity as a basis of information storage in the brain. Hardly any other central nervous system function has attracted more attention than our ability to learn and remember both as a basic mechanism but also from the view of ageing and disease. As outlined in this chapter our present knowledge comes from many models, ranging from comparatively simple systems as that in *Aplysia* to analysis of events in the mammalian hippocampus. A fundamental question is how relevant concepts in simple system are for our understanding of these processes in the human brain. For example, is the increase in transmitter release related to sensitization in *Aplysia* also applicable to higher forms of synaptic plasticity? The focus on hippocampus is a consequence of earlier work carried out in humans with specific lesions in this brain area. In the center of much of this work is, at present long-term potentiation (LTP), a mechanism first described more than 20 years ago which consists of an activity-dependent synaptic plasticity. However, its significance for acquisition is still uncertain, and not infrequently this topic evokes strong emotions among scientists in the field. All these aspects and many more are thoroughly and thoughtfully discussed and challenged.

Purves et al., among earlier contributions, has described morphological plasticity over longer periods by analysing in vivo the exact distribution of synapses in peripheral tissues and studying the living brain. However, in Chapter 8 he and his colleagues are concerned with another tantalizing problem in neuroscience, the relationship between the size of a given system and its functional capacity, ultimately the question to what extent brain size reflects 'intelligence'. This question has been dealt with for more than 100 years going through different phases but such a relation is according to Purves et al. 'simplistic and ultimately untenable'. However, upon more detailed examination of neural circuitries it seems likely that activity during ontogeny can lead to stable developmental changes in terms of size of circuitry and subsequent increase in capacity of such neuron systems.

In the last contribution in this part (Chapter 9), Edelmann & Tononi approach neuronal development from a conceptual point of view, seen in the context of the global theory of neuronal group selection developed by Edelmann. In this theory several fundamental processes are encompassed including developmental variation and selection, pointing to the fact that the apparent similarity at the macroscopic scale is contrasted by genetically and developmentally unconstrained process when it comes to detailed connectivity. Moreover, during development behavior and experience including changes in synaptic activity will vary and select particular subsystems leading to secondary repertoires. Finally, the bidirectional interaction between parallel subsystems, a process termed reentry, has a major impact in this theory. This concept is supported by sophisticated and extensive simialtion experiments in which computers and mathematical modeling form an important basis.

6 Neurotransmitter receptors in the changing brain: allosteric transitions, gene expression and pathology at the molecular level

JEAN-PIERRE CHANGEUX

Chemical synaptic transmission is the dominant mechanism by which nerve cells communicate with each other and with sensory and effector cells. More than 20 neurotransmitters and a larger number of neuro-peptides serve as chemical signals and several of them may coexist within a single neuron (review, Hökfelt, 1991) thus offering a particularly rich and flexible system of information transfer in the nervous system.

Many of these first messengers are primarily engaged in a fast and robust mechanism of synaptic transmission, sometimes referred to as 'wiring' transmission, where the neurotransmitter is released in the synaptic cleft as a discrete and brief ($<$ 1 msec) high local concentration pulse (around 1 mM). After rapid diffusion through the cleft ($<$0.2 msec), the neurotransmitter reaches the postsynaptic membrane, when it binds to complementary *receptor molecules*, thereby causing the collective, all-or-none opening, or 'activation' of *ion selective channels* (Katz & Miledi, 1977). When the neurotransmitter activates a cation-selective channel, a depolarization results, the transmission is *excitatory*; when, instead, an anion selective channel opens, a hyperpolarization takes place, the transmission is *inhibitory*. Such fast 'wiring' transmission accounts for information processing in the brain in the psychological (0.1 sec) timescale.

Another mode of communication, named 'volume' or 'paracrine' transmission results from a longer range and slower diffusion of the neurotransmitter through intercellular spaces, reaching sometimes targets far distant from their release site within the brain (review, Fuxe & Agnati, 1991). At their level, the neurotransmitter initiates a cascade of intracellular enzymatic processes often referred to as 'metabotropic' effects. The neurotransmitter binds to receptors which are no longer linked with ion channels, but interact with specialized *G-proteins* (because they bind guanine nucleotides). The second messenger produced ultimately causes a change of the electrophysiological properties of the cell membrane but within hundreds of milliseconds to several seconds. Therefore, most often (yet, with notable exceptions, e.g., visual transduction) metabotropic receptors contribute to the 'modulation' of fast information processing in the brain.

The receptors for neurotransmitters thus play a central role in brain chemical communications since they 'decode' intercellular chemical signals into electrical and/or enzymatic responses of the target cell. Their identification, nevertheless, took almost three-quarters of a century after the initial formulation of the concept of 'receptor' by Langley & Ehrlich at the turn of the century. In the late 1950s, neurotransmitter receptors were compared with enzymes (Nachmansohn, Del Castillo & Katz). Until work on regulatory enzymes and hemoglobin (review, Perutz, 1989), led to the proposal that the elementary process of signal recognition and transduction by neurotransmitter receptors belong to the general category of *allosteric interactions* (review, Changeux, 1990) between topographically distinct sites which are mediated by discrete all-or-none conformational transitions of the target protein. The recent developments of our knowledge on the biochemistry, physiology and molecular biology of both ionotropic and metabotropic receptors are consistent with this notion.

Moreover, neurotransmitter receptors appear of particular importance in modern medicine because they represent the site of action for many pharmacological and therapeutic agents but also because their alteration is probably involved in the pathophysiology of various global psychiatric and/or neurological disease states as a consequence of genetic, developmental, autoimmune, and/or degenerative processes.

MOLECULAR ORGANIZATION AND ALLOSTERIC TRANSITIONS OF RECEPTORS COUPLED TO IONIC CHANNELS AND G-PROTEINS

Ia – Ion channel-linked neurotransmitter receptors

The ion channel that the classical neurotransmitters, acetylcholine, glutamate, serotonin, glycine and GABA, rapidly open when they bind to the receptor is an integral component of the receptor protein. Following the initial work done on the acetylcholine nicotinic receptor from fish electric organ (review, Devillers-Thiéry et al., 1993; Karlin, 1993; Galzi & Changeux, 1994), a large number of these neurotransmitter-gated ion channels have been identified as proteins in brain (review, Cockcroft et al., 1990). They form hetero-oligomers of about 300,000 daltons (or more) with five membrane-spanning subunits assembled into a barrel-like structure, which possesses a quasi-fivefold axis of symmetry perpendicular to the plane of the membrane (Figure 6.1A, B and C) (see Unwin, 1993).

For each 'ionotropic' neurotransmitter receptor, various isoforms (or subtypes) of subunits have been identified in the nervous system and shown to assemble into a wide diversity of functional hetero-oligomers with different distribution and distinct pharmacological specificity for agonists and antagonists, ion channel selectivity and response kinetics (review, Cockcroft et al., 1990; Sargent, 1993). In the electric organ and muscle, the nicotinic

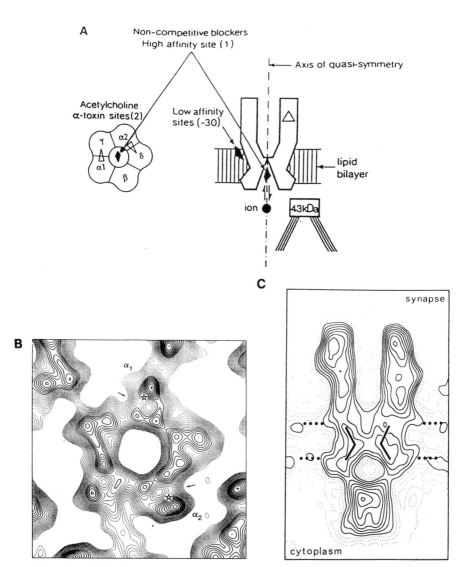

Figure 6.1. Molecular architecture of neurotransmitter receptors linked to ionic channels. (A) Quarternary structure of the nicotinic acetylcholine receptor from fish electric organ and vertebrate muscle. The five subunits $[2\alpha\ \beta\gamma\delta]$ are organized in a pseudo-symmetrical manner like the staves of a barrel. Each acetylcholine binding site overlaps one α- and one non-α-subunit. The non-competitive blockers bind, (1) with high affinity to a unique site located in the axis of rotational symmetry within the ion channel and (2) with low affinity to multiple sites distributed at the interface between the receptor protein and the lipid bilayer (from Changeux et al., 1992). (B) and (C) Front view and side view of the nicotinic receptor from *Torpedo* by high resolution electron microcopy (from Unwin, 1993); the two putative active sites are tentatively indicated by an arrow in B, the two broken segments in C are tentatively assigned to the transmembrane segments MII known to line the ion channel.

acetylcholine receptor molecule is composed of four different subunits with the fixed stoichiometry $[2\alpha.1\beta.1\gamma.1\delta]$ (review, Karlin, 1993; Galzi and Changeux, 1994). In the brain, eight different nicotinic α-subunits and three β-subunits have been identified by molecular cloning yielding functional hetero-pentamers, which may incorporate up to four different subunits with diverse stoichiometries (review, Sargent, 1993). In the case of the other neurotransmitter-gated ion channels, molecular cloning studies have resulted in the identification of at least 16 subunits (6α, 4β, 3γ, 1δ and 2 rho) for the $GABA_A$ receptor (MacDonald & Olsen, 1994), four for the glycine receptor (Betz, 1992), 16 for the various glutamate receptors* (Gasic & Heinemann, 1992; Seeburg, 1993). Most of these subunits alone form homo-oligomeric ion channels, although sometimes rather inefficiently. Incorporation of other subunits, however, by coexpression of several gene sequences dramatically alter their physiological and pharmacological properties and in particular their sensitivity to allosteric effectors (for instance benzodiazepines for the GABA receptor, see Chapter 2), (MacDonald & Olsen, 1994). In the case of the glycine receptor, the hetero-pentamers formed by coexpression of α- and β-subunits have tentatively a $[3\alpha.2\beta]$ subunit stoichiometry (that of the glutamate and $GABA_A$ receptors is not known).

Comparison of the amino acid sequences of the subunits from all known ligand-gated ion channels has led to the distinction of two families. The acetylcholine, serotonine $5HT_3$, $GABA_A$ and glycine-gated channels share striking homologies with fully conserved (or 'canonical') amino acids (Cockcroft et al., 1992; Devillers-Thiéry et al., 1993) and compose what we shall refer to as the *acetylcholine receptor subfamily*. On the other hand, the subunits of the known glutamate-gated ion channels display homologies between themselves but less with the above mentioned receptors (Seeburg, 1993; Gasic & Heinemann, 1992) and constitute the *glutamate receptor subfamily*.

In the acetylcholine receptor subfamily, quantitative analysis of the distribution of hydrophilic and hydrophobic amino acids along the aligned sequences (Devillers-Thiéry et al., 1993; Cockcroft et al., 1992; Karlin, 1993) delineate several discrete regions (Figure 6.1D and E): (1) a signal peptide which is removed from the polypeptide chain during translocation; (2) an NH2 terminal large hydrophilic domain; (3) a compact hydrophobic domain split into three segments of 19–27 uncharged amino acids termed MI, MII, MIII; (4) a small hydrophilic domain; (5) an hydrophobic C terminal segment about 20 amino acids long (MIV).

---

* The 16 glutamate I-receptor subunits known have been regrouped into three main classes (Seeburg, 1993); AMPA (α-amino-3-hydroxy-5-methyl-4-isoxazole propionic acid) receptors (referred to as GluR1 to GluR7) activate channels with fast activation and desensitization kinetics and low Ca^{++} permeability; NMDA (N-methyl-d-aspartate) receptors gate channels with slow kinetics, high Ca^{++} permeability and voltage dependent block by Mg^{++}; the potent neurotoxin kainate activates, in addition to AMPA receptors, high affinity kainate receptors which desensitize rapidly.

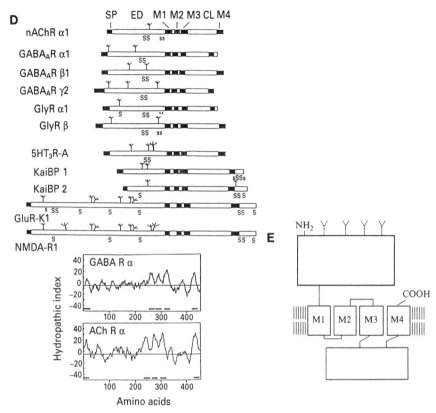

Figure 6.1. (D) Compared diagrammatic representation of the primary structure of a variety of neurotransmitter receptors linked to ion channels; the solid line represents polypeptide segments with a highly hydrophobic hydropathy index (M1 to M4 and signal peptide SP) (from Betz, 1990 and Schofield et al., 1987). (E) Model for the transmembrane organization of receptors from the nicotinic receptor subfamily with *four* transmembrane segments M1 to M4. The NH2 terminal hydrophilic domain faces the synaptic cleft and carries the neurotransmitter binding site. (From Galzi et al., 1991.)

The most plausible model (Figure 6.1E) for the folding of the subunit through the membrane (review, Devillers-Thiéry et al., 1993) is that: (1) the large hydrophilic domain faces the synaptic cleft and carries at least part of the acetylcholine binding site; (2) the small hydrophilic domain is exposed to the cytoplasm where it can be phosphorylated; (3) the four hydrophobic stretches span the membrane as α helices and/or β-plated sheets [still, there is not complete agreement about the number of segments or even residues in either conformation (review, Unwin, 1993; Karlin, 1993; Galzi & Changeux, 1994)]; (4) one of these transmembrane segments MII is in an α-helical

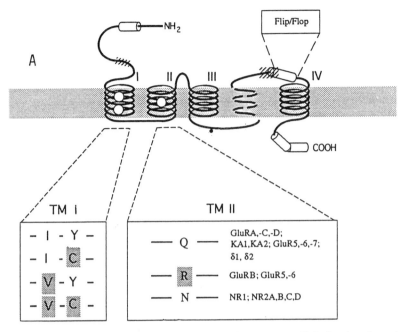

Figure 6.2. Molecular architecture of neurotransmitter receptors linked to ion channels
(*continued*). (A) Model of transmembrane topology and functional domains
of glutamate receptor subunits as proposed by Seeburg (1993). Five
transmembrane segments are postulated and the alternatively spliced 'flip'
and 'flop' modules exposed to the synaptic cleft on AMPA receptors,
differentially affect desensitization; channel determinants in MII and MI
are indicated by open circles and the amino acids concerned listed below,
the stippled residues are introduced by RNA editing; presence of an
arginine (R) in MII is associated with a low Ca^{++} permeability of the
channel, presence of a glutamate (Q) or of an arginine (N) with a high
Ca^{++} permeability; editing within MI conditions the influence of Q/R
editing within MII on Ca^{++} permeability (from Seeburg, 1993) (for
abbreviations, see footnote n° 1).

conformation and contributes to the lining of the ion channel (Giraudat et
al., 1986, 1987; Hucho et al., 1986).

The folding of the subunits in the glutamate receptor subfamily remains
conjectural; yet a putative topology with five transmembrane segments has
been suggested (review, Seeburg, 1993) (Figure 6.2A).

The nicotinic receptor from electric organ and muscle carries two acetylcholine binding sites with structural differences, most likely related to the
contribution of non α-subunits (γ and δ) to the sites and thus plausibly located
at the interface between subunits (as found with typical allosteric enzymes,
such as aspartate transcarbamylase or phosphofructokinase, see Perutz, 1989).
Furthermore, in agreement with the allosteric scheme (review, Changeux,

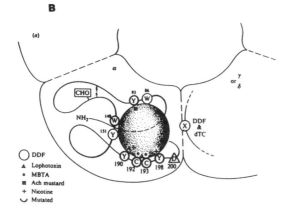

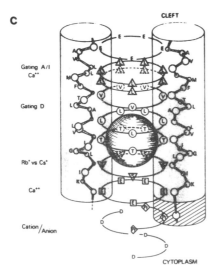

Figure 6.2. (B) Multiple-loop model of the binding site for nicotinic ligands of the acetylcholine receptor from *Torpedo*; the sphere represents the molecule of the affinity labeling reagent DDF in all positions possible; the amino acids labeled by DDF, lophotoxin, MBTA, acetylcholine mustard or nicotine are circled; bold circles indicate mutated residues in muscle or brain α7 neuronal receptor; the residues labeled by d-tubocurarine on the γ and δ-subunits are respectively Trp 55 and Trp 57 in *Torpedo* (from Changeux et al., 1992). (C) Model of the amino acid rings critical in ion channel functions in the MII segment from brain α7-neuronal receptor; the sphere indicates by analogy with *Torpedo* receptor, the putative position of chlorpromazine acting as a channel blocker. Mutations in the equatorial Val, Leu, Thr rings permeabilize the ion channel in the desensitized D state; mutation of the intermediate anionic ring E alters Ca^{++} permeability; the introduction of a proline ring Pr at the cytoplamic end of MII is necessary for the conversion of the selectivity of the ion channel from cationic to anionic. (From Galzi et al., 1992 and Bertrand et al., 1993b.)

1990) both sites interact in a positively cooperative manner, yielding a molecular switch.

Affinity labeling and site directed mutagenesis experiments (review, Galzi & Changeux, 1994; Karlin, 1993) performed with *Torpedo* electric organ α1-, muscle α1- and neuronal α7* subunits of the nicotinic receptor have led to the identification of amino acids which contribute to the *neurotransmitter binding site*. They belong to *three loops* (*A, B and C*) (Figure 6.2B) which, as expected, are part of the large N-terminal hydrophilic domain. As in other choline binding proteins (e.g. acetylcholine esterase), these residues are predominantly aromatic (with, in addition, a characteristic Cys-Cys pair in loop C), the electronegative character of the side chains being thought to suffice for complexing large organic ammonium ions (like acetylcholine, nicotine or curare) exhibiting a diffuse positive charge (Galzi et al., 1990). All of these residues are conserved at homologous positions in all known α-subunits from *Torpedo* electric organ to muscle and neuron (except α5) and in all vertebrate species investigated (including humans). Additional evidence supports the view that the three-loop model applies to other members of the acetylcholine receptor family, yet with amino acid side chain differences (GABA$_A$ and glycine receptors) (review, Devillers-Thiéry et al., 1993; Galzi & Changeux, 1994).

Affinity labeling also contributed to the identification of the amino acids which border the *ion channel* (Figure 6.2). Local anesthetics and other noncompetitive blockers (such as chlorpromazine or triphenylmethylphosphonium) were selected on the basis of their ability to block the open ion channel and were found to label residues in *Torpedo* receptor, which all belong to the MII membrane spanning segment from all four types of subunits. The pattern of labeled amino acids (Giraudat et al., 1986, 1987; Hucho et al., 1986; Révah et al., 1990; White & Cohen, 1992) indicates that: (1) the site for channel blockers is unique and located within the ion channel along the axis of quasi-symmetry of the protein and (2) the walls of the ion channel are made up of MII segments coiled into α helices.

In agreement with this scheme, site-directed mutagenesis experiments with electric organ or muscle nicotinic receptor further showed that mutations within MII of three rings of mostly negative charge (named outer, intermediate and inner) (Imoto et al., 1988) or of serine (or threonine) rings (Leonard et al., 1988) altered conductance, and, for one of them (but to a slight extent) ion selectivity (Villaroel et al., 1991).

Neuronal nicotinic receptors exhibit a significantly higher (about tenfold) permeability to Ca^{++} than skeletal muscle receptors (review, Bertrand et al., 1993a) and mutations at two distinct sites within the channel domain MII of chick α7 receptor (which include the 'intermediate ring') abolish Ca^{++}

---

* The α7 subunit from chick (or rat) brain forms functional homo-oligomers in frog oocyte (see ref. in Devillers-Thiéry et al., 1993).

transport without affecting the relative permeabilities for Na^+ and K^+ (Bertrand et al., 1993a). The acetylcholine receptor family includes inhibitory receptors with a selective channel gated by the neurotransmitter (glycine or GABA). Introduction by site-directed mutagenesis of three amino acids from MII of the glycine (or $GABA_A$) receptor into the MII segment of $\alpha 7$ nicotinic receptor, nevertheless, suffices to convert the cation selective channel into an anion selective channel gated by acetylcholine (Galzi et al., 1992). Thus MII contributes to both ion selectivity and ion transport.

In the glutamate receptors subfamily (Seeburg, 1993; Gasic & Heinemann, 1992), the AMPA receptors* (which include GluR2, GluR5 and GluR6) have a cationic channel with a low Ca^{++} permeability. On the other hand, channels formed *in vitro* from GluR1, 3 or 4 subunits show high Ca^{++} permeability. The difference can be traced to a single residue from a segment homologous to MII, which, in the first group, is a glutamine (Q) and in the second an arginine (R) (review, Seeburg, 1993; Gasic & Heinemann, 1992). The NMDA receptor channel is highly permeable to Ca^{++} but blocked by Mg^{++} ions in a voltage-sensitive manner. Interestingly, this difference is determined by an asparagine residue at the same Q/R position in MII within the AMPA receptor channel (review, Seeburg, 1993; Nakanishi, 1992). Thus, as for the neurotransmitter binding site, the selectivity of the ion channel relies on a few amino acid differences within a common backbone.

The distance between the acetylcholine binding sites and the high affinity site for channel blockers is in the range of 21–40 Å (Herz et al., 1989). As a consequence, the interaction between these sites must be 'indirect' or allosteric. The signal transduction mechanism which causes the opening of the ion channel thus involves changes of conformation which are propagated over distances larger than 20 Å with rates of up to 10,000 s^{-1}. The relevant structural changes have not yet been resolved. On the other hand, the construction of functional chimeras (Eiselé et al., 1993) which combine distinct ligand binding (from $\alpha 7$ nicotinic receptor) and channel specificities (from $5HT_3$) is consistent with the view that despite differences in amino acid sequences, the different members of the acetylcholine receptor family share a highly conserved architectural framework designed to mediate signal transduction.

Ic – G-protein-coupled neurotransmitter receptors

The G-protein coupled receptors compose another large family of receptors that link a wide diversity of extra cellular signals to a relatively small number of intracellular second messenger pathways. These signals include classical neurotransmitters (such as acetylcholine, norepinephine, dopamine, serotonin, glutamate), neuropeptides (such as substances P and K, opioids, somatostatin,

---

* See footnote on page 110.

angiotensin and many other peptide hormones) but also single photons, odorants, ions like Ca^{++} and even proteases like thrombin (review, Baldwin, 1993; Savarese & Fraser, 1992). The binding of a signalling molecule to the extracellular side of the membrane modifies the reversible interaction of the receptor protein with a regulatory protein intracellularly. These regulatory proteins are guanine nucleotide-binding-proteins (or G-proteins) which are *not* intrinsic moieties of the receptor molecule. Several signalling agents that bind to G-protein-coupled receptors are also known to interact with ligand-gated ion channels (for example, acetylcholine, glutamate, GABA serotonin ATP) and the same neurotransmitter may also bind to different iso-types of receptors coupled to G-proteins. For example, there exists at least 10 types of adrenergic receptors (α_1A to C, α_2A to C, B1 to 3), 5 types of muscarinic acetylcholine (m_1 to m_5) or dopaminergic (D1 to 5) receptors and many other examples of receptor isoforms can be found (Savarese & Fraser, 1992). To date, more than 100 G-protein coupled-receptors have been cloned and sequenced. There might be as many as 1000 types of such receptors, including a large number of odorant receptors.

G-proteins are heterotrimeric molecules made up of α, β and γ-subunits which are encoded by a large superfamily of genes (review, Iyengar & Birnbaumer, 1990). In the resting state, the G-protein trimer forms a stable complex with GDP. Binding of the agonist to the receptor facilitates an exchange of GTP for bound GDP on the cytoplasmic side of the membrane at a site located on the G-protein α-subunit. Subsequently, binding of GTP to the α-subunit causes the dissociation of this subunit from the β and γ-subunits. The GTP-α-subunit complex (and sometimes the $\beta\gamma$-subunits) subsequently modulates the activity of effector systems, themselves regulating second messenger levels (Figure 6.3a). These types of regulation may be as diverse as the activation (Gs) or inhibition of (Gi) adenylate cyclase, the activation (G_T) of a cGMP phosphodiesterase or of phospholipase C, or the mobilization of intracellular Ca^{++}. The cleavage of GTP into GDP by a phosphodiesterase intrinsic to the α-subunit terminates the reaction cascade. The GDP α-subunit complex then reassociates with the $\beta\gamma$-subunit complex released earlier, and a new cycle can begin. In other words, the G-protein serves as a catalytic subunit in the reversible transmembrane allosteric complex and as a transfer and amplification device within the cell.

The sequence homology between all known members of the G-protein-coupled receptor family (review, Baldwin, 1993) and their common interaction with G-proteins, supports the view that they share a common three-dimensional organization in the membrane-embedded region of the protein. Even more striking is the observation that a purple protein from *Halobacterium halobium* named bacteriorhodopsin also displays similar patterns of amino acid distribution in its sequence despite the absence of overall sequence identity and its function as a proton pump which does *not* require coupling with a G-protein.

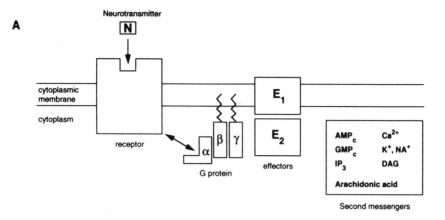

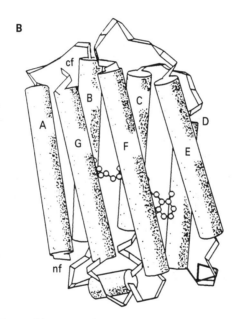

Figure 6.3. Molecular architecture of neurotransmitter receptors coupled to G-
proteins. (A) Diagrammatic representation of the complex receptor
G-protein–effector. The effectors can be a transmembrane (E_1, adenylate
cyclase, ionic channel) or a cytoplasmic (E_2) molecule. Several second
messengers are boxed. (B) Overall chain trace of bacteriorhodopsin
determined at a minimal resolution of 3.5 Å by high-resolution electron
cryo-microscopy; the seven transmembrane α-helices are represented as
solid rods (from Henderson et al., 1990); the C terminal (cf) is at the top
facing the cytoplasm; the position of the molecule of bound retinal is
shown.

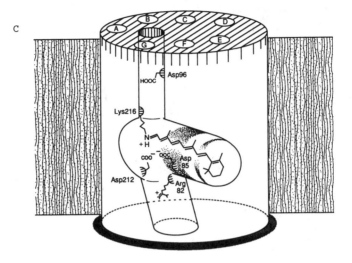

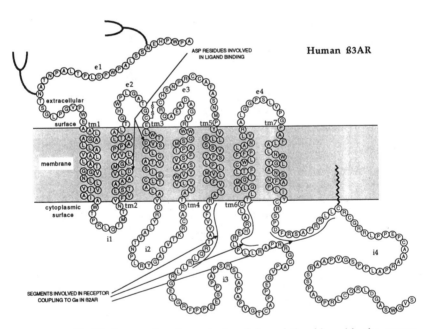

Figure 6.3. (C) Binding pocket for retinal and its relationship with the proton channel connecting the two surfaces of the membrane (from Henderson et al., 1990). (D) Proposed topology of the β-adrenergic receptor (βAR) as a typical member of the G-protein coupled receptors family. (From Strosberg, 1991.)

The distinctive pattern of amino acid sequence common to all these membrane receptors is the occurrence of seven stretches of 20–28 hydrophobic amino acids (MI to MVII) assumed to span the lipid bilayer (review, Henderson & Schertler, 1990; Baldwin, 1993). Interestingly, within the purple membrane, bacteriorhodopsin makes perfect two dimensional crystals with associated lipid in the ratio of ten lipids to one protein molecule, thus making possible structural studies. Electron diffraction patterns and high-resolution electron cryo-microscopy have given a three-dimensional density map of the structure at near atomic resolution (3.5 Å parallel and 10 Å perpendicular to the membrane) (Henderson & Schertler, 1990). It consists of a bundle of seven α-helices orientated roughly perpendicular to the plane of the lipid bilayer with the N-terminus on the extra-cellular side and the C-terminus on the intracellular side of the membrane (Figure 6.3B). The seven domains are tightly packed in a sequential counterclockwise manner (when observed from the extracellular side) and define a central pocket where the retinal molecule binds, almost half-way between the cytoplasmic and extracellular surfaces of the protein (Henderson & Schertler, 1990).

On the basis of the similarity of their primary structure, it has been widely assumed that the G-protein-coupled receptors possess a tertiary organization similar to that of bacteriorhodopsin. The recent establishment of bovine rhodopsin projection structure at 9 Å resolution (Schertler, Villa & Henderson, 1993) supports this assumption, yet with differences (review, Baldwin, 1993). The binding site for the retinal chromophore (Figure 6.3C) or for the neurotransmitter involves, despite differences in the structure of the ligands, closely related domains of α helices MIII, V, VI and VII (ref. in Table III of Baldwin, 1993). The extracellular half of the molecule appears more 'open' than the cytoplasmic half and thus gives access to the ligand binding pocket from the outside environment. Ligands, such as acetylcholine and noradrenaline which are smaller than retinal, would occupy only one part of its binding pocket, while peptides may occupy distinct extracellular domains (Figures 6.4A and B).

Site-directed mutagenesis experiments and receptor chimeras constructions show that the seven membrane spanning segment receptors interact with G-proteins on their cytoplasmic face by a defined set of polypeptide loops (Figure 6.3D) referred to as loop 2, loop 3 and C-terminal peptide. These loops cooperatively form a folded structure which determines G-protein binding specificity and G-protein activation.

The distance between the ligand binding pocket and the G-protein binding site on the cytoplasmic face is of a minimum of 20 Å. Transduction of the signal thus takes place, as in the case of ligand-gated ion channels between topographically distinct binding sites and is thus *allosteric*. Structural studies with bacteriorhodopsin have paved the way to the identification of the conformational change involved (Subramaniam et al., 1993). The main intermediate formed upon light absorption (trapped by rapidly freezing the

A

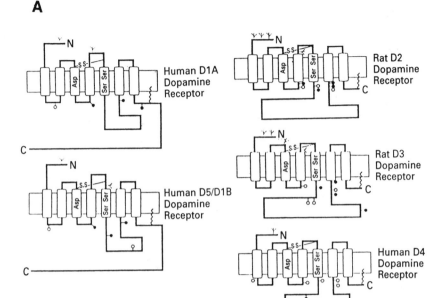

Figure 6.4. (A) Comparison of the transmembrane organization of the dopamine receptor subtypes. The vertical boxes represent putative transmembrane α-helices; branch-like structures represent N-linked glycosylation consensus sites; the *dark circles* represent the presence of a *protein kinase A* consensus site and *open circles* the presence of *protein kinase C* consensus site (from Gingrich & Caron, 1993).

crystals in liquid ethane following illumination) differed in the projection maps at 3.5 Å from the ground state at the level of MVII and MVI which moved away from the central position of the protein. As a consequence, a 'widening' of the structure at the level of the cytoplasmic half results. Interestingly, the cytoplasmic loops and the C-terminal end are also crucial for G-protein activation in rhodopsin, adrenergic and muscarinic receptors. This raises the intriguing possibility that similar allosteric changes underlie signal transduction in bacteriorhodopsin and in the G-protein coupled receptors.

THE MULTIPLE ALLOSTERIC TRANSITIONS OF NEUROTRANSMITTER RECEPTORS AT THE REGULATION OF SYNAPSE EFFICACY

A general feature of neurotransmitter receptor and sensory systems is that prolonged exposure to the stimulus causes a progressive, slow and reversible decline of the response amplitude, often referred to as 'desensitization' or

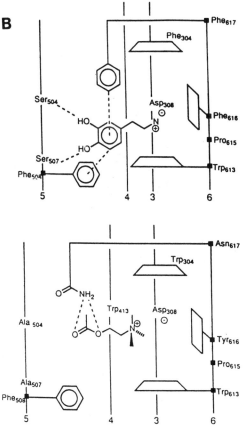

Figure 6.4. (B) Schematic representation of the interaction between D2 dopamine receptor (top) and m2 muscarinic receptor (bottom) recognition sites with their corresponding neurotransmitter, inferred from mutagenesis and labeling studies and computer generated three-dimensional models. (From Hibert et al., 1991.)

'adaptation', which follows the 'activation' of the biological response (opening of an ion channel or enhanced interaction with a G-protein).

In the case of ligand-gated ion channels, the activation and desensitization transition have been extensively analysed, *in vivo* by electrophysiological techniques (Katz & Thesleff, 1957; Sakmann, Patlak & Neher, 1980) and *in vitro* by chemical methods (review, Changeux, 1990). The data are consistent with a generalized and more complex version of the two-state allosteric scheme postulated for 'activation' (review, Changeux, 1990). The model (ref. in Léna & Changeux, 1993) assumes that the receptor protein may spontaneously exist in a minimum of *four* interconvertible states (Figure 6.5 A): the *resting* state (R), the *active* open channel state (A) and two *desensitized*

A

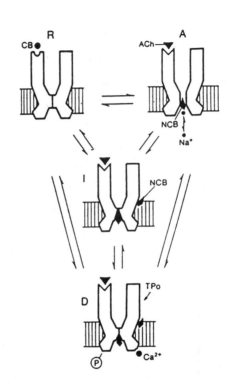

Figure 6.5. Models for activation and desensitization of: (A) the acetylcholine nicotinic receptor as a prototype of ligand-gated ion channel and of (B) G-protein-linked receptors (rhodopsin or β_2-adrenergic receptor). The minimal four-state model for the allosteric transitions of the acetylcholine receptor shows that, among the four states, the channel is open only in A. The affinity for the agonists and for some competitive antagonists increases from R-A to I to D (from Changeux, 1990). A cascade of G-protein interactions, phosphorylation and dephosphorylation reactions regulate activation and desensitization of the G-protein coupled receptors. (From Palczewski & Benovic, 1991.)

closed channel states (I and D) that are refractory to activation. The R and A states display a *low apparent affinity* for acetylcholine, while the I and D states exhibit a *high affinity* (K_D ranging from about 10 µM to 1 nM) for nicotinic ligands (agonists and some antagonists). The kinetics of the transition between several of these states has been resolved *in vitro* with *Torpedo* acetylcholine receptor. The rate of isomerisation between R and A lies in the µs to ms time scale, toward I in the ms to 100 ms range and toward D up to the minute-time range (review, Changeux, 1990).

The 'concerted allosteric' scheme of allosteric transition posits that an equilibrium between discrete conformations is stabilized prior to ligand

B

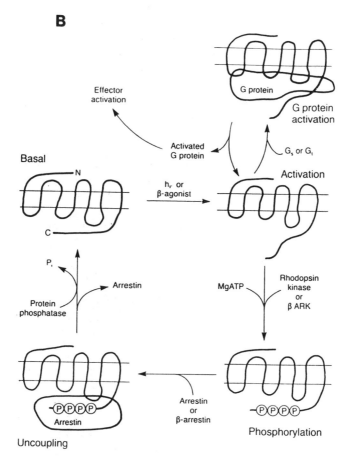

Figure 6.5. (*continued*).

binding. Indeed, 20% of the nicotinic receptor molecules from *Torpedo* receptor-rich microsacs are present in the high affinity desensitized D state in the absence of ligand, and spontaneous openings of the channel are detected, though at a low frequency, in embryonic mouse muscle cells (see Changeux & Edelstein, 1994). The nicotinic ligands may then be viewed as differentially stabilizing the conformational state(s) to which they preferentially bind.

The agonists (e.g. acetylcholine, nicotine) transiently stabilize the active A state under conditions that are those of the high local concentration 'pulse' of neurotransmitter in the synaptic cleft during fast 'wiring' transmission (Katz & Miledi, 1977). On the other hand, the low concentrations of neurotransmitter present in the intercellular space, for instance during 'volume' transmission, match the high affinity of the desensitized state, thereby making possible regulation of the amount of receptor in the R state available for activation. In other words, the R/D ratio sets the *efficacy* of the synapse at the postsynaptic level (review, Changeux, 1990).

Torpedo and muscle nicotinic receptors, undergo desensitization in the absence of phosphorylation but phosphorylation (at defined residues within the cytoplasmic loop) by protein kinases A or C or by tyrosine kinases, strikingly enhances their rate of desensitization (ref. in Huganir & Greengard, 1990). Phosphorylation also enhances desensitization of $GABA_A$ and AMPA receptors, but in other systems, phosphorylation potentiates glutamate receptors responses.

In the case of the G-protein linked receptors, the word desensitization covers a number of rather different processes which, *a priori*, appear distinct from the desensitization of ligand-gated ion channels. First of all, it is clear from studies with rhodopsin and with the β_2-adrenergic receptor (review, Palczewski & Benovic, 1991) that the reversible short-term desensitization which takes place (less than 0.5 sec for rhodopsin or within seconds and minutes for the β_2 adrenergic receptor), differs from long-term 'down-regulation', which is characterized by a decrease in the total *number* of cell receptors over several hours and by a requirement for *de novo* protein synthesis for recovery of receptor number. Moreover, short-term desensitization and its recovery comprises a set of biochemical reactions which are plausibly mediated by at least three distinct proteins, in addition to the receptor-G protein pair: (1) a kinase which phosphorylates light-activated rhodopsin (rhodopsin kinase) or agonist-activated β_2 adrenergic receptor (β-adrenergic receptor kinase or βARK); (2) arrestin or β-arrestin which interact with the phosphorylated rhodopsin or β_2-adrenergic receptor; (3) a protein phosphatase which dephosphorylates the phosphorylated receptors. According to Palczewski and Benovic (1991) (see Figure 6.5B), receptor activation by light or agonist binding, promotes, in addition to G-protein and effector activation, its own phosphorylation which is mediated by rhodopsin kinase or by βARK. Phosphorylation partially uncouples the receptor from the G-protein but also promotes its interaction with arrestin (or β arrestin) which further uncouples the receptor from the G-protein. It is known that regeneration of native rhodopsin with 11-cis retinal is required for dephosphorylation of rhodopsin and arrestin dissociation. The exact conformation of the receptor which becomes phosphorylated in this process of densensitization is often referred to as an activated form of the receptor. But, is this the case?

Recently, an interesting series of mutations has been identified in rhodopsin and several G-protein coupled receptors which alter signal transduction in a manner which seems relevant to this question (review, Lefkowitz et al., 1993). Distributed in diverse domains of the molecule, these mutations result in persistent (agonist independent) activation of the G-protein and of the linked second messenger pathways, supporting the view that normally the receptor is spontaneously constrained into an inactive resting conformation, in agreement with the allosteric scheme. Another important outcome is that these constitutively active mutant receptors, which *do not desensitize*, cause a variety of pathologies in humans (including *retinitis pigmentosa*), hyper-thyroidism and precocious puberty.

The structural changes which occur in the course of desensitization have been explored mostly in the case of the nicotinic receptor. In the acetylcholine binding regions affinity labeling experiments (Galzi et al., 1991) reveal changes in the differential contribution of the non-α-subunits and of the three loops from the α-subunit consistent with a reorganization of the interface between subunits where the active sites lie. Also, cryomicroscopy experiments show that under conditions which promote desensitization, the δ-subunit becomes more inclined tangentially around the channel and the γ-subunit is displaced slightly outward (Unwin et al., 1988). Furthermore, in α7 neuronal nicotinic receptor, mutations of several rings of amino acids, all located in the equatorial region of MII result in remarkable pleiotropic effects (loss of desensitization, increased apparent affinity, presence of a new channel type, agonistic effect of some competitive antagonists) which are interpreted as the 'unblocking' of the ion channel in a desensitized state (Révah et al., 1991; Galzi & Changeux, 1994). In other words, the molecule possesses a sophis-ticated architectural design which selectively accounts for its regulation by desensitization (see Figure 6.2C).

Heterologous desensitization may result in the desensitization of a given receptor by the activation of another receptor. Such 'cross-talk' between receptors has been documented in the case of the G-protein linked receptors: for instance, desensitization of the β-adrenergic receptor may be caused by the stimulation of any receptor that activates adenylyl cyclase, such as protaglandin E1 receptor. But, interaction between G-protein-linked receptors and ligand-gated ion channels may also be mediated by a similar mechanism. For instance, stimulation of adenylyl cyclase linked CGRP receptor enchances desensitization of the nicotinic receptor most likely indirectly via its phos-phorylation by protein kinase A. Interactions between ligand-gated ion channels themselves may also occur and be mediated, for instance, by changes of internal ionic concentration, for example, Ca^{++} relayed (or not) by phosphorylation (review, Léna & Changeux, 1993).

In the neuronal nicotinic receptor, external Ca^{++} potentiates the response to agonists at both negative and positive potentials at sites located outside the ion channel (Mulle et al., 1992) by increasing opening frequency without changing channel opening duration. Also in the glutamate receptor family, Zn^{2+}, which is released from the mossy fibers in the hippocampus together with excitatory amino acids, inhibits the NMDA- and GABA-evoked currents in a voltage-independent manner and potentiates the AMPA/kainate-evoked currents. In addition, the neurotransmitter glycine behaves as a positive allosteric effector of the NMDA receptor (review, Léna & Changeux, 1993).

In the case of the $GABA_A$ receptor, benzodiazepines (vs β-carbolines) behave as positive (vs negative) allosteric effectors and endogenous molecules

(endozepines) which compete with diazepam and potentiate GABA$_A$ response
have been isolated from brain extracts (review, MacDonald & Olsen, 1994).
There are approximately 8 categories of allosteric sites for pharmacological
ligands carried by GABA receptors. Any GABA receptor formed from a single
(or two or three) subunit is consistently enhanced by barbiturates, but not
by benzodiazepines. Coexpression of α-, β- and γ_2- subunits is, on the other
hand, required for benzodiazepine modulation (MacDonald & Olsen, 1994).

In conclusion, signalling molecules interact with neurotransmitter receptors
at the level of multiple specific sites (including allosteric sites) and, via their
conformational transitions, regulate the efficacy of synaptic transmission.

GENE REGULATION OF NEUROTRANSMITTER RECEPTORS

The isolation and sequencing of the genes and cDNAs encoding the multiple
subunits of various receptor types has provided tools to localize precisely the
cells that express particular receptor subunit gene(s), thus opening a new field
of investigation. *In situ* hybridization techniques, for example, have revealed
distinct patterns of expression for each subunit of a particular neurotransmitter
receptor family, with frequent overlaps (see Sargent, 1993; Zoli et al., 1994
for the nicotinic receptor; Wisden & Seeburg, 1992 for the GABA$_A$ receptor;
Nakanishi, 1992 for the glutamate ionotropic and metabotropic receptors;
Sibley & Monsma, 1992 for the dopamine metabotropic-receptors). Some
subunit mRNAs appear widely expressed in the brain (e.g. the β2-subunit of
the nicotinic receptor) others are highly restricted to some areas (e.g. α2- or
α3-subunit of the same receptor) (see Zoli et al., 1994). Immunocytochemistry
studies complement in *in situ* hybridization by providing topological information about the receptors present on cell bodies or located on dendrites (or
axon terminals).

In the case of the monomeric G-protein linked receptors, correlation
between subunit distribution in the brain and pharmacological specificity for
defined therapeutical agents (and G-proteins) sheds new light on their function
and pathology (review, Sibley & Monsma, 1992). For example, in the case
of the dopamine receptors, the D$_3$ receptor mRNA is more narrowly
distributed than that of the D$_2$ receptor; it is predominantly expressed in
limbic brain areas thus leading to the hypothesis that it mediates dopaminergic
control of emotional functions (relevant to dopamine antagonist antipsychotic
therapy). On the other hand, the area of highest expression of the D$_4$ receptor
includes the frontal cortex, midbrain and amygdala, and this receptor possesses
a high affinity for a typical antipsychotic clozapine, suggesting a link with
schizophrenia and offering new tools of analysis for this disease (Sibley &
Monsma, 1992).

The adult pattern of expression of neurotransmitter receptor subunit
mRNAs arises from complex developmental regulation which differentially

affects each type of receptor subunit. In the case of the neuromuscular junction, developmental changes in ion channel kinetics, conductance and pharmacological specificity, which take place (in some species) during synapse formation and maturation, results from a switch of expression from the γ to the ε-subunit (Numa, 1989). Similar genetic switches may also occur in brain synapses as in the case of the glycine receptor (from $\alpha 2$ to $\alpha 1$ isoform). In many cases, several receptor subunit mRNAs are detected very early in development (as early as embryonic day E11 for nicotinic receptor $\alpha 3$, $\alpha 4$, $\beta 2$, $\beta 4$-subunits and E12 for $GABA_A$-receptor $\alpha 4$, $\beta 1$ and $\gamma 1$-subunits) and are often found colocalized in the same cells. Subsequently, they evolve according to developmental profiles which depend on the brain region, some subunits reaching their maximum level postnatally, others peaking transiently, before birth. The widespread occurrence of neurotransmitter receptors at early stages of neural development, long before functional synaptic contacts are established, suggest that neurotransmitters (and neuropeptides) possess an '*ontogenetic function*' and serve as trophic factors for neuronal differentiation and/or formation of brain circuits (see Lauder, 1993; Duclert & Changeux, 1994). For instance, they may induce retraction of neurites, turning of nerve growth cones, causing restriction of an initially widespread distribution into a focal localization of the receptor in the postsynaptic membrane.

Alternate splicing of exons giving rise to different receptor protein isoforms has been recognized for several G-receptors (in particular the dopamine D_2 and D_3 receptors). The resulting amino acid sequence insertions (or deletions) alter the extracellular region, thus modifying ligand binding specificity or generating (or eliminating) cytoplasmic phosphorylation sites, or domains implicated in G-protein binding (Sibley & Monsma, 1992). Splice variants also exist in ligand-gated ion channels. A particularly striking example is that of the AMPA/kainate glutamate receptors (GluRA to GluRD, sometimes termed GluR1 to GluR4), which occur in two major forms (*flip* and *flop*) with respect to an alternatively spliced exonic sequence of 38 residues which precedes the last putative transmembrane region MIV (Figure 6.2A). The prenatal brain expresses mostly flip forms of the four GluRA to D receptors which display desensitization to finite steady-state at variance with the flop forms. The adult brain contains both flip and flop forms, the latter one appearing only from early postnatal ages onward and being coexpressed with flip forms in many cells (review, Seeburg, 1993). Moreover, as mentioned earlier, in several non-NMDA glutamate-receptors single amino acid exchanges within transmembrane segments MII (and/or MI) give rise to channels with high/low Ca^{++} permeability which result from developmentally regulated RNA editing (Seeburg, 1993).

Transcriptional regulation appears to be a key step in the differential control of gene expression within the central nervous system in space and time. It may thus be viewed as part of a particularly sophisticated morphogenetic process which may be analyzed at the level of the DNA *cis* acting regulatory sequences and promoters. In this respect, the evolution of the postsynaptic distribution of the nicotinic receptor in muscle cells in the course of the development of the motor endplate appears as a rather simple, yet, relevant experimental model (review, Duclert & Changeux, 1994). In the embryonic myotube, the nicotinic receptor protein (and the mRNA for the α, β and δ subunits) are initially dispersed over the *entire* surface of the muscle fiber while, in the adult, they are present exclusively in the postsynaptic membrane (the ε-subunit mRNA replacing the γ-one after birth directly at the endplate) and *the electrical activity* of the developing postsynaptic muscle fiber as *neural factors* released by the ingrowing motor nerve contribute to this compartmentalization. Identification and functional analysis of the promoters and upstream regulatory sequences of the α- and other subunits using *in vitro* transfection techniques and *in vivo* transgenic mouse models, lead to the conclusion that different DNA elements are involved in subneural expression of the ε-subunit and in the activity-dependent elimination of transcription (e.g. E-Box which bind myogenic proteins) by the extrajunctional nuclei. Finally, investigation of the putative first and second messengers involved in this compartmentalized gene expression strongly support the concept that different signalling cascades are involved in the regulation by the motor nerve at the endplate (CGRP and cAMP, or acetylcholine receptor-inducing-activity (ARIA) and tyrosine kinase) and by electrical activity in extrajunctional areas (Ca^{++} ions and activation of protein kinase C) (review, Duclert & Changeux, 1994).

Transposition of this model to developing neurons cannot be achieved without caution since nerve cells are mononuclear and the topology investigated three-dimensional in the brain and in the neuron. Only a few promoters of genes encoding brain receptors have been identified and their regulatory elements analysed (e.g. nicotinic neuronal α_7, α_2 and β_2 subunits, review, Bessis et al., 1994). In all these cases, *cis* acting regulatory elements in the $5'$ flanking region direct reporter gene expression. Of particular interest is the presence within this region of the α_2- and of the β_2-subunit gene of *silencers* raising the attractive possibility that negative regulation of transcription contributes to the compartmentalized pattern of expression of these genes (review, Bessis et al., 1994).

Moreover, mRNAS encoding receptor subunits can be regulated by electrical activity, such as the up-regulation of NMDA-R2 subunit by K^+ induced depolarization in cultured cerebellar cells or the increase in a presynaptic glutamate receptor GR33 mRNA after induction of LTP. Extension of the promoter approach to the analysis of these mechanisms both *in vitro* and *in vivo* by the available methods of transfection, transgenesis and/or gene inactivation opens new perspectives in the analysis of these processes and of the long-term learning traces (see Kandel, 1993; Changeux, 1993) laid down in the developing or adult brain at the gene level.

In addition to regulation at the transcriptional level, a cascade of post-transcriptional processes play a critical role in the formation and maturation of the endplate including mRNA stabilization, assembly, targeting and clustering of the receptor protein, interaction with the cytoskeleton and basal lamina, metabolic stabilization of the receptor protein. In all these processes, the activity of the network may play a critical regulatory role (review, for the motor endplate, Cartaud & Changeux, 1993). A particularly intriging and still unresolved issue is the mechanism by which receptor molecules of particular subunit composition become sorted and localized in neurons at the dendritic, somatic or axon terminal level. Such fine placement and location of receptor aggregates may play a critical role in the plasticity of the nerve cell and of neuronal networks.

NEUROTRANSMITTER RECEPTORS AND PATHOLOGY

The principal targets for drug action on mammalian cells have been subdivided by Rang & Dale (1991) into four main categories: receptors, ion channels, enzymes and carrier molecules. The ionotropic and G-protein coupled receptors for neurotransmitters compose the large majority of the first category in the nervous system and many psychotropic drugs act at this level, thus suggesting a direct contribution of neurotransmitter receptors to mental diseases as important as depression or schizophrenia (see Gershon & Rieder, 1992; Sedvall et al., 1994). Indeed, anxiolytic and hypnotic drugs are either positive allosteric effectors of the $GABA_A$ ionotropic receptor (benzodiazepines, barbiturates) thus enhancing the neuronal inhibitory effect of GABA or agonists of the $5\text{-}HT_{1A}$ G-protein coupled receptor (buspirone, sumatriptan); neuroleptic drugs are, in general, antagonists of dopamine D2 G-protein coupled receptors but may also block other monoamine G-protein coupled receptors. Also, some anti-epileptic drugs are positive effectors of $GABA_A$ receptors and some anti-parkinsonian (benzotropine) drugs are antagonists of muscarinic G-protein linked receptors. Finally, analgesic morphine-like drugs act as agonists of opioid G protein coupled receptors (μ and δ).

Consistent with these interpretations, *in vivo* brain imaging techniques by positron emission tomography (which offer means to estimate brain receptors density and occupancy) did not reveal alterations of dopamine receptor subtypes density in drug naive schizophrenic patients but showed that conventional anti-psychotic drugs markedly reduce the binding of specific radiolabeled ligands of the D_1 and D_2 dopamine receptors (Sedvall et al., 1994).

Many of the main drugs of abuse also act on neurotransmitter receptors: morphine on the opioid receptors; nicotine on the acetylcholine (nicotinic) receptors; ethanol among several cellular mechanisms potentiates $GABA_A$ receptors and inhibits NMDA receptors; LSD acts as a mixed agonist/antagonist at 5HT G-protein coupled receptors; cannabis interacts with specific G-protein coupled receptors, possibly for anandamide; phencyclidine acts on opiate receptors and blocks glutamate NMDA gated ionic channels (see Barinaga, 1992).

General anesthetics, until recently, were thought to influence nerve activity by indirectly perturbing membrane lipids. Yet, according to Franks & Lieb (1994), at surgical concentrations, their principal effects are on ionotropic receptors. Some agents act predominantly as blockers of excitatory receptors (such as ketamine on NMDA receptors), but allosteric potentiation of inhibitory synaptic ionotropic receptors (mainly $GABA_A$) would give the best match for the pharmacological profile of a wide variety of agents in producing general anesthesia in mammals. On the other hand, voltage-gated ion channels are much less sensitive to general anesthetics. The differential sensitivity of particular classes of neurons would result from their particular composition of receptors and ion channel subunits (Franks & Lieb, 1994).

The elucidation of the structure of channel-linked and G-protein linked receptors offers novel possibilities for drug discovery and design. Indeed, recombinant DNA technologies have resulted in information on the sequence of multiple types of subunits existing for a given neurotransmitter receptor, on the key amino acids responsible for ligand-binding specificity and allosteric transitions (see Chapters 1 and 2, and on the distribution of these various combinations of subunits in the brain. The availability of expression systems (such as frog oocyte or cells in culture) also facilitates pharmacological assays and gives hope for a more selectively 'targeted' pharmacology. As a consequence, a new domain of investigation, referred to as computer-aided drug design, has been created on the basis of possible models of ligand binding pockets (see Chapters 1 and 2).

The structure–function studies carried out on these receptors has resulted in several new notions: (1) a single receptor molecule may be the target of *several* different series of pharmacological agents binding to topographically distinct sites, for instance allosteric sites in addition to the neurotransmitter binding sites (e.g. glycine and glutamate on the NMDA receptor, benzodiazepines and GABA on the $GABA_A$ receptor); (2) some of these drug binding sites might not be standard binding pockets but, instead might be located in the axial cleft of pseudo-symmetrical oligomers (such as chlorpromazine, phencyclidine and various local anesthetics on the nicotinic receptor) and/or overlap the boundaries between subunits (for instance d-tubocurarine on the nicotinic receptor); (3) the interaction between pharmacological agents binding to these diverse categories of sites may not be 'steric' but allosteric, taking place between topographically distinct sites and being mediated by conformational transitions of the receptor molecule.

Models of drug addiction, which rely upon biochemical alteration of receptors and signal transduction, have also been proposed in the case of opiate action (see Nestler et al., 1993). In the *locus ceruleus* opiates acutely inhibit neuronal activity by directly increasing the conductance of a K^+

channel (via coupling with G-proteins) and indirectly decreasing Na^+-dependent inward current via inhibition of adenylate cyclase. On the other hand, chronic morphine administration causes an up-regulation of cAMP pathway (G-proteins, adenylate cyclase and protein kinase A), yielding an increased excitability of *locus coeruleus* neurons and a marked elevation of their firing rate upon withdrawal. Tolerance, then, would result from greater levels of opioid receptor desensitization through its enhanced phosphorylation.

An alternative view not incompatible with the former one, is that drugs of abuse (morphine, cocaine, ethanol) act as positive reinforcers at the level of the mesolimbic dopaminergic system (at least in *nucleus accumbens*) via an up-regulation of the cAMP pathway and an enhanced sensitivity of dopamine D1 receptor (Nestler et al., 1993).

In a general manner, chronic treatment by pharmacological agents acting on neurotransmitter receptors are expected to affect their allosteric states (see Chapter 2) and/or their biosynthesis, for instance via their activity-dependent regulation of gene expression (see Chapter 3). Indeed, chronic treatment with antidepressants and neuroleptics has been claimed to alter catecholamine receptors gene expression (Creese & Sibley, 1981). Also, nicotine exposure over time causes an increase (approximately doubling) in brain nicotinic receptor sites, plausibly as a consequence of their sustained desensitization.

Specific instances exist where a disease can be causally linked to altered receptor function. The most studied is *myasthenia gravis* (Oosterhuis, 1993) which develops as an auto-immune disease directed against muscle nicotinic receptors. Also, as already mentioned, *retinitis pigmentosa* is caused, in humans by mutations in rhodopsin genes (review, Lefkowitz, et al., 1993). Patients suffering from hereditary hyperekplexia (or familial startle disease) have point mutations in the gene encoding the $\alpha 1$ subunit of the glycine ionotropic receptor (Shiang et al., 1993). In a selectively outbred alcohol nontolerant rat line, a benzodiazepine-induced impairment of postnatal reflexes is linked to point-mutation in granule cell specific $GABA_A$ receptor ($\alpha 6$) from cerebellum (Korpi et al., 1993).

Recently, animal models of neurological and/or psychiatric diseases have been developed by receptor genes inactivation or antisense oligodeoxy nucleotide inhibition of their expression. For instance, inactivation of the $5HT_{1B}$ receptor in the mouse causes enhanced aggressive behavior and less fear under stress. Also, antisense oligodeoxynucleotide against D2-dopamine receptor inhibits rotational behavior induced by the D2-dopamine agonist quinpirole. Consistent with the notion that the activity of the developing nervous system contributes to its epigenesis by the selective stabilization of synapses (see Changeux & Danchin, 1976; Edelman, 1978, 1987), NMDA receptor, knockout mice fail to develop whiskers related neuronal patterns in the trigeminal brainstem nuclei (Li et al., 1994). More diseases associated with deficits of neurotransmitter receptors are expected to be discovered both in humans and in animal model systems.

Neuronal death following cerebral vascular occlusion has been assigned to Ca^{++} influx consecutive to glutamate acting upon NMDA-receptor (Meldrum, 1985). Antisense oligodeoxynucleotides to NMDA-R_1-receptor indeed protect cortical neurons *in vivo* from excitotoxicity and reduce focal ischaemic infarctions (Wahlestedt et al., 1993). In addition, patients suffering from Alzheimer's disease have a large reduction in nicotine binding sites in both neocortex and hippocampus (Perry et al., 1986). The identification of neurotransmitter receptors as well as the analysis of the regulation of their gene expression has opened new fields of investigation in human pathology.

CONCLUSIONS

Since the proposal of the receptor concept by Langley at the turn of the century, our knowledge of the biochemical and structural properties of the transmembrane macromolecular complexes engaged in neurotransmitter recognition and signal transduction has made considerable progresss. The introduction of automated microsequencing, genetic engineering and high-resolution structural methods has led to the recognition of two main 'prototypes' of molecular architecture under which one can regroup most known neurotransmitter receptors. The ion channel-forming receptors are single molecular entities which contain all the structural elements responsible for the conversion of the neurotransmitter signal into an electrical response. Members of this family share putative *four* (or *five*) membrane spanning domain structures. On the other hand, the *seven*-membrane spanning receptors reversibly interact, on their cytoplasmic side, with an heterotrimeric G-protein which mediates a cascade of intracellular reactions. In both instances, the ligand binding site and the biologically active site are topographically distinct; their physiological interaction is therefore allosteric and mediated by a change of conformation.

Rapid kinetic methods, protein phosphorylation studies and mutagenesis experiments have further demonstrated that slower adaptation reactions (often referred to as densensitization) occur upon prolonged exposure to the physiological signal and result from transitions between distinct conformations (phosphorylated or not) and ligand binding properties. The balance between these activatable and refractory conformations may contribute to the short-term regulation of the efficiency of signal transmissions across synapses.

Most ion channel and G-protein coupled receptor genes display different patterns of expression in different brain regions which unfold over the course of embryonic and postnatal development. In addition to the occurrence of multiple genes encoding receptor subtypes, heterogeneity in receptor molecules may result from alternative splicing, RNA editing and combinational association of diverse subunits into multimeric receptors (in the case of the ion channel coupled receptors). Knowledge of the structural, pharmacological and physiological properties of these multiple receptors species and of their precise distribution within the brain offers new tools and methods for the development of a more targeted modern pharmacology. Also the analysis of receptor gene structure, of the promoter elements which govern their transcription and of their post-transcriptional processing, provides a novel experimental and theoretical framework to analyse long-term plasticity of developing and adult neuronal networks, to understand genetically inherited and acquired neurological and psychiatric diseases and to suggest models for individual psychological variability.

ACKNOWLEDGMENTS

We thank Dr Marina Picciotto and Nicolas Le Novère for constructive comments on the manuscript.

This work was supported by grants from the Association Française contre les Myopathies, the Collège de France, the Centre National de la Recherche Scientifique, the Ministère de la Recherche, the Institut National de la Santé et de la Recherche Médicale (contract number 872004), the Direction des Recherches Etudes et Techniques (contract number 90.142), The Human Frontiers Program (contact number RG 415/93 B) and the EEC (contracts CT 93 0518, 94 1060).

REFERENCES

Baldwin, J. M. (1993) The probable arrangement of the helices in G protein-coupled receptors. *EMBO Journal*, **12**, 1693–703.

Barinaga, M. (1992) Pot, heroin unlock new areas for neuroscience. *Science*, **258**, 1882–4.

Bertrand, D., Galzi, J. L., Devillers-Thiéry, A., Bertrand, S. & Changeux, J. P. (1993a) Mutations at two distinct sites within the channel domain MII alter calcium permeability of neuronal alpha 7 nicotinic receptor. *Proceedings of the National Academy of Science of the USA*, **90**, 6971–5.

Bertrand, D., Galzi, J. L., Devillers-Thiéry, A., Bertrand, S. & Changeux, J. P. (1993b) Stratification of the channel domain in neurotransmitter receptors. *Current Opinion in Cell Biology*, **5**, 688–93.

Bessis, A., Salmon, A. M., Zoli, M., Le Novère, N., Picciotto, M. & Changeux, J. P. (1994) Promoter elements conferring neuron specific expression of the β2-subunit of the neuronal nicotinic acetylcholine receptor studied *in vitro* and in transgenic mice. *Neuroscience*, in press.

Betz, H. (1990) Ligand-gated ion channels in the brain: the amino acid receptor superfamily. *Neuron*, **5**, 383–92.

Betz, H. (1992) Structure and function of inhibitory glycine receptors. *Quarterly Review of Biophysics*, **25**, 381–94.

Cartaud, J. & Changeux, J. P. (1993) Posttranscriptional compartmentalization of acetylcholine receptor biosynthesis in the subneural domain of muscle and electrocyte junctions. *European Journal of Neuroscience*, **5**, 191–202.

Changeux, J. P. & Danchin, A. (1976) Selective stabilization of developing synapses as a mechanism for the specification of neuronal networks. *Nature*, **264**, 705–12.

Changeux, J. P. (1990) Functional architecture and dynamics of the nicotinic acetylcholine receptor: an allosteric ligand-gated ion channel. In Changeux, J. P., Llinas, R. R., Purves, D. & Bloom, F. E. (eds.) *Fidia Research Foundation Neuroscience Award Lectures, Vol. 4.* New York: Raven Press, pp. 21–168.

Changeux, J. P. (1993) A critical view of neuronal models of learning and memory. In Andersen, P., Hvalby, O., Paulsen, O. & Hökfelt, B. (eds.) *Memory Concepts. Basic and Clinical Aspects. Novo Nordisk Foundation Symposium No. 7.* Copenhagen: Elsevier, pp. 413–33.

Changeux, J. P. & Edelstein, S. (1994) On allosteric mechanisms and acetylcholine receptors. *Trends in Biochemical Science*, **19**, 399–400.

Changeux, J. P., Galzi, J. L., Devillers-Thiéry, A. & Bertrand, D. (1992) The functional architecture of the acetylcholine nicotinic receptor explored by affinity labeling and site-directed mutagenesis. *Quarterly Review of Biophysics*, **25**, 395–432.

Cockcroft, V. B., Osguthorpe, D. J., Barnard, E. A. & Lunt, G. G. (1990) Modeling of agonist binding to the ligand-gated ion channel superfamily of receptors. *Proteins: Structure, Function and Genetics*, **8**, 386–97.

Cockcroft, V. B., Osguthorpe, D. J., Barnard, E. A., Friday, A. E. & Lunt, G. G. (1992) Ligand-gated ion channels: homology and diversity. *Molecular Neurobiology*, **4**, 129–69.

Creese, I. & Sibley, D. R. (1981) Receptor adaptations to centrally acting drugs. *Annual Reviews of Pharmacology and Toxicology*, **21**, 357–91.

Devillers-Thiéry, A., Galzi, J. L., Bertrand, S., Changeux, J. P. & Bertrand, D. (1992) Stratified organization of the nicotinic acetylcholine receptor channel. *NeuroReport*, **3**, 1001–4.

Devillers-Thiéry, A., Galzi, J. L., Eiselé, J. L., Bertrand, S., Bertrand, D. & Changeux, J. P. (1993) Functional architecture of the nicotinic acetylcholine receptor: a prototype of ligand-gated ion channels. *Journal of Membrane Biology*, **136**, 97–112.

Duclert, A. & Changeux, J. P. (1995) Acetylcholine receptor expression at the developing neuromuscular junction. *Physiological Review*, **75**, 339–68.

Edelman, G. (1978) *The Mindful Brain: Cortical Organization and the Group-Selective Theory of Higher Brain Function.* Cambridge, Mass.: MIT Press.

Edelman, G. (1987) Neural Darwinism. New York: Basic Books.

Eiselé J. L., Bertrand, S., Galzi, J. L., Devillers-Thiéry, A., Changeux, J. P. & Bertrand, D. (1933) Chimaeric nicotinic-serotonergic receptor combines distinct ligand binding and channel specificities. *Nature*, **366**, 479–83.

Franks, N. P. & Lieb, W. R. (1994) Molecular and cellular mechanisms of general anaesthesia. *Nature*, **367**, 607–14.

Fuxe, K. & Agnati, L. F. (1991) Two principal modes of electrochemical communication in the brain: volume versus wiring transmission. In Fuxe, K. & Agnati, L. F. (eds.) *Volume Transmission in the Brain: Novel Mechanisms for Neural Transmission.* New York: Raven Press, pp. 1–9.

Galzi, J. L., Revah, F., Black, D., Goeldner, M., Hirth, C. & Changeux, J. P. (1990) Identification of a novel amino acid α-Tyr 93 within the active site of the acetylcholine receptor by photoaffinity labeling: additional evidence for a three-loop model of the acetylcholine binding site. *Journal of Biochemical Chemistry*, **265**, 10430–7.

Galzi, J. L., Revah, F., Bouet, F., Ménez, A., Goeldner, M., Hirth, C. & Changeux, J. P. (1991) Allosteric transitions of the acetylcholine receptor probed at the amino acid level with a photolabile cholinergic ligand. *Proceedings of the National Academy of Science of the USA*, **88**, 5051–5.

Galzi, J. L., Devillers-Thiéry, A., Hussy, N., Bertrand, S., Changeux, J. P. & Bertrand, D. (1992) Mutations in the ion channel domain of a neuronal nicotinic receptor convert ion selectivity from cationic to anionic. *Nature*, **359**, 500–5.

Galzi, J. L. & Changeux, J. P. (1994) Neurotransmitter-gated ion channels as unconventional allosteric proteins. *Current Opinion in Cell Biology*, **4**, 554–65.

Gasic, G. P. & Heinemann, S. (1992) Determinants of the calcium permeation of ligand-gated cation channels. *Current Opinion in Cell Biology*, **4**, 670–7.

Gershon, E. & Rieder, R. (1992) Major disorders of mind and brain. *Scientific America*, **267**, 127–33.

Gingrich, J. A. & Caran, M. G. (1993) Recent advances in the molecular biology of dopamine receptors. *Annual Reviews of Neuroscience*, **16**, 299–321.

Giraudat, J., Dennis, M., Heidmann, T., Chang, J. Y. & Changeux, J. P. (1986) Structure of the high affinity site for noncompetitive blockers of the acetylcholine receptor: serine-262 of the delta subunit is labeled by [3H]-chlorpromazine. *Proceedings of the Natural Academy of Science of the USA*, **83**, 2719–23.

Giraudat, J., Dennis, M., Heidmann, T., Haumont, P. Y., Lederer, F. & Changeux, J. P. (1987) Structure of the high-affinity binding site for noncompetitive blockers of the acetylcholine receptor: [3H] chlorpromazine labels homologous residues in the beta and delta chains. *Biochemistry*, **26**, 2410–18.

Henderson, R. & Schertler, G. (1990) The structure of bacteriorhodopsin, and its relevance to the visual opsins and other seven helix G-protein coupled receptors. *Philosophical Transactions of the Royal Society of London*, **B326**, 379–89.

Henderson, R., Baldwin, J. M., Ceska, T. A., Zemlin, F., Beckmann, E. & Downing, K. H. (1990) A model for the structure of bacteriorhodopsin based on high resolution electron cryo-microscopy. *Journal of Molecular Biology*, **213**, 899–929.

Herz, J. M., Johnson, D. A. & Taylor, P. (1989) Distance between the agonist and noncompetitive inhibitor sites on the nicotinic acetylcholine receptor. *Journal of Biological Chemistry*, **264**, 12439–48.

Hibert, M., Trump-Kallmeyer, S. T., Bruinvels, A. & Hoflak, J. (1991) Three-dimensional models of neurotransmitter G-binding protein-coupled receptors. *Molecular Pharmacology*, **40**, 8–15.

Hökfelt, T. (1991) Neuropeptides in perspective: the last ten years. *Neuron*, **7**, 867–79.

Hucho, F., Oberthür, W. & Lottspeich, F. (1986) The ion channel of the nicotinic acetylcholine receptor is formed by the homologous helices M2 of the receptor subunits. *FEBS Letters*, **205**, 137–42.

Huganir, R. L. & Greengard, P. (1990) Regulation of neurotransmitter receptor desensibilization by protein phosphorylation. *Neuron*, **5**, 555–67.

Imoto, K., Busch, C., Sackmann, B., Mishina, M., Konno, T., Nakai, J., Bujo, H., Mori, Y., Fukuda, K. & Numa, S. (1988) Rings of negatively charged amino acids determine the acetylcholine receptor channel conductance. *Nature*, **335**, 645–8.

Iyengar, R. & Birnbaumer, L. (eds.) (1990) *G Proteins*. New York: Academic Press.

Johnson, J. W. & Ascher, P. (1987) Glycine potentiates the NMDA response in cultured mouse brain neurons. *Nature*, **325**, 529–31.

Kandel, E. R. (1993) The switch from short- to long-term facilitation at the connections between sensory and motor neurons of the Gill-withdrawal reflex in *Aplysia*. In Andersen, P., Hvalby, O., Paulsen, O. & Hökfelt, B. (eds.) *Memory Concepts: Basic and Clinical Aspects*. BV International Congress Series, Copenhagen: Elsevier, pp. 93–7.

Karlin, A. (1993) Structure of nicotinic acetylcholine receptors. *Current Opinion in Neurobiology*, **3**, 299–309.

Katz, B. & Miledi, R. (1977) Transmitter leakage from motor nerve endings. *Proceedings of the Royal Society of London*, **B196**, 59–72.

Katz, B. & Thesleff, S. (1957) A study of the desensitization produced by acetylcholine at the motor end-plate. *J. Physiol.*, **138**, 63–80.

Korpi, E. R., Kleingoor, Kettenmann, H. & Seeburg, P. H. (1993) Benzodiazepine-induced motor impairment linked to point mutation in cerebellar $GABA_A$ receptor. *Nature*, **361**, 356–9.

Lauder, J. M. (1993) Neurotransmitters as growth regulatory signals: role of receptors and second messengers. *Trends in Neuroscience*, **16**, 233–40.

Lefkowitz, R. J., Cotecchia, S., Samama, P. & Costa, T. (1993) Constitutive activity of receptors coupled to guanine nucleotide regulatory proteins. *Trends in Pharmacological Science*, **14**, 303–7.

Léna, C. & Changeux, J. P. (1993) Allosteric modulations of the nicotinic acetylcholine receptor. *Trends in Neuroscience*, **16**, 181–6.

Leonard, R. J., Labarca, C. G., Charnet, P., Davidson, N. & Lester, H. A. (1988) Evidence that the M2 membrane-spanning region lines the ion channel pore of the nicotinic receptor. *Science*, **242**, 1578–81.

Li, X. M., Zoli, M., Finnman, U. B., Le Novère, N., Changeux, J. P. & Fuxe, K. (1995) A single ($-$)-nicotine injection causes change with a time delay in the affinity of striatal D_2 receptors for antagonist, but not for agonist, nor in the D_2 receptor mRNA levels in the rat substantia nigra. *Brain Research*, **679**, 157–167.

Macdonald, R. L. & Olsen, R. W. (1994) $GABA_A$ receptor channels. *Annual Reviews of Neuroscience*, **17**, 569–602.

Meldrum, B. (1985) Possible therapeutic applications of antagonists of excitatory amino acid neurotransmitters. *Clinical Science*, **68**, 113–22.

Mulle, C., Léna, C. & Changeux, J. P. (1992) Potentiation of nicotinic receptor response by external calcium in rat central neurons. *Neuron*, **8**, 937–45.

Nakanishi, S. (1992) Molecular diversity of glutamate receptors and implications for brain function. *Science*, **258**, 597–603.

Nestler, E. J., Hope, B. T. & Widnell, K. L. (1993) Drug addiction: a model for the molecular basis of neural plasticity. *Neuron*, **11**, 995–1006.

Numa, S. (1989) A molecular view of neurotransmitter receptors and ionic channels. *Harvey Lecuture Series*, **83**, 121–65.

Oosterhuis, H. J. G. H. (1993) Clinical aspects. In De Baets, M. H. & Oosterhuis, H. J. G. H. (eds.) *Myasthenia Gravis*. Boca Raton: CRC Press, pp. 14–42.

Palczewski, K. & Benovic, J. L. (1991) G-protein-coupled receptor kinases. *Trends in Biochemical Science*, **16**, 387–91.

Perry, E. K., Perry, R. H., Smith, C. J., Purohit, D., Bonham, J., Dick, D. J., Candy, J. M., Edwardson, J. A. & Fairbairn, A. (1986) Cholinergic receptors in cognitive disorders. *Can. J. Neurol. Sci.*, **13**, 521–7.

Perutz, M. F. (1989) Mechanisms of cooperativity and allosteric regulation in proteins. *Quarterly Reviews of Biophysics*, **22**, 139–236.

Rang, H. & Dale, M. (1991) *Pharmacology*. Churchill Livingstone. Edinburgh.

Révah, F., Bertrand, D., Galzi, J. L., Devillers-Thiéry, A., Mulle, C., Hussy, N., Bertrand, S., Ballivet, M. & Changeux, J. P. (1991) Mutations in the channel domain alter desensitization of a neuronal nicotinic receptor. *Nature*, **353**, 846–9.

Sakmann, B., Patlak, J. & Neher, E. (1980) Single acetylcholine-activated channels show burst-kinetics in presence of desensitizing concentrations of agonist. *Nature*, **286**, 71–3.

Sargent, P. B. (1993) The diversity of neuronal nicotinic acetylcholine receptors. *Annual Reviews of Neuroscience*, **16**, 403–43.

Savarese, T. M. & Fraser, C. M. (1992) *In vitro* mutagenesis and the search for structure-function relationships among G protein-coupled receptors. *Biochemical Journal*, **283**, 1–19.

Schertler, G. F. X., Villa, C. & Henderson, R. (1993) Projection structure of rhodopsin. *Nature*, **362**, 770–72.

Schofield, P. R., Darlison, M. G., Fujita, N., Burt, D. R., Stephenson, F. A., Rodriguez, H., Rhee, L. M., Ramachandran, J., Reale, V., Glencorse, T. A., Seeburg, P. H. & Barnard, E. A. (1987) Sequence and functional expression of the GABA$_A$ receptor show a ligand-gated receptor super-family. *Nature*, **328**, 221–7.

Sedvall, G., Karlsson, P., Lundin, A., Anvret, M., Suhara, T., Halldin, C. & Farde, L. (1994) Dopamine D1 receptor number – a sensitive PETT marker for early brain degeneration in Huntington disease. *European Archives of Psychiatry and Clinical Neuroscience*, **243**, 249–55.

Seeburg, P. H. (1993) The TINS/TIPS Lecture: the molecular biology of mammalian glutamate receptor channels. *Trends in Neuroscience*, **16**, 359–65.

Shiang, R., Ryan, S., Zhu, Y. Z., Hahn, A., O'Connell, P. & Wasmuth, J. J. (1993) Mutations in the α1 subunit of the inhibitory glycine receptor cause the dominant neurologic disorder, hyperekplexia. *Nature Genetics*, **5**, 351–8.

Sibley, D. R. & Monsma, Jr. F. J. (1992) Molecular biology of dopamine receptors. *Trends in Pharmacological Science*, **13**, 61–9.

Strosberg, A. D. (1991) Structure function relationship of proteins belonging to the family of receptors coupled to GTP binding proteins. *European Journal of Biochemical*, **196**, 1–10.

Subramaniam, S., Gerstein, M., Oesterhelt, D. & Henderson, R. (1993) Electron diffraction analysis of structural changes in the photocycle of bacteriorhodopsin. *EMBO Journal*, **12**, 1–8.

Unwin, P. N. T. (1993) Nicotinic acetylcholine receptor at 9 Å resolution. *Journal of Molecular Biology*, **229**, 1101–24.

Unwin, P. N. T., Toyoshima, C. & Kubalek, E. (1988) Arrangement of the acetylcholine receptor subunits in the resting and desensitized states, determined by cryoelectron microscopy of crystallized *Torpedo* postsynaptic membranes. *Journal of Cell Biology*, **107**, 1123–38.

Villarroel, A., Herlitze, S., Koenen, M. & Sakmann, B. (1991) Location of the threonine residue in the alpha-subunit M2 transmembrane segment that determines the ion flow through the acetylcholine receptor channel. *Proceedings of the Royal Society of London*, **B243**, 69–74.

Wahlestedt, C., Golanov, E., Yamamoto, S., Yee, F., Ericson, H., Yoo, H., Inturrisi, C. E. & Reis, D. J. (1993) Antisense oligodeoxynucleotides to NMDA-R1 receptor channel protect cortical neurons from excitotoxicity and reduce focal ischaemic infarctions. *Nature*, **363**, 260–3.

White, B. J. & Cohen, J. B. (1992) Agonist-induced changes in the structure of the acetylcholine receptor M2 regions revealed by photoincorporation of an uncharged nicotinic noncompetitive antagonist. *Journal of Biological Chemistry*, **267**, 15770–83.

Wisden, W. & Seeburg, P. H. (1992) GABA$_A$ receptor channels: from subunits to functional entities. *Current Opinion in Neurobiology*, **2**, 263–9.

Zoli, M., Le Novère, N., Hill, J. A. & Changeux, J. P. (1995) Developmental regulation of nicotinic receptor subunit mRNAs in the rat central and peripheral nervous system. *Journal of Neuroscience*, **15**, 1912–39.

7 Learning, memory and synaptic plasticity: cellular mechanisms, network architecture and the recording of attended experience

R. G. M. MORRIS

INTRODUCTION

Most neuroscientists suspect that synaptic plasticity – the capacity for synapses to change in efficacy – is the basis of information storage in the brain. Altering neurons at their points of contact with one another is a suitable locus for achieving a change in their functional interrelationship. In its simplest form, the idea is that an increase in synaptic efficacy causes the firing of neuron A to be more likely to cause the firing of a neuron B onto which it is afferent. Given that learning often involves a change in the likelihood of one stimulus to evoke the memory of another, such an alteration in the functional connectivity of neurons should be useful in implementing information storage within the brain. Moreover, a synaptic locus has the merit of affording, at least in principle, greater information storage capacity than a mechanism based solely on changes in cell excitability because the many thousands of synapses on an individual neuron could participate in many different memories. Indeed, if information is represented in the vertebrate brain as distributed spatio-temporal patterns of neural activity, individual synapses can potentially participate in many overlaid memories.

However, achieving a full understanding of the relationship between learning, memory and synaptic plasticity is a much taller order. The existence of multiple types of memory and several types of synaptic plasticity raises immediately the question of specificity. Understanding how information is stored and retrieved by circuits in the nervous sytem will require a detailed account of the process (or processes) of learning that a particular neural circuit implements, how information is represented as patterns of neural activity within it, when synaptic changes are induced, and how they are expressed and maintained through the lifespan. Memory, particularly what has come to be known as autobiographical memory (McCarthy & Warrington, 1990), is an active process in which stored information is retrieved creatively to give the phenomenological experience that we think of as conscious remembrance. We are still a long way from understanding whether and, if so, how changes in synaptic efficacy allow the memories of scenes, facts or events to be reconstructed in the mind's eye during the process of memory retrieval.

THE ARGUMENT

This chapter is divided into three main parts. First, I shall discuss certain conceptual issues about the relationship between learning and synaptic plasticity, illustrating these with reference to classic work on the marine mollusc *Aplysia* which provides a benchmark against which other studies may be assessed. I shall argue that while research on *Aplysia* has given and continues to offer deep insights into mechanisms of neuronal plasticity that may be conserved through evolution (particularly the relationship between short-term and long-term changes), it is unlikely that studies of the up and down-regulation of synaptic throughput in sensorimotor reflex pathways could alone lead to a general theory of the role of synaptic plasticity in memory. Within higher vertebrates, other types of memory exist, different neural circuits, and novel ways of representing information as distributed spatiotemporal patterns of neuronal activity. These have radical implications for the way in which the up and down-regulation of synaptic efficacy contributes to the processing and storage of information.

Secondly, any explanation of the contribution that synaptic plasticity makes to memory within a given brain area is predicated on an understanding of the function(s) of that brain area and of its interaction with other interconnected areas. It follows that, to have a theoretical understanding of the role of synaptic plasticity in, for example, the hippocampal formation, we must also have an adequate systems-level theory of hippocampal function. In this chapter, I shall advance the specific hypothesis that the hippocampal formation contains circuitry involved in the automatic registration of attended experience, that this information is encoded as discrete scenes, and that it is stored temporarily for periods ranging from as short as a few hours up to longer periods, the duration of which cannot yet be specified. Via neural activity in other circuits interacting with the hippocampal formation (both cortical and subcortical), this scene-based information is then used to construct mental models of experience which constrain both our perception of the world and the encoding of discrete episodic and semantic memory traces in long-term memory. According to this hypothesis, which clearly owes much to the ideas of O'Keefe & Nadel (1978), Johnson–Laird (1983), and Gaffan (1991, 1992a), the registration of experience within the hippocampus, specifically of the scenes where noticed events or actions take place, may be likened to successive snapshots of day-to-day experience.

Thirdly, I shall propose that the encoding of information about scenes is achieved as alterations in synaptic weights between neurons in the hippocampal formation. The hippocampus displays a prominent form of activity-dependent synaptic plasticity, called long-term potentiation (LTP; Bliss & Lømo, 1973), having the properties of associativity, synapse-specificity and persistence. These properties are, respectively, ideal for linking events to their context, for encoding a large amount of information, and for holding onto that information temporarily. The implications of this idea, which is a specific version of the generic 'LTP and learning' hypothesis, will be discussed with reference to various functionally orientated studies.

THE MAPPING BETWEEN TYPES OF LEARNING AND TYPES OF PLASTICITY

One-to-one mapping

At least at a descriptive level, there are many types of learning and memory. There are also several types of synaptic plasticity. Their relationship may sometimes be a relatively straightforward 'one-to-one' mapping between type of learning P, Q or R and type of plasticity X, Y or Z respectively. For example, in an influential paper, Kandel & Schwartz (1982) proposed that *habituation* and *sensitization* of the gill and siphon withdrawal reflexes in the marine mollusc *Aplysia* are mediated by distinct forms of plasticity, namely *use-dependent presynaptic depression* (for habituation) and *presynaptic facilitation* (for sensitization). This elegantly simple scheme accounts remarkably well for the expression of these 'simple' forms of learning that are carried out, at least in part, by the circuitry of the abdominal ganglion in this animal. Studies of habituation and sensitization at a behavioural, physiological, anatomical and cell-biological level, primarily by Kandel and his colleagues over the past 20 years, have produced a large body of data indicating that short- and long-lasting alterations in transmitter release at defined synapses between identified neurons can mediate aspects of the appropriate behavioural changes across a comparable timescale. Strikingly, the relationship between learning and plasticity may be perceived as parallel in the mind's eye: habituation, a *waning* of behavioural responsiveness, is implemented by a *decrease* in neurotransmitter release; sensitization, an *augmentation* of behavioural responsiveness, is implemented by an *increase* in transmitter release. In addition, more complex forms of learning, such as classical alpha-conditioning, may be mediated by an activity-dependent amplification of presynaptic facilitation, namely a dual calcium-dependent and G-protein mediated allosteric modification of adenylate cyclase augmenting its synthesis of cyclicAMP (Abrams & Kandel, 1988; Anholt, 1994). Detecting the contiguity of the conditional (CS) and unconditional stimulus (US) in this way sets in train a cascade of biochemical changes that cause the augmented sensitization of the CS–CR pathway thought to underly this form of associative conditioning. There is no need to appeal to any additional complications concerning the way information is represented in the neural circuitry of the abdominal ganglion to perform the job of detecting stimulus contiguity. A cell-biological mechanism, in which the CS is represented quantitatively as the level of intracellular calcium at synaptic terminals, the US as activation of a G-protein, and their contiguity as the allosteric interaction at a specific enzyme, can apparently suffice. An additional feature of work on *Aplysia* is that habituation, sensitization and classical conditioning may be either short- or long-lasting. There is now clear evidence that the development of long-term memory depends upon protein synthesis and recent work implicates the activation of transcriptional regulatory elements in the nucleus (such as CREB, Kandel, 1993; Nguyen et al., 1994). Taken together, these findings reveal a beautifully straightfoward relationship between learning and synaptic plasticity in the sensorimotor reflex pathways of *Aplysia,* encompassing several 'simple' types of learning and including both short- and long-term changes.

The generality of the one-to-one mapping principle

The question arises, however, of the generality of this one-to-one mapping principle to other forms of learning and to other species, notably vertebrates. Vertebrates are capable of a wider variety of learning processes than *Aplysia*. It does not seem likely that each of these more complex processes will be underpinned by ever more complex types of synaptic plasticity in a strictly one-to-one manner; there will not be a type of plasticity for episodic memory, another for semantic memory, and so on. Indeed, there is even some doubt in my mind whether our understanding of the cell-biological mechanisms modulating presynaptic transmitter release in *Aplysia* can be generalized to provide a complete explanation of habituation, sensitization and classical conditioning in other species. Dishabituation can, for example, sometimes occur in response to decreases in stimulus strength or to the omission of a regularly repeating stimulus, implying that the inhibition of responsiveness may sometimes be guided by an 'internal model' of the pattern of stimulus presentation (Gray, 1982). Moreover, Kandel's ingenious 'differential facilitation' theory of associative conditioning (see Carew et al., 1983), which supposes that every CR that any CS can ever elicit is prewired but subthreshold, is not without difficulties (see Morris, 1990).

A more likely mapping is that different types of *information processing and storage* will turn out to be mediated by a restricted set of types of synaptic plasticity, differing with respect to their physiological and biochemical characteristics to be sure, but equally importantly, organised such that a single type of plasticity can have a different functional role in distinct neural circuits. The physiological characteristics would include the associativity versus non-associativity of the induction or 'learning-rule', whether the expression of the functional change in synaptic efficacy is homosynaptic, heterosynaptic or local volume, and the temporal persistence for which the synaptic change can last (minutes, hours, days). However, while characterizing these different types of plasticity – physiologically, biochemically and structurally – is an important and tractable task, it will not be enough. The involvement of synaptic plasticity in multiple forms of memory must also be a function of the differing neural circuitry in which it is embedded, of the types of information presented to each circuit, and of the dynamic neuronal code in which that information is represented. For example, a single type of plasticity (such as N-methyl-D-asparate receptor-dependent LTP in vertebrates – currently a focus of particular attention) could mediate different processes of learning in different circuits.

Synergistic action of multiple types of plasticity within a single circuit – the concept of the cellular alphabet

In addressing these systems-level complications, I hasten to point out that Hawkins & Kandel (1984) have themselves proposed that a small set of different types of plasticity – a *cellular alphabet* – could be put together in novel ways to mediate ever more complex forms of learning. According to this hypothesis, the distinct forms of plasticity are the 'letters' and the various types of learning are the 'words' – there being more of the latter than the former. Hawkins & Kandel (1984) illustrate how, armed with certain assumptions about how information is represented within the reflex pathways of the abdominal ganglion, together with the principles of homosynaptic depression, presynaptic facilitation and activity-dependent amplication of presynaptic facilitation, it may be possible to explain a variety of learning phenomena ranging from spontaneous recovery through to complex conditioning phenomena, such as overshadowing and blocking (see also Hawkins, 1990 for a quantitative treatment). Thus, a restricted number of types of plasticity can be combined to explain a wide variety of learning phenomena.

Although this hypothesis takes us rightly away from a strict one-to-one mapping principle, it retains the sense that the neurobiology of learning can be largely understood in terms of the combined action of a restricted set of cell-biological mechanisms. The argument runs as follows: words (types of learning) consist of letters (types of plasticity). Thus, if the letters can be identified and understood (i.e. at the cell-biological and molecular level), perhaps we can then spell out the words they make. One consequence of this way of looking at things has been the enormous emphasis upon understanding the cell-biological mechanisms of synaptic plasticity with, until recently, less regard to other levels of analysis. Pursuing the cellular alphabet hypothesis for a moment, it is as if a reductionist understanding of the 'letters' is implicitly taken to be both a *necessary* (I agree) and a *sufficient* (I disagree) prerequisite for understanding the neurobiology of learning and memory. This bottom-up focus is by no means peculiar to work on *Aplysia*, being also a characteristic of research on hippocampal LTP. Thus, LTP is now routinely studied in brain slices *in vitro* whose capacity for learned behaviour and conscious memory is, at best, limited. The overwhelming majority of papers on LTP are concerned with addressing its underlying mechanisms; relatively few have, until recently, addressed the wider functional relevance of this form of plasticity in the real circuits of behaving animals.

However, if we are to understand the relationship between synaptic plasticity and memory, we must come to grips with how synaptic plasticity actually operates in neural circuits (see also Hooper et al., 1994). A specific type of synaptic plasticity (P) may have no unique relationship to a particular form of learning (X), not only because it can be combined with another type of plasticity (Q) to mediate a distinct form of learning (Y2), but because what it does depends critically upon other systems-level parameters. That is, type of plasticity P may be part of the mechanisms of form of learning X, or of forms of learning Y2 or Z2, as a function of the type of information being processed, the way that information is represented and the local circuitry in which this type of plasticity occurs. This 'systems-level' perspective is logically different from that of supposing that different types of learning only become possible when different types of plasticity are combined with one another. The cellular alphabet can only be part of the story.

Expression of a single type of synaptic plasticity in different neural circuits can mediate different types of learning

An example of the principle that one type of synaptic plasticity may mediate different forms of learning in different circuits is with reference to the synaptic enhancement triggered by activation of a specific type of glutamate receptor – the N-methyl-D-aspartate (NMDA) receptor. This type of synaptic plasticity is found in the hippocampus (in the form of NMDA-receptor dependent LTP), in the amygdala, and the intermediate region of the hyperstriatum ventrale (IMHV) region of the newly hatched chick brain. Blocking it in each of these structures impairs spatial learning (Morris et al., 1986a), fear-potentiated startle conditioning (Miserendino et al., 1990) and filial imprinting (McCabe & Horn, 1991), respectively. These are clearly different types of learning, at least in the sense that the information processing involved in each is different and they have a regionally distinct anatomical substrate, but interestingly, they all depend upon an associative process (see Morris & Davis, 1994). It is perhaps because of this latter shared property that the NMDA receptor is involved in each. If this argument is correct, to understand more fully exactly what role a given type of synaptic plasticity is carrying out within a given circuit, it is essential to establish first the type of memory in which that brain area is involved. That is, analysis of the *relationship* between plasticity and learning must involve a 'top-down' component. Once that step is accomplished, one can then begin another interesting phase of the brain/behavior analysis, namely that of working out how the local circuits of that brain area compute the appropriate information processing algorithms for learning.

THE HIPPOCAMPUS AS A SYSTEM FOR THE AUTOMATIC RECORDING OF ATTENDED EXPERIENCE

The hippocampus has been implicated in various types of memory but, despite argument about which theoretical description is correct, there is at least general agreement that its function does not include what Squire (1992) has characterized as 'non-declarative' learning. As this category is said to include simple forms of associative and nonassociative learning, such as those shown by *Aplysia*, we may infer that synaptic plasticity in the hippocampus is unlikely to be involved in such types of learning. So what does the hippocampus do?

There are many theories of hippocampal function. The best known are the proposals that it is involved in spatial and cognitive mapping (O'Keefe & Nadel, 1978), declarative memory and consolidation (Squire, 1992), or is part of a larger neural system (consisting of several brain areas) responsible for episodic memory (Gaffan, 1992a). From the perspective of mapping synaptic plasticity to memory, a difficulty with each of these theories is that they are cast in a form that do not naturally lend themselves to thinking about its function with reference to its striking and prominent form of activity-dependent synaptic plasticity, namely LTP. I shall now sketch out the gist of an alternative idea about what the hippocampus does that points to a specific role that NMDA-receptor dependent synaptic plasticity could play in its function.

Most neuropsychologists today subscribe to the notion that memory comes in many forms. For example, a long established distinction between *short-term working memory* (consisting of both a central executive and both verbal and visual short-term storage devices – Baddeley, 1992) and *long-term memory,* consisting of a number of semi-independent information processing systems. Within long-term memory, psychological distinctions have been drawn between explicit and implicit memory (Schacter, 1987), spatial and nonspatial memory (O'Keefe & Nadel, 1978), declarative and non-declarative memory (Squire 1992), and so on. These binary categories may themselves be subdivided, such as that between episodic and semantic memory (Tulving, 1983), both of which are usually considered as types of explicit (or declarative) memory. The proposal below, drawing upon Gaffan (1992a), is that the creation of long-term memories is preceded by an intermediate 'scene-based' stage of storage.

Scene memory and the creation of mental models

The encoding of information into long-term memory is still poorly understood although many factors have been identified as determinants. One possibility is that the formation of discrete long-term memory traces, probably laid down in the neocortex, depends upon the prior registration of successive experiences each of which is retained for a short time as an isolated 'scene'. For example, all of us can picture today quite well including, specifically, the non-habitual aspects of this day. Most of us could say whether someone else was waiting at the bus stop on the way to work, whether someone had parked in our favorite spot in the car-park, or whether, when we went out for lunch, we had to open the front door of the department ourselves or someone opened it for us, and so on. Such events are unique to today and the scenes in which they occurred are easily reconstructed in the mind's eye. But remembering this kind of inconsequential detail is not something that any of us could do for an arbitrarily chosen day as short as a month ago unless a remembered event of that day was in some way special and so merited the formation of a discrete long-term memory. It therefore seems likely that embedded somewhere in our brains is a device that keeps track of the events of each day – *a system for the automatic recording of attended experience*. The capacity of this intermediate memory system would be substantially greater than that of working memory, being able to record whole scenes and the events occurring within them such as who did what and to whom. We may think of these scenes, to borrow Worden's (1992) metaphor, as the temporarily remembered 'fragments' of experience. The persistence of information within this memory system is probably on the order of a day, perhaps a week, although I would not rule out that it might occasionally be longer. This is long enough for selected aspects of information to be extracted or abstracted from this record of experience and stored as discrete long-term memories elsewhere in the brain before they fade and are lost. The long-term memories that are eventually formed may be of specific scenes and the events that occurred within them (episodic memories). However, they may also be facts that only arise by virtue of some noticed similarity between an element of one scene and of that in another. For example, if it turned out that the stranger waiting as the bus stop was the same person who opened the door to the department at lunchtime, the system could creatively combine these two isolated experiences into a single unique 'fact' about the day and remember it as such. Notice, in this example, that the fact that is eventually stored never pre-exists as a discrete 'stimulus' or even as a single 'event' within a single scene, but is *created* from separate episodes within the day that share some common feature.

There are two separate points here. First, following Gaffan (1992a), I am suggesting that information in the putative temporary record of attended experience is probably stored as a succession of whole scenes. An implication is that the content of an explicitly remembered experience is inextricably part of the temporarily stored information and it is always possible to ask where you learned a particular recently acquired fact or when you last saw a particular person. Scene-encoding provides a straightforward way of categorizing experience and a way of resolving ambiguity (e.g. of remembering that the significance of a stimulus in one scene may be different from its significance in another).

Secondly, I am supposing that there exists some kind of machinery for comparing successive scenes, in the mind's eye so to speak, prior to the creation of discrete long-term memories. This comparison or abstraction process is an essential step in the construction of mental models of experience, models that can be generalized from one set of events to others of a similar kind (Johnson–Laird, 1983). The simplest kind of mental model is a spatial 'map' of an environment, sometimes referred to as a cognitive map (O'Keefe & Nadel, 1978), in which the common features in one scene and those in another are identified and then used to build a geometric representation of the world 'out there', a representation that makes sense from the perspective of the person moving through the world and experiencing successive scenes. The stability of the real world is an essential prerequisite for building such a representation (Biegler & Morris, 1993). The capacity to retrieve information from long-term memory into such a system could, in addition, make possible yet more complex models. Long after the specific details are lost, mental models enable us to remember what kinds of things tend to occur, or not to occur, in a particular context, such as at a lecture or at a football game. We build these models through experience by recalling the events or patterns of behaviour that are common to particular situations – that is, by comparing current experience with that which occurred in a categorically similar scene. Thus, we sit quietly at a lecture but cheer at a football match because our expectations of these situations reflect our past experience.

In summary, the system used for recording experience would require both a substantial but temporary memory capacity and an information processing capacity able to create models of the world by noticing similarities between a current scene and that of similar ones recalled from memory. Such a capacity for comparing and relating events would provide a mental framework for understanding the regularities of the world around us and help us to identify unusual events.

The role of the hippocampal formation in recording experience

The neuroanatomical aspect of this hypothesis is the proposal that the hippocampal formation is the specific part of a larger neural circuit in the brain that provides the automatic but temporary register of attended experience. Activity-dependent synaptic plasticity in the hippocampus (i.e. the neural mechanisms underlying LTP) is the mechanism by which we stored successive scenes.

This hypothesis is compatible with (although not demanded by) evidence concerning human amnesia. Thus, human amnesics, some of whom have damage to the hippocampal formation or certain nuclei of the thalamus, commonly show a disproportionate deficit in remembering recent events but their access to general knowledge is unaffected (McCarthy & Warrington, 1990). However, the memory deficit after damage to the hippocampal formation is unlikely to be specific to all instances of episodic memory, because some amnesic patients (e.g. H. M.-Scoville & Milner, 1957; R. B.-Zola–Morgan, Squire & Amaral, 1986) have a time-limited retrograde amnesia with apparently normal access to episodic memories for events occurring long before the onset of amnesia. Interestingly, amnesics can sometimes show good recognition of isolated stimuli (e.g. magazine pictures) if required only to indicate whether they are familiar, but are unable to indicate where or when they saw these pictures before. This suggests that input to the system for recording experience may be via modality specific intermediate memory systems that can encode the identity and familiarity of a stimulus, but not the context in which it was presented (see also Eichenbaum, Otto & Cohen, 1994).

A large body of animal experiments conducted using both rats and primates has investigated whether recognition memory is impaired by damage to areas within the medial temporal lobe (Squire, 1992; Mishkin & Murray, 1994). The usual procedure in such experiments is to present an object A as a 'sample' and, then, after a delay, present a 'choice' trial in which A is presented with another object B. The rule for solution may be either delayed matching-to-sample (i.e. choose A to secure reward), or delayed non-matching-to-sample (i.e. choose B). In either case, the animal is required to make a judgement about the absolute familiarity of an object. The balance of evidence at present suggests that the integrity of the perirhinal and parahippocampal cortex, rather than the hippocampal formation, is critical for recognition memory. However, the hypothesis outlined above implies that there can be more to explicit recognition than merely indicating *that* an object has been seen before. It can also be relevant to ask *where* the object was seen before or *when* it was seen, that is in what scene it occurred. One of several reconstructive features of memory is that of recreating in the mind's eye the scene in which an object or event occurred. Gaffan (1991) has proposed that remembering an object within a scene is neuropsychologically dissociable from merely recognising that a specific object is familiar. In support of this view, he has shown that fornix lesions (that are likely to disrupt normal hippocampal function, although the extent to which they do is still unclear) impair a monkey's ability to remember that a complex visual scene is rewarded or non-rewarded (Gaffan, 1992b) or to learn that object A (but not B) is rewarded in scene X, while object B (but not A) is rewarded in scene Y (Gaffan & Harrison, 1989). It would be good to follow up these intriguing observations with a study of the context-specificity of recognition memory after discrete hippocampal lesions.

Clearly there are several features of this automatic recording of experience hypothesis that need to be fleshed out more than space permits. A key difficulty, similar to that confronting theories that posit a difference between explicit and implicit memory, is to identify the boundaries between tasks that require the operation of the putative recording system and those that do not. Without this being specified, the hypothesis makes no hard and fast predictions. However, given the specific claim is that the hippocampal formation is constantly and automatically registering attended experience in the form of scenes, one implication is that it would certainly need to have the capacity for storing, albeit temporarily, a large amount of information derived from multiple sensory modalities and for building associations between disparate inputs. Associative activity-dependent synaptic plasticity in the hippocampus is precisely the kind of mechanism by which this might be achieved.

HIPPOCAMPAL LONG-TERM POTENTIATION (LTP)

The phenomenon of LTP and its principal characteristics

LTP is a long-lasting increase in the capacity of afferent neuronal activity to activate postsynaptic neurons and consists of both synapse-specific and cell-specific components (Bliss & Lømo, 1973).

Several characteristics of LTP have been apparent since its discovery, while others have emerged in the course of research on the phenomenon over the past 20 years (Bliss & Collingridge, 1993). Those attracting particular interest as properties desirable of a memory mechanism are persistence, synapse specificity and associativity. *Persistence* refers to the fact that LTP lasts for at least an hour, although certain methods of inducing it result in an increase of synaptic efficacy lasting substantially longer. *Synapse specificity* refers to the fact that not all the synapses on a neuron, or set of neurons, will demonstrate the increase – only those activated by high-frequency presynaptic activity. *Associativity* refers to the fact that synapses which are stimulated too weakly to cause an increase in their own right can, if stimulated at the same time as other stronger afferents to the same neuron, nevertheless show potentiation. Taken together, these properties are suggestive of a possible underlying neural mechanism that could be useful for associative learning. Whatever the cell-biological mechanism is in detail, it enables the temporal conjunction of a weak stimulus (s) with a strong one (S) to be detected by a neuron (N) and then expressed as an alteration in connectivity in a stimulus specific way (i.e. s can more easily activate N). Such a cellular mechanism of detection and expression cannot, on its own, enable a neural representation of S to be evoked by that of s, but, embedded into an appropriate neural architecture, this simple property of associative learning might be realised (see McNaughton & Morris, 1987).

If information about events, stimuli, and the scene in which they occur are projected to the hippocampus from relevant association areas of the neocortex, the *associativity* of LTP might perform the job of linking these elements such that the memory of one could activate the memory of another. For example, a recent event would be remembered as having occurred in a particular context (or vice versa). The *synapse specificity* of LTP would ensure there is substantial storage capacity, but it should be noted that the extent of the specificity to individual synapses is still in doubt (Bonhoeffer, Staiger & Aertsen, 1989) and its existence does not preclude neurons from making other cell-specific as well as synapse-specific alterations. A 'ball-park' calculation might be to suppose that an animal could record experience at the maximum rate of (say) 1 scene per second (although it would often be much slower than this). Doing so would require a system with the capacity to store, in a 12-hour day, up to 40,000 memories. The rodent hippocampus has approximately 500,000 CA3 cells (only 10 times less than the human), each with approximately 10,000 synapses per cell. If individual memories are stored in an overlaid, spatially distributed manner, using changes in synaptic weights for storage, there might be adequate storage capacity for numerous quite complex scenes each of which would involve the activity of many neurons (see Treves & Rolls, 1994). It is, however, impossible to be precise about such calculations in the absence of detailed knowledge about exactly what information is projected into the system from the entorhinal cortex and the sparsity of the coding in which it is represented. In any event, the *persistence* of LTP implies that synaptically stored information could last at least an hour and, in some cases, for several days. However, the fact that LTP has been seen to decay in all cases in which it has been studied is compatible with other evidence that the hippocampus is unlikely to be a site of long-term storage. This raises the intriguing question of how the hippocampus interacts with cortex in the creation of stable long-term memories about which we remain somewhat ignorant (see Barnes, 1994).

Synaptic learning rules and the encoding of variance and invariance

The empirical study of LTP has been accompanied by a range of theoretical proposals about so-called synaptic learning rules specifying the circumstances in which synaptic changes are to take place. An interesting feature of many such rules is that they attempt to capture the regularities or conditional probabilities of one event given another. They are, therefore, rules in which increases and decreases of associative strength are necessary to represent consistency in the world, i.e. *invariance*. To be implemented in neural hardware one would (probably) need both activity-dependent synaptic potentiation and activity-dependent synaptic depression. Interestingly, the proposed system for the temporary registration of attended experience may *not* need this. Such a system would be used to register stimuli that might, in their conditional relations with other stimuli, temporarily contradict the invariant associations stored in long-term memory. Such a system would be immensely useful for encoding the unusual and often inconsequential events of everyday life (i.e. *variance*) and could be implemented with very rapid ('1-trial') synaptic potentiation together with strictly time-dependent decay – such as the type of synaptic potentiation displayed in experiments on LTP. The system would not necessarily need activity-dependent LTD because saturation of synaptic weights may not occur – the storage limit of the system not often being approached given the usual rate at which most events occur, and, in general, are conveniently forgotten. Interestingly, the evidence to date indicates that, *in vivo,* the hippocampus shows robust LTP which decays over time but, as yet, no strong indication of activity-dependent homosynaptic LTD. The system would, of course, still need to have the potential to alter long-term memory in the neocortex, but how this might be accomplished is still an open question.

IS HIPPOCAMPAL SYNAPTIC PLASTICITY OF FUNCTIONAL SIGNIFICANCE?

I have argued that the hippocampal formation is involved in the automatic recording of attended experience and that this information is somehow abstracted from the record to create long-term episodic and semantic memories in the neocortex. This abstraction of experience is also part of the process of creating mental models of the world. Essentially no work on the functions of LTP has been done from quite this perspective, although many experiments have utilized spatial learning which, at least during its earliest stages of acquisition, surely depends upon registering successive scenes and abstracting from them to encode the invariant geometric relationships between landmarks. Accordingly, I shall review aspects of the literature from the perspective of examining whether the neural mechanisms underlying hippocampal LTP occur during, and are necessary for, certain kinds of spatial memory. Three predictions follow:

(1) Changes in hippocampal synaptic efficacy will occur continuously in association with exploration and spatial learning.
(2) Saturation of LTP should interfere with existing recent memories but not older ones, and occlude new learning.
(3) Blockade of LTP should cause a selective impairment of certain types of learning.

Do changes in hippocampal synaptic efficacy occur in association with exploration or spatial learning?

If increases in synaptic efficacy are involved in the temporary information storage responsible for recording recent scenes, an increase in field excitatory post-synaptic potentials (fEPSPs) to afferent stimulation within the hippocampal formation should be observed in association with exploratory behavior or spatial learning. The problem with this 'simple' prediction is that such changes in synaptic efficacy might be very difficult to detect because, if a brain structure has significant storage capacity (as the hippocampus almost certainly does), an individual learning experience would not be expected to cause changes in synaptic efficacy at any but a small proportion of synapses.

Sharp, McNaughton & Barnes (1989) discovered what appeared to be a striking short-term up-regulation of hippocampal fEPSPs in the dentate gyrus during spatial exploration. Subsequent work by Moser, Mathiesen & Andersen (1993) has indicated, however, that part of the increase reported by Sharp, McNaughton & Barnes (1989) may be explained in terms of a behaviourally induced alteration in brain temperature. They implanted miniature thermistors in the brain at approximately the same dorso-ventral level to that of the dentate-gyrus recording electrode and found that changes in the magnitude of the measured fEPSP occurred in association with an increase in brain temperature as the animals explored. When the rats were placed instead into a pool of cold water, brain temperature declined and fEPSPs decreased.

Moser, Moser & Andersen (1994) have taken a step in the direction of unconfounding temperature-associated from 'real' changes in fEPSPs. They first worked out the calibration functions between brain temperature and fEPSP for individual animals under conditions in which the rats sat undisturbed in a box and were either warmed or cooled. They then placed them into an environment containing landmarks that the animals were allowed to explore. Recordings of fEPSPs were taken prior to and during this exploration period, and during a later exploration period in which the location of two of the landmarks was interchanged. The latter period of exploration did, of course, trigger an increase in brain temperature, but Moser and his colleagues were able to use the calibration functions to identify a temperature-independent enhancement of the field potential. This component was maximal within 5 sec of the start of exploration and declined gradually to baseline over approximately 15 min. This change may be a true learning-related alteration in synaptic efficacy triggered by, and relating to, the changed scene in front of the animal. Further work using this or a related paradigm could focus on the underlying mechanism of this brief period of enhanced synaptic efficacy and then, by blocking or enhancing it, establish whether it is encoding information.

Does saturation of LTP interfere with stored information or occlude subsequent learning?

If information were temporarily stored in the hippocampus as distributed patterns of synaptic weights, direct physiological activation of as many synapses as possible with LTP-inducing patterns of stimulation should have two effects. First, it should disrupt recently stored information (although not information that had already been 'consolidated' in neocortex). Secondly, if the experimentally induced LTP reaches its physiological asymptote, it should occlude new learning. The logic underlying the second of these predictions is that when an animal's brain attempts to alter synaptic weights in the hippocampus during learning, it would be unable to do so if the prior experimentally induced LTP had saturated the biochemical machinery that mediates such changes.

McNaughton et al. (1986) and Castro et al. (1989) both reported data bearing out both of these predictions. However, subsequent research has been fraught by a number of failures to replicate these earlier findings (Cain et al., 1993; Jeffery & Morris, 1993; Korol et al., 1993; Sutherland, Dringenberg & Hoesing, 1993). Our own study (Jeffrey & Morris, 1993) included both as near an exact replication as we could achieve of part of Castro et al's (1989) experiment and a second experiment using somewhat different experimental conditions. In neither of our experiments was a reliable learning deficit observed. Of the several others that have also failed to find a positive effect of saturation, it is noteworthy that one of the recent papers (Korol et al., 1993) comes from the same laboratory as that of the original positive findings.

The reasons for this irreproducibility of results is unclear (see Bliss & Richter–Levin, 1993 for a commentary). Clearly, it could be that the hypothesis is wrong and that LTP is not involved in spatial learning and its saturation is therefore without effect. Alternatively, the hypothesis might be rescued: (1) because the only synapses of the hippocampal formation that were saturated were those of the perforant path input to the dentate gyrus (but not those of other extrinsic or intrinsic hippocampal pathways); (2) due to failure to saturate the full septo-temporal axis of the hippocampus (see Barnes et al., 1994). With respect to the second of these possibilities, if saturation of LTP were to be restricted to a small part of the dentate gyrus, a substantial resource of modifiable dentate synapses would still be available. Interestingly, the extent of saturated potentiation then measured could, rather than occluding learning, serve instead as an index of synaptic modifiability in individual animals. Perhaps animals with different degrees of plasticity will learn at different rates? In this vein, it is noteworthy that while Jeffrey & Morris (1993) found no difference in rate of watermaze spatial learning in either of their two experiments between animals given LTP-inducing or non-LTP inducing stimulation they did find, again in both experiments, a significant correlation within the high-frequency group between the magnitude of LTP and performance in the watermaze. Animals showing good LTP tended to persist in searching in the correct quadrant of the pool during a post-training retention test, whereas animals showing weak LTP performed more poorly.

Two predictions follow from the index of plasticity idea. First, the correlation between LTP magnitude and learning should still be present if the order of behavioral training and LTP induction were to be reversed such that the behavioral phase preceded the electrophysiology rather than *vice versa*. Jeffrey (1995) has recently completed such an experiment and finds the prediction upheld. However, she also ran into the complication that the correlation between magnitude of LTP and extent of spatial learning is *positive* at high intensities of test stimuli to the perforant path, but *negative* at weak intensities. The reason for this paradoxical reversal of the correlation with variation in the strength of perforant path stimulation remains unclear. A second prediction is that the correlation should break down and the saturation-induced learning impairment be readily observed in a 'reduced preparation' in which the synaptic resource is independently made smaller. Such a preparation might be an animal in which lesions have been made to many parts of the hippocampus leaving only an island or 'lamella' (Andersen, 1983) of intact tissue.

Does blockade of LTP impair certain types of learning?

Arguably the most persuasive evidence to date that the neural mechanisms of LTP underly the registration of recent experience has come from experiments in which LTP is blocked and spatial learning has been shown to be compromised. There are several ways in which the associative form of LTP has been (or might be) blocked *in vivo*: (1) application of NMDA-receptor antagonists (such as the drug AP5); (2) inhibition of enzymes putatively involved in the expression of LTP, such as those responsible for the synthesis of candidate intercellular messengers (such as nitric oxide synthase); (3) targeted deletion of genes encoding receptors or enzymes involved in the expression of LTP (so-called gene 'knock-outs'). I shall here consider only the first of these approaches.

Morris et al. (1986a) found that chronic infusion of the selective NMDA receptor antagonist, AP5, impaired the acquisition of spatial learning in a watermaze. AP5 was infused continuously over two weeks into the lateral ventricle of the brain via subcutaneously implanted minipumps (this drug does not easily cross the blood–brain barrier). These pumps, which work by osmosis, cause the slow steady infusion (0.5 µl/hr) of a small quantity of the drug (or artificial cerebrospinal fluid vehicle solution) into the ventricular space from which it can readily spread throughout the forebrain. The advantage of this method of applying the drug is that its concentration is relatively well restricted to the forebrain (i.e. does not infiltrate the spinal cord very much) and relatively uniform through the 14-day infusion period. Using this technique, and at a drug concentration found in separate animals to be sufficient to block hippocampal LTP without affecting baseline fEPSPs mediated by AMPA receptors, spatial learning in a watermaze was impaired while acquisition of a visual discrimination task was unaffected. The spatial task involved searching for an escape platform hidden at one place in the pool, while the visual discrimination task involved distinguishing between a visible black-and-white platform providing escape from the water and a visible grey platform which did not (or vice versa). The apparent selectivity of the learning impairment induced by AP5 is important for two reasons: (1) it suggests that the drug did not impede spatial performance by virtue of some gross sensorimotor disturbance (e.g. impaired vision), and (2) it points to a functional parallel between the effects of blocking hippocampal synaptic plasticity and those of lesions (Morris et al., 1982; Sutherland, Whishaw & Kolb, 1983; Morris, Hagan & Rawlins, 1986b; Morris et al., 1990). It should also be noted that the spatial task is more likely to be dependent upon the proposed hippocampal mechanism of recording successive experiences in the watermaze (being placed in, swimming around, climbing onto the platform, etc.) than the visual discrimination task. The latter requires for its solution only that the rats learn to associate a particular pattern with escape; it does not require the animal to remember specific experiences of having done this or the context in which this learning took place.

These findings have been both criticized and followed up in a number of ways. A major problem is the possibility that the apparent impairment of spatial learning is an artifact of disturbed sensorimotor function – and such disturbances are pronounced at high drug concentrations with multiple training trials per day (Davis, Butcher & Morris, 1992). However, such disturbances are actually quite subtle at intracerebral concentrations just sufficient to block LTP *in vivo* and, contrary to the notion that sensorimotor disturbances are inevitable, AP5 has no effect on performance in the watermaze if learning precedes the start of drug infusion (Morris, 1989). Nonspatial pretraining can also reduce the incidence of even the more subtle sensorimotor disturbances (such as occasional falling off the escape platform) without interacting statistically with the drug-induced impairment of spatial learning. Studies following up the original observations include Davis, Butcher & Morris's (1992) discovery that the dose-response profile of the learning impairment exactly parallels the dose-response profile of the blockade of LTP *in vivo* and, strikingly, that the measured intrahippocampal concentrations of AP5 are comparable to those concentrations that block LTP in the *in vitro* hippocampal slice. However, it is clear that AP5 causes only a modest impairment in the rate of spatial learning, not the complete block that might be expected if the induction of associative LTP was an absolute pre-requisite of information storage. Whether this represents a problem for the theory or a reflection of task ambiguity is still unresolved.

The dissociation between hippocampal-dependent spatial learning and hippocampal-independent visual discrimination learning has also been substantiated by the finding that intracortical infusion of AP5 into a site just anterior to visual cortex does not impair visual discrimination learning despite giving rise to a cortical concentration of the drug exactly comparable to that which, in hippocampus, does impair spatial learning (Butcher, Hamberger & Morris, 1991). In addition, acute intrahippocampal infusion of AP5 (restricting the drug to the hippocampus) is sufficient to cause the impairment of spatial learning (Morris, Halliwell & Bowery, 1989). Work by others has established that the similarities between the deleterious effects of AP5 and hippocampal lesions also extend to various nonspatial tasks such as the operant schedule called 'differential reinforcement of low rates of responding' (Tonkiss, Morris & Rawlins, 1989) and delayed matching to sample with trial repeating stimuli (Lyford et al., 1993), each of which would require an intact system for recording recent experience and have been shown to depend on hippocampal function.

There are, however, many problems with the strategy of blocking NMDA receptors. One is that the intraventricular route of administration of AP5 does not restrict the drug to the hippocampus and thus NMDA receptor function is likely to be compromised in a number of brain areas. These would include such areas as the striatum, thalamus and neocortex where NMDA receptors participate in diverse aspects of brain function including, but not restricted to, synaptic plasticity (Draw, Stein & Fox, 1992). It is, therefore, an oversimplification to suppose that the major, still less the only effect of AP5 administration is to block synaptic plasticity. The problem can, in part, be obviated by using acute intra-structure drug administration which, as we have seen, is apparently sufficient to cause a spatial learning impairment in the watermaze following intrahippocampal infusion. This does not, however, get round all the difficulties: even if the only (or major) effect of acute intra-structure AP5 administration is to block NMDA receptors in a regionally specific way, there can be no guarantee that doing so would not also disrupt aspects of the dynamic 'system properties' of the hippocampus in addition to blocking LTP. If this were to happen, the fact that AP5 blocks LTP could be beside the point; the hippocampus may be electrophysiologically dysfunctional and hippocampal-dependent learning could be impaired for that reason alone (Leung & Desborough, 1988). This is an immensely difficult ambiguity to break apart experimentally. One route to tackling it might be to attempt to block LTP at a point biochemically downstream of the NMDA receptor such that system properties of the hippocampus that depend upon normal NMDA receptor function are ostensibly unaffected. This is part of the thinking behind the use of enzyme-inhibitors and gene knockouts to investigate the issue further, although these techniques are not without problems of their own that may limit their ease of interpretation.

CONCLUSION

The argument of this chapter has been in three parts. First, I have suggested that the relationship or mapping between learning, memory and synaptic plasticity involves several different levels of analysis. For certain ostensibly simple forms of learning, such as sensitization in *Aplysia*, there is a beautiful one-to-one mapping between an increase in transmitter release and an augmentation of subsequent behavioural responsiveness to previously innocuous stimuli. But it is far from clear that this principle applies generally to the relationship between memory and other forms of synaptic plasticity. More specifically while it seems likely that synaptic plasticity is a mechanism for storing information in the central nervous system, what is stored can depend critically on the network architecture within which a given type of plasticity is embedded.

Secondly, I have argued that the hippocampal formation plays a role in the automatic registration of attended experience – specifically of the successive scenes where the events of our life take place. A key difficulty with this speculative hypothesis is to establish a formal link between the automatic encoding of experience and the kinds of learning tasks, such as spatial learning, that benefit from it or, better still, definitively require it. This requires conceptual work and then the development of relevant memory tasks. Recent work by Gaffan (1991, 1992a,b) has begun to do this, but his studies need to be developed in a variety of ways – to be adapted for the rat in which synaptic plasticity is more easily studied, examined with other kinds of brain lesions, and so on. Related to this is the larger problem of how the registration of experience provides the basis for constructing mental models that guide our perception of the world and the long-term storage of information elsewhere in the brain.

Thirdly, I have proposed that hippocampal synaptic plasticity is the basis by which recent experience is temporarily stored as scenes. At present, we can ask only the relatively crude 'empirical' question of whether there is any evidence that LTP or an LTP-like mechanism is continually being activated to encode experience in a hippocampal-dependent fashion. The brief review presented in the latter half of this chapter has indicated the following: (1) There are no convincing indications that persistent LTP-like changes in synaptic potentials occur during any of the forms of exploration or learning with which it has so far been studied. Short-lasting temperature-independent electrophysiological changes do occur during spatial exploration, but we do not know if these last for sufficient time for a long-term trace to be set up elsewhere in cortex; (2) while the prediction that saturation of LTP should impair spatial learning has proved hard to uphold, there are grounds for thinking the experiment is very difficult to do properly. Interestingly, an unexpected consequence of one study was a highly significant positive correlation between the cumulative extent of LTP in individual animals and their performance in a spatial learning task. Understanding this correlation, particularly its reversal at low test-pulse intensities, will require a great deal of further work; (3) blocking LTP by NMDA receptor blockade impairs spatial learning as predicted, but there are several grounds to be guarded about the interpretation of the experiments that have demonstrated this.

Sensorimotor disturbances are also induced by the competitive NMDA antagonist that has been used, and, even at concentrations that definitively block LTP, learning is impaired but not blocked. Thus, numerous outstanding problems confront the functional analysis of the most prominently studied type of activity-dependent synaptic plasticity in the vertebrate brain in both the neurobiological and psychological domains.

ACKNOWLEDGEMENTS

This work was supported by an MRC Programme Grant and a grant from the Human Frontiers Science Programme. I am grateful to many colleagues for discussion and, particularly Tim Bliss, David Gaffan, Kate Jeffery, John O'Keefe, Rick Lathe and Edvard Moser who criticised earlier versions of the manuscript.

REFERENCES

Abrams, T. W. & Kandel, E. R. (1988) Is contiguity detection in classical conditioning a system of a cellular property? Learning in Aplysia suggests a possible molecular site. *Trends in Neuroscience,* **11**, 128–35.

Andersen, P. (1983) Operational principles of hippocampal neurons – a summary of synaptic physiology. In Siefert, W. (ed.) *Neurobiology of the Hippocampus.* London: Academic Press, pp. 81–5.

Anholt, R. R. H. (1994) Signal integration in the nervous system: adenylate cyclases as molecular coincidence detectors. *Trends in Neuroscience,* **17**, 37–41.

Baddeley, A. D. (1992) Working memory. *Science,* **255**, 556–9.

Barnes, C. A. (1994) Group report: relating activity-dependent modifications of neuronal function to changes in neural systems and behaviour. In Selverston, A. I. & Ascher, P. (eds.) *Cellular and Molecular Mechanisms Underlying Higher Neural Functions,* Dahlem Workshop Reports. Chichester: John Wiley, pp. 81–110.

Barnes, C. A., Jung, M. W., McNaughton, B. L., Korol, D. L., Andreasson, K. & Worley, P. F. (1994) LTP saturation and spatial learning disruption: effects of task variables and saturation levels. *Journal of Neuroscience,* **14**, 5793–5806.

Biegler, R. & Morris, R. G. M. (1993) Landmark stability is a prerequisite for spatial but not discrimination learning. *Nature,* **361**, 631–3.

Bliss, T. V. P. & Collingridge, G. L. (1993) A synaptic model of memory: long-term potentiation in the hippocampus. *Nature,* **361**, 31–9.

Bliss, T. V. P. & Lømo, T. (1973) Long-lasting potentiation of synaptic transmission in the dentate area of the anaesthetized rabbit stimulation of the perforant path. *Journal of Physiology (London)* **232**, 331–56.

Bliss, T. V. P. & Richter–Levin, G. (1993) Spatial learning and the saturation of long-term potentiation. *Hippocampus,* **3**, 123–6.

Bonhoeffer, T., Staiger, V. & Aertsen, A. (1989) Synaptic plasticity in rat hippocampal slice cultures: Local Hebbian conjunction of pre- and postsynaptic stimulation leads to distributed synaptic enhancement. *Proceedings of the National Academy of Science of the USA,* **86**, 8112–17.

Butcher, S. P., Hamberger, A. & Morris, R. G. M. (1991) Intracerebral distribution of D,L-2-amino-phosphonopentanoic acid (AP5) and the dissociation of different types of learning. *Experimental Brain Research,* **83**, 521–6.

Cain, D. P., Hargreaves, E. L., Boon, F. & Dennison, Z. (1993) An examination of the relations between hippocampal long-term potentiation, kindling, afterdischarge, and place learning in the watermaze. *Hippocampus,* **3**, 153–63.

Carew, T. J., Abrams, T. W., Hawkins, R. D. & Kandel, E. R. (1983) The use of simple invertebrate systems to explore psychological issues related to associative learning. In Alkon, D. L. & Farley, J. (eds.) *Primary Neural Substrates of Learning and Behavioural Change.* Cambridge: Cambridge University Press, pp. 169–83.

Castro, C. A., Silbert, L. H., McNaughton, B. L. & Barnes, C. A. (1989) Recovery of spatial learning following decay of experimental saturation of LTE at perforant path synapses. *Nature,* **342**, 545–8.

Davis, S., Butcher, S. P. & Morris, R. G. M. (1992) The NMDA receptor antagonist, D-2 amino-5-phosphonpentanoate (D-AP5) impairs spatial learning and LTP *in vivo* at intracerebral concentrations comparable to those that block LTP *in vitro. Journal of Neuroscience,* **12**, 21–34.

Daw, N. W., Stein, P. S. G. & Fox, K. (1992) The role of NMDA receptors in information processing. *Annual Review of Neuroscience,* **16**, 207–22.

Eichenbaum, H., Otto, T. & Cohen, N. J. (1994) Two functional components of the hippocampal memory system. *Behavioral and Brain Sciences,* **17**, 449–518.

Gaffan, D. (1991) Spatial organisation of episodic memory. *Hippocampus,* **1**, 262–4.

Gaffan, D. (1992a) The role of the hippocampus-fornix-mammillary system in episodic memory. In Squire, L. R. & Butters, N. (eds.) Neuropsychology of Memory. New York: Guilford Press, pp. 336–46.

Gaffan, D. (1992b) Amnesia for complex naturalistic scenes and for objects following fornix transection in the rhesus monkey. *European Journal of Neuroscience,* **4**, 381–8.

Gaffan, D. & Harrison, S. (1989) Place memory and scene memory: effects of fornix transection in the monkey. *Experimental Brain Research,* **74**, 202–12.

Gray, J. A. (1982) *Elements of a Two-process Theory of Learning.* London: Academic Press.

Hawkins, R. D. (1990) A biologically realistic neural network model for higher order features of classical conditioning. In Morris, R. G. M. (ed.) *Parallel Distributed Processing: Implications for Psychology and Neurobiology.* Oxford: Oxford University Press, pp. 214–46.

Hawkins, R. D. & Kandel, E. R. (1984) Is there a cell-biological alphabet for simple forms of learning? *Psychological Review,* **91**, 375–91.

Hooper, S. L. (1994) What are the mechanisms for state-dependent changes? In Selverston, A. I. & Ascher, P. (eds.) *Cellular and Molecular Mechanisms Underlying Higher Neural Functions,* Dahlem Workshop Reports. Chichester: John Wiley, pp. 171–88.

Jeffrey, K. J. (1995) Paradoxical enhancement of long-term potentiation in poor-learning rats at low test stimulus intensities. *Experimental Brain Research,* **104**, 55–69.

Jeffrey, K. J. & Morris, R. G. M. (1993) Cumulative long-term potentiation in the rat dentate gyrus correlates with, but does not modify, performance in the watermaze. *Hippocampus,* **3**, 133–40.

Johnson-Laird, P. N. (1983) *Mental Models.* Cambridge University Press, Cambridge.

Kandel, E. R. (1993) The switch from short- to long-term facilitation at the connections between sensory and motor neurons of the gill-withdrawal reflex in

Aplysia. In Andersen, P., Hvalby, Ø, Paulsen, O. & Hökfelt, B. (eds.) *Memory Concepts: Basic and Clinical Aspects.* Amsterdam: Excerpta Medica.

Kandel, E. R. & Schwartz, J. H. (1982) Molecular biology of learning: modulations of transmitter release. *Science,* **218**, 433–43.

Korol, D. L., Abel, T. W., Church, L. T., Barnes, C. A. & McNaughton, B. L. (1993) Hippocampal synaptic enhancement and spatial learning in the Morris swim task. *Hippocampus,* **3**, 127–32.

Leung, L.-W. S. and Desborough, K. A. (1988) APV, an N-methyl-D-aspartate receptor antagonist, blocks hippocampal theta rhythm in behaving rats. *Brain Research,* **463**, 148–52.

Lynford, G. L., Gutnikov, S. A., Clark, A. M. & Rawlins, J. N. P. (1993) Determinants of non-spatial working memory deficits in rats given intra-ventricular infusions of the NMDA antagonist, AP5. *Neuropsychologia,* **31**, 1079–98.

McCabe, B. J. & Horn, G. (1991) Synaptic transmission and recognition memory: time course of changes in N-methyl-D-aspartate receptors after imprinting. *Behavioural Neuroscience,* **105**, 289–94.

McCarthy, R. A. & Warrington, E. R. (1990) *Cognitive Neuropsychology.* London: Academic Press.

McNaughton, B. L., Barnes, C. A., Rao, G., Baldwin, J. & Rasmussen, M. (1986) Long-term enhancement of synaptic of hippocampal synaptic transmission and the acquisition of spatial information. *Journal of Neuroscience,* **6**, 563–71.

McNaughton, B. L. & Morris, R. G. M. (1987) Hippocampal synaptic enhancement and information storage within a distributed memory system. *Trend in Neuroscience,* **10**, 408–15.

Miserendino, M. J. D., Sananes, C. B., Melia, K. R. & Davis, M. (1990) Blocking of acquisition but not expression of conditioned fear-potentiated startle by NMDA antagonists in the amylgdala. *Nature,* **345**, 716–18.

Mishkin, M. & Murray, E. A. (1994) Stimulus recognition. *Current Opinion in Neurobiology,* **4**, 200–7.

Morris, R. G. M. (1989) Synaptic plasticity and learning: selective impairment of learning and blockade of long-term potentiation in vivo by the N-methyl-D-aspartate receptor antagonist, AP5, *Journal of Neuroscience,* **9**, 3040–57.

Morris, R. G. M. (1990) Synaptic Plasticity, Neural Architecture and Forms of Memory. In McGaugh, J. L., Wienberger, N. M. & Lynch, G. (eds.) *Brain Organisation and Memory: Cells, Systems and Circuits,* New York: Oxford University Press, pp. 52–76.

Morris, R. G. M. & Davis, M. (1994) The role of NMDA receptors in learning and memory. In Watkins, J. C. & Collingridge, G. L. (eds.) *The NMDA Receptor.* Oxford: Oxford University Press.

Morris, R. G. M., Anderson, E., Lynch, G. & Baudry, M. (1986a) Selective impairment of learning and blockade of long-term potentiation by an N-methyl-D-aspartate receptor antagonist, AP5. *Nature,* **319**, 774–6.

Morris, R. G. M., Hagan, J. J. & Rawlins, J. N. P. (1986b) Allocentric spatial learning by hippocampectomised rats: A further test of the spatial-mapping and working-memory theories of hippocampal function. *Quarterly Journal of Experimental Psychology,* **38B**, 365–95.

Morris, R. G. M., Garrud, P., Rawlins, J. N. P. & O'Keefe, J. (1982) Place navigation impaired in rats with hippocampal lesions. *Nature*, **297**, 681–3.

Morris, R. G. M., Halliwell, R. & Bowery, N. (1989) Synaptic plasticity and learning II: do different kinds of plasticity underlie different kinds of learning? *Neuropsychologia* **27**, 41–59.

Morris, R. G. M., Schenk, F., Tweedie, F. & Jarrard, L. E. (1990) Ibotenate lesions of the hippocampus and/or subiculum: dissociating components of allocentric spatial learning. *European Journal of Neuroscience*, **2**, 1016–28.

Moser, E., Mathiesen, I. & Andersen, P. (1993) Association between brain temperature and dentate field-potentials in exploring and swimming rats. *Science*, **259**, 1324–6.

Moser, M.-B., Moser, E. I. & Andersen, P. (1994) Potentiation of dentate synapses initiated by exploratory learning in rats: dissociation from brain temperature, motor activity, and arousal. *Learning and Memory*, **1**, 55–73.

Nguyen, P. V., Alberini, C. M., Huang, Y.-Y., Ghiradi, M., Abel, T. & Kandel, E. R. (1994) Genes, synapses and long-term memory. *Wenner-Gren Symposium*, Stockholm.

O'Keefe, J. & Nadel, L. (1978) *The Hippocampus as a Cognitive Map*. Oxford: Oxford University Press.

Schacter, D. L. (1987) Implicit memory: history and current status. *Journal of Experimental Psychology*, **13**, 591–618.

Scoville, W. B. & Milner, B. (1957) Loss of recent memory after bilateral hippocampal lesions. *Journal of Neurology Neurosurgery and Psychiatry*, **20**, 11–21.

Sharp, P. E., McNaughton, B. L. & Barnes, C. A. (1989) Exploration-dependent modulation of evoked response in fascia dentata: fundamental observations and time-course. *Psychobiology*, **17**, 257–69.

Squire, L. R. (1992) Memory and the hippocampus: a synthesis from findings with rats, monkeys and humans. *Psychological Review*, **99**, 195–231.

Sutherland, R. J., Whishaw, I. Q. & Kolb, B. (1983) A behavioral analysis of spatial localisation following electrolytic, kainate or colchicine induced damage to the hippocampal formation in the rat. *Behavioural Brain Research*, **7**, 133–53.

Sutherland, R. J., Dringenberg, H. C. & Hoesing, J. M. (1993) Induction of long-term potentiation at perforant path dentate synapses does not affect place learning or memory. *Hippocampus*, **3**, 141–8.

Tonkiss, J., Morris, R. G. M. & Rawlins, J. N. P. (1989) Intraventricular infusion of the NMDA antagonist AP5 impairs DRL performance in the rat. *Experimental Brain Research*, **73**, 181–8.

Treves, A. & Rolls, E. T. (1994) Computational analysis of the role of the hippocampus in memory, *Hippocampus*, **4**, 1–18.

Tulving, E. (1983) *Elements of Episodic Memory*. Oxford: Clarendon Press.

Worden, R. P. (1992) Navigation by fragment fitting: a theory of hippocampal function. *Hippocampus*, **2**, 165–88.

Zola-Morgan, S., Squire, L. R. and Amaral, D. G. (1986) Human amnesia and the medial temporal region: enduring memory impairment following a bilateral lesion limited to field CA1 of the hippocampus. *Journal of Neuroscience*, **6**, 2950–7.

8 Brain size, behavior and the allocation of neural space

DALE PURVES, LEONARD E. WHITE, DAKE ZHENG,
TIMOTHY J. ANDREWS AND DAVID R. RIDDLE

INTRODUCTION

Humans – and other animals – vary greatly in their talents and predispositions for a wide range of behaviors. A long-standing question in neurology and neurobiology concerns the relationship between the amount of brain substance devoted to the execution of a given behavior and the special abilities of individuals. Does a particular talent imply a greater amount of neural space in the service of that function? And if so, what are we to make of the manifest differences in the size of brains (or homologous brain regions) among species, among the members of a species, and even between the two hemispheres of a particular brain? The observations we review here explore a broad neurological principle that may apply to each of these circumstances: whether comparing the sides of an individual brain, the brains of different individuals, or the brains of different species, especially competent behavior is based on the development of a commensurately greater amount of relevant neural circuitry.

EARLY EFFORTS TO UNDERSTAND THE RELATIONSHIP BETWEEN PERFORMANCE AND NEURAL SPACE

Historically, the most popular approach to the issue of neural space and behavior has been to relate the absolute size of brains to a nominally broad index of performance, such as 'intelligence' tests in humans. This way of studying the relationship between brain space and behavior has caused considerable trouble. In general terms, the idea that the size of an animal's brain reflects its intelligence represents a simple and apparently valid idea. The ratio of brain weight to body weight for fish is 1 to 5000, for reptiles about 1 to 1500, for birds 1 to 220, for mammals 1 to 180 and for man 1 to 50 (Waller, 1891).* If intelligence is defined as the full scope of mental

---

* The ratio of brain and body size has itself generated a long-running controversy about how to interpret the fact that intelligence does not sort out strictly according to brain size. Whales and elephants have larger brains than humans; although these animals are very smart, they are not as intelligent as humans. This anomaly is conventionally explained by pointing out the need to refine the principle that bigger brains are better by factoring in body size (usually considered in terms of an 'encephalization quotient'; see Jerison, 1973).

performance, surely no one would dispute that a man is more intelligent than a mouse, or that this difference is explained in large part by the three-thousandfold difference in the size of the brains of these species. Does it follow, however, that relatively small differences in the size of brains among related species, strains, genders, or individuals are also a valid indication of mental abilities? Certainly no issue in neuroscience has provoked a more heated debate than the notion that alleged differences in brain size among races – or the demonstrable differences in brain size between men and women – engender differences in performance (see, for example, Gross, 1990; Maddox, 1992; Fausto-Sterling, 1993). The passion attending this controversy has been generated not only by the scientific issues involved, but equally, or perhaps predominantly, by the specter of racist or misogynist mischief.

Nineteenth-century enthusiasm for brain size as a simple metric of human performance was championed by some remarkably astute scientists (e.g. Galton, 1883, 1889; Broca 1861a, 1885), as well as others whose motives and methods are now suspect (e.g. Morton, 1849; see Gould, 1978 for an interesting commentary). Broca – one of the great neurologists of his day and a gifted observer – not only thought that brain size reflected intelligence, but was of the opinion (as was almost every other nineteenth-century scientist who considered the matter) that white European males had larger and better developed brains than anyone else (Broca, 1861a). Based on what was known about the human brain in the late nineteenth century, it was reasonable for him to consider it an organ comparable to the liver or the lung, that is, a structure having a largely homogenous function. Ironically, it was Broca himself who laid the groundwork for the modern view that the brain is a heterogeneous collection of highly interconnected but functionally discrete systems (Broca, 1861b). Nevertheless, the nineteenth-century approach to brain size and intelligence has persisted in some quarters (Rushton, 1991a; 1992; 1994). Using modern databases and statistical methods, the contemporary psychologist J. P. Rushton has also concluded that brain size differs among races, and that such measurements reflect differences in intelligence and other aspects of behavior such as reproductive strategy (Rushton, 1991b). Although Rushton's critics have generally sought to impeach him on ideological, political, or sociological grounds (see Gross, 1990; Maddox, 1992; Fausto-Sterling, 1993), his conclusions are equally dubious as neurobiology.

There are at least two reasons why measures such as brain weight (or cranial capacity) are not easily interpretable indices of intelligence (even though small observed differences may be statistically valid) (Figure 8.1). First is the obvious difficulty of defining and accurately measuring intelligence among animals, particularly among humans with different educational and cultural back-grounds. Second is the functional diversity and connectional complexity of the brain. Imagine assessing the relationship between body size and athletic ability, which might be considered the somatic analog of intelligence. Body

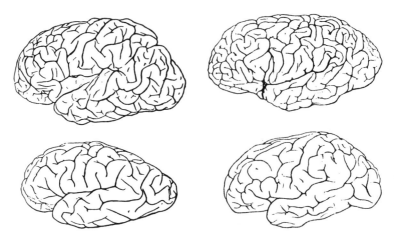

Figure 8.1. The brains of accomplished individuals were thought to be grossly larger than average by most late nineteenth-century neuroscientists. This drawing, taken from the work of E. Spitzka compares the brains of H. Helmholtz (upper left), and that of K. F. Gauss (upper right) to the brains of two unidentified individuals from 'primitive' cultures (a Papuan on the left, and a Bushwoman on the right). The opinion that individuals accomplished in a particular field have larger brains has never been confirmed by more extensive normative studies, and seems unlikely to be true in the light of present knowledge. (From Spitzka, 1907.)

weight, or any other global measure of somatic phenotype, would be a woefully inadequate index of athleticism. Although the evidence would presumably indicate that bigger is better in the context of sumo wrestling, more subtle somatic features would be correlated with extraordinary ability in ping pong, gymnastics or figure skating. The diversity of somatic function *vis-à-vis* athletic ability confounds the interpretation of any simple metric such as body size.

The implications of this analogy for the brain are straightforward. It makes no more sense to consider the brain as a whole with respect to its many functions than to consider a global measure of somatic development a useful predictor of performance in athletic endeavors. Any program that seeks to relate brain weight, cranial capacity or some other measure of overall brain size to individual performance ignores the reality of the brain's functional diversity. Thus, quite apart from the political or ethical probity of attempts to measure intelligence by brain size, by the yardstick of modern neuroscience – or just commonsense – this approach will inevitably generate more heat than light (see also Tobias, 1970).

This pessimistic conclusion should not, however, be taken to mean that macroscopic measurements of the brain have no value, or that they cannot be importantly related to human performance. Quite the contrary, making such measurements may be extraordinarily useful to the progress of modern neuroscience. In what follows, we argue that bigger is indeed better when this principle is applied to particular brain regions whose function can be surmised and related to a measurable behavior.

SPECIALIZED BEHAVIOR AND THE ALLOCATION OF NEURAL SPACE AMONG SPECIES

That extraordinary amounts of neural circuitry can, in this more limited sense, instantiate extraordinary performance is perhaps obvious when one considers how the specialized abilities of particular species are realized in brain structure. Comparisons across species show that special behavioral talents are invariably based on commensurately sophisticated brain circuitry, which means more neurons, more synapses, more supporting glial cells, and therefore the occupancy of more space in the brain.

In echolocating bats, for example, much of the cerebral cortex is allocated to the analysis of auditory information (Grinnell, 1963; Griffin, 1974). Indeed, a remarkably large fraction of the auditory cortex is devoted to processing the narrow range of signal frequencies used to navigate and locate prey (Suga & Jen, 1976; Suga & O'Neill, 1980; Suga, Kujisai & O'Neill, 1981; Suga, 1984). Similarly, the size of various representations in the primary somatic sensory and motor cortices reflects the nuances of a species' behavioral predilections regarding mechano-sensory discrimination and motor control. Thus, the representations of the hands are disproportionately large in the human and raccoon sensorimotor cortex (Penfield & Boldrey, 1937; Penfield & Rasmussen, 1950; Woolsey, 1958; Johnson, 1980), whereas many rodents devote a great deal of space in this region of the cortex to the representations of the mystacial vibrissae, specializations that are used by these largely nocturnal animals to move about in the dark (Woolsey & Van der Loos, 1970; Dawson & Killackey, 1987 – see also below) (Plate 8.1). By the same token, a large fraction of the somatic sensory cortex in the star-nosed mole is given over to the representation of the elaborate nasal appendages that provide a major source of mechano-sensory information for this subterranean animal (Catania, et al., 1993). Not surprisingly, when a species shows a particularly well developed behavior, a large fraction of the animal's brain is allocated to that task.

The relationship between behavioral competence and the allocation of space in the nervous system is equally apparent in the neural 'underrepresentation' evident in species in which a special ability has been lost (or never evolved). For instance, most subterranean rodents have limited visual abilities, since this sensory modality is of little use during a life spent almost entirely underground. In such animals (e.g. moles and mole-rats), the visual centers are markedly reduced in size compared to species that live above ground and therefore make more use of information conveyed by light (Burda, Bruns &

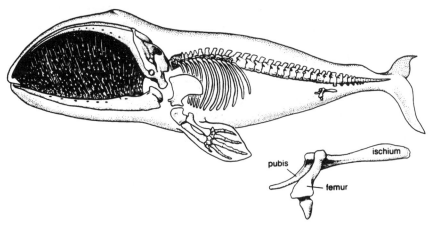

Figure 8.2. Rudimentary hindlimbs of a Greenland right whale (*Balaenoptera mysticetus*). Enlargement of the major bones is shown below. Somatic adaptations during the course of evolution are accompanied by commensurate decreases in the size of the corresponding regions of the nervous system, in this case the lumbar spinal cord. Such examples provide dramatic evidence that rudimentary behaviors are supported by correspondingly meager neural representations. (From Purves, 1988; after Romanes, 1895.)

Müller, 1990). Another example is the absence of significant olfactory ability in cetaceans, which have rudimentary olfactory nerves and olfactory bulbs (Jacobs, McFarland & Morgane, 1979). Similarly, the loss of the hindlimbs in the evolution of aquatic mammals is reflected in the decreased size of the lumbar enlargement of the spinal cord (Figure 8.2) (Morgane & Jacobs, 1972). The cortical (and subcortical) 'overrepresentation' of extraordinary talents – and the 'underrepresentation' of vestigial behaviors – underscores the general principle that specialized functions entail the allocation of a corresponding amount of neural space.

SPECIALIZED BEHAVIOR AND THE ALLOCATION OF NEURAL SPACE WITHIN A SPECIES

The relationship between behavior and the allocation of neural space suggested by these phylogenetic examples may be equally pertinent to the neural basis of differential behavior among individual members of a species. Just as extraordinary abilities of different species are reflected in a disproportionate allocation of the relevant neural circuitry, the idiosyncratic talents and behavioral predilections of individuals seem likely to be realized in a greater – or lesser – amount of related neural space.

A fundamental question in this regard is whether there are substantial differences in the size of well-defined neural regions. An indication of variability in the human brain has been provided by physicians interested in determining, for clinical purposes, the location of brain regions devoted to a particularly important function. For example, when a portion of the brain is to be removed, the neurosurgeon must meticulously delineate regions which, if damaged, would leave the patient with a significant deficit. One such region is that devoted to language in the left hemisphere of right-handed (and most left-handed) patients. Careful electrophysiological mapping of such cortical representations during surgery performed under local anesthesia shows a great deal of variation in the arrangement of the language areas in different individuals (Ojemann, 1983). A similar degree of variability has been reported in the human somatosensory and motor cortices (Penfield & Boldrey, 1937; Penfield & Rasmussen, 1950; Woolsey, Erickson & Gilson, 1979), as well as in visual cortex (Stensaas, Eddington & Dobelle, 1974).

Inter-individual variation in the regional allocation of brain space has been amply confirmed by more detailed experimental work on sub-human primates. Thus, there are often marked differences among individual monkeys in the extent of the primary visual cortex and other visual areas (Van Essen, Maunsell & Bixby, 1981; Van Essen, Newsome & Maunsell, 1984; LaMantia & Purves, 1993). Careful mapping of the cortical areas that subserve particular somatosensory modalities in the monkey has also shown substantial variation in the arrangement of the same functions from animal to animal (Figure 8.3; Merzenich, 1985; Merzenich et al., 1987). Nor is such variation limited to primates: differences in the size of the major somatic representations in the rat primary somatosensory cortex can be as much as twofold to threefold (Riddle & Purves, 1995).

In short, relating the size of well-defined cortical (or subcortical) regions to specific sensory or motor abilities is a much more plausible goal than relating overall brain size to the limited and ill-defined abilities assessed by 'intelligence' tests.

SPECIALIZED BEHAVIOR AND THE ALLOCATION OF NEURAL SPACE IN THE TWO HEMISPHERES OF INDIVIDUAL BRAINS

Another context in which to explore the proposition that extraordinary performance is based on the allocation of a correspondingly greater amount of neural space is a comparison of the right and left cerebral hemispheres in an individual brain. Neurologists and neurobiologists have known for more than a century that the two hemispheres of the human cerebral cortex are similar but not identical. Functional asymmetry of the hemispheres was first noted by Broca when he observed that lesions of the left frontal cortex often cause severe language dysfunction, whereas lesions of the right hemisphere usually do not (Broca, 1861b; 1885; see also Berker, Berke & Smith, 1986).

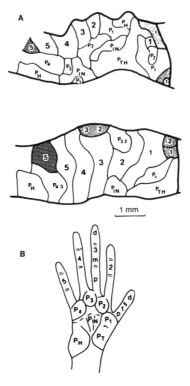

Figure 8.3. Regions of the somatosensory cortex responding to tactile stimulation of the hand in two different squirrel monkeys. (A) These maps were made by recording the location of electrical responses in the cortex evoked by stimulating various parts of the contralateral hand. (B) Regions on the palmar surface that elicited the responses are indicated in the cortical maps (the stippled sectors in A represent responses to touching the dorsal surface of the hand). Variations of this magnitude among different individuals of the same species were typical of the other monkeys examined in the study. (After Merzenich et al., 1987.)

More recent studies have directly confirmed the lateralization of language functions (Sperry, 1982), and have identified a corresponding structural asymmetry of the superior aspect of the posterior temporal lobes (Geschwind & Levitsky, 1968; Wada, Clarke & Hamm, 1975). Despite these intriguing observations, language, which is an extraordinarily complex behavior, has proven difficult to relate more specifically to cortical regions that can be reliably measured.

An alternative domain in which to explore the relationship of cerebral space to human behavior is handedness – the most obvious and arguably the simplest lateralized behavior in man. Approximately nine out of 10 of us are right-handed, a proportion that appears to have been stable over thousands of years and across all cultures in which handedness has been examined (Coren & Porac, 1977; Coren, 1992). This consistency allows one to ask whether handedness, an apparently straightforward model of preferred behavior, is based on the asymmetrical elaboration of neural centers devoted to the representation of the favored limb.*

In order to explore the neurological basis of hand preference, we measured the somatic and neural structures most clearly related to handedness, starting with the hands themselves (Purves, White & Andrews, 1994). The reason for beginning with this simple determination is the well-established link between peripheral somatic structures and corresponding neural centers: the size of neural representations and their constituent nerve cells generally reflects the amount of peripheral machinery that such centers must monitor and motivate (reviewed in Purves, Snider & Voyvodic, 1988; Purves, 1988, 1994). Accordingly, we solicited a group of right-handed adults and measured the hands of each subject by an easy water displacement technique. Among right-handers, the right hand was consistently larger than the left, the average difference being 3.5% (Figure 8.4).†

The larger size of the right hand (and presumably the entire right upper limb) among right-handers suggested that there might be some asymmetry of the related neural apparatus. We therefore proceeded to examine the extent of the cortical surface within the central sulcus of each cerebral hemisphere. The central sulcus is formed by the pre- and post-central gyri, which contain the primary motor and somatosensory representations of the contralateral body (Penfield & Boldrey, 1937; Penfield & Rasmussen, 1950; Woolsey, 1958; Woolsey et al., 1979). The portion of the central sulcus in the dorsolateral convexity of the hemisphere harbors the sensorimotor representations of the upper extremity in most individuals (Figure 8.5). Our initial measurements in 22 brains suggested that the primary sensori-motor representation of the upper extremity is on average larger in the left hemisphere (which controls the right hand) (White et al., 1994). A more detailed cytoarchitectonic study of additional brains, however, showed no significant lateral difference in the amount of primary sensory or motor cortex in the region of the hand representation (L. White et al., unpublished). Nor were any lateral differences apparent at the level of the medullary pyramids or the cervical enlargement of the spinal cord (Andrews et al., unpublished).

---

* Although several anatomical observations have been correlated with handedness, these have not been proposed as an explanation of manual bias. For example, the corpus callosum has been reported to be larger in left-handers than right-handers (Witelson, 1985; Habib, 1989), and the horizontal segment of the Sylvian fissure is larger in right-handed men (Witelson & Kigar, 1992).

† The larger size of the right hand among right-handers presumably arises at least in part by differential use. Nevertheless, not all measurements of somatic asymmetry support the view that lateral differences develop in this manner (Garn, Mayor & Shaw, 1976; Plato, Wood & Norris, 1980; Holt, 1968).

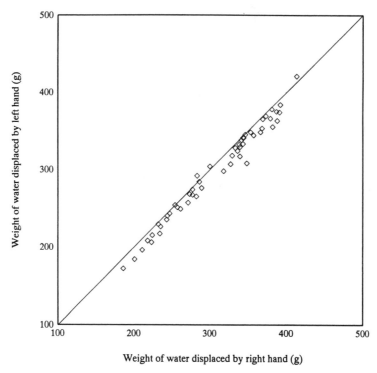

Figure 8.4. Hand size asymmetry among right-handers. Graph showing left-hand water displacement plotted against right-hand displacement for 52 right-handed subjects; the diagonal line represents perfect symmetry. For most individuals, the right hand is larger than the left (mean percentage difference = 3.5%). (From Purves et al., 1994.)

THE ALLOCATION OF NEURAL SPACE DURING DEVELOPMENT

The idea that behavioral predilections are realized in a disproportionate allocation of neural circuitry raises the question of how brain space is determined in the course of development. To a predominant degree, this distribution must occur according to an intrinsic developmental plan, the rules of which have evolved to suit the needs of each species. In some measure, however, the allocation of neural space seems likely to be influenced by experience and practice, which have such obvious effects on the outcome of development (reviewed in Purves & Lichtman, 1985; Purves, 1988, 1994). An attractive hypothesis in this regard is that experience modulates brain growth, causing the more active regions of the brain to grow relatively more than the less active ones. Since brain growth ultimately slows and then ceases, this consequence of experience would permanently affect the ultimate allocation of neural space.

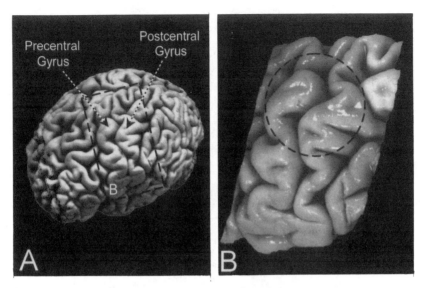

Figure 8.5. The human central sulcus, indicating the region of the hand representation. (A) Superficial appearance of the left hemisphere in an intact brain; the photograph was taken at an oblique angle roughly orthogonal to the dorsolateral convexity of the cerebrum. (B) Photograph of the pre- and post-central gyri after isolation from the rest of the brain shown in A. The region of the hand representation is marked by the dotted circle.

It is obvious, but not often remarked upon, that the brains of mammals, including humans, increase gradually and progressively in size during the postnatal period (Figure 8.6) (see, for example, Pakkenberg & Voight, 1964; Dekaban & Sadowsky, 1978; Pomeroy, LaMantia & Purves, 1990). Ideally, the analysis of the growth of functionally discrete cortical regions should proceed in humans; however, the logistics of such studies make this aim a difficult one. Fortunately, in some rodents the primary somatic sensory cortex (S1) can be visualized and measured with sufficient precision to analyze the pattern of growth in this region of the brain (Riddle et al., 1992). Comparison of juvenile and adult brains shows that the postnatal growth of the rat cortex is surprisingly heterogeneous (Plate 8.2). For example, S1 barrels – the functional units in cortical layer IV that represent special sensors such as whiskers and digital pads – grow about twice as much postnatally as the intervening cortex. Moreover, 'overrepresented' areas within the somatotopic map, such as the head representation, grow more than 'underrepresented' areas, such as the paw regions. Thus, although a disproportionate allocation of neural circuitry is already present at the first appearance of the S1 map within the first few days of postnatal life, such differences are augmented during postnatal growth.

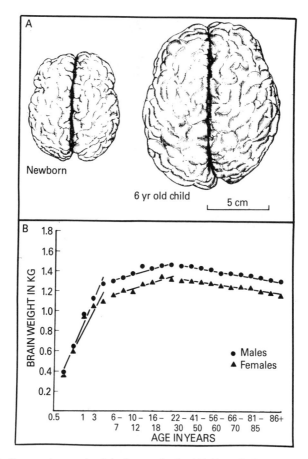

Figure 8.6. Postnatal growth of the human brain. (A) Dorsal view of a normal brain at birth (left) and at age 6 years (right). (B) The duration of human brain growth (according to brain weight). The growth of the brain (here based on 2603 neurologically normal subjects) continues for a decade or more. (From Purves, 1994; (A) after Conel, 1939–67; (B) after Dekaban and Sadowsky, 1978.)

Are the cortical regions that grow the most in fact the most active? To answer this question, we assessed the regional metabolic and electrical activity of the developing rat brain by measuring the distribution of mitochondrial enzymes, Na^+/K^+ ATPase (which reflects ion pumping), microvessel density, electrical activity and 2-deoxyglucose uptake (Riddle et al., 1993).* By each of these techniques, systematic variations in the average levels

---

* Since most of the energy demand on neurons is generated by synaptic signaling, local levels of energy metabolism reflect regional differences in the brain's electrical activity (Ingvar & Lassen, 1975; Sokoloff, 1977; Mata et al., 1980; Yarowsky & Ingvar, 1981).

of neural activity across the cortex correlated well with regional patterns of differential postnatal cortical growth (Plate 8.3 and Riddle et al., 1993).

The relationship between enhanced neural activity and increased growth in normal development does not, however, demonstrate a causal link between these phenomena. We therefore asked whether cortical growth is increased by an experimental augmentation of neural activity, as might occur normally by use (practice) during development. Previous studies in rodents had shown that the growth of one neural system (e.g. the primary somatic sensory cortex) can be enhanced by impairing the function of a different modality (e.g. vision) (Rauschecker et al., 1990; Bronchti et al., 1992; Gelhard, Tian & Rauschecker, 1993). Thus, eye removal at birth induces an enlargement of the cortical modules and neurons that represent the mystacial vibrissae. We confirmed that individual barrels in the rat whisker pad representation are consistently larger in enucleated rats compared to the corresponding barrels in littermate controls (Zheng & Purves, 1995) (Figure 8.7A).

Next we asked whether this experimental expansion of S1 and its component parts is associated with increased neural activity. Blood vessel density in S1 and the surrounding cortex was measured to assess the activity in those cortical regions with enhanced growth following enucleation (see Plate 8.3). The average vascular density in S1 was indeed higher in the enucleated rats; moreover, the increase was limited to barrels – the regions of greatest growth (Figure 8.7B). Neither microvessel density nor the growth of the non-barrel S1 and interbarrel cortex were significantly different in the experimental and control animals.

The observation that postnatal growth is greatest in the most active cortical regions, and that enucleation enhances both the activity and growth of S1, provides additional evidence that increased levels of neural activity promote the growth of neural circuitry in the developing brain. Such modulation of brain growth by activity during postnatal maturation may explain how the effects of early experience are stored in the nervous system.

CONCLUSION

The historical enthusiasm for the idea that overall brain size is a valid measure of 'intelligence' is simplistic and ultimately untenable. It is, however, possible to relate disproportionate allocations of neural space to specific behaviors in more limited domains. A wealth of comparative evidence shows that animals exhibiting an especially well-developed behavior invariably reflect that talent in the amount of corresponding neural circuitry. Although largely determined by phylogeny, the amount of space devoted to a particular behavior is evidently modulated by activity during ontogeny, such that the effects of early experience are stably encoded in the adult nervous system.

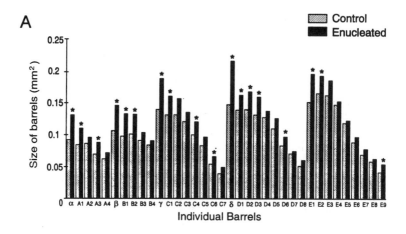

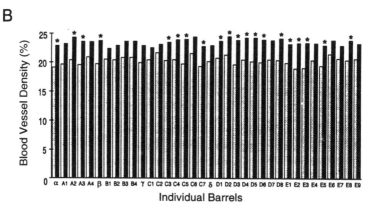

Figure 8.7. Correlation of chronic regional differences in neural activity and cortical growth in the somatic sensory cortex of rats enucleated since birth. (A) Blood vessel density in each of the whisker pad barrels in normal and enucleated rats. (B) Size of each of the whisker pad barrels in normal and enucleated rats. Both vascular density and growth are augmented in the experimental animals compared to littermate controls, implying that chronically increased activity during development foments cortical growth. (From Zheng and Purves, 1995.)

REFERENCES

Berker, E. A., Berke, A. H. & Smith, A. (1986) Translation of Broca's 1885 report: localization of speech in the third left frontal convolution. *Archives of Neurology*, **43**, 1065–72.

Broca, P. (1861a) Sur le volume et la forme du cerveau suivant les individus et suivant les races. *Bulletins et Memoires de la Societe Anthropologie de Paris*, **2**, 139–207, 301–22.

Broca, P. (1861b) Remarques sur le siege de la faculte du langage articule, suivies d'une observation d'aphemie. *Bull. Soc. Anat. Paris, 2nd Series*, **6**, 398–407.

Bronchti, G., Schönenberger, N., Welker, E. & Van der Loos, H. (1992) Barrelfield expansion after neonatal eye removal in mice. *NeuroReport*, **3**, 489–92.

Burda, H., Bruns, V. & Müller, M. (1990) Sensory adaptations in subterranean mammals. In Nevo, E. & Reig, O. A. (eds.) *Evolution of Subterranean Mammals at the Organismal and Molecular Levels*. New York: Wiley-Liss, pp. 269–93.

Catania, K. C., Northcutt, R. G., Kaas, J. H. & Beck, P. D. (1993) Nose stars and brain stripes. *Nature*, **364**, 493.

Conel, J. L. (1939–67) *The Postnatal Development of the Human Cerebral Cortex. Vols 1–8*. Cambridge: Harvard University Press.

Coren, S. (1992) *The Left-Hander Syndrome: The Causes and Consequences of Left-Handedness*. New York: The Free Press.

Coren, S. & Porac, C. (1977) Fifty centuries of right-handedness: the historical record. *Science*, **198**, 631–2.

Corsi, P. (ed.) (1991) *The Enchanted Loom: Chapters in the History of Neuroscience*. New York: Oxford University Press.

Dawson, D. R. & Killackey, H. P. (1987) The organization and mutability of the forepaw and hindpaw representations in the somatosensory cortex of neonatal rat. *Journal of Comparative Neurology*, **256**, 246–56.

Dekaban, A. S. & Sadowsky, D. (1978) Changes in brain weights during the span of human life: relation of brain weight to body heights and body weights. *Annals of Neurology*, **4**, 345–56.

Fausto-Sterling, A. (1993) Sex, race, brains and calipers. *Discover*, **14**, 32–7.

Galton, F. (1883) *Inquiries into Human Faculty and its Development*. London: Macmillan.

Galton, F. (1889) *Natural Inheritance*. London: Macmillan.

Garn, S. M., Mayor, G. H. & Shaw, H. A. (1976) Paradoxical bilateral asymmetry in bone size and bone mass in the hand. *American Journal of Physical Anthropology*, **45**, 209–10.

Gelhard, R., Tian, B. & Rauschecker, J. P. (1993) Increased soma size underlies compensatory expansion of whisker barrels in somatosensory cortex of neonatally enucleated mice. *Society of Neuroscience Abstracts*, **23**, 47.

Geschwind, N. & Levitsky, W. (1968) Human brain: left-right asymmetries in temporal speech region. *Science*, **161**, 186–7.

Gould, S. J. (1978) Morton's ranking of races by cranial capacity. *Science*, **200**, 503–9.

Griffin, D. R. (1974) *Listening in the Dark: the Acoustic Orientation of Bats and Men*. New York: Dover Publications.

Grinnell, A. D. (1963) The neurophysiology of audition in bats. *Journal of Physiology (London)*, **167**, 38–127.

Gross, B. R. (1990) The case of Phillipe Rushton. *Academic Questions*, **3**, 35–46.

Habib, M. (1989) Anatomical asymmetries of the human cerebral cortex. *International Journal of Neuroscience*, **47**, 67–79.

Holt, S. B. (1968) *The Genetics of Dermal Ridges*. Springfield: Charles C. Thomas.

Ingvar, D. H. & Lassen, N. A. (eds.) (1975) Brain work 1: the coupling of function metabolism and blood flow in the brain. *Proceedings of the Alfred Benzon Symposium*. Copenhagen: Munksgaard.

Jacobs, M. S., McFarland, W. L. & Morgane, P. J. (1979) The anatomy of the brain of the bottlenose dolphin (*Tursiops truncatus*). Rhinic lobe (rhinen-cephalon): the archicortex. *Brain Research Bulletin*, **4** (suppl. 1), 1–108.

Jerison, H. J. (1973) *Evolution of the Brain and Intelligence*. New York: Academic Press.

Johnson, J. I., Jr. (1980) Morphological correlates of specialized elaborations in somatic sensory cerebral cortex. In Ebbesson, S. O. E. (ed.) *Comparative Neurology of the Telencephalon*. New York: Plenum Press, pp. 423–47.

LaMantia, A.-S. & Purves, D. (1993) Development of blobs in the visual cortex of macaques. *Journal of Comparative Neurology*, **334**, 169–75.

Maddox, J. (1992) How to publish the unpalatable? *Nature*, **358**, 187.

Mata, M., Fink, D. J., Gainer, H., Smith, C. B., Davidsen, L., Savaki, H., Scwarts, W. J. & Sokoloff, L. (1980) Activity-dependent energy metabolism in rat posterior pituitary primarily reflects sodium pump activity. *Journal of Neurochemistry*, **34**, 213–15.

Merzenich, M. M. (1985) Sources of intraspecies and interspecies cortical map variability in mammals: Conclusions and hypotheses. In Cohen, M. J. & Strumwasser, F. (eds.) *Comparative Neurobiology: Modes of Communication in the Nervous System*, New York: John Wiley, pp. 105–16.

Merzenich, M. M., Nelson, R. J., Kaas, J. H., Stryker, M. P., Jenkins, W. M., Zook, J. M., Cynader, M. S. & Schoppmann, A. (1987) Variability in hand surface representations in areas 3b and 1 in adult owl and squirrel monkeys. *Journal of Comparative Neurology*, **258**, 281–96.

Morgane, P. J. & Jacobs, M. S. (1972) Comparative anatomy of the cetacean nervous system. In Harrison, R. J. (ed.) *Functional Anatomy of Marine Mammals*. New York: Academic Press pp. 117–244.

Morton, S. G. (1849) Observations on the size of the brain in various races and families of man. *Proceedings of the National Academy of Natural Science of the USA*, **4**, 221–4.

Ojemann, G. A. (1983) Brain organization for language from the perspective of electrical stimulation mapping. *Behavioral Brain Science*, **2**, 189–230.

Pakkenberg, H. & Voight, J. (1964) Brain weight of the Danes. *Acta. Anat.* **56**, 297–307.

Penfield, W. & Boldrey, E. (1937) Somatic motor and sensory representation in the cerebral cortex of man as studied by electrical stimulation. *Brain*, **60**, 389–443.

Penfield, W. & Rasmussen, T. (1950) Sensorimotor representation of the body. In *The Cerebral Cortex of Man: A Clinical Study of Localization of Function*. New York: Macmillan, pp. 12–65.

Plato, C. C., Wood, J. L. & Norris, A. H. (1980) Bilateral asymmetry in bone measurements of the hand and lateral hand dominance. *American Journal of Physical Anthropology*, **52**, 27–31.

Pomeroy, S. L., LaMantia, A.-S. & Purves, D. (1990) Postnatal construction of neural circuitry in the mouse olfactory bulb. *Journal of Neuroscience*, **10**, 1952–66.

Purves, D. (1988) *Body and Brain: A Trophic Theory of Neural Connections*. Cambridge: Harvard University Press.

Purves, D. (1994) *Neural Activity and the Growth of the Brain*. Cambridge: Cambridge University Press.

Purves, D. & Lichtman, J. W. (1985) *Principles of Neural Development*. Sunderland: Sinauer Associates, Inc.

Purves, D., Snider, W. D. & Voyvodic, J. T. (1988) Trophic regulation of nerve cell morphology and innervation in the autonomic nervous system. *Nature*, **336**, 123–8.

Purves, D., White, L. E. & Andrews, T. J. (1994) Manual asymmetry and handedness. *Proceedings of the National Academy of Science of the USA*, **91**, 5030–2.

Rauschecker, J. P., Tian, B., Korte, M. & Egert, U. (1990) Crossmodal changes in the somatosensory vibrissa/barrel system of visually deprived animals. *Proceedings of the National Academy of Science of the USA*, **89**, 5063–7.

Riddle, D., Richards, A., Zsuppan, F. & Purves, D. (1992) Growth of the rat somatic sensory cortex and its constituent parts during postnatal development. *Journal of Neuroscience*, **12**, 3509–24.

Riddle, D. R., Gutierrez, G., Zheng, D., White, L., Richards, A. & Purves, D. (1993) Differential metabolic and electrical activity in the somatic sensory cortex of the developing rat. *Journal of Neuroscience*, **13**, 4193–213.

Riddle, D. R. & Purves, D. (1995) Individual variation and lateral asymmetry of the rat primary somatosensory cortex. *Journal of Neuroscience*, **15**, 4184–4195.

Romanes, G. J. (1895) *Darwin and After Darwin*. London: Open Court Publishing Co.

Rushton, J.-P. (1991a) Do r-K strategies underlie human race differences? A reply to Weizmann et al. *Canadian Psychology*, **32**, 29–42.

Rushton, J.-P. (1991b) Mongoloid-Caucasoid differences in brain size from military samples. *Intelligence*, **15**, 351–9.

Rushton, J.-P. (1992) Cranial capacity related to sex, rank and race in a stratified random sample of 6,325 US Military personnel. *Intelligence*, **16**, 401–13.

Rushton, J.-P. (1994) Sex and race differences in cranial capacity from International Labour Office data. *Intelligence*, **19**, 281–94.

Sokoloff, L. (1977) Relation between physiological function and energy metabolism in the central nervous system. *Journal of Neurochemistry*, **29**, 13–26.

Sperry, R. W. (1982) Some effects of disconnecting the cerebral hemispheres. *Science*, **217**, 1223–6.

Spitzka, E. A. (1907) A study of the brains of six eminent scientists and scholars belonging to the American Anthropometric Society, together with a description of the skull of Professor E. D. Cope. *Transactions of the American Philosophical Society*, **21**, 175–308.

Stensaas, S. S., Eddington, D. K. & Dobelle, W. H. (1974) The topography and variability of the primary visual cortex in man. *Journal of Neurosurgery*, **40**, 747–55.

Suga, N. (1984) Neural mechanisms of complex-sound processing for echolocation. *Trends in Neuroscience*, **7**, 20–7.

Suga, N. & Jen, P. H.-S. (1976) Disproportionate tonotopic representation for processing species specific CF-FM sonar signals in the mustache bat auditory cortex. *Science*, **194**, 542–4.

Suga, N., Kujisai, K. & O'Neill, W. E. (1981) Biosonar information is represented in the bat cerebral cortex. In Syka, J. & Aitken, L. (eds.) *Neural Mechanisms of Hearing*. New York: Plenum, pp. 197–219.

Suga, N. & O'Neill, W. E. (1980) Auditory processing of echoes: Representation of acoustic information from the environment in the bat cerebral cortex. In Busnel, R. G. & Fish, J. F. (eds.) *Animal Sonar Systems*. New York: Plenum, pp. 589–611.

Tobias, P. V. (1970) Brain size, grey matter and race – fact or fiction? *American Journal of Physical Anthropology*, **32**, 3–25.

Topinard, L. D. P. (1885) Chapter. In A. Delahaye & E. Lecrosnier (eds.) *Elements d'Anthropologie Generale*. Paris, p. 591.

Van Essen, D. C., Maunsell, J. H. R. & Bixby, J. L. (1981) The middle temporal visual area in the macaque: Myeloarchitecture, connections, functional properties and topographic organization. *Journal of Comparative Neurology*, **199**, 293–326.

Van Essen, D. C., Newsome, W. T. & Maunsell, J. H. R. (1984) The visual field representation in striate cortex of the macaque monkey: Asymmetries, anisotropies, and individual variability. *Vision Research*, **24**, 429–48.

Wada, J. A., Clarke, R. & Hamm, A. (1975) Cerebral hemispheric asymmetry in humans: cortical speech zones in 100 adult and 100 infant brains. *Archives of Neurology*, **32**, 239–46.

Waller, A. D. (1891) *Human Physiology*. London: Longmans, Green.

White, L., Lucas, G., Richards, A. & Purves, D. (1994) Cerebral asymmetry and handedness. *Nature*, **263**, 197–9.

Witelson, S. F. (1985) The brain connection: the corpus callosum is larger in left-handers. *Science*, **229**, 665–8.

Witelson, S. F. & Kigar, D. L. (1992) Sylvian fissure morphology and asymmetry in men and women: Bilateral differences in relation to handedness in men. *Journal of Comparative Neurology*, **323**, 326–40.

Woolsey, C. N. (1958) Organization of somatic sensory and motor areas of the cerebral cortex. In Harlow, H. F. & Woolsey, C. N. (eds.) *Biological and Biochemical Bases of Behavior*. Madison, Wisc.: University of Wisconsin Press, pp. 63–82.

Woolsey, C. N., Erickson, T. C. & Gilson, W. E. (1979) Localization in somatic sensory and motor areas of human cerebral cortex as determined by direct recording of evoked potentials and electrical stimulation. *Journal of Neurosurgery*, **51**, 476–506.

Woolsey, T. A. & Van der Loos, H. (1970) The structural organization of layer 4 in the somatic sensory region (SI) of mouse cerebral cortex. *Brain Research*, **17**, 205–42.

Yarowsky, P. J. & Ingvar, D. H. (1981) Symposium summary. Neuronal activity and energy metabolism. *Federation Proceedings*, **40**, 2353–62.

Zheng, D. & Purves, D. (1995) The effects of increased neural activity on brain growth. *Proceedings of the National Academy of Science of the USA*, **92**, 1802–1806.

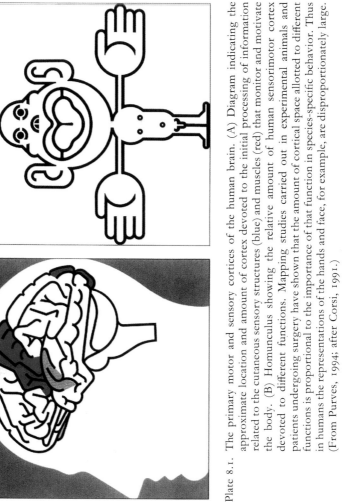

Plate 8.1. The primary motor and sensory cortices of the human brain. (A) Diagram indicating the approximate location and amount of cortex devoted to the initial processing of information related to the cutaneous sensory structures (blue) and muscles (red) that monitor and motivate the body. (B) Homunculus showing the relative amount of human sensorimotor cortex devoted to different functions. Mapping studies carried out in experimental animals and patients undergoing surgery have shown that the amount of cortical space allotted to different functions is proportional to the importance of that function in species-specific behavior. Thus in humans the representations of the hands and face, for example, are disproportionately large. (From Purves, 1994; after Corsi, 1991.)

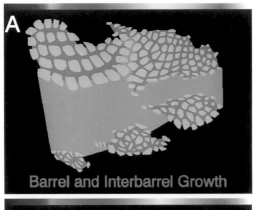

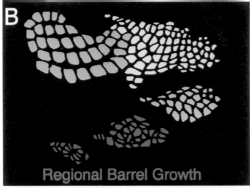

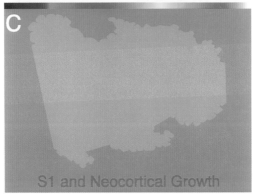

Plate 8.2. Differential pattern of postnatal growth in the primary somatic sensory cortex of the rat. The average amount of postnatal growth (represented here as the percentage increase in area from 1 to 10 weeks of age) is color coded for each region; warmer colors indicate greater growth. Barrels grow more than other areas of S1 (A), barrels in the head representations grow more than those in the paw representation (B), and S1 as a whole grows more than the surrounding cortex (C). (From Riddle et al., 1993.)

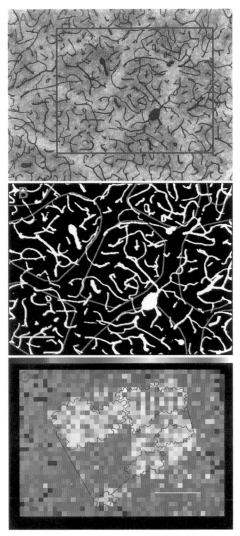

Plate 8.3. Microvessel distribution in and around the rat primary somatic sensory cortex. (A) Photomicrograph of ink-filled microvessels and barrels (revealed by cyto-chrome oxidase staining) in the anterior snout representation. (B) Digitized and processed image of microvessel profiles in (A); red lines indicate barrel borders. Such images were used to measure microvessel density in the barrel and interbarrel regions of S1. Scale bar = 100 μm. (C) Distribution of microvessel density in layer IV of the primary somatic sensory cortex of a representative juvenile rat. Microvessel density across S1 as a whole was determined by sequential analysis of 1400 in 200 × 200 μm squares; the density of each square was converted to gray levels from 1 to 255, color coded, and then projected onto a map of the S1 barrels reconstructed from the same sections. Scale bar = 2 mm. (From Riddle et al., 1993.)

9 Commentary **Selection and development: the brain as a complex system**

G. M. EDELMAN AND G. TONONI

What differentiates developing systems from those following orderly physical laws, such as crystals and dilute gases? And, in particular, what developmental properties do brains have that can give rise to motor, sensory, and cognitive behavior of a high order? In this brief paper we want to consider some of these properties. We shall focus on selection and a particular kind of complexity as essential. Our goal will be to hint at how functional segregation of parts can coexist with integration of the whole without any need to invoke direct information transfer from genes or the world, or any detailed explicit program in which computation occurs.

GENERAL LESSONS OF DEVELOPMENT

Since Darwin, evolutionists have known that there is an intimate relationship between animal form, animal behavior, and the workings of the mind. This relationship is perhaps most evident in the study of the development of the nervous system. The understanding of such development must account not only for the morphological characteristics of the brain, but also for the ability to learn and for the emergence of behavioral and cognitive patterns. In the perceptual and in the motor domain, respectively, Gestalts (Wertheimer, 1923) and gestures (Bernstein, 1967) bear the hallmarks of form. Finally, form and function are inextricably linked in the working of the brain and they are subject together to natural selection. It is therefore not surprising that, in discussing the development of morphology, one encounters many principles that are essential for the understanding of the mind.

Whenever the most classic of the questions concerning development is asked – that of the relative contribution of nature versus nurture – the inevitable answer seems to be that the truth lies somewhere in between. Yet an answer partly in terms of nature, partly in terms of nurture, is deeply unsatisfactory. As we will argue, there is no simple apportionment of genetic determinism on one side and environmental instructions on the other that can explain the development of brain and mind.

Genetic determinism assumes that genes directly control development, morphology, and behavior and that the genome as a whole contains a program for development. Development, in this view, would be purely a process of programmed maturation, contaminated perhaps occasionally by a certain amount of noise. This notion is often coupled to the idea that maturation goes through discrete stages that are also specified by the genome. Molecular genetics and embryology have shown, however, that development, like evolution, is both multiply determined and degenerate (Edelman, 1988). Development is epigenetic: many different components have to come together at the right place at the right time, and in the right proportions. Conversely, as shown dramatically by gene knock-out experiments, a biological organism can often develop quite normally without some genetic ingredient considered to be essential in the adult, presumably because several regulatory loops can self-adjust in a redundant fashion. This is just another example of the fact that, in a system composed of multiple interacting elements and loops, it is generally not possible to assign control to any one variable in isolation (Ashby, 1966), except on rare occasions. Moreover, there is also very little evidence to support the idea that the genome contains any information 'coding' directly for a precise sequence of events. On the contrary, the sequence of gene activation in development is the result of temporal and spatial interactions that are context-dependent (Edelman, 1988). The insistence on the demarcation of discrete stages of motor or cognitive development, each supposed to correspond to specific structural constructs (Piaget, 1980), has also been criticized (Thelen & Smith, 1994). Indeed, attempts to impose the observer's perspective, whether it is a staged structural order onto developmental processes (Piaget, 1980), a universal grammar onto language (Chomsky, 1986), or universal problem solving capabilities onto the workings of the mind (Newell & Simon, 1972), all ignore the importance of natural selection and epigenetic development. Unlike biological systems themselves, they all fail when forced to confront the variability of the fine structure and function of the brain and the ambiguity and novelty of an 'unlabelled' environment (Edelman, 1987). Indeed, the world of stimuli encountered by a newborn animal cannot be described adequately as pre-existing, unambiguous information. Although the real stimulus world certainly obeys the laws of physics, it is not uniquely partitioned into 'objects' and 'events' (Smith & Medin, 1981).

The alternative view, *environmental instructionism*, according to which the instructions do not come from the genome but from the outside world, is also fraught with problems. A recent version of such 'tabula rasa' environmental determinism has reappeared in the so-called neural-network community. To account for learning, there has been an attempt to devise general purpose algorithms which, if implemented on a generic architecture, would enable it to solve any sort of problem, that is acquire any sort of knowledge. Solutions to problems would thus be obtained by universal means that consist essentially of a search through a very high-dimensional space and require no additional constraints. As discussed elsewhere (Reeke & Edelman, 1988), many of these approaches can be discounted on the grounds that they are based on supervised learning strategies. They assume the existence of an instructor or teacher who already knows the answers (the correct outputs), or who carefully selects and precategorizes the sets of inputs to be used during training.

Yet other, so-called unsupervised approaches to neural network learning, assume that learning is possible provided that a suitable algorithm is used to extract the statistical structure of the inputs. In this sense, these methods represent a particular implementation of statistical procedures of nonparametric inference. When this has been recognized (Geman, Bienenstock & Doursat, 1992), it has been pointed out that these approaches are susceptible to the so-called bias/variance dilemma: in all of these procedures, either there must be a strong bias, such as a set of constraints that limit the search in parameter space, or, for all practical purposes, there will never be sufficient time or precision to determine the statistical regularities in a set of inputs. Despite some success in tasks in which the training set was carefully prepared, such general purpose learning algorithms do not appear to be able to achieve satisfactory performance in real-world problems, such as learning how to walk, to recognize objects, and to speak. It is becoming apparent that a major part of the problem in all these cases is to discover an appropriate set of biases or constraints. *Pari passu*, it is also slowly being recognized that this is exactly what natural selection has done, over millions of years. It follows that it is essential to study and try to understand all of those constraints that manifest themselves in the ontogenesis of the brain, i.e. to study the lessons of development.

In marked contrast to instructionist theories such as genetic determinism, tabula rasa environmentalism, or any compromise struck between the two, our view is that two quite different processes are required to account for how development gives rise to morphology and mind. These two processes are epigenesis and selection.

The *epigenetic* nature of development implies the coexistence of both regularities and variability. Genetic constraints and place-dependent inter-actions are responsible for the relative constancy of the macroscopic structure and of many microscopic features of organisms. Yet development is not the precise unfolding of a genetic program. Rather, it necessarily entails a large amount of individual variability, especially at the microscopic level. In the brain, this variability is not merely noise, but is the prerequisite source of diversity for the subsequent process of neural selection. *Neural selection*, like clonal selection in the immune system, occurs during the lifetime of the organism. Both neural and clonal selection represent effective strategies, discovered through natural selection, through which higher vertebrates can adapt to a world full of novelty and change at a timescale that natural selection itself could not negotiate directly. Thus, epigenetic events are considered to be a source of both regularity and variability, while neural selection is seen as the main process through which the functioning of the brain can be rapidly matched to short-term regularities in the environment that are unpredictable in the timescale of natural selection. The two processes are strictly coupled, at many different levels: epigenetic aspects of the structure and functioning of the nervous system significantly constrain or bias the kind of adaptations that neural selection can bring about.

This view of the development of brain and mind has been framed in the context of a global theory of the functioning of the nervous system, called the theory of neuronal group selection (Edelman, 1978; Edelman, 1987; Edelman, 1993). This developmental theory explains regularity at the macro level as a result of epigenetic processes, emphasizes variability at the micro-level as a substrate for selection, envisions neural adaptation to short-term regularities of the internal and external environment as resulting from processes of neural selection, and recognizes that there is a continuum between development and experience.

THE THEORY OF NEURONAL GROUP SELECTION

There are two key questions that any theory of neural development must answer. One is how a one-dimensional string of nucleotides can specify the shape of a three-dimensional animal, including its brain. The second is how morphological and behavioral patterns exhibiting constancy characteristic of a species arise given the astonishing diversity in the anatomy and functioning of an individual's nervous system. The theory of neuronal group selection (TNGS) was proposed as a theoretical framework sufficiently broad to connect biology and psychology in a fashion consistent with developmental and evolutionary mechanisms. Like the theories of natural selection and of clonal selection in immunity, the TNGS is a population theory. It argues that the ability of organisms to categorize an unlabeled world and behave in an adaptive fashion arises not from instruction or information transfer but from processes of selection upon variation. Instead of ignoring the observed variance and fluctuations in neuroanatomy and neural dynamics, these are treated as key features that are essential to the functioning of the nervous system.

The TNGS considers that there is continual generation of diversity in the brain, with selection occurring at various levels. In the embryonic and maturing brain, for example, variation and selection occur in migrating cellular populations and during cell death, as well as during synapse formation; both processes are dramatically reflected in enormous synaptic loss during development, as well as in the appearance of new anatomical structures (Edelman, 1988). Variation and selection in the mature brain are reflected mainly, but not exclusively, in the differential amplification of synaptic efficacies. This results in the formation of neuronal groups and is a process that is continually modified by reentrant signaling. To understand neuronal groups and reentrant signaling requires a closer look at the postulates of the

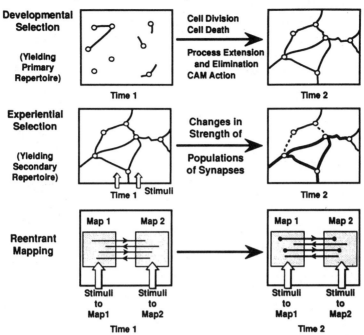

Figure 9.1. Basic tenets of the theory of neuronal group selection, a global theory of brain function. *Top: Developmental selection.* This occurs as a result of the molecular effects of CAM and SAM regulation, growth factor signaling, and selective cell death to yield variant anatomical networks in each individual. These networks make up the *primary repertoire. Center: Experiential selection.* Selective strengthening or weakening of populations of synapses as a result of behavior leads to the formation of various circuits constituting a *secondary repertoire* of neuronal groups. The consequences of synaptic strengthening are indicated by bold paths; of weakening, by dashed paths. *Bottom: Reentry.* Binding of functionally segregated maps occurs in time through parallel selection and the correlation of the various maps' neuronal groups. This process provides a fundamental basis for perceptual categorization. Dots at the ends of some of the active reciprocal connections indicate parallel and more or less simultaneous strengthening of synapses facilitating certain reentrant paths. Synaptic strengthening (or weakening) can occur in both the intrinsic and extrinsic reentrant connections of each map.

TNGS and at its proper mechanisms: developmental selection, experiential selection, and reentry (Figure 9.1).

Developmental variation and selection

According to the TNGS, although many features of the development of a brain, especially at a macroscopic spatial and temporal scale, are governed by evolutionarily constrained processes of self-organization, the detailed connectivity among its neural elements is relatively unconstrained genetically and developmentally. In other words, at the finest ramifications of neuroanatomical networks, a large amount of variation occurs despite the fact that the overall pattern in any particular specialized region is similar from individual to individual.

In the absence of a precise determination of individual cell position by the genetic code, the structural diversity of neuroanatomical organization at the finest ramifications of the nervous system is an unavoidable consequence of the epigenetic regulation of cell division, adhesion, migration, death and neurite extension and retraction (Changeux & Danchin, 1973; Cowan, 1978; Edelman, 1988; Rakic, 1988). Neuronal adhesion and migration are constrained by a series of morphoregulatory molecules called CAMs, or cell adhesion molecules, and SAMs, or substrate adhesion molecules (Edelman, 1988). These molecules interact at neuronal surfaces and affect the dynamics of cellular interactions as they occur at particular neural sites. The temporal patterns and levels of expression of morphoregulatory molecules are transcriptionally regulated. While characteristic of a given anatomical area, they are nevertheless dynamically regulated and subject to epigenetic influences. In certain regions, there is also a large amount of cell death which occurs stochastically in particular developing neuronal populations. Such processes result in the formation by selection within a given anatomical region of *primary repertoires* containing large numbers of variant neuronal groups or local circuits. A great deal of evidence has now accumulated suggesting that, during development, such preexisting variant connectivity is pruned, strengthened, and selectively amplified in an activity-dependent way, largely through synaptic change.

It should be stressed that the structures and mechanisms brought about by epigenesis strongly constrain the adaptations that can be achieved through processes of neural selection. This bias is essential in allowing neural selection to be fast and effective. As we have seen, if variation and selection were unconstrained by preexisting biases or values developed during natural selection, it would be almost impossible to reach any satisfactory degree of adaptation in somatic time, as we already indicated in discussing the relative inefficacy of general purpose neural network strategies.

Examples of interactions of natural and neural selection in neural adaptation range from the anatomical segregation of different sensory modalities, to the rough topographic arrangement within many sensory and motor pathways, to the great variety of inborn reflexes and behavioral patterns, to the modality-specific aspects of conditioning, and to the innate responsiveness of neuronal value systems (see below) to particular stimuli. In other words, although the nervous system is born with specific limitations on what it can adapt to, these limitations are precisely what allow it to tune in and adapt to short-term regularities in the environment in a fast and reliable way.

Experiential variation and selection

After most of the anatomical connections of the primary repertoires have been established, the activities of particular functioning neuronal groups continue to be dynamically selected by ongoing mechanisms of synaptic change driven by behavior and experience. Unlike natural selection in evolution, which results from differential reproduction, experiential selection results from differential amplification of synaptic populations, strengthening some and weakening others without major changes in anatomy. Continued experiential selection leads to the formation of *secondary repertoires* of neuronal groups in response to particular patterns of signals. The consequence is that certain patterns of neural activity that happen to match or fit better than others as a given set of input signals become progressively more frequent and specific.

It should be emphasized that processes giving rise to local variation also occur in the adult brain. These may include the generation and breaking of synaptic contacts (Darian-Smith & Gilbert, 1994; Doubell & Stewart, 1993; Greenough & Chang, 1988; Keller, Arissian & Asanuma, 1992) as well as changes in synaptic efficacies due to rearrangements of the many interacting components that contribute to it. The large number of neurotransmitters and neuromodulators as well as the great diversity of receptors and channels that continue to be discovered (see Changeux, Chapter 6) offer striking demonstrations of the bases for local diversity in the central nervous system. Such a profusion is embarrassing or inexplicable in terms of either genetic determinism or functionalism, both of which require precise and reliable wiring diagrams and channels for information processing. In contrast, the existence of an increasing diversity of transmitters, receptors and signaling modes varying from cell to cell is fully consistent with a selectional model of brain function. An increase in the number of neurotransmitters and neuromodulators greatly increases the number of functional circuits that are combinatorially possible within a given anatomical network. A kind of 'transmitter logic' can be defined in which combinations of transmitters, operating in a particular anatomical context, provide part of the diversity required for selection of interactive secondary repertoires (Finkel & Edelman, 1987). A rich pharmacology of the kind described by Changeux thus assures a very rich set of functional network variants.

Reentry

Reentry is the third major component of the TNGS. It is defined as ongoing parallel signaling occurring between separate neuronal groups along large numbers of ordered anatomical connections in a bidirectional and recursive fashion. It is the existence of the dynamic process of reentry that allows the nervous system to deal with spatiotemporal correlation of inputs and with integration of disparate maps. Although it can occur within a single map, reentry usually involves signaling between at least two maps (which can form a so-called classification couple), and it acts through the ordered connections that sample these maps in both space and time. Reentrant signaling can take place via reciprocal connections between and within maps (as seen in cortico-cortical, corticothalamic, and thalamocortical radiations) as well as via more complex arrangements seen in the connections among cortex, basal ganglia, and cerebellum (Edelman, 1989). Reentrant signaling has several general properties that are of fundamental importance to the function of the brain. These properties can be schematically subdivided into constructive, correlative and associative. As we will show, the overall result is that reentry allows the integration, at many different levels, of functionally segregated maps.

The *constructive properties* of reentry refer to the ability of reciprocal and recursive interactions across multiple areas to influence the response properties of neurons within each area. Reentry can give rise to new properties of the system such as simultaneous satisfaction of multiple constraints; cross-modal construction, as when one area uses the outputs of another area, which may be specialized for a different function, for its own operation; conflict resolution, for example between the responses of different areas to the same stimulus; and recursive synthesis, as when a stable response pattern requires several cycles of reentry between specialized areas (Finkel & Edelman, 1989).

In many cases, rather than radically altering the response properties of neuronal units, reentry may primarily act to *correlate* their activity, both within and between areas. This is of fundamental importance in the brain, because there are no specific tags or labels that could possibly indicate whether disjunct signals in different brain areas refer to the same object. Nor is there evidence for a master area where the many attributes of a scene are synthesized. By allowing the establishment of specific patterns of correlations across multiple areas, reentry is the key process that guarantees the unity of a perceptual scene.

The *associative properties* of reentry refer to the consequences of reentrant signaling on the plastic synaptic changes that are constantly occurring in the brain. We have suggested that, in general, differential amplification of populations of synapses leads to the selection of local activity patterns of neuronal groups that happen to match well with a set of input signals. This is typically the case when a group of neurons receives strongly correlated inputs. Considered from this perspective, the exchange of signals through reentry is advantageous because distant groups of neurons become sensitive to correlations over different modalities and submodalities, both motor and perceptual. Thus, during interactions with the environment, functionally segregated perceptual and motor maps, which allow a disjunctive sampling of both environmental and intrinsic signals, undergo coordinated synaptic changes reflecting intermodal correlations that are due to invariances in the environment. In addition, reentrant loops allow the effects of previous activity to influence synaptic changes, thus assuring the integration of behavioral and perceptual sequences. Ultimately, these statistical correlations must reflect the spatiotemporal properties of signals arising in the real world and can thus serve adaptive behavior.

The importance of plastic changes that are sensitive to correlations sampled across different sensory modalities and submodalities, across perceptual and motor activities, and between past and present events emerges vividly in the study of infant development (Thelen & Smith, 1994). It has been repeatedly demonstrated that multimodal, sensory-motor correlations help reduce the number of degrees of freedom in the otherwise impossible dynamical problem that any infant is able to solve when he learns to grasp, to recognize objects, and to walk. Thus, reentrant signaling ensures that experimental selection involves statistical signal correlations at many different levels within the nervous system.

Value and value systems

Although reentry guarantees that differential amplification at the level of populations of synapses reflects multimodal correlations existing among functionally segregated areas, the resulting selectional events if unconstrained would purely reflect the changes in the patterns of correlated neural activity that occur during the interaction with the environment. They would lack reference to the saliency of events or their significance to the organism. According to the TNGS, a further set of mechanisms constrain *value-dependent selection*. By these means, evolutionarily selected phenotypic structures can exert a global influence on local synaptic events depending on the adaptive value of a situation (Reeke et al., 1990; Tononi, Sporns & Edelman, 1992b; Friston et al., 1994). *Values* reflect structures that have been selected during evolution because they have contributed to adaptive behavior and to phenotypic fitness. Examples of low-level values are: 'eating is better than not eating' or 'seeing is better than not seeing'. From a selectionist perspective, there are no programs, sets of instructions, or teachers explicitly controlling synaptic changes in neuronal systems (Edelman, 1978; Edelman, 1987). In the absence of specific detailed instructions, evolution has endowed organisms with several means to sense the occurrence of behaviors having adaptive value and to select the neural events that bring them about.

Certain specialized structures in the brain, for example the cholinergic and aminergic neuromodulatory systems, seem particularly well suited to serve as neural *value systems* (Friston et al., 1994; Tononi et al., 1992b). Much evidence indicates that these neuromodulatory systems possess certain properties that would be expected of value systems, such as the ability to give a transient but strong response to the occurrence of events having adaptive value, both innate and acquired, to signal such an occurrence to wide areas of the brain through diffuse projections, and to release substances that modulate changes in synaptic strength. The modulation of local synaptic changes by global signals that are associated directly or indirectly with evolutionarily selected values constitutes a major means of ensuring value-dependent selection. Indeed, according to the TNGS, value-dependent learning is essential in the selection of adaptive behaviors in somatic time. To show how this might operate, we choose a recently analyzed example – perceptual integration in the operation of the cerebral cortex.

FUNCTIONAL SEGREGATION, INTEGRATION, AND THE BINDING PROBLEM

Among the extraordinary variety of phenomena demanding explanation in terms of fundamental principles of brain organization, perhaps one of the most challenging is the problem of figure-ground segregation and cortical integration during perception. Any global theory of brain function must deal with this central problem in a way that is consistent with both anatomical and physiological facts. Providing a solution to it represents a particularly telling test, because many different levels of explanation, as well as many different mechanisms, are simultaneously required. For this reason, here we choose to discuss this problem in order to illustrate and probe the self-consistency of the TNGS.

The organization of the cerebral cortex is characterized by functional segregation: even within a single sensory modality such as vision, there is a multitude of specialized areas and functionally segregated maps (aspects of this are considered in Purves, et al., Chapter 8). More recently, neurophysiology has demonstrated finer and finer parcellations within each cortical area; for example, neighboring neuronal groups tend to be specialized for different stimulus attributes: in vision, for example, one may name spatial position, shape, color, texture, and depth, or different values of the same attribute. While the presence of areas consisting of specialized neuronal groups is advantageous from a functional point of view, it is evident that the activity of these specialized groups and areas has to be integrated to yield a coherent perceptual scene. Considered in terms of phenomenology, this is quite obvious: despite the diversity of elements and relations, each perceptual scene has an undeniable unity and coherence. Functionally, a unified perceptual scene is essential to drive adaptive motor behavior, which is necessarily integrated if survival is to be assured.

A key question is how the integration of functionally segregated elements takes place. A glance at the anatomical organization of the brain, especially of the cerebral cortex, reveals that reciprocal and parallel connectivity is the rule rather than the exception, indicating that ongoing mutual interactions among neuronal groups and areas are not just possible but unavoidable. Yet there is no overriding executive program, no superordinate area regulating integration, and no homunculus analyzing the scene. How does the brain 'bind' together the attributes of objects and events in space and time? In what follows, we will briefly describe how computer models based on the TNGS have addressed this problem and proposed a solution that is based on the notion of reentry. These models will illustrate at once the constructive, correlative, and associative properties of reentry as well as the role of value systems in neural selection.

Reentry, occurring both locally and between maps, is the basic means by which integration occurs in the absence of any single cortical 'master map'. It is essential to realize that neural integration must occur at many different levels of organization. Within a single cortical area, 'linking' must occur among the responses of neuronal groups that belong to the *same* sensory feature domain. Perceptual grouping within a single submodality such as color or movement provides an example of integrative linking at an early level. At a higher level, 'binding' must take place among the responses of neuronal groups found in *different* feature domains that are distributed in different cortical areas. An example is the integration of neuronal responses to a particular object contour with its color, position, and direction of movement. Such perceptual and behavioral integration across functionally segregated maps can occur in times ranging from 50–500 msec, placing strong temporal constraints on any proposed mechanism.

The self-consistency of this proposal has been tested extensively in a series of computer models (Sporns et al., 1989; Sporns, Tononi & Edelman, 1991; Tononi et al., 1992b). It has been shown that reentrant interactions within a single cortical area can give rise to temporal correlations between neighboring as well as distant groups with a near-zero phase lag as observed in cats and monkeys (Engel et al., 1991; Gray & Singer, 1989; Kreiter & Singer, 1992). An early computer simulation (Sporns, et al., 1989) showed how linking can be mediated by reentry. In agreement with experimental data, when a continuous long bar was presented as a moving stimulus to the model, correlations were found between units in groups with non-overlapping receptive fields. These distant correlations disappeared if two collinear short bars that are separated by a gap are moved with the same velocity. A more extended model (Sporns et al., 1991) was presented with several bars moving coherently together but embedded in a background of vertical and horizontal bars that were moving at random to the right and left, or up and down. The neuronal groups responding to the bars that moved in the same direction were rapidly linked by coherent oscillations through reentry even though the lateral spread of the anatomical connections from each neuronal group was much smaller than the projected size of the 'object'. This model was shown to segregate a Gestalt – a figure from another overlapping figure or from a coherent background of identical texture moving in a different direction (Figure 9.2).

All of these simulations that resulted in linking depended strongly upon the occurrence of rapid changes in synaptic efficacy. The neural mechanism for integration and segregation of elementary features into objects and

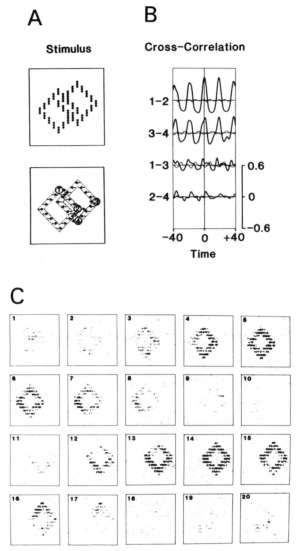

Figure 9.2. Consequences of reentry in a neural model of perceptual grouping and segregation (Sporns et al., 1991). (A) A stimulus consisting of two identical patterns each composed of vertically oriented bars is presented to the model. The two patterns overlap in visual space but move in different directions. In the top panel, the bars are shown at their starting positions; in the bottom panel, their corresponding directions of movement are indicated by arrows. Encircled numbers with arrows in the bottom panel refer to the locations of recorded neuronal activity; corresponding cross-correlations are displayed in (B). 'Electrodes' 1 and 2 recorded from neurons responding to pattern 1, and 'electrodes' 3 and 4 from neurons responding to pattern 2. (B) Cross-correlograms computed

background appears to be based on the pattern of temporal correlations and phase relationships among neuronal groups. These correlations depended critically upon reentry and disappeared when the underlying reciprocal connectivity was disrupted. The resulting figural grouping and segregation are consistent with the Gestalt laws (Köhler, 1947) of continuity, proximity, similarity, common orientation, and common motion, and this work thus suggests that synchronization through reentry provides a neural basis for these laws.

In a much larger simulation (Tononi et al., 1992b), it has been shown that a model with inter-areal reentry among nine functionally segregated areas, divided into three anatomical streams for form, color, and motion (Figure 9.3), could distinguish two or more objects present in the same visual scene regardless of position. Reentry and temporal correlation were shown to be sufficient to solve the 'binding' problem, without any need to call upon a superordinate executive area. Consistent with functional segregation in the visual cortex, units within each separate area of the model responded to different properties (motion, form and color) of the stimuli. Reentrant interactions within and between the multiple areas gave rise to short-term temporal correlations between the units responding to different attributes of the same stimulus, while units responding to attributes of different stimuli were less correlated. In this way, several features of a single object were 'bound' together across different streams and hierarchical levels and at the same time that object was differentiated (Figure 9.4) from other objects present in the same visual scene. The model also suggests that such *correlative properties* of reentry are at the

---

Figure 9.2. (*Continued*).
over a 100 msec sample period and subsequently averaged over 10 trials. Numbers refer to the locations of responding direction-selective repertoires containing neuronal groups that are analyzed for their correlations (see A). Four correlograms computed between msec 201 and 300 after stimulus onset are shown. The correlograms are scaled, and shift-predictors (thin lines; averages over nine shifts) are displayed for comparison. (C) Frames taken from a movie showing the responses of direction selective groups in the model to the stimulus in (A). The frames show a continuous period of 20 msec (20 iterations) recorded about 150 msec after stimulus onset. Each frame displays the model's entire array of neuronal groups (16 × 16 for a total of 50,720 cells) selective for motion to the right and to the left, and arranged in an interleaved fashion (this accounts for the striped pattern). Each small dot within the array is an active neuron. For the first 10 msec (frames 1–10) groups responding to the pattern moving right are mainly active; subsequently these groups are silent and groups responsive to the other pattern become active (frames 11–20). Note that neuronal activity is strongly correlated both within groups as well as over the entire extent of each pattern. (A and B: modified from Sporns et al., 1991, reproduced with permission; C: modified from Tononi, et al., 1992a, reproduced with permission.)

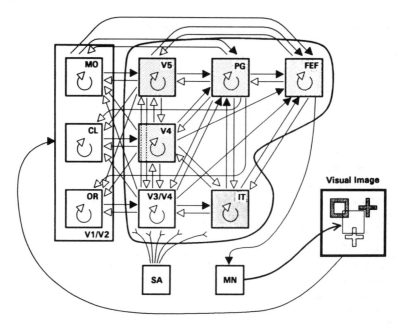

Figure 9.3. Architecture of the visual cortex model. Segregated visual maps are
indicated as boxes, pathways (composed of many thousands of individual
connections) are indicated as arrows. The model comprises three parallel
streams involved in the analysis of visual motion (top row), color (middle
row), and form (bottom row). Areas are finely (no shading) or coarsely
topographic (light shading), or nontopographic (heavy shading). The
visual image (sampled by a color camera) is indicated at the extreme right.
The output of the system (simulated foveation movements under the
control of eye motorneurons MN) is indicated at the bottom. Filled arrows
indicate voltage-independent pathways, unfilled arrows indicate voltage-
dependent pathways. Curved arrows within boxes indicate intra-areal
connections. Box labeled SA refers to the diffusely projecting saliency
system used in the behavioral paradigm; the general area of projection is
outlined. The complete system contains a total of about 10,000 neuronal
units and of about 1,000,000 connections. (From Tononi et al., 1992b,
reproduced with permission.).

basis of an entire class of perceptual illusions, such as motion capture and
other capture phenomena (Ramachandran, 1990).

These simulations have also been used to make specific suggestions about
the *constructive properties* of reentry. Although neuronal response properties
can be determined by a hierarchical arrangement of forward connections,
various backward, lateral, intra-areal and recursive interactions may be equally
important. For instance, reciprocal and recursive interactions between multiple
visual areas can influence the response properties of neurons within each area,
and give rise to new properties of the system. The constructive aspect of
reentry is particularly evident when reentrant signals from a hierarchically

'higher' area (V_5) interact with signals coming from the periphery to construct responses consistent with form from motion in the area V_1/V_2; these responses disappear when reentrant inputs are cut. Some experimental evidence consistent with this prediction has been recently provided by PET studies in humans (Zeki, 1993).

Finally, this model of functional segregation and integration in the visual system (Tononi et al., 1992b) can also be used as an illustration of some of the points made earlier about the importance of selectionist principles in accounting for behavioral adaptation, in this case in the adult. In the simulations, the specific patterns of activity and correlations determined by reentrant interactions across functionally segregated neuronal groups and areas produced a focus of synchronous activity in an area controlling eye movements. This activity often gave rise to a foveation response towards one of the objects presented. Such a response was used as a basis for conditioning the model to foveate an object that was characterized by a certain conjunction of shape and color, for example, a red cross, in any position of the visual field. Operant conditioning was achieved, whenever the model foveated the red cross, through the activation of diffusely projecting units of the value system that signaled saliency (e.g. the delivery of a reward in a conditioning paradigm) and thereby influenced the modifications of cortico-cortical connections. After the training period, the model foveated the red cross almost exclusively, although that simulation was presented simultaneously with other objects sharing the same attributes, e.g. a red square and a green cross. The correct response, which depended on the integration of color, form, and location, was achieved without the need for a hierarchically superordinate area, for units that responded to that particular conjunction, or for a preexisting program.

The way this simulated visual system was able to learn to respond to the reinforced object illustrates several of the points raised before. Firstly, the model was based on a local selectionist rule. There was no supervised mechanism to measure an error gradient at each synapse and to dictate the sign or magnitude of each synaptic change. Learning a correct response was instead based on an initial, highly variant, repertoire of firing patterns. From this variant repertoire, a subset of firing patterns was eventually selected, through local synaptic mechanisms, that consistently led to a rewarding response.

Secondly, given the huge number of parameters of the model (tens of thousands of neurons and millions of connections), an exploration of the entire parameter space would have been impossible. Nevertheless, the model could rapidly learn to discriminate among different objects because it incorporated many important structural features of the organization of the visual system (Felleman & Van Essen, 1991; Zeki, 1981). This demonstrates the importance of intrinsic value constraints that 'bias' what and how fast the system can or cannot learn. Because of these constraints, the brain is far from being a general purpose learning machine implementing some

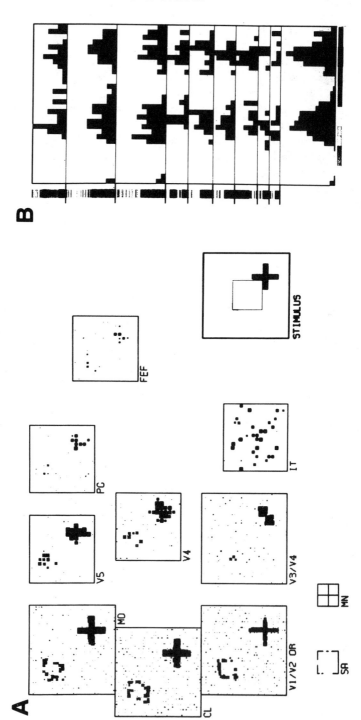

learning algorithm; on the other hand, these very constraints, developed and refined through natural selection, allow the brain to adapt rapidly and efficiently.

Third, the model illustrates the *associative properties* of reentry. Thanks to reentry, each functionally segregated group or map can sample correlations across different modalities and submodalities. Selective events can thus occur at several different levels in terms of differential amplification of synapses. For example, a correct response requires the registration of intermodal correlations between color (red) and shape (cross). There are no units that are directly selective for such an arbitrary conjunction of properties. However, specialized units selective for red can respond to such a correlation if reentrantly connected to specialized units selective for cross-like patterns. Fast local synaptic changes occurring at one functionally specialized area will thus be influenced by events occurring in some other specialized part of the system. In this way, both a high specificity of response and a wide range of associations are accommodated.

The advantages that such an arrangement provides are obvious. For example, the task presented to the model required the discrimination of a red cross, no matter at which location. It would take a very long time for the system to learn from scratch to respond to a particular configuration of pixels, irrespective of their location in the visual field, but only if they are red. In addition, the required connectivity would be practically useless (actually harmful) if the system were retrained to respond to green crosses, or to red squares. The strategy followed by the brain, and modelled here, is based

---

Figure 9.4. Responses of the complete system to two objects at iteration 10 during a typical trial. (A) Display of activity and correlation patterns during presentation of two objects, a red cross (shown in black) and a red square (shown in gray). Units responding to the same object are correlated both within and between (topographic or non-topographic) areas forming a cohort. The two cohorts corresponding to the two different objects are segregated by having different mean phases. Each small filled square represents one active unit, with the size of the square indicating the activation value and its gray level indicating the phase value (for gray scale see B). Binding occurs across three hierarchical levels, between topographically and nontopographically organized areas, and with little or no phase lag despite conduction delays. (B) Histograms of phase distributions (for units with high activity values) at the same iteration displayed in A. There is one histogram for each area as well as a cumulative histogram for the complete system on the bottom. The column on the left represents the phase of the units in each area. Units within and between areas are strongly correlated and there is little or no systematic phase shift from 'lower' (top) to 'higher' (bottom) areas, despite inter-areal delays of 10 phase bins. Note the segregation of units responding to different objects into two cohorts. A gray scale for the phase is given at the bottom. (From Tononi et al., 1992b, reproduced with permission.)

instead on the development and selection of functionally specialized neuronal groups and areas that respond to statistical regularities in the environment, for example, different shapes (crosses and squares) and different colors (red and green). It thus becomes easy to identify a particular, arbitrary conjunction of these regularities. The actual synaptic changes, occurring among specialized units communicating by reentry, are relatively minor and can easily be reversed.

Finally, these simulations strongly illustrate the role of a value system in providing a global saliency signal that modulates local synaptic events in a way that depends upon the adaptive value of the response. By these means, selective events over a relatively short time scale can be constrained in the direction of evolutionarily selected values. By projecting to the entire cortical mantle, and by releasing neuromodulatory signals, neural value systems can affect whatever complex set of interactions leads to an adaptive response.

The required cooperation of all these factors in determining the model's performance is a strong reminder that memory is a property of the dynamics of the entire system: it is a system property and it refers to the enhanced ability of the animal to categorize stimuli in its environment. Memory, in short, is recategorization (Edelman, 1987).

As pointed out also by Morris (Chapter 7), memory cannot be reduced to synaptic changes, since, for example, the same synaptic rules lead to very different results in different anatomical structures. More generally, synaptic changes are as necessary as the presence of spontaneous variant patterns of activity, of particular anatomical structures, of reentrant interactions in an integrated, functionally specialized system, and of global, evolutionarily adaptive saliency signals transmitted by value system. It is only through the interaction of all of these components in a particular arrangement that the brain can achieve the degenerate repetition of a performance that we call memory. Paraphrasing Morris, there are as many types of memory as there are types of neuroanatomical structures, phenotypes, and behaviors.

Even with respect to synaptic changes, the neural models discussed here also illustrate that, in general, there is no place where a 'memory trace' is located. Changes in synaptic weights occur in many different locations, but generally it is difficult if not impossible to attribute a specific memorial function to any particular synapse or cell. The model's memory is expressed as increased behavioral performance, for example the increased ability to re-categorize the surrounding world of stimulus objects, but it is not replicative or localized in a precise fashion. Behavioral performance (i.e. the measurable effect of memory) can be degraded in various ways and to various extents by 'lesions' in different parts of the model (some of them far removed from sites of synaptic change). This may not sound surprising: neural network models have often been used to show the distributed nature of memory. However, in the present models, memory is not just the delocalized property of a single network, but is distributed among several functionally distinct brain areas. In addition, because of the incorporation of actual behavioral output, memory becomes directly measurable as increased or decreased levels of performance.

Functional segregation and integration reconciled

One of the recurring themes of this paper has been the multiplicity of levels that need to be considered to understand brain function and behavior. In particular, we have seen that a general principle of brain organization emerging through neural development seems to be functional segregation and specialization at a small scale, coupled with integration and cooperative interactions at a larger scale. That is, individual areas or neuronal groups are functionally segregated, yet the cortex as a whole gives rise to an integrated and cooperative activity. While the chosen modality to illustrate these points in the computer simulations was visual, there is every reason to expect that similar principles operate in other modalities throughout the brain.

In order to be able to make some experimental predictions, for example about the consequences of neural development on functional segregation and integration, we have recently attempted to provide a more general theoretical perspective as well as a measure of functional segregation and integration in the brain (Tononi, Sporns & Edelman, 1994). By making certain simplifying assumptions, we have shown that these two organizational aspects can be formulated within a unified framework. In such a framework, functional segregation and integration are characterized in terms of deviations from statistical independence among the components of a neural system, measured using the concepts of statistical entropy and mutual information (Papoulis, 1991). We will consider these notions briefly here to give some of the flavor of the approach.

Consider a bipartition of a neural system X into a jth subset X_j^k composed of k components (which can be taken to represent neuronal groups) and its complement $X - X_j^k$. The deviation from statistical independence between X_j^k and $X - X_j^k$ is measured by their mutual information MI:

$$MI(X_j^k; X - X_j^k) = H(X_j^k) + H(X - X_j^k) - H(X)$$

where $H(X_j^k)$ and $H(X - X_j^k)$ are the entropies of X_j^k and $X - X_j^k$ considered independently, and $H(X)$ is the entropy of the system considered as a whole. $MI = 0$ if X_j^k and $X - X_j^k$ are statistically independent and $MI > 0$ otherwise.

The *integration* $I(X)$ of a neural system is then defined as the total deviation from independence among all its n components and can be measured through a single measure that is a generalization of the notion of mutual information. $I(X)$ is defined as the difference between the sum of the entropies of all individual components $\{x_i\}$ considered independently and the entropy of X considered as a whole:

$$I(X) = \sum_{i=1}^{n} H(x_i) - H(X)$$

If the n components of the system are completely independent, as when neuronal groups are completely desynchronized, integration is zero. If, on the other hand, such groups show strong deviations from independence, as when they are fully synchronized, integration is high.

Measuring integration in terms of deviation from statistical independence allows us simultaneously to characterize functional segregation and integration within a neural system, by considering the average integration for subsets of increasing size. Functional segregation is expressed by the relative statistical independence of the activity of individual neuronal groups if these groups are considered in small subsets, that is a few at a time (low average integration for small subsets). Conversely, functional integration is expressed by a high degree of statistical dependence when neuronal groups are considered in large subsets, that is many at a time (high average integration for large subsets).

This leads to the formulation of a measure, called *neural complexity* (C_N), which reflects the interplay between functional segregation and integration within a neural system, and which is defined as follows:

$$C_N(X) = \sum_{k=1}^{n} ((k/n)I(X) - \langle I(X_j^k) \rangle)$$

where we consider all subsets X^k composed of k-out-of-n components of the system ($1 \leq k \leq n$) and the average integration for subsets of size k is denoted as $\langle I(X_j^k) \rangle$ (the index j indicates that the average is taken over all $n!/(k!(n-k)!)$ combinations of k components). In essence, C_N measures how much the increase of average integration with increasing subset size deviates from linearity, that is, roughly speaking, how much the whole is more integrated than its parts. C_N can be shown to be equivalent to the mutual information between each part of a neural system and the rest, summed over all possible bipartitions:

$$C_N(X) = \sum_{k=1}^{n/2} \langle MI(X_j^k; X - X_j^k) \rangle.$$

Thus, for complexity to be high, the average mutual information between each component and the rest of the brain must be high, indicating that the system is very integrated. At the same time, the average mutual information must be higher the larger the subset being considered. This indicates that each component has a rather specialized function, in that considering more components provides additional mutual information. Thus, consistent with intuitive notions and with current attempts in physics and biology to conceptualize complex systems, C_N is high for systems such as the vertebrate brain that conjoin local specialization with global integration. On the other hand, C_N is low for systems that are composed either of completely independent parts or of parts that show completely homogeneous behavior.

As an illustration, we calculated the complexity associated with the primary visual area used in our model of perceptual grouping and figure-ground segregation (Sporns et al., 1991). Neuronal activity was triggered by un-correlated Gaussian noise rather than by patterned external input. We observed that certain structural characteristics of cortical connectivity, as incorporated in the model, are associated with high values of C_N (Figure 9.5). These characteristics include a high density of connections, strong local connectivity helping to organize cells into neuronal groups, patchiness in the connectivity among neuronal groups, and a large number of short reentrant circuits.

It can also be anticipated that a measure of neural complexity should be able to reflect important changes in neural organization that take place during processes of neural selection occurring during development. As an example, the work of Callaway & Katz (1990) indicates that, in the primary visual cortex of the cat, the distribution of horizontal intra-areal connections is marked, in the first postnatal days, by uniformity and apparent randomness. This stage is followed by a substantial pruning and rewiring of these connections, such that, in the adult, the uniform connectivity is replaced by a more specific connectivity scheme according to which specialized groups of neurons are selectively connected. This process seems to be activity-dependent and to result from the tendency of axons carrying correlated signals to group together and segregate from other axons (what fires together, wires together). Such process of grouping and segregation seems to be a key organizational principle that allows temporal correlations in the input to be converted into spatial proximity of synaptic terminals resulting in the formation of axonal patches.

We have simulated these two patterns of immature and adult connectivity in a primary visual area and measured their respective neural complexity. Under the assumption that the total amount of input received by each neuron does not change (which may not be the case), we found that the complexity of the adult pattern (Figure 9.5, case b) was almost twice that of the immature pattern. Interestingly, the overall integration was higher for the immature pattern (Figure 9.5, case c).

This prediction is not restricted to intra-areal interactions. There is anatomical evidence that, in newborn animals, there is a much larger degree of anatomical multisensory convergence than in adult animals (Asanuma et al., 1988; Frost, 1984; Innocenti & Clarke, 1984; Roe et al., 1990). Physiologically, areas that are unimodal in the adult are multimodal in the newborn or fetal brain (Stein & Meredith, 1993). Thus, it may be hypothesized

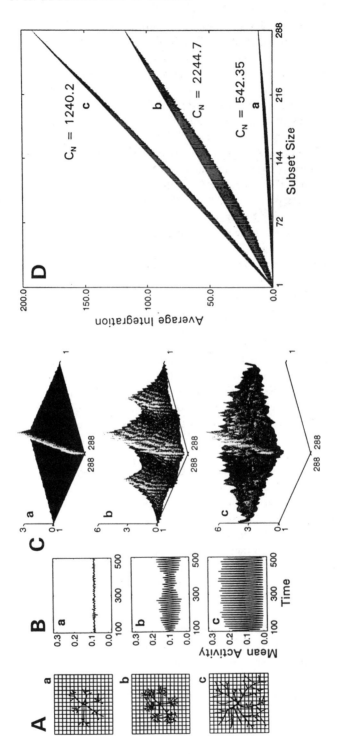

that even at the level of cortical areas one should observe, during development, a similar increase in complexity, most likely associated with an increase in functional specialization. Imaging studies could hopefully be used in assessing whether global measures, such as neural complexity, can serve as an overall and objective indication of perceptual, motor, and cognitive development.

CONCLUSION

In this chapter, we have mentioned several times the enormous variability in development at the microscopic scale. Microscopic events are highly variable in every developmental or behavioral context, from gastrulation to locomotion to speech. At higher levels of organization, however, the variability is greatly diminished and is replaced by relatively constant, species-specific macroscopic patterns. In structural terms, a high variability at the cellular level coexists with high regularity at the level of tissues or organs. The same dichotomy between functional segregation and global integration is seen in the organization of the adult brain, both in time and in space. There is also great constancy in what in general can be learned by organisms, but this constancy is accompanied by a great variability in what precisely will be learned and how it will be learned by a given individual. The coexistence of

---

Figure 9.5. Integration and complexity obtained from simulations of a primary visual area for different patterns of connectivity. All cases shown contain 512 neuronal groups in two arrays (16 by 16) and were modeled as collections of 40 excitatory and 20 inhibitory neurons that are mutually interconnected (Sporns et al., 1991). No external input is provided to the network; neuronal group activity is triggered by intrinsic Gaussian noise. The groups tend to discharge in an oscillatory fashion. To compute C_N, we sampled the mean activity traces of groups forming the central 12 by 12 portion of the two arrays (one for each orientation preference) for 10,000 time steps (discarding an initial transient) and derived the covariance matrix. (A) Schematic connectivity patterns. (B) Mean activity traces of the entire array for the first 400 time steps following the initial transient. Large amplitude is an indicator of coherent activity within the array. (C) Covariance matrices. (D) Average integration and complexity derived from the covariance matrices. Cases (a), (b), and (c) (compare Figure 9.1) explore the variation of $C_N(X)$ with different patterns of inter-group connections. In case (b) intergroup connections are clustered in local patches around the group of origin (details in (Sporns et al., 1991)); connections are spread within a 5 by 5 region for the same orientation domain, and within a 3 by 3 region for a different orientation domain. Case (a) is identical to (b), but the connection density is reduced twofold. In case (c), the same amount of inter-group connections as in (b) are distributed uniformly within the array. Although $I(X)$ increases from case (a) to (b) to (c), $C_N(X)$ is highest for case (b) and lower for both cases (a) and (c).

local variation and global coherency, of short-term unpredictability and long-term regularity is thus one of the hallmarks of complex systems. Not surprisingly, such complexity is both the substrate and the result of selectional processes. It is this that distinguishes biological developmental systems from those in the non-biological domain.

REFERENCES

Asanuma, C., Ohkawa, R., Stanfield, B. B. & Cowan, W. M. (1988) Observations on the development of certain ascending inputs to the thalamus in rats. I. Postnatal development. *Developmental Brain Research*, **41**, 159–70.

Ashby, W. B. (1966) *An Introduction to Cybernetics*. New York: John Wiley.

Bernstein, N. (1967) *The Coordination and Regulations of Movements*. Oxford: Pergamon Press.

Callaway, E. M. & Katz, L. C. (1990) Emergence and refinement of clustered horizontal connections in cat striate cortex. *Journal of Neuroscience*, **10**, 1134–53.

Changeux, J.-P. & Danchin, A. (1973) Selective stabilization of developing synapses as a mechanism for the specification of neuronal networks. *Nature*, **264**, 705–11.

Chomsky, N. (1986) *Knowledge of Language: Its Nature, Origin, and Use*. New York: Praeger.

Cowan, W. M. (1978) Aspects of neural development. *International Review of Physiology*, **17**, 150–91.

Darian-Smith, C. & Gilbert, C. D. (1994) Axonal sprouting accompanies functional reorganization in adult cat striate cortex. *Nature*, **368**, 737–40.

Doubell, T. P. & Stewart, M. G. (1993) Short-term changes in the numerical density of synapses in the intermediate and medial hyperstriatum ventrale following one-trial passive avoidance training in the chick. *Journal of Neuroscience*, **13**, 2230–6.

Edelman, G. M. (1978) Group selection and phasic re-entrant signalling: a theory of higher brain function. In Edelman, G. M. & Mountcastle, V. B. (eds.) *The Mindful Brain*. Cambridge, Mass.: MIT Press.

Edelman, G. M. (1987) *Neural Darwinism: The Theory of Neuronal Group Selection*. New York: Basic Books.

Edelman, G. M. (1988) *Topobiology: An Introduction to Molecular Embryology*. New York: Basic Books.

Edelman, G. M. (1989) *The Remembered Present: A Biological Theory of Consciousness*. New York: Basic Books.

Edelman, G. M. (1993) Neural Darwinism: selection and reentrant signalling in higher brain function. *Neuron*, **10**, 1–20.

Engel, A. K., König, P., Kreiter, A. K. & Singer, W. (1991) Interhemispheric synchronization of oscillatory neuronal responses in cat visual cortex. *Science*, **252**, 1177–9.

Felleman, D. J. & Van Essen, D. C. (1991) Distributed hierarchical processing in the primate cerebral cortex. *Cerebral Cortex*, **1**, 1–47.

Finkel, L. H. & Edelman, G. M. (1987) Population rules for synapses in networks. In Edelman, G. M., Gall, W. E. & Cowan, W. M. (eds.) *Synaptic Function*. New York: Wiley, pp. 711–57.

Finkel, L. H. & Edelman, G. M. (1989) The integration of distributed cortical systems by reentry: a computer simulation of interactive functionally segregated visual areas. *Journal of Neuroscience*, **9**, 3188–208.

Friston, K. J., Tononi, G., Reeke, G. N., Jr., Sporns, O. & Edelman, G. M. (1994) Value-dependent selection in the brain: simulation in a synthetic neural model. *Neuroscience*, **59**, 229–43.

Frost, D. O. (1984) Axonal growth and target selection during development: retinal projections to the ventrobasal complex and other 'nonvisual' structures in neonatal Syrian hamsters. *Journal of Comparative Neurology*, **230**, 576–92.

Geman, S., Bienenstock, E. & Doursat, R. (1992) Neural networks and the bias/variance dilemma. *Neural Computation*, **4**, 1–58.

Gray, C. M. & Singer, W. (1989) Stimulus-specific neuronal oscillations in orientation columns of cat visual cortex. *Proceedings of the National Academy of Science USA*, **86**, 1698–702.

Greenough, W. T. & Chang, F.-L. F. (1988) Plasticity of synapse structure and pattern in the cerebral cortex. In Jones, E. G. & Peters, A. (eds.) *Development and Maturation of Cerebral Cortex*. New York: Plenum Press, pp. 391–440.

Innocenti, G. M. & Clarke, S. (1984) Bilateral transitory projection to visual areas from auditory cortex in kittens. *Developmental Brain Research*, **14**, 143–8.

Keller, A., Arissian, K. & Asanuma, H. (1992) Synaptic proliferation in the motor cortex of adult cats after long-term thalamic stimulation. *Journal of Neurophysiology*, **68**, 295–308.

Köhler, W. (1947) *Gestalt Psychology*. New York: Liverwright.

Kreiter, A. K. & Singer, W. (1992) Oscillatory neuronal responses in the visual cortex of the awake macaque monkey. *European Journal of Neuroscience*, **4**, 369–75.

Newell, A. & Simon, H. A. (1972) *Human Problem Solving*. Englewood Cliffs, NJ: Prentice-Hall.

Papoulis, A. (1991). *Probability, Random Variables, and Stochastic Processes*, 3rd edn. New York: McGraw-Hill.

Piaget, J. (1980) *Psychology and Epistemology*. New York: Norton.

Rakic, P. (1988) Specification of cerebral cortical areas. *Science*, **241**, 170–6.

Ramachandran, V. S. (1990) Visual perception in people and machines. In Blake, A. & Troscianko, T. (eds.) *AI and the Eye*. New York: John Wiley, pp. 21–77.

Reeke, G. N., Jr. & Edelman, G. M. (1988) Real brains and artificial intelligence. *Daedalus*, **117**, 143–73.

Reeke, G. N., Jr., Finkel, L. H., Sporns, O. & Edelman, G. M. (1990) Synthetic neural modeling: A multilevel approach to the analysis of brain complexity. In Edelman G. M., Gall, W. E. & Cowan, W. M. (eds.) *Signal and Sense: Local and Global Order in Perceptual Maps*. New York: John Wiley.

Roe, A. W., Pallas, S. L., Hahm, J.-O. & Sur, M. (1990) A map of visual space induced in primary auditory cortex. *Science*, **250**, 818–20.

Smith, E. E. & Medin, D. L. (1981) *Categories and Concepts*. Cambridge, Mass: Harvard University Press.

Sporns, O., Gally, J. A., Reeke, G. N., Jr. & Edelman, G. M. (1989) Reentrant signaling among simulated neuronal group leads to coherency in their oscillatory activity. *Proceedings of the National Academy of Science of the USA*, **86**, 7265–9.

Sporns, O., Tononi, G. & Edelman, G. M. (1991) Modeling perceptual grouping and figure-ground segregation by means of active reentrant conditions. *Proceedings of the National Academy of Science of the USA*, **88**, 129–33.

Stein, B. E. & Meredith, M. A. (1993) *The Merging of the Senses.* Cambridge, Mass. MIT Press.

Thelen, E. & Smith, L. B. (1994) *A Dynamic Systems Approach to the Development of Cognition and Action.* Cambridge, Mass.: MIT Press.

Tononi, G., Sporns, O. & Edelman, G. M. (1992a) The problem of neural integration: induced rhythms and short-term correlations. In Basar, E. & Bullock, T. (eds.) *Induced Rhythms in the Brain.* Boston: Birkhäuser, pp. 365–93.

Tononi, G., Sporns, O. & Edelman, G. M. (1992b) Reentry and the problem of integrating multiple cortical areas: simulation of dynamic integration in the visual system. *Cerebral Cortex*, **2**, 310–35.

Tononi, G., Sporns, O. & Edelman, G. M. (1994) A measure for brain complexity: relating functional segregation and integration in the nervous system. *Proceedings of the National Acacemy of Science of the USA*, **91**, 5033–7.

Wertheimer, M. (1923). Untersuchungen zur Lehre von der Gestalt II. *Psychologische Forschung*, **4**, 301–50.

Zeki, S. (1981) The mapping of visual functions in the cerebral cortex. In Katsuki, Y., Norgren, R. & Sato, M. (eds.) *Brain Mechanisms of Sensation: The Third Taniguchi Symposium on Brain Sciences.* New York: John Wiley, pp. 105–28.

Zeki, S. (1993) *A Vision of the Brain.* Oxford: Blackwell Scientific.

PART III

COGNITION AND BEHAVIOR

The earliest research on cognitive aspects of individual development was conducted at the end of the last century and early this century. Much has happened since then. The four chapters of this part take on to explore some of the classical questions in developmental research in the light of recent technological discoveries, contemporary empirical findings and theoretical development.

With few exceptions the developmental studies from the turn of the century were limited to descriptions of developmental trends. Little effort was put into integrating empirical findings and facts to general theories specifying processes and mechanisms underlying cognitive development. Even the ambition to develop conceptual tools for further understanding of the individual development was very limited. All four chapters included in this part show a clear theoretical orientation with an explicit support to the notion that the maturity of a given discipline to a large extent consists in the development of scientific concepts in this field.

In addition to an emphasis on theory, current research on cognitive development parts company with previous approaches in that it focuses on longitudinal rather than cross-sectional studies. Weinert & Perner (Chapter 10) are clear on this point in claiming that many topics in developmental research cannot be explored satisfactorily unless a longitudinal approach is taken. In retrospect, and in comparison to the research undertaken a century ago, it can be appreciated that much has been gained with the current interest in longitudinal methods. However, much remains to be done in this regard. At most, cross-sectional studies can make statements about developmental differences – not about developmental changes. Whether early person-and-environmental factors account for later cognitive characteristics can only be evaluated when it is possible to describe how particular individuals change and differ from one point in development to another.

Individual differences constitute another aspect of developmental research that has been more thoroughly investigated in recent years than before. Again, much more is to be gained by pursuing the approach of individual differences as a complement to the notion of general principles. In this context the contribution by Bellugi, Klima & Wang (Chapter 11) emphasizes the dimension of individual differences by the studies of children with genetic disorders, Williams syndrome and Down syndrome, for the development of language and other cognitive behavior. It is obviously the case that the particular nature of the cognitive development in these children need to be specified and related to the features of the cognitive development in children without such a handicap. However, in focusing on individual development in general, as this volume does, and the role of cognitive factors for this development, as this part does, it might be rewarding to explore the role of other interindividual differences as well. It might prove fruitful even to consider individual differences that are less dramatic than those between various patient groups and normal controls. For example, gender differences in cognitive functioning might prove valuable to explore more thoroughly, not only as a single independent variable, but perhaps in interaction with various environmental factors occurring at different stages of life.

The role of cross-cultural differences for individual development constitutes another main factor that has been explored to some degree in earlier research – mostly as an independent variable in solving a particular cognitive task suitable for the laboratory. In a similar vein as for gender, culture and other large-scale variables in the society might play major roles in interaction with other factors (psychological and biological), that are of importance for the development of various cognitive capabilities fostering the individual development. In his contribution to this section Klein (Chapter 12) pays tribute to several such general factors affecting cognitive properties that are of importance for language development, in particular for second-language acquisition in comparison to first-language acquisition.

Finally, Damasio & Damasio (Chapter 13), point to a trend in contemporary research on cognitive development, that was not present at all in research in this area a century ago. This is the integration of psychological and neurobiological factors in development. The interaction between psychology and biology is also covered in the chapters by Bellugi et al. and by Klein. This integration, which is the result of findings, discoveries and new concepts primarily during the 1980s and 1990s, has coined the term cognitive neuroscience. Damasio and Damasio sketch how difficult the development of this new field of investigation would have been without several recent technological developments and without the theoretical development that has taken place in recent years. This new area of research is at the forefront in research on development. It has also become an area of primary interest for all those who engage in exploring the human mind.

10   Cognitive development

FRANZ E. WEINERT AND JOSEF PERNER

We organize our arguments around the question, 'How general are the observed regularities in cognitive development and what is their source?' This question highlights an important shift in dominance of research paradigms over the last decade in the field from a 'generalist' perspective (laws of cognitive development hold for all people, across the lifespan and for any content of knowledge) to a 'domain specific' view (regularities differ for different areas of knowledge, aspects of development and, perhaps, subpopulations, even individuals).

SOURCE OF REGULARITIES

The main sources of observed regularities are three: (1) the structure of the present, ontogenetically encountered environment emphasized by the empiricists, (2) the ancestral environment relayed by the genetic program (emphasized by nativists), and (3) the interaction between existing internal structures (e.g. genetic outfit) and new input through encounters with the environment (interactionism).

   Although it is now uncontroversial that strong genetic factors are at work, current discussion centers around exactly what and in which form knowledge is innately specified. Chomsky's (1965) original claim of an innate universal grammar may not entail much detailed linguistic knowledge (Klein, Chapter 12), whereas Fodor's (1981) claim that all our concepts and the core of folk theories are genetically specified amounts to strong genetic preformationism. Such strong preformationist positions face the problem of how to account for the fact that not all allegedly innate knowledge is apparent from birth. There are several strategies to account for this: (a) the competence in question is present at birth but its successful application in diagnostic tasks is hampered by *limited information processing capacities* which are only gradually overcome through maturation (e.g. Case, 1995); (b) competencies are not present at birth but emerge at different ages due to *genetically timed maturation*; (c) competencies are present at birth but they need to be *triggered* through sustained environmental stimulation (Fodor, 1981).

   These nativist strategies raise certain questions that are often not adequately addressed. Recourse to increasing processing capacities would be more convincing if there were a completely knowledge-independent specification of processing capacity, for example, in terms of brain maturation. Unfortunately, although the size of specific brain regions relates to a species' sophistication with the function located in that region (Purves *et al.*, Chapter 8), correlations between periods of rapid brain growth and cognitive advances (Case, 1995; Fischer & Rose, 1994) is still very speculative.

Similarly, claims about timed maturation (e.g. Leslie & Roth 1993, that an innately specified theory of mind module matures at the age of $1\frac{1}{2}$ years) are hardly more than a redescription of the observed cognitive changes, unless they can be supported with a plausible argument that timed maturation serves an evolutionary purpose. Such explanations can be given (e.g. for the delayed onset of sexual maturity) but are hardly ever used to bolster such claims about the maturation of cognitive abilities.

Finally, Fodor's (1981) explanatory reliance on environmental triggers of innately specified structures puts the nativist position in danger of becoming empirically equivalent to its environmentalist counterpart. It was originally put forward in reaction to the lack of a satisfactory theory of concept formation within the traditional cognitive science framework. However, until a satisfactory theory of the nature of concepts and how concepts could be encoded in genes is provided, the nativist option is no real advance in our understanding of the origin of concepts.

In contrast to genetic preformationism biological adaptation theorists (Oyama, 1989; Symons, 1992) emphasize that every apparent developmental regularity is the product of the interaction between existing internal structures and the structure of the environment. One case in point is the *epigenetic process* of a particular phenotype emerging from particular genetic specifications in interaction with a particular environment.

A somewhat different type of interactionism extends the interaction between genes and environment in terms of an interaction between existing knowledge and new environmental information. Again, a generalist variant can be discerned, that of Piaget, who saw the interaction between existing internal structures and environment governed by domain general laws of *equilibrium*, that is a necessity to achieve mathematical group structures for mental transformations. In contrast, domain dependent interactions are also conceivable on the basis of prerequisite structures between different bodies of knowledge. For instance, certain environmental regularities can only be abstracted if prerequisite knowledge structures have already been built.

Carey (1985) for instance, proposed that conceptual development, is constrained by the hierarchy of basic to more specific theories (theory view of concept formation, e.g., Keil, 1989) and that this hierarchy can explain the stage-like acquisition of different knowledge domains without having to adopt the completely domain general laws of Piagetian theory.

By way of summary the currently dominant explanations of observed developmental regularities are (1) nativism in conjunction with processing limitations, (2) nativism with maturational timing, (3) nativism with limited empiricism (e.g. triggering of preformed concepts), (4) interactionism with prerequisite hierarchies, (5) environmentalism.

COGNITIVE CONTENT

The appeal of each theoretical position about the source of observed developmental regularities varies with the type of cognitive content under consideration. Content matters along at least two dimensions: its specificity and its domain.

Specificity of knowledge content

Even the staunchest environmentalists agree that some general content must be innately specified. On the other side, even the most stringent nativists agree that knowledge of specific facts is environmentally determined. Controversy exists mostly about the intermediate region between the most general and most specific content.

This issue can be illustrated with the finding that by 10 weeks of age infants understand objects by the general principles of being continuous in space and time, and solid (besides other features such as being rigid, bounded, cohesive, and of moving as a unit; Spelke, 1991). This early competence may mean that infants are born with these principles that define the object concept. However, the other, for adults equally obvious, principle of gravity (that unsuspended objects fall) cannot be demonstrated until some months later despite use of the exact same methodology.

Spelke is inclined to assume that fundamental concepts, like the object concept, are innate, but that less central regularities, like that of falling bodies, are left for the child to discover by experience (nativism with limited empiricism). However, there are two aspects to this explanation. One aspect is the relatively early emergence of the object concept around 10 weeks. The available evidence leaves it open as to whether this is a reflection of methodological difficulties demonstrating innate knowledge at birth or whether it is a reflection of very fast learning. The other aspect concerns the lag between the earlier development of the object principles and the later emergence of understanding gravity. The explanation for this lag is basically that understanding objects is a prerequisite for understanding gravity, that is, one needs first a concept of objects before one can discover that unsuspended objects fall (interactionism with prerequisite hierarchies).

It is difficult to see how other positions can explain the observed lag. Nativism with timed maturation would need an argument for why late maturation of understanding gravity is adaptive. Also, since the testing methods were kept constant, nativism cannot draw on changes in processing capacity to explain the observed lag. Pure environmentalist assumptions are not sufficient either since it is not obvious that, for example, the principle of space-time continuity is more often encountered than failure of unsuspended objects to fall. Interestingly, the same is a problem for Fodor's nativist suggestion that preformed concepts are being environmentally triggered.

Our illustrations of these theoretical issues with an example from early infancy can be extended to later developments. For instance, Piaget & Inhelder's (1941/1974) famous conservation experiments have been criticized on methodological grounds as valid tests of children's acquisition of the concept of quantity around the age of about 6 or 7 years (concrete operational period). By devising smarter, more child-adequate methods experimentally orientated researchers were intent to demonstrate ever earlier competence. The logical consequence of this research strategy is a tacit commitment to a nativist position of innate conceptual competence and explaining the observed changes with the increasing mastery of semantic and pragmatic aspects of language use.

Domains of knowledge

Carey (1985) once suggested that the child might be born with two basic theories, a naive physics and a naive psychology. As an example we concentrate on children's naive psychology. As 'social cognitive development' this field was concerned with how the general structural and logical changes predicted by Piagetian theory enable children to take another person's point of view (role-taking). Under the heading of 'children's theory of mind', the focus is on how children come to acquire the conceptual framework within which they conceive of other people's as well as their own mind (Perner, 1991).

Again, in opposition to the original Piagetian domain-general program, increasingly domain-specific theories have been proposed. However, there is no clear definition of what defines a domain. Views range from the very narrow suggestion of extremely specific, evolved skills to large bodies of theories. In particular, Cosmides & Tooby (1992) suggest that specific evolutionary pressures define domains. For instance, vampire bats who cooperate by sharing blood are specifically adapted for detecting blood-sharing cheaters. In contrast, humans whose cooperative efforts stretch across many domains have developed a general cheater detector. For this reason, they can solve Wason's (1966) conditional reasoning task when the stated conditions express a social contract for which cheaters can be suspected but not when the stated conditions express any other, albeit, logically equivalent rule.

Most theorists, however, assume that domains are more broadly defined for humans. For instance, Leslie and Roth (1993) speak of a 'theory of mind module' responsible for dealing only with mental states. Damage to this module is seen as the core intellectual deficit of children with autism. In contrast, Leekam & Perner (1991) suggest that the domains are defined by the field of common conceptual distinctions. Thus the mental is a domain insofar as it requires conceptual distinctions surrounding the concept of intentionality (the defining feature of the mental according to Brentano, 1924). Hence the domain of the mental should also include public representations, like pictures, linguistic expressions, and so on, which are not mental states in any traditional sense, since they are also characterized by intentionality. Indeed, normal children's problems in understanding false belief extend to their understanding of misleading direction signs. For instance, Parkin & Perner (1994) found a remarkable concordance in children's ability to answer a question about where a person *thinks* an object is, when the person mistakenly thinks that the object is in a different place than where it really is, and to answer a question about where a direction sign *shows* the object is, when the sign points in the wrong direction.

INDIVIDUAL DIFFERENCES

The observation by Kluckhohn & Murray (1948: 53) seems trivial that 'EVERY MAN is in certain respects

a. like all other men [universal perspective],
b. like some other men [differential perspective],
c. like no other man [individual perspective].'

However, the fact that of these three perspectives only the first one has dominated cognitive and cognitive developmental research during the first century of scientific psychology is not trivial. Despite complaints from researchers and practitioners about this bias, retrospectively it could prove a wise research strategy on grounds of evolutionary considerations since 'individual differences cannot be understood apart from human nature mechanisms' (Buss, 1994: 42).

Tooby & Cosmides (1990) give an evolution-theoretic argument for why human nature should provide for largely universal cognitive functions. In sexual reproduction, their argument begins, genes from two parents are randomly combined to form genetically unique offspring. Such a genetic mixing would be very disruptive to offspring viability unless the exchange of parental genes is carefully coordinated (see Bateson, Chapter 1, about the dangers of excessive outbreeding). The simplest solution to this coordination problem is to make the genes from all humans functionally equivalent, that is, regardless of whose gene is placed in a certain locus it has the same epigenetic effect as any other person's gene. This leads to *functional monomorphism* (as borne out in the uniform functions of human physiology) unless there is selection pressure to build different functional types (*functional polymorphism*, for example, functional physiological differences between sexes). Without this pressure there would be few genetic differences between individuals. However, strong pressure for polymorphism does exist at the genetic level itself. In fact, the pathogenic theory of sexual reproduction says that sexual reproduction leads to a maximum of individual variation at the molecular level of genetic material to provide maximum immunological protection against parasites. In sum, there is monomorphism of design properties, but polymorphism at the material levels at which parasites operate (genetic level and level of protein sequences).

These considerations lead to the following points about the origin and nature of individual differences in cognitive development:

(1) The polymorphism at the genetic and material level can be expected to result in quantitative variation at the functional level (e.g. body size, speed of processing, maturation rate).

(2) Unless there is selection pressure for different functional types (e.g. physiological differences between sexes) we can expect that most people will be equipped with the same essential cognitive functions.

(3) Despite the universal functional mechanism to process environmental information, different experiences will lead to individual differences in knowledge.

These evolution-based speculations are compatible with Anderson's (1992) model of individual differences in cognitive development and with evidence from longitudinal studies. Cognitive development depends on three aspects according to Anderson's model:

(1) Cognitive development depends on the genesis of thinking algorithms (Route 1) which is limited through the knowledge free 'speed of the basic processing mechanism' which is unchanging with cognitive development. Speed of the basic mechanism can be seen as a quantitative variation due to the molecular differences between individuals which forms the basis for individual differences in general intelligence.

(2) Cognitive development is the consequence of the maturation of domain specific knowledge modules (Route 2) which uniformly makes information available to all developing organisms (i.e. functionally panspecific, except members recognized as abnormal). However, the speed of maturation of modules (another quantitative variation) differs between individuals allowing for individual variation in the rate of cognitive development independently from individual differences in general intelligence.

(3) Cognitive development is a function of the *acquisition* and *elaboration* of knowledge. These processes depend on partly culturally determined individual experiences and on the stable differences in intelligence and the maturation level of knowledge modules.

Excursion: modules vs. implicit learning

While acknowledging the explanatory power of Anderson's model we question the necessity of having to rely on innate modules as the IQ-independent route to basic domain-specific knowledge. Innate modules that specify whole bodies of structured knowledge ('theories') revitalize the dichotomy between nature and nurture, which has been thought of as an issue of the past (Bateson, Chapter 1) that has been put to rest (Hinde, Chapter 18). Thus it is of interest that implicitly acquired knowledge (Reber, 1993) and the allegedly modular knowledge share many of their characteristics. Hence, by replacing the innately maturing knowledge modules in Anderson's model by implicitly learned bodies of knowledge, the explanatory power of his model can be preserved without having to buy into the evolutionarily undesirable features of modules.

Two of the empirically critical features of knowledge acquired by the modular route are its independence of IQ and, in distinction to the stable individual differences in IQ, it is supposed to be largely universal. In Reber's (1993) characterization implicit knowledge differs from explicit knowledge in similar ways. Implicit acquisition of knowledge is IQ independent and it shows much less individual variation than explicit acquisition of knowledge (IQ related) more or less independent of the state of cognitive development.

On the face of it a problematic point is that the mechanism for implicit knowledge is usually not treated as domain specific but most of the relevant developmental studies are domain specific (syntax development, Weinert 1992). However, there is no reason why domains need to be internally defined rather than externally by the domain itself. So a general learning mechanism differentiates domains by detecting that certain things cohere structurally while others do not do so across domains. This is demonstrated in implicit acquisition of artificial grammars where people can acquire two different grammars and employ them differentially (e.g. Dienes et al., 1994).

By replacing modules with implicitly acquired knowledge about domains we gain the advantage of being able to make sense of a rapidly increasing body of evidence that much knowledge is first acquired implicitly before it becomes explicit (conscious and verbalizable). Karmiloff-Smith (1992) gives examples from many domains, in particular, how language knowledge manifests itself at first implicitly as successful comprehension and production procedures before it becomes gradually explicit as shown by spontaneous corrections of errors and later explicit talk about it. Goldin-Meadow, Alibali & Church (1993) review their research on the fact that understanding of Piagetian conservation concepts and algebraic knowledge often emerges several months earlier in children's manual gestures before it enters their conscious verbalizations about the problem. Clements & Perner (1994) found that even as abstract a concept as false belief is first understood implicitly. Almost a year in advance children correctly look in anticipation for a story character in a video display where that character will mistakenly search for an object before they can give an answer to a question about where the character will search for the object.

Inspection of *existing longitudinal studies* reveals patterns of individual differences and stability with age that are compatible with Anderson's model:

(A) When averaged over individuals almost all cognitive measures show the typical monotonic increase in childhood and more or less steep decrease in old age (Brody, 1994; Schaie, 1983; Weinert & Helmke, in press). Thus longitudinal studies replicate the results of cross-sectional studies almost perfectly. In addition to cross-sectional studies, longitudinal results make clear that this increase in mean performance during childhood is due to a steady increase of individual contributions. This can be interpreted as a reflection of the largely universal human nature at the functional level.

(B) Despite the parallelity of improvements with age between individuals there is only a small- to medium-sized correlation between achievements in different domains. The small size of these correlations could have many causes, for example, domain-specific differences in interests, interest driven activities, environmental incentives and rewards, exposures (inherited) abilities, maturation rate between knowledge acquisition modules, and the related individual learning processes.

(C) The stability of differences in cognitive achievements on complex tasks between individuals is surprisingly low during childhood as well as during adulthood. This can be taken as a reflection of individual differences in content-specific learning experiences and of a high variability of behavior and performance in solving cognitive tasks (Siegler, 1994).

(D) In contrast, individual differences for highly aggregated measures of content free abilities (IQ or other indicators of factor g) tend to be very stable (Bloom, 1964). Despite the drastic increase in cognitive competence during childhood and decrease in old age individual differences persist over relatively long periods; at the same time there is a small group of individuals with significant changes. But: 'the reliable change that does take place appears to be idiosyncratic; it is not systematically associated with environmental change'.   (Moffitt et al., 1993: 499)

This pattern of data teaches us that one should not, as the many cross-sectional studies tempted us to do, infer from consistent replications of apparently systematical changes in group means that general causal mechanisms are at work. As a cautionary point one should add that from the lack of strong correlations between cognitive variables one cannot infer their functional independence (Howe, Rabinowitz & Grant 1993). Similarly, the low stability over time is not a reliable indicator for the total absence of causal factors of multicausally determined changes in cognitive performance.

On a more positive note, the pattern of longitudinal findings is interpretable within the framework of the evolutionary considerations and Anderson's model. The rather stable individual differences in IQ (point D) can be interpreted as kinds of quantitative differences due to individual differences in genetic make up. The other individual differences (points B and C), too, can be attributed to quantitative variations. More specifically, the low correlations between cognitive measures (point B) can be explained by the different acquisition rates for different knowledge domains and the low stability (point C) by the fact that these differences between acquisition rates differ across individuals. In contrast to the individual differences in rate of acquisition, developmental uniformity is observed in that almost all individuals acquire all the cognitive contents, that are functionally essential.

This interpretation of findings may help solve an apparent contradiction between two important lines of modern developmental research: behavioral genetics (heritability research) and the novice–expert paradigm. Although there was prolonged resistance to accept genetic influence on human cognition, most social scientists now believe in such a link (Snyderman & Rothman, 1987).

In apparent contradiction research on the novice–expert paradigm is based on the assumption that it is the dogged application to acquiring knowledge about a particular domain that turns novices into experts:

'We agree that expert performance is qualitatively different from normal performance. . . However, we deny that these differences are immutable, that is, due to innate talent. Instead, we argue that the differences between expert performance and normal adults reflect a life-long persistence of deliberate effort to improve performance in specific domains.'   Ericsson, Krampe & Tesch-Römer 1993: 400)

The apparent contradiction between these two positions can be resolved by considering the following facts. Heritability of intelligence is likely to influence the acquisition of expertise through a mechanism that has often been overlooked: 'The proximal cause of most psychological variance probably involves learning through experience, just as radical environmentalists have always believed. The effective experiences, however, to an important extent are self-selected, and that selection is guided by the steady pressure of the genome (a more distal cause).' (See Bouchard, et al., 1990: p. 227; see also Plomin, 1994, for the contribution of the genetic approach to identifying environmental influences.) Hence, Ericsson may be right that, once one has decided to become an expert, the main factor for achieving this goal is the time and effort spent. Yet, the decision and willingness to endure this effort may be highly dependent on successful learning experiences in the early stages (Bloom, 1985) and this motivation-sustaining success may in turn depend on heritable preferences ('attitude') for particular domains (Teser, 1993), heritable ability, and will.

In sum, we tried to develop a coherent argument from basic evolutionary considerations that individual differences are by and large limited to quantitative variations in cognitive functioning (differences in processing speed affecting IQ, different maturation rates of modules or domain specific learning preferences, processes and learning opportunities) while qualitatively most cognitive functions are panspecific. Although we also tried to adduce relevant empirical evidence for this view, at present it is an attempt to theoretically integrate apparently discrepant findings rather than an empirically validated theory.

LIFESPAN

The evolution theoretic considerations about individual differences, as outlined at the beginning of the last section, also yield predictions for age dependent changes. Although there is strong pressure for a uniform functional human nature it is possible to be in limited ways functionally polymorph (genetically programmed functional differences). In the human physiology two kinds of morphs are clearly pronounced: sexual differences and differences with age (i.e. bodily changes at certain ages are genetically programmed). As far as physiology gives us some hint of what can be expected psychologically (although, when considering sex, the very apparent physiological differences do not seem to be reflected in equally profound psychological or neural differences; cf. Gorski, Chapter 16), we would expect that intellectual changes in childhood are partly, if not largely, governed by genetically programmed qualitative functional differences (e.g. most easily but not necessarily correctly conceived of as different maturation rates of modules) since there may be selection pressure to ensure an optimal (or at least sufficient) acquisition of necessary cognitive skills. In contrast, since no such selection pressure is likely to operate on postreproductive organisms, we would not expect genetically programmed qualitative changes in old age. Rather, changes of aging are more likely to be caused by deterioration of genetic and other material, hence result in quantitative changes in functioning, akin to genetic differences between individuals.

Support for this assumption is reflected in a list of attributes put forward by Flavell (1970) in order to highlight how development in childhood markedly differs from cognitive change in adulthood. The intellectual advances in childhood are typically, says Flavell, species-specific uniform, *general, inevitable, momentous, directional, irreversible* and *sequential*, while few changes in adulthood are of this kind. Although changes in old age might have some of these characteristics they do not conform to all of them.

Some support for cognitive age morphs (i.e. genetically programmed age-dependent qualitative functional differences) is provided by evidence for sensitive periods in language acquisition (e.g. Newport, 1991). For instance, deaf individuals with at least 30 years of daily exposure to American sign language (ASL) showed no decrement in basic word order but increasingly clear qualitative deficiencies in morphology the later their exposure began, in particular, if their first exposure was not until the age of 12 years (but see Snow, 1989; Klein, Chapter 12).

In contrast, the best documented cognitive changes in old age concern loss of general, content free (information processing) capacities and decrease in *fluid* intelligence, whereas *crystallized* intelligence, which depends heavily on education, experience and breadth of knowledge content, is relatively resistant to aging (Horn & Donaldson, 1980). Moreover, expertise helps cognitive performance at every age (Salthouse, 1989), but the greater expertise of later life cannot quite compensate for the age-dependent losses of fluid intelligence, reduction in working memory and learning capacity, which particularly affect testing-the-limits tasks (Baltes & Kliegl 1992; Knopf, Preussler & Stefanek, in press).

A particularly interesting hypothesis about developments across the lifespan is that the order of acquisition (emergence) of abilities is reversed in old age ('first in – last out'). This reversal was originally claimed by Ribot (1982) to hold for memory contents. It has also been claimed to hold for Piagetian stages of development (Bäckman, 1987), and has recently found a new field of application.

Implicit memory is functional from early infancy and does not improve over early childhood whereas there is no evidence for explicit memory in early infancy and it improves over the childhood years. In contrast, in old age explicit memory declines noticeably while loss in implicit memory is relatively minor (Graf, 1990). This is particularly interesting since the same pattern of loss is also found in amnesia through brain injury. Amnesiacs tend to lack explicit memory but can have implicit memory intact (Tulving, Hayman & MacDonald, 1991). Typically no clear cases of intact explicit memory without implicit memory are documented (Schacter et al. 1993; Squire, Knowthon & Musen 1993). This helps distinguish between different developmental explanations. One is that implicit memory is more important initially for acquiring basic procedural skills and, hence, there is an evolutionary adaptation that this type of memory is present from the beginning while explicit memory matures later. However this explanation would not quite account for the reversed pattern of loss due to old age or due to brain insult. Another explanation is that explicit memory is functionally dependent on implicit memory (not in terms of individual memories but in terms of general ability: for instance that implicit memory requires the ability to represent certain properties of the stimulus, while explicit memory requires to represent these properties and in addition to attribute these properties to a representation of the stimulus as a particular event. That would explain why implicit memory can function before explicit memory becomes functional and after explicit memory has become impossible or severely impaired.

INDIVIDUAL DEVELOPMENT

In psychology one should distinguish between the 'differential perspective on development' (description and explanation of individual differences) and 'individual development' (description and explanation of how individuals develop). However, attempts at making this distinction have led to much theoretical controversy and into empirical impasses. For instance, William

Stern, one of the founding fathers of differential psychology, considered 'individuality as the asymptote of science looking for laws'. (Stern, 1911: 4, our translation). Consequently, decades of controversy ensued over whether scientific knowledge about individuals and their development is intrinsically tied to the phenomenological-hermeneutic method and only the universal and differential perspectives are amenable to nomothetic approaches. Such a position seems somewhat obsolete these days in view of the existence of several good examples of how the lawfulness of individual development can be analyzed. Three methodological approaches, in particular, have proven fruitful:

(1) The *tradition of learning theory* assumes on principle that the regulation of behaviour is governed by universal laws. However, given the practically infinite variety of environmental conditions under which the universal laws of learning operate, an equally infinite variety of individual learning histories is possible (Skinner, 1953). Biographical studies of experts provide convincing support for the fruitfulness of this theoretical position (Bloom, 1985).

(2) In the tradition of *research on individual differences (differential perspective)* the individual is seen as the respective value of intersecting personality variables. A typical example is the attempt to operationalize a person's cognitive control system as a pattern of strength of different cognitive styles (levelling-sharpening, impulsivity-reflexivity, field dependency-field independency, etc.; Gardner et al., 1959). Similarly, individual profiles of intelligence can be defined within the n-dimensional space of different cognitive abilities. It is assumed that in the course of development a change occurs in the number of independent intelligence factors which are necessary to explain the pattern of ability specific to a particular age and/or a particular individual (hypothesis of increasing differentiation in childhood and decreasing differentiation in old age). However, the validity, theoretical interest, and practical utility of such factor-analytic models for describing cognitive development are still the focus of persistent criticism.

(3) In contrast to the previous two positions, the person-centered approach assumes that individuals are not just the idiosyncratic intersection of variables but emphasizes people as carriers of individually organized patterns as a theoretically significant fact (Magnusson, 1988). In other words, while the differential perspective investigates the distribution of particular variables or sets of variables in populations and subpopulations of persons, the person centered approach is concerned with the patterning of a large number of variables within a particular person. Individual development is then seen as the change or constancy of such patterns over age.

Unfortunately, the individual approach has so far been neglected in the cognitive area – in contrast to personality development (e.g. use of the Q-sort paradigm). We lack models and instruments for measuring the developmental changes in the (a) individual organization of knowledge domains,

(b) individual varieties of intuitive theories of physics, biology and psychology, and (c) structure of individual thinking habits and problem-solving heuristics. The only candidate for such an approach, Kelly's (1955) concept of 'personal constructs' failed to engender a lasting tradition within developmental psychology.

CONCLUSION

We have been heavily relying on evolutionary arguments in our attempt to gauge the likely generality of developmental regularities. However, by doing so, we did not want to create the impression that most of what is of interest in cognitive development is innate, that is, that all interesting aspects of cognitive development are genetically preprogrammed. Rather, an evolutionary perspective does not prejudge the issue of what is innately programmed and what is programmed to be acquired through interaction with the environment. It is perhaps as a reaction to the past dominant empiricism in the 'biological' or 'evolutionary' conjures up fears of everything being innate.

ACKNOWLEDGMENTS

The authors express their gratitude to Jens Asendorpf, Paul Baltes, Gerd Gigerenzer, Lars-Göran Nilsson, and Bob Siegler for helpful comments on an earlier draft.

REFERENCES

Anderson, M. (1992) *Intelligence and Development. A cognitive Theory.* Oxford: Blackwell.

Bäckman, L. (1987) Applications of Ribot's law to life span cognitive development. In G. L. Maddox and E. W. Busse (eds.) *Aging: The Universal Human Experience,* New York: Springer-Verlag, pp. 403–10.

Baltes, P. B. & Kliegl, R. (1992) Further testing of limits of cognitive plasticity: negative age differences in a mnemonic skill are robust. *Developmental Psychology,* **28,** 121–5.

Bloom, B. S. (1964) *Stability and Change in Human Characteristics.* New York, London, Sydney: John Wiley.

Bloom, B. S. (ed.) (1985) *Developing Talent in Young People.* New York: Ballantine Books.

Bouchard, T. J. Jr., Lykken, D. T., McGue, M., Segal, N. L. & Tellegen, A. (1990) Sources of human psychological differences: the Minnesota study of twins reared apart. *Science,* **250,** 223–8.

Brentano, F. (1924). *Psychologic vom empirischen Standpunkt* [Psychology from an empirical standpoint]. Leipzig: Felix Meiner.

Brody, N. (1994) 0.5 + or −0.5: Continuity and change in personal dispositions. In Heatherton, T. F. & Weinberger, G. J. L. (eds.) *Can Personality Change?* Washington, DC: American Psychological Association, pp. 59–81.

Buss, D. M. (1994) Personality evoked: the evolutionary psychology of stability and change. In Heatherton, T. F. & Weinberger, G. J. L. (eds.) *Can Personality Change?* Washington, DC: American Psychological Association, pp. 41–57.

Carey, S. (1985) *Conceptual Change in Childhood.* Cambridge: MIT Press.

Case, R. (1995) Capacity based explanations of working memory growth: a brief history and a reevaluation. In Weinert, F. E. & Schneider, W. (eds.) *Memory Performance and Competencies: Issues in Growth and Development.* Hillsdale, NJ: Erlbaum.

Chomsky, N. (1965) *Aspects of the Theory of Syntax.* Cambridge, Mass. MIT Press.

Clements, W. & Perner, J. (1994) Implicit understanding of belief. *Cognitive Development,* **9,** 377–397.

Cosmides, L. & Tooby, J. (1992) Cognitive adaptations for social exchange. In Barkow, J. H., Cosmides L. & Tooby, J. (eds.) *The Adapted Mind.* Oxford: Oxford University Press, pp. 163–228.

Dienes, Z., Altmann, G. T. M., Kwan, L. & Goode, A. (1994) *Unconscious Knowledge of Artificial Grammars is Applied Strategically.* Unpublished manuscript, University of Sussex.

Ericsson, K. A., Krampe, R. T. & Tesch-Römer, C. (1993) The role of deliberate practice in the acquisition of expert performance. *Psychological Review,* **100,** 363–406.

Fischer, K. W. & Rose, S. P. (1994) Dynamic development of coordination of components in brain and behavior. In Dawson, G. & Fischer, K. E. (eds.) *Human Behavior and the Developing Brain.* New York: Guildford Press, pp. 3–66.

Flavell, J. H. (1970) Cognitive changes in adulthood. In Goulet, L. R. & Baltes, P. (eds.) *Life-Span Developmental Psychology.* New York: Academic Press.

Fodor, J. A. (1981) *Representations.* Cambridge, Mass.: MIT Press.

Gardner, R. W., Holzman, Ph.S., Klein, G. S., Linton, H. B. & Spence, D. P. (1959) Cognitive control. *Psychological Issues,* **1,** 1–185.

Goldin-Meadow, S., Alibali, M. W. & Church, R. B. (1993) Transitions in concept acquisition: using the hand to read the mind. *Psychological Review,* **100,** 279–97.

Graf, P. (1990) Life-span changes in implicit and explicit memory. *Bulletin of the Psychonomic Society,* **28,** 353–8.

Horn, J. L. & Donaldson, G. (1980) Cognitive development in adulthood. In Brim, Jr., O. G. & Kagan, J. (eds.) *Constancy and Change in Human Development.* Cambridge, MA: Harvard University Press, pp. 445–529.

Howe, M. L., Rabinowitz, F. M. & Grant, M. J. (1993) On measuring (in)dependence of cognitive processes. *Psychological Review,* **100,** 737–47.

Karmiloff-Smith, A. (1992) *Beyond Modularity: A Developmental Perspective on Cognitive Science.* Cambridge, Mass.: MIT Press.

Keil, F. C. (1989) *Concepts, Kinds and Cognitive Development.* Cambridge, Mass.: MIT Press.

Kelly, G. A. (1955) *The Psychology of Personal Constructs.* New York: Norton.

Kluckhohn, C. & Murray, H. A. (1948) Personality formation: the determinants. In Kluckhohn, C., Murray, H. A. & Schneider, D. M. (eds.) *Personality in Nature, Society and Culture.* New York: A. A. Knopf, pp. 53–67.

Knopf, M., Preussler, W., and Stefanek, J. (in press). '18, 20, 2 . . .' – Kann Expertise im Skatspiel Defizite des Arbeitsgedächtnisses älterer Menschen kompensieren? *Schweizerische Zeitschrift für Psychologie.*

Leekam, S. R. & Perner, J. (1991) Does the autistic child have a metarepresentational deficit? *Cognition,* **40,** 203–18.

Leslie, A. M. & Roth, D. (1993) What autism teaches us about metarepresentation. In Baron-Cohen, S., Tager-Flusberg, H. & Cohen, D. (eds.) *Understanding other minds: Perspectives from Autism.* Oxford: Oxford University Press, pp. 83–111.

Magnusson, D. (1988) *Individual Development from an Interactional Perspective: A Longitudinal Study.* Hillsdale, NJ: Erlbaum.

Moffitt, T. E., Caspi, A., Harkness, A. R. & Silva, P. A. (1993) The natural history of change in intellectual performance: who changes? How much? Is it meaningful? *Journal of Child Psychology and Psychiatry,* **34,** 455–506.

Newport, E. L. (1991) Contrasting conceptions of the critical period for language. In Carey, S. & Gelman, R. (eds.) *The Epigenesis of Mind: Essays in Biology and Knowledge.* Hillsdale, NJ: Erlbaum, pp. 111–30.

Oyama, S. (1989) Ontogeny and the central dogma: do we need the concept of genetic programming in order to have an evolutionary perspective? In Gunnar, M. R. & Thelen, M. (eds.) *Systems and Development: The Minnesota Symposia on Child Psychology, Vol. 22.* Hillsdale, NJ: Erlbaum, pp. 1–34.

Parkin, L. & Perner, J. (1994) Wrong directions in children's theory of mind: what it means to understand belief as representation. Unpublished manuscript, Experimental Psychology, University of Sussex.

Perner, J. (1991) *Understanding the Representational Mind.* Cambridge, Mass.: MIT Press.

Piaget, J. & Inhelder, B. (1941/1974) *The Child's Construction of Quantities: Conservation and Atomism.* (Pomerans, A. J. trans.) New York: Basic Books.

Plomin, R. (1994) The Emanuel Miller Memorial Lecture 1993. Genetic research and identification of environmental influences. *Journal of Child Psychology and Psychiatry,* **35,** 817–34.

Reber, A. S. (1993) *Implicit Learning and Tacit Knowledge.* Oxford: Oxford University Press.

Ribot, T. (1982) *Diseases of Memory.* New York: Appleton.

Salthouse, T. A. (1989) Aging and skilled performance. In Colley, A. M. & Beech, J. R. (eds.) *Acquisition and Performance of Cognitive Skills.* Chichester: John Wiley, pp. 247–64.

Schacter, D. L., Chiu, C.-Y.P. & Ochsner, K. N. (1993) Implicit memory: a selective review. *Annual Review of Neuroscience,* **16,** 159–82.

Schaie, K. W. (1983) The Seattle longitudinal study: a 21-year exploration of psychometric intelligence in adulthood. In Schaie, K. W. (ed.) *Longitudinal Studies of Adult Psychological Development.* New York, London: Guildford Press, pp. 64–135.

Siegler, R. S. (1994) Cognitive variability: a key to understanding cognitive development. *Current Directions in Psychological Science,* **3,** 1–5.

Skinner, B. F. (1953) *Science and Human Behavior.* New York: Macmillan.

Snow, C. (1989) Relevance of the notion of a critical period to language acquisition. In Bornstein, M. H. (ed.) *Sensitive Periods in Development.* Hillsdale, NJ: Erlbaum, pp. 183–209.

Snyderman, M. & Rothman, S. (1987) Survey of expert opinion on intelligence and aptitude testing. *American Psychologist,* **42,** 137–44.

Spelke, E. S. (1991) Physical knowledge in infancy: Reflections on Piaget's theory. In Carey, S. & Gelman, R. (eds.) *The Epigenesis of Mind: Essays in Biology and Knowledge.* Hillsdale, NJ: Erlbaum, pp. 133–69.

Squire, L. R., Knowlton, B. & Musen, G. (1993) The structure and organization of memory. *Annual Review of Psychology*, **44**, 453–95.

Stern, W. (1911) *Die differentielle Psychologie in ihren methodischen Grundlagen*. Leipzig: Barth.

Symons, D. (1992) On the use and misuse of Darwinism in the study of human behavior. In Barkow, J. H., Cosmides, L. & Tooby, J. (eds.) *The Adopted Mind*. Oxford: Oxford University Press, pp. 137–59.

Teser, A. (1993) The importance of heritability in psychological research: the case of attitudes. *Psychological Review*, **100**, 129–42.

Tooby, J. & Cosmides, L. (1990) On the universality of human nature and the uniqueness of the individual: the role of genetics and adaptation. *Journal of Personality*, **58**, 17–67.

Tulving, E., Hayman, C. A. G. & MacDonald, C. (1991) Long-lasting perceptual priming and semantic learning in amnesia: a case experiment. *Journal of Experimental Psychology, Learning, Memory and Cognition*, **17**, 595–617.

Wason, P. (1966) Reasoning. In Foss, B. M. (ed.) *New Horizons in Psychology*. Harmondsworth: Penguin.

Weinert, F. E., & Helmke, A. (in press). The neglected role of individual differences in theoretical models of cognitive development. *Learning and Instruction (Special Issue)*.

Weinert, S. (1992) Deficits in acquiring language structure: The importance of using prosodic cues. *Applied Cognitive Psychology*, **6**, 545–71.

11 Cognitive and neural development: clues from genetically based syndromes

URSULA BELLUGI, EDWARD S. KLIMA AND PAUL P. WANG

Cognitive neuroscience is the new research enterprise that studies the mind and its workings. It draws on the theoretical, experimental, and analytical traditions of fields such as neurobiology, psychology, linguistics and computational science, using results from each to constrain theories in the others. It also draws on powerful new experimental methods, such as those being developed in the field of neuroimaging.

The field of developmental cognitive neuroscience focuses on the biological and psychological determinants of the development of cognitive functions. The long-term goal of much of cognitive neuroscience is to understand the brain mechanisms that underlie language and other domains of cognition. The study of development requires examination of trajectories over time, and may help clarify the determinants of brain organization for language and other cognitive functions. The study of normal development is important, and the use of specific 'experiments of nature' may allow new perspectives on these central issues. In one approach, studies of specific well-defined neurodevelopmental disorders may provide some insights into these complex issues. We report here on significant attempts to forge links between neurodevelopmental disorders, development of specific neuropsychological abilities, and the functional establishment of patterns of brain organization. Such research programs are providing converging evidence for the coherence or dissociability of components of cognition and inform theoretical explanations of the underlying architecture of human cognition.

BACKGROUND

Cognitive neuroscience is inherently multidisciplinary, examining processes of development from diverse perspectives, all of which converge on the central issue of the development of higher cognitive functions in man. This field examines the cascade of events from the genetic to the neurobiological level, using different modes of brain imaging which would not have been possible a decade ago, and coordinates studies of brain structure, brain function, and brain cytoarchitectonics.

Some of the central issues of cognitive neuroscience are exemplified by contrasting the development of language and other higher cognitive functions in normal children with the development in children with abnormal phenotypes. Children with autism, deaf children, children with focal lesions to the right or the left hemisphere, and children with genetically-based disorders such as Williams syndrome and Down syndrome provide revealing, striking examples.

Two genetic disorders, Williams syndrome and Down syndrome, result in abnormalities of language and other cognitive behavior, and of neurobiological development (e.g. Coyle, Oster-Granite & Gearhart, 1986; Korenberg, 1993, 1994; Bellugi, Wang & Jernigan, 1994). In this chapter, we examine cognitive and neural development using some 'experiments of nature' to illustrate this new field. While Down syndrome is well-known, Williams syndrome until very recently has been relatively obscure. Recognized as a distinct entity only since 1961 (Williams, Barratt-Boyes & Lowe, 1961), it has an estimated incidence of 1 in 25,000 live births. Diagnosis to date has rested on a distinctive facies in conjunction with mental retardation and abnormalities of cardiac and vascular structures, typically a specific heart defect (supravalvular aortic stenosis), abnormalities of calcium metabolism, and failure to thrive in infancy, among others. Culler, Jones & Deftos (1985) and Jones (1995) suggest that an impaired calcitonin response to calcium may serve as an endocrine marker for Williams syndrome, even in the absence of known hypercalcemia. Molecular geneticists have recently made a major discovery with respect to the pathogenesis of Williams syndrome in their identification of a major part of the specific defect responsible for Williams syndrome, a hemizygosity around the elastin locus on chromosome 7. Consequently, genetic diagnosis is now possible (Bellugi & Morris, 1995; Morris, 1995). In a large number of sporadic cases studied, it has been found that Williams syndrome results from the deletion of one copy of the elastin gene and adjacent gene or genes (Morris, 1995).

Researchers have therefore undertaken systematic sets of studies across matched subjects with Williams syndrome and Down syndrome who are contrasted with normal controls, and children with focal lesions to the right or the left hemisphere. Down syndrome, in particular, provides a relatively homogeneous and well-defined contrast group from the larger population of adolescents with mental retardation, and active research on the neurobiology and genetic basis of Down syndrome make it another exciting area for investigations of the biological basis of cognition. In our research studies reported in this chapter, Williams syndrome and Down syndrome subjects were selected to match for age, full-scale intelligence quotient (IQ), and educational background. Each of the Williams syndrome and Down syndrome subjects were studied across a comprehensive battery of neuropsychological, linguistic, neurobiological, neuroanatomic and neurophysiologic measures.

DECOUPLING BETWEEN LANGUAGE AND OTHER COGNITIVE FUNCTIONS

The precise relationship between language structure (grammar) and other aspects of cognitive functions is a strongly debated theoretical issue. Major theoretical models of language acquisition present alternative views bearing on the relationship of cognitive and linguistic domains. The study of normal development sheds little light on this issue in that linguistic and nonlinguistic cognitive functions are so intimately intertwined that it is difficult to separate these functions. Studies with atypical populations such as Williams syndrome and Down syndrome can be critical in addressing these issues which bear on the domains of higher cognitive capacities and their underlying neural substrate.

Equal impairment of general cognition in two genetically-based syndromes

Both the Williams syndrome subjects and the comparison cohort of Down syndrome subjects are classified as mentally retarded, as defined by the American Association on Mental Deficiency, with IQ scores ranging between about 40 and 70. Studies have found that fewer than 5% of the Williams syndrome adults surveyed had obtained open employment or had the skills necessary to maintain an independent household; the remainder lived or studied in sheltered environments (Udwin, 1990). These difficulties are consistent with marked impairment of general cognitive abilities in Williams syndrome and form the context for the comparative studies of language and other cognitive skills in the two genetically-based disorders. The groups of subjects studied are well-matched on age and on overall measures of cognitive function. On other probes of general intelligence, subjects with Williams syndrome and Down syndrome turn out to be equally impaired. Across an array of conceptual and problem-solving tasks, both groups demonstrate a consistent equivalent impairment in general cognitive functioning.

Cognitive prerequisites and linguistic correlates dissociated

Both Williams syndrome and Down syndrome adolescents characteristically score poorly on other cognitive probes; for example on Piagetian tests of conservation, including conservation of number, weight and substance (Bellugi et al., 1994). These tasks which probe general cognitive abilities are normally mastered early in the course of cognitive development. Both Williams syndrome and Down syndrome adolescents fail completely on cognitive tasks of conservation easily mastered by young normal children. In contrast, adolescents with Williams syndrome perform nearly perfectly on a

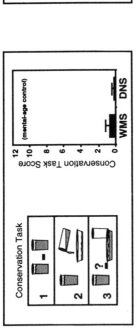

Figure 11.1. Decoupling between language and cognition in Williams syndrome.

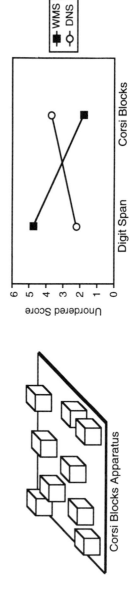

Figure 11.2. Double dissociation between phonological and Visual-Spatial short-term memory in Williams syndrome and Down syndrome.

linguistic task of comprehension of passive sentences, while Down syndrome subjects are close to chance (Figure 11.1). These findings challenge important theoretical models of cognitive abilities.

Differences in memory and learning

The examination of memory and learning abilities provides a direct avenue by which one can address the developmental route that children have traversed on the way toward their current state. Exploration of memory and learning and their neurobiological substrates is critical to understanding the specific cognitive and neurobiological profiles of Williams syndrome and Down syndrome subjects.

While on global measures of cognitive function Williams syndrome and Down syndrome adolescents score equivalently, there are specific cognitive functions (e.g. learning and memory) where the two cohorts are significantly different. There is a double dissociation between phonological and visual spatial stores in *explicit memory* with the Down syndrome subjects better on the visual-spatial stores than the phonological stores. The Williams syndrome subjects show the reverse pattern (Figure 11.2) (Wang & Bellugi, 1994). There is differential impairment of *implicit memory* on a rotor pursuit task with Down syndrome subjects showing better performance than Williams syndrome subjects (Bellugi, Wang & Jernigan, 1994).

REMARKABLY SPARED LINGUISTIC ABILITIES IN WILLIAMS BUT NOT DOWN SYNDROME SUBJECTS

In the setting of general cognitive impairment, the expressive language of adolescent subjects with Williams syndrome is dramatically distinct from the language of matched Down syndrome subjects, and the language of other groups of mentally retarded children as well. Indeed, one of the hallmarks of Williams syndrome subjects may be their remarkably competent language processing, given their severe level of cognitive impairment. We investigate many aspects of language processing (phonological, morphological, semantic, syntactic, as well as discourse and narrative capacities). Our new studies are also illuminating the interplay between language and affect (Reilly, Klima & Bellugi, 1990; Reilly, Harrison & Klima, 1995).

Grammar

The grammatical facility of adolescents with Williams syndrome, as well as their difference from IQ- and age-matched Down syndrome subjects, is apparent on formal tests of comprehension and production. The Williams syndrome adolescents perform much better than their Down syndrome matches, and nearly at ceiling, for example, on certain tests of comprehension of passive sentences, negation and conditionals (Bellugi et al., 1992). On a test of comprehension of passive sentences, the Williams syndrome adolescent subjects score near ceiling. The ability to detect and correct anomalies in the syntax of a sentence depends on knowledge of syntactic constraints and the ability to reflect upon grammatical form. These are sophisticated metalinguistic abilities that can be mastered considerably after the acquisition of grammar and may never fully develop in certain at-risk populations. We find that the Williams syndrome subjects' linguistic proficiency extends to tests of metalinguistic abilities as well (Wang & Bellugi, 1993). Moreover, analysis of the spontaneous expressive language of adolescent Williams syndrome subjects shows that they typically produce well-formed, grammatically correct sentences. They characteristically employ a rich variety of grammatically complex forms, including passive sentences, conditional clauses and embedded relative clauses, although there are occasional errors, and even some systematic ones (Rubba & Klima, 1991).

Importantly, the Williams syndrome subjects are able to manipulate, process and comprehend complex grammatical structures, and they are also able to monitor and correct ungrammatical sentences. Despite the occasional errors, Williams syndrome subjects generally use morphological markers appropriately and correctly, including markers for tense and aspect, as well as auxiliaries and articles. By contrast, the language of the matched Down syndrome subjects is more simple and less varied in construction, often with errors and omissions in both morphology and syntax. These differences in linguistic competence, on both production and comprehension tasks, evidence a remarkable preservation of linguistic ability in Williams syndrome, in the context of otherwise widespread general cognitive impairment.

Unusual semantics: a characteristic of Williams syndrome

Across a realm of studies, Williams syndrome adolescent subjects appear to show a *proclivity* for unusual words, not typical of normal or Down syndrome subjects. Despite their low IQ scores, adolescents with Williams syndrome were typically correct on matching such words as 'canine', 'abrasive', and 'solemn' with a picture (see Figure 11.3, left side). In a task of semantic organization, subjects were asked to name all the animals they could think of in a minute. The Williams syndrome adolescents gave quantitatively more responses than the Down syndrome cohort, in fact, as many as matched normal controls. The Down syndrome group gave fewer responses and did not always stay within the category of animals ('ice cream'). Older Williams syndrome subjects produced many animal names, not just typical category members but also low-frequency, non-prototypical choices (see Figure 11.3, right side). Adolescent and adult subjects included choices such as 'yak', 'Chihuahua', 'ibex', 'condor', 'vulture', 'unicorn', 'saber-tooth tiger', far more often than controls matched for mental age. Thus, it appears that unusual word knowledge, processing and choice is characteristic of adolescent and adult Williams syndrome subjects. Note that this is unlike the semantic disturbances that accompany other and clinical disorders (the aphasias, the dementias), unlike errors occasionally committed by normal subjects (slips of the tongue), and decidedly unlike the semantic limitations characteristic of other mentally retarded groups (Bellugi, et al., 1992; Bellugi et al., 1994; Rossen, et al., in press).

Once more with feeling: infusion of linguistic affect in Williams syndrome
We have begun to investigate the interaction of language and affect in Williams syndrome subjects with a series of narrative tasks. In one, subjects were asked to tell a story from a wordless picture book, with no framework provided beyond the pictures themselves. We found marked differences between the matched Williams syndrome, Down syndrome, and control subjects. The spontaneous language displayed by Williams syndrome subjects was phonologically and syntactically sophisticated, as well as effective in using subordinate clauses to foreground and background information, in stark contrast to language samples from the matched Down syndrome counterparts (Figure 11.4). Williams syndrome (but not Down syndrome) subjects characteristically provided well-structured narrations, establishing a clear orientation, introducing time, characters and their states and behaviors ('Once upon a time, when it was dark at night'), stating the problem ('Next morning . . . there was no frog to be found'), and including a resolution ('Lo and behold, they find him. . .') (Reilly, Klima & Bellugi, 1990; Reilly, Harrison & Klima, 1995).

Language may be emotionally enriched by affective prosody as well as through the use of lexically encoded affective devices. In their narrations, Williams syndrome subjects were found to use affective prosody (pitch change, vocalic lengthening, modifications in volume) *far* more frequently than either Down syndrome matches, or even normal children. The affective richness of the Williams syndrome subjects' narratives was also reflected in their lexical choices. Their narratives included frequent comments on the affective state of the characters in the stories (e.g. 'And ah! He was amazed' or 'The dog gets worried and the boy gets mad'), as well as the use of dramatic devices such as character speech and sound effects ('And BOOM, millions of bees came out and tried to sting him'). Their use of exclamatory phrases and other audience engagement devices is evident throughout many of the stories, for example: 'Suddenly splash! The water came up'; 'Lo and behold, they found him with a lady'; and 'Gadzooks! The boy and the dog start flipping over.' These devices were far less frequent in normal subjects and were notably absent in the Down syndrome subjects' stories. In sum, not only are the Williams syndrome adolescents' stories replete with narrative enrichment devices, they use proportionately more affective prosody and make greater

Word Fluency (60 sec timed test): "Name all the animals you can."

WMS: BRONTASAURUS, TYRANDON, BRONTASAURUS REX, DINOSAURS, ELEPHANT, DOG, CAT, LION, BABY HIPPOPOTAMUS, IBEX, WHALE, BULL, YAK, ZEBRA, PUPPY, KITTEN, TIGER, KOALA, DRAGON

DNS: DOGS, CATS, FISH, BIRD, FISH

WMS: TIGER, OWL, SEA LION, ZEBRA, HIPPPOPOTAMUS, TURTLE, LIZARD, REPTILE, FROG, BEAVER, GIRAFFE, CHIHUAHUA

DNS: GOATS, RABBITS, BUNNIES, HORSEY, FRENCH FRIES, GOATS, MONKEYS, HORSEY, ICE CREAM

WMS name many more, and more unusual animals, than DNS.

Figure 11.3. Rich but deviant semantics in Williams syndrome.

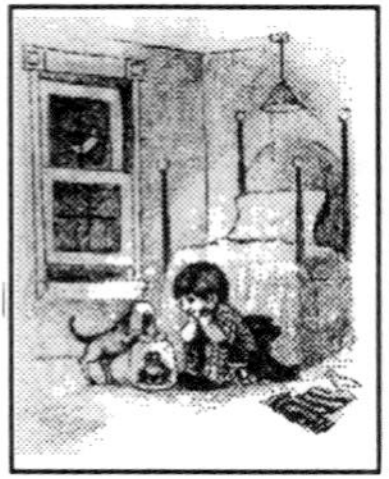

WMS Age 17, IQ 50:
Once upon a time when it was dark at night...the boy had a frog. The boy was looking at the frog...sitting on the chair, on the table, and the dog was looking through....looking up to the frog in a jar. That night he sleeped and slept for a long time, the dog did. But, the frog was not gonna go to sleep. The frog went out from the jar. And when the frog went out...the boy and the dog were still sleeping. Next morning it was beautiful in the morning. It was bright and the sun was.nice and warm. Then suddenly when he opened his eyes...he looked at the jar and then suddenly the frog was not there. The jar was empty. There was no frog to be found.

DNS Age 18, IQ 55:
The frog is in the jar. The jar is on the floor. The jar on the floor. That's it. The stool is broke. The clothes is laying there.

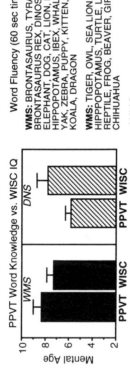

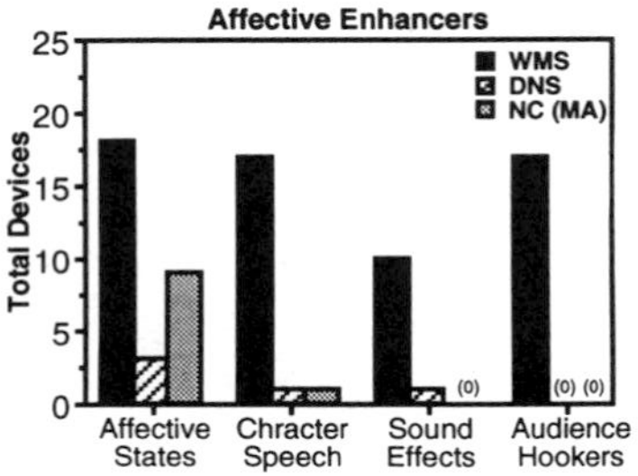

Figure 11.4. Enriched linguistic affect in Williams syndrome.

use of linguistic affective devices than do Down syndrome or even matched normal children (Figure 11.4) (Bellugi et al., 1995).

Despite their cognitive impairments, subjects with Williams syndrome are not only sociable and affectively sensitive, but also they appear to be consciously able to manipulate affective linguistic devices for the purposes of story-telling. However, these subjects appear to use the same level of expressivity regardless of how many times they have told the story and irrespective of their audience. This suggests that their extreme expressivity may turn out to be aberrant (Reilly et al., 1990; Wang & Bellugi, 1993). Research is revealing that the abundance of affectivity, both in prosody and in linguistic devices, may be characteristic of many subjects with Williams syndrome, distinctly different from subjects with right hemisphere damage and markedly different from some autistic subjects. Indeed, in some respects, individuals with Williams syndrome, and individuals with autism appear to be socially, cognitively and neurally opposites (Courchesne, Bellugi & Singer, 1995). Hypersociability, without underlying social judgment, may turn out to be characteristic of Williams syndrome, not unlike certain patients with frontal lesions described in Damasio, 1994.

PEAKS AND VALLEYS IN SPATIAL COGNITION IN WILLIAMS SYNDROME

Like language, spatial cognition may also be fractionated into components. However, the identity of those components has been difficult to establish. Studies of Williams syndrome and Down syndrome have illuminated one of the ways in which visual-spatial abilities may fractionate as a result of genetic anomaly (Bihrle et al., 1989; Bellugi et al., 1990; Bihrle, 1990; Bellugi et al., 1992). We review some of these results in this chapter.

Unique patterns of spatial deficits in Williams versus Down syndrome subjects

Drawings by subjects with Williams syndrome often lack cohesion and overall organization. That is, a drawing of a house might include windows, a door and a roof, but the parts would not be in the correct relationship to each other, for example, 'windows' stretched out across the page outside of the boundaries of the house. By contrast, a comparable Down syndrome subject's drawing might be very simplified, yet show good closure and form, with appropriate relationships among elements. Tested on the Block Design subtest of the WISC-R, the two groups scored equally poorly. However, examination of the *process* by which they arrived at their scores reveals striking differences. Although they failed to provide correct designs, the subjects with Down syndrome generally adhered to the global conformation of the block arrangements, with the internal configurations of the designs incorrect. Williams

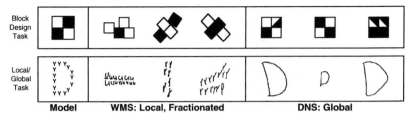

Figure 11.5. Differential spatial processing in Williams and Down syndrome.

subjects, by contrast, failed to adhere to the global conformation of the designs, appearing biased to the details of the designs. Instead, they placed the blocks in apparently haphazard, non-contiguous arrangements. In a process analysis comparing Williams syndrome and Down syndrome adolescents, we found that Williams syndrome subjects made far more moves, and almost invariably moved in continuously fragmented patterns (Figure 11.5, top section).

An experimental task that distinguishes local and global features more rigorously was employed to investigate and characterize these different visual cognitive impairments. Items were composed of local components that together constituted a global form (i.e. a big *D*) made up of little *Y*'s). In these tasks, we found characteristic deficits in Williams syndrome versus Down syndrome that superficially mirrored differences between right- and left-lesioned brain damaged subjects (Bihrle et al., 1989). When asked to draw the designs, both groups failed, but in distinctively different ways. In these paradigms, Williams syndrome subjects typically produced only the local forms sprinkled across the page and were impaired at producing the global forms. Subjects with Down syndrome showed the opposite pattern; they tended to produce the global forms without the local forms (see Figure 11.5, bottom section). This was true whether subjects had to reproduce forms from memory (after a five-second delay) or whether they were asked to copy the form placed in front of them. In perceptual matching tasks as well, Williams syndrome subjects showed a local bias. These results suggest an unusual processing pattern in Williams syndrome, a bias toward attention to detail at the expense of the whole (Wang, Doherty, Rourke & Bellugi, in press).

Preservation of facial processing in Williams syndrome

Despite their severe spatial cognitive dysfunctions, there are realms where Williams syndrome subjects display selective sparing of abilities. The Williams subjects (but not the Down subjects) demonstrate a dramatic ability at recognizing, discriminating and remembering unfamiliar and familiar faces (Rossen 1995, in press). These include abilities related to the perception of faces, such as recognizing the same face in various conditions of lighting and orientation. Subjects with Williams syndrome show remarkable abilities, performing much better than subjects with Down syndrome, and as proficiently as normal age-matched controls on face recognition tasks. Thus, while there are gross deficits in general cognitive ability, subjects with Williams syndrome exhibit a unique pattern of peaks and valleys in spatial cognition: the preference for local over global processing; extreme fractionation in drawing; yet an island of sparing for processing, recognizing and remembering faces (Bellugi et al., 1994).

Neurocognitive probes suggest that Williams syndrome, but not Down syndrome, results in a highly uneven neurobehavioral profile of specific deficits, preservation and anomalies both within and across domains of higher cognitive functioning. Williams syndrome thus presents a rare pattern of dissociations providing an unusual opportunity to forge links to neural substrates and to the genetic basis of the syndrome.

STAGES OF DEVELOPMENT IN WILLIAMS SYNDROME

Interestingly, the neurocognitive profile we find in adolescent and adult Williams and Down syndrome subjects is in some ways quite different from that exhibited during development. Studies of the acquisition of first words and grammar in large groups of subjects with Williams syndrome and Down syndrome reveal that aspects of language are quite late in both cohorts. Although both groups of children are equally delayed as compared to normally developing children, differential trajectories of language and communication emerge. In particular, children with Down syndrome exhibit an early advantage for communicative gestures, while children with Williams syndrome display an advantage for grammar later in development. These findings are striking given the marked differences observed between adolescents and adults with Williams syndrome and Down syndrome, where subjects with Williams syndrome exhibit linguistic skills superior to those of matched Down syndrome controls despite their significant cognitive deficits (Singer et al., 1994; Jones, Rossen & Bellugi, 1995). Other differences emerge in a comparison of three domains across developmental ages (vocabulary, visuospatial abilities, and face processing). Down syndrome children showed similar depressed scores across the three domains. On the other hand, the Williams syndrome developmental profile is different across the domains: visuospatial functions are significantly below the Down syndrome level at all ages and never go beyond the equivalent level of five years of age. In language development there is an initial delay in Williams syndrome subjects equivalent to that of the Down syndrome subjects, and a distinct but late continuing rise in linguistic processing as grammar emerges. Face processing is excellent from very early on, with Williams syndrome subjects tending to score above their mental age regardless of chronological age. Thus the profile of linguistic

Table 11.1. *Williams and Down syndrome profiles*

Neuropsychological profiles

	Williams syndrome	Down syndrome
Preschoolers		
Vocabulary acquisition	Delayed	Delayed
Motor milestones	Delayed	Delayed
Adolescents/young adults		
Grammar	Correct, complex	Poor, simple
Semantics	Larger vocabulary, unusual word	Small vocabulary
Linguistic affect	Rich	Diminished
Visuomotor ability	Poor, fragmented	Simple, cohesive
Hierarchical processing	Local	Global
Processing of faces	Remarkably strong	Impaired

Brain morphometry

Brain region	Williams syndrome	Down syndrome
Cerebrum (and regional proportions)		
Overall volume	↓	→
Anterior cerebrum	↕	→
Temporal limbic	↕	→
Subcortical nuclei (proportional sizes)		
Caudate	↕	↕
Lenticular/diencephalon	↕	←
Cerebellum (volumes)		
Overall	↕	→
Paleocerebellar vermis	↕	↑
Neocerebellar vermis	←	↕
Neocerebellar tonsils	↕	→

↓ less than controls, ↔ similar to controls, ↑ greater than controls preservation in the face of severe cognitive deficits found in older children with Williams syndrome is not evident initially. Table 11.1 summarizes aspects of the distinctive neuropsychological profile of Williams syndrome in contrast to Down syndrome children.

THE NEUROBIOLOGICAL BASIS OF WILLLIAMS SYNDROME

In addition to insights on the organization of cognitive abilities, we are interested in the neurobiological bases of language and thought. This effort has been spurred recently by the development of unprecedented methods for evaluating brain structure and function in living, thinking subjects. For the study of human subjects, the development of neurophysiological studies using event-related potentials (ERPs), positron emission tomography (PET) and the new techniques for three-dimensional visualization and analysis of magnetic resonance imaging (MRI) are currently the most important.

Neurophysiological characterization of Williams syndrome

A series of studies has been undertaken using event-related potential techniques (ERPs) to assess the timing and organization of neural systems active during sensory, cognitive and language processing in Williams syndrome subjects (Bellugi et al., 1992; Neville, Mills & Bellugi, 1994). Two of the notable characteristics of the Williams syndrome behavioral profile have so far been investigated. First, the auditory recovery cycle has been tested for indices of hyperexcitability at any stage along the auditory pathway that might provide clues to the basis of the sensitivity to auditory stimuli shown by many Williams syndrome subjects. Secondly, auditory sentence processing which includes semantic anomalies has been assessed as to whether such processing is mediated in Williams syndrome by the same pathways that are active in normal age-matched controls.

Auditory brainstem evoked responses turn out to be normal in Williams syndrome subjects, indicating that auditory hyperexcitability does not occur at the brainstem level. However, data from an auditory recovery paradigm suggest a possible cortical mechanism subserving the apparent sensitivity to sounds. This is only evident over the temporal cortex and is specific to auditory input; Williams syndrome subjects are indistinguishable from normal controls on a visual recovery paradigm. Taken together, these studies suggest that the hyperacusis observed in Williams syndrome may be mediated by hyperexcitability specifically within the cortical areas that are utilized in processing acoustic information (Figure 11.6a).

ERPs have also been recorded of Williams syndrome subjects' responses to auditorally presented words in sentences (Nevill et al., 1994). One half of the sentences were highly contextually constrained, ending with a

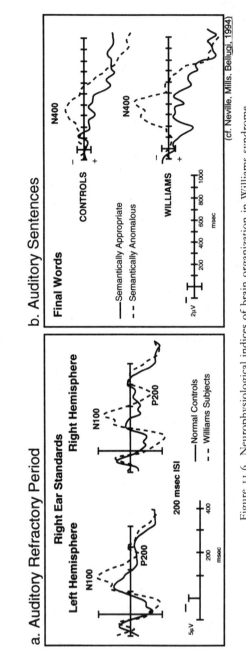

Figure 11.6. Neurophysiological indices of brain organization in Williams syndrome.

semantically appropriate word, whereas the other half ended with an anomalous word (e.g. 'I take my coffee with cream and paper'). Previous research has shown that normal subjects indicate a large negative response at 400 msec (N400) to semantically unprimed words and this is considered an index of how the mental lexicon is organized. Williams syndrome subjects displayed responses that were highly abnormal within the first 200–300 msec following word onset. The abnormality consisted of a large positivity, not seen in normal control subjects at any age. This effect, only apparent over temporal brain regions, may relate to Williams syndrome hyperacusis. The effect of the semantic anomaly is larger in Williams syndrome than in the controls, which may be related to the unusual semantic proclivities shown by Williams syndrome subjects in certain tasks (Bellugi et al., 1992). Moreover, the Williams syndrome responses did not show the expected left-hemisphere asymmetries that are typical for normal children and adults, suggesting that there may be an unusual pattern of brain organization underlying the Williams syndrome language capacities (Figure 11.6).

The neuroanatomical basis of Williams syndrome

New techniques of brain imaging permit visualization and analysis of structures within the brain that were not possible in the past. Techniques developed by Damasio and Frank (1992) for example, now permit an unprecedented visualization and three-dimensional analysis of the living brain of subjects. Our studies have been revealing that both Williams syndrome and Down syndrome leave a distinctive morphological stamp on specific brain regions. Morphometric MRI studies of the brain have been performed on a group of adolescents and young adults with Williams syndrome and Down syndrome (Jernigan & Bellugi, 1990; Wang et al., 1992; Jernigan & Bellugi, 1994). Figure 11.6 shows results of the neuromorphological characterization of Williams syndrome versus Down syndrome subjects, with comparable overall reductions of cerebral volume in both syndromes, in comparison to age-matched normal controls. Analyses reveal important regional differences in brain volume between the two groups of subjects. First, anterior brain volume is disproportionately reduced in Down syndrome subjects but proportionately preserved in subjects with Williams syndrome. Secondly, limbic structures in the temporal lobe show essentially equal volumes in Williams syndrome and control subjects, but are significantly reduced in Down syndrome subjects. On the other hand, the volume of the thalamus and lenticular nuclei are much better preserved in subjects with Down syndrome than those with Williams syndrome. We are also finding that the anterior parts of the corpus callosum, like the anterior hemispheres, are preserved in Williams syndrome subjects, but diminished in Down syndrome subjects (Figure 11.7).

Quantitative analysis of cerebellar volumes also suggests differences, with

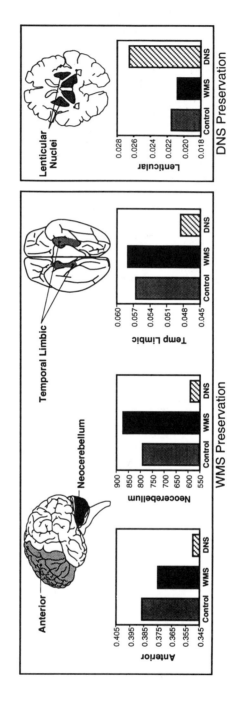

Figure 11.7. Differential brain morphology in Williams syndrome and Down syndrome.

cerebellar volume well-preserved in Williams syndrome subjects but diminished in Down syndrome subjects. Closer regional analyses are enlightening: we find that the locus of preservation in Williams syndrome is the neocerebellum. Of the two parts of the neocerebellum that are subjected to analysis, the neocerebellar vermis and the neocerebellar tonsils, both show volumetric preservation or even increases in Williams syndrome as compared to controls, whereas both are volumetrically diminished in Down syndrome (Figure 11.7). Importantly, the specific regions of the neocerebellum that may be enlarged in Williams syndrome have been shown to be dysplagic in autism (Courchesne et al., 1988; Bellugi, Wang & Jernigan, 1994; Courchesne, Bellugi & Singer, 1995).

Results of related research suggest that the expansive pre-frontal cortex and the neocerebellum, both selectively preserved in Williams syndrome, are thought to be closely related. These two regions of the brain are most highly developed in *homo sapiens*, and are thought to have evolved contemporaneously (Deacon, 1990). Furthermore, the neocerebellum has more extensive connections to pre-frontal and other association areas of the cortex, than do the older parts of the cerebellum (Leiner, Leiner & Dow, 1993). The third area of preservation in Williams syndrome, the mesial temporal lobe, may include portions of auditory association cortex, which also projects to Broca's and other pre-frontal areas. The neuroanatomic profile of Williams syndrome emerging from our new methods of neuroimaging thus is beginning to contribute to the understanding of the brain's organization, by exhibiting a morphological pattern that can result from genetic bias. The finding that anterior, temporal limbic and neocerebellar regions are selectively preserved in Williams syndrome suggests that they all may come under the influence of a single genetic, developmental factor, or that their development is mutually interactive, or both (Bellugi et al., 1994). These issues bearing on the relationship of brain to behavior are fundamental to central questions of cognitive neuroscience (Bellugi & Morris, 1995).

Brain cytoarchitectonic studies of Williams syndrome

Over the past decade there has been an explosion in knowledge about the biological basis of many mental retardation syndromes. It is now possible to attribute these syndromes to factors acting prenatally or postnatally and linked to abnormal environmental influences such as toxins, deprivations, or asphyxia, or to abnormalities in the chromosomes or mitochondrial genes. In a small number of mental retardation syndromes it is possible to understand the steps between the environmental or innate factors and resultant brain malformations. With the possible exception of Trisomy 21 and a few cases of malformation affecting the brain focally, however, it has not been possible to understand the neuropsychological findings in terms of the cyto-architectonic findings in the brain. Study of Williams syndrome, which consists of focal rather than generalized cognitive deficits, offers an un-precedented opportunity for linking brain findings to specific atypical cognitive profiles.

The brain of a 31-year-old male autopsied individual with Williams syndrome was donated for the purpose of scientific investigation. Cytoarchi-tectonic brain findings revealed that posterior forebrain areas were markedly diminished in volume (Galaburda, Wang, Rossen & Bellugi, 1994; Galaburda, Wang, Bellugi & Rossen, 1995). Other findings include exaggerated hori-zontal organization of neurons within layers, most striking in the occipital lobe, area 17, in which the upper layers assumed a rippled, horizontal alignment reminiscent of layering neurons of a much younger developmental cortical stage. There was also increased cell packing density throughout brain regions and unusually clustered and orientated neurons. The results may relate to the unusual visuospatial processing in Williams syndrome. Such cases provide opportunities for linking brain findings to cognitive deficits and their genetic underpinnings.

IMPLICATIONS FOR DEVELOPMENTAL COGNITIVE NEUROSCIENCE

In the studies reported in this chapter, we consider a line of investigation in cognitive neuroscience which provides clues to long-standing theoretical issues in language and brain organization, and additionally may forge links between specific metabolic disorders, specific neuropsychological profiles and abnormal brain organization. We investigate a major dissociation between language and cognitive functions in Williams syndrome subjects who exhibit selectively spared grammatical capacity in the face of marked cognitive deficits. Furthermore, Williams syndrome results in a distinctive cleavage *within* spatial cognition, in which there is selective attention to details of a configuration at the expense of the whole. These dissociations are explored in terms of their implications for the understanding of normal language and cognitive functions and their underlying neural network, allowing us to address issues such as the basis for cerebral specialization in humans. Our studies combine several approaches that include the inter-relationship of neurolinguistics, neuropsychology, cognitive psychology and studies of brain structure as well as function. One of the greatest challenges in understanding the brain and cognition lies in being able to link inves-tigations across disciplines within the neurosciences. Up to now this goal has remained elusive. These studies with a specific neurodevelopmental disorder, which presents a rare fractionation of higher cortical functioning, may provide opportunities to explore some of the central issues of cognitive neuroscience that tie cognitive functions to brain organization.

ACKNOWLEDGMENTS

The research described here was supported by grants to Dr Ursula Bellugi from the National Institutes of Health (R01 HD26022, P50 NS22343, and P01 DC01289), a grant from the Oak Tree Philanthropic Foundation, as well as a grant from the March of Dimes Foundation to the Salk Institute for Biological Studies.

REFERENCES

Bellugi, U., Bihrle, A., Jernigan, T., Trauner, D. & Doherty, S. (1990) Neuropsychological, neurological, and neuroanatomical profile of Williams syndrome. *American Journal of Medical Genetics*, **6**, 115–25.

Bellugi, U., Bihrle, A., Neville, H., Jernigan, T. & Doherty, S. (1992) Language, cognition and brain organization in a neurodevelopmental disorder. In Gunnar, M. R. & Nelson, C. A. (eds.) *Developmental Behavioral Neuroscience*. Hillsdale, NJ: Erlbaum, pp. 201–32.

Bellugi, U. & Morris, C. A. (eds.) (1995) Williams syndrome: From cognition to gene. Abstracts from the Williams Syndrome Association professional conference. *Genetic Counseling*, Special Issue, **6**(1), 131–92.

Bellugi, U., Wang, P. P. & Jernigan, T. L. (1994) Williams syndrome: an unusual neuropsychological profile. In Broman, S. & Grafman, J. *Atypical Cognitive Deficits in Developmental Disorders: Implications for Brain Function*. Hillsdale, NJ: Erlbaum, pp. 23–56.

Bihrle, A. M. (1990) Visuospatial processing in Williams and Down syndromes. Unpublished Doctoral Dissertation. University of California, San Diego.

Bihrle, A. M., Bellugi, U., Delis, D. & Marks, S. (1989) Seeing either the forest or the trees: Dissociation in visuospatial processing. *Brain and Cognition*, **11**, 37–49.

Courchesne, E., Bellugi, U. & Singer, N. (1995). Infantile autism and Williams syndrome: social and neural worlds apart. Abstract. In Special Issue, *Genetic Counseling*, **6**(1), 144–5.

Courchesne, E., Yeung-Courchesne, R., Press, G. A., Hesselink, J. R. & Jernigan, T. L. (1988). Hypoplasia of cerebellar vermal lobules VI and VII in autism. *New England Journal of Medicine*, **318**, 1349–1354.

Coyle, J., Oster-Granite, M. & Gearhart, J. (1986). The neurobiologic consequences of Down syndrome. *Brain Research Bulletin*, **16**, 773–87.

Culler, F. L., Jones, K. L. & Deftos, L. J. (1985) Impaired calcitonin secretion in patients with Williams syndrome. *Journal of Pediatrics*, **107**, 720–3.

Curran, M. E., Atkinson, D. L., Ewart, A. K., Morris, C. A., Leppert, M. F. & Keating, M. T. (1993) The elastin gene is disrupted by a translocation associated with supravalvular aortic stenosis. *Cell*, **73**, 159–68.

Damasio, A. R. (1994) *Descartes' Error: Emotion, Reason, and the Human Brain*. New York: G. P. Putnam's Sons.

Damasio, H. & Frank, R. (1992) Three-dimensional in vivo mapping of brain lesions in humans. *Archives of Neurology*, **49**, 137–43.

Deacon, T. W. (1990) Rethinking mammalian brain evolution. *American Zoology*, **30**, 629–705.

Galaburda, A., Wang, P. P., Bellugi, U. & Rossen, M. 1994. Cytoarchitectonic anomalies in a genetically based disorder: Williams syndrome. *Neuroreport*, **5**, 753–7.

Galaburda, A., Wang, P. P., Rossen, M. L. & Bellugi, U. (1995) Cytoarchitectonic and immunohistochemical findings in Williams syndrome. Abstract. In Special Issue, *Genetic Counseling*, **6**(1), 142–4.

Jernigan, T. L. & Bellugi, U. (1990) Anomalous brain morphology on magnetic resonance images in Williams syndrome and Down syndrome. *Archives of Neurology*, **47**, 529–33.

Jernigan, T. L. & Bellugi, U. (1994) Neuroanatomical distinctions between Williams and Down syndromes. In Broman, S. & Grafman, J. (eds.) *Atypical Cognitive Deficits in Developmental Disorders: Implications for Brain Function*. Hillsdale, NJ: Erlbaum, pp. 57–66.

Jones, K. L. (1995) Williams syndrome and calcium metabolism. Abstract. In Special Issue, *Genetic Counseling*, **6**(1), 151–2.

Jones, W., Rossen, M. L. & Bellugi, U. (1995) Distinct developmental trajectories of cognition in Williams syndrome. Abstract. In Special Issue, *Genetic Counseling*, **6**(1), 178–9.

Korenberg, J. (1993) Down syndrome: a molecular understanding of the origin of phenotypes. In Epstein, C. (ed.) *The Phenotypic Mapping of Down Syndrome and Other Aneuploid Conditions*. New York: Wiley-Liss, pp. 87–115.

Korenberg, J. (1994) Down syndrome phenotypes: the consequences of chromosomal imbalance. *Proceedings of the National Academy of Science of the USA*, 91: 4997–5001.

Leiner, H. C., Leiner, A. L. & Dow, R. S. (1993) Cognitive and language functions of the human cerebellum. *Trends in Neurosciences*, **16**(11), 444–7.

Morris, C. A. (1995) The search for the genetic etiology of Williams syndrome and supravalvular aortic stenosis. Abstract. In Special Issue, *Genetic Counseling*, **6**(1), 153–5.

Neville, H. J., Mills, D. L. & Bellugi, U. (1994) Effects of altered auditory sensitivity and age of language acquisition on the development of language-relevant neural systems. Preliminary studies of Williams syndrome. In Broman, S. & Grafman, J. (eds) *Atypical Cognitive Deficits in Developmental Disorders: Implications for Brain Function*. Hillsdale, NJ: Erlbaum, pp. 67–83.

Reilly, J. S., Harrison, D. & Klima, E. S. (1995) Emotional talk and talk about emotions. Abstract, Special Issue, *Genetic Counseling*, **6**(1), 158–9.

Reilly, J. S., Klima, E. S. & Bellugi, U. (1990) Once more with feeling: affect and language in atypical populations. *Developmental Psychopathology*, **2**, 367–91.

Rossen, M. L., Jones, W., Wang, P. P. & Klima, E. S. (1995) Face processing: remarkable sparing in Williams syndrome. Abstract, Special Issue, *Genetic Counseling*, **6**(1), 138–40.

Rossen, M. L., Klima, E. S., Bellugi, U., Bihrle, A. & Jones, W. (in press) Interaction between language and cognition: evidence from Williams syndrome. In Beitchman, J. H., Cohen, N., Konstantareas, M. & Tannock, R. (eds.) *Language Learning and Behaviour*. New York: Cambridge University Press.

Rubba, J. & Klima, E. S. (1991) Preposition use in speakers with Williams syndrome: some cognitive grammar proposals. In *Center for Research in Language Newsletter*. San Diego, Calif.: University of California, pp. 3–12.

Singer, N. G., Bellugi, U., Bates, E., Jones, W. & Rossen, M. (1994) Contrasting profiles of language development in children with Williams and Down syndromes.

Project in Cognitive and Neural Development, Technical Report 9403, University of California, San Diego, Calif.

Udwin, O. (1990) A survey of adults with Williams syndrome and idiopathic infantile hypercalcemia. *Developmental Medicine and Child Neurology*, **32**, 129–41.

Wang, P. P. & Bellugi, U. (1993) Williams syndrome, Down syndrome and cognitive neuroscience. *American Journal of Diseases of Children*, Special Contribution, **147**, 1246–51.

Wang, P. P. & Bellugi, U. (1994) Evidence from two genetic syndromes for a dissociation between verbal and visual-spatial short-term memory. *Journal of Clinical and Experimental Neuropsychology*, **16**, 317–22.

Wang, P. P., Doherty, S., Rourke, S. B. & Bellugi, U. (in press) Unique profile of visuo-perceptual skills in a genetic syndrome. *Brain and Cognition*.

Wang, P. P., Hesselink, J. R., Jernigan, T. L., Doherty, S. & Bellugi, U. (1992) The specific neurobehavioral profile of Williams syndrome is associated with neocerebellar hemispheric preservation. *Neurology*, **42**, 1999–2002.

Williams, J., Barratt-Boyes, B. & Lowe, J. (1961) Supravalvular aortic stenosis. *Circulation*, **24**, 1311–18.

12 Language acquisition at different ages

WOLFGANG KLEIN

1. INTRODUCTION

Among the various properties in which humans differ from any other species, it is perhaps the ability to convert thoughts, feelings and wishes into soundwaves, to transmit those to others and thus to influence their thoughts, feelings and wishes, and eventually their behaviour, which is most fundamental. It is *language* which allows human beings an orientation in their environment different from that of a monad in a world defined by the laws of prestabilised harmony, different from that of an ant in a world ruled by the rigid interaction principles of the ant heap. The verbal transmission of all sorts of theoretical and practical knowledge handed down from one generation to the next, on the one hand, and of rapidly changing, situation-bound information, on the other, sets the stage for that particular type of behaviour which we consider to be human. It is language that makes possible all higher forms of cognition as well as that particular kind of interaction between members of a species which is characteristic of human beings. We can imagine a 'mind' without language, but surely not a human mind without language. We can imagine a society without language but not a human society without language.

We are not born with a language in our head. No new-born child knows English, Chinese, or Mopan. At birth, the child is literally an 'infans' – someone who does not speak. But every new-born is able to learn English, Chinese, Mopan, or any other language spoken in the social environment in which he (or she) grows up. Thus, the individual's capacity to speak and to understand a particular language – the *linguistic competence* – has two quite different but equally indispensable sources:

(1) The innate, genetically transmitted *language capacity*, which
  (a) distinguishes us from any other species;
  (b) seems to be more or less the same for all human beings; and
  (c) is neutral with respect to the properties of any particular language.
(2) The socially transmitted knowledge of what is particular to, for example, English as compared to any other language: the child's innate language capacity has to be applied to a particular 'input' –

the structured and meaningful sound waves produced by parents, siblings, and other people in the social environment.

There is no doubt that both components are necessary conditions for the acquisition of a language. Opinions vary, however, with respect to their precise nature and their relative weight in the course and final outcome of this process.

We all learn one language in the first years of our life – our mother tongue. But the capacity to acquire a language does not disappear with childhood. In fact, most people on earth know more than one language. It is common, therefore, to distinguish between *first language acquisition* (abbreviated FLA) and *second language acquisition* (SLA). This simple opposition is a gross simplification, however, for at least two reasons. First, whereas first language acquisition normally has a clear onset defined by biological factors, this is not the case for the acquisition of a second language: it may start at any age and, more importantly perhaps, at any point during the acquisition of the first language – including the borderline case in which two languages rather than one are learned right from the beginning ('bilingual first language acquisition'). Since we are here mainly interested in potential differences of language acquisition over the lifespan, we will, apart from a few side remarks, exclude all cases of temporal overlapping and contrast the child's normal FLA with SLA by the adult. In fact, it is not entirely clear when FLA really comes to an end. The answer varies with the particular linguistic features considered. Phonology is normally fully mastered at school age,whereas there is evidence that important syntactic regularities are not mastered before age nine or 10, and the acquisition of individual lexical items only ends with death. It seems fair, however, to assume that FLA is completed at puberty. In what follows, we shall therefore consider puberty to be the dividing line between first and second language acquisition.

Secondly, whereas FLA is relatively uniform in that it is always directly based on the child's exposure to real language in everyday situations, this is not so for SLA. It may occur, too, in everyday interaction with the speakers of the language to be learned – as in the case, for example, of a Moroccan worker coming to Holland without knowing a single word of Dutch. But it may also be the result of explicit teaching in the classroom – as in the case of Latin classes, to give a particularly extreme example. There are all sorts of transitions between these extremes of 'spontaneous' or 'nonguided' acquisition and 'tutored' or 'guided' acquisition. Most research on SLA deals with learning in the classroom. This is mainly for practical reasons. It is much easier to record and to analyse the performance of students than to follow the erratic ways of an adult foreign worker struggling with an often hostile social and linguistic environment, and it is also felt that the results of this research are particularly useful for educational purposes. But classroom acquisition reflects not so very much the normal functioning and the regularities of the human language learning capacity rather than the effect of particular teaching procedures. The child as well as the nonguided adult learner develop their growing knowledge by an interpretation of sound waves in context. This is a complex process which leads, among others, to a certain order in which the various linguistic properties are learned. The classroom learner is faced with a fixed syllabus that defines the order of acquisition – perhaps totally against the 'natural order'. Therefore, if we want to understand the nature of the human language capacity and its functioning at various ages, we must compare first language acquisition with 'natural' SLA outside the classroom.

Everyday experience tells us that there is at least one salient difference between first language acquisition and second language acquisition (in the narrower sense explained above; henceforth, I shall use it only in this sense, unless said otherwise). The child normally attains 'full mastery' – not in the sense that no more could be learned (not every fluent speaker of English is a Shakespeare) but in the sense that there is no noticeable difference to the language of the social environment.* This is hardly ever the case for the adult second language learner: normally, his/her acquisition stops at a level which is still very far from the language of the 'natives'. Typically, SLA 'fossilises' at some stage whereas fossilisation in FLA is considered to be pathological. How is this difference to be explained?

Apparently, it must have to do either with age – child versus adult – or with the fact that in SLA there is already the first language which, in one way or another, blocks full acquisition of another one. The latter assumption is not very appealing, given what we know about almost unlimited storage capacities of the human brain, and it is clearly falsified by the fact that SLA *before* puberty, say at the age of six, normally does not fossilise. Hence, the difference seems to be a clear age effect – the 'LA age effect': the language learning capacity does not disappear after puberty, but it changes, and apparently becomes much less efficient.

As any other cognitive capacity, the capacity to learn and to use languages is stored in the brain. Therefore, it seems most natural to relate the LA age effect to changes in the brain. The most radical claim to this effect is probably Lenneberg's theory of a 'critical period' during which the brain is receptive for language acquisition (Lenneberg, 1967). Later research did not confirm this theory (see, for example, Lamendella, 1977; Long, 1990; Pulvermüller & Schumann, 1994) and, in fact, any account in terms of purely biological changes in the brain faces a number of problems. First, there is clear evidence that it is atypical but not impossible to learn a second language to perfection after puberty – in the sense that the natives do not notice any difference (for

---

* Even within a small social group, the linguistic competence of its members is usually not fully homogeneous; there are differences in vocabulary size, in discourse rules, even in grammatical features. Therefore, the notion of 'full mastery' should rather be understood in the sense that the linguistic competence of the speaker is within a certain range observed within and tolerated by the social environment.

a recent discussion, see Birdsong, 1992). For more than one thousand years, all European scholars had to learn Latin in school – as a second language. Not all of them did well: there are many medieval jokes about the bad Latin of the clergy. But very many indeed attained 'full mastery'. Cicero would have frowned when reading the writings of St Thomas Aquinas or Newton, because of the content, not because of their language (except a few new words perhaps).* Secondly, there are many biological changes in the brain during the lifespan, but it is difficult to relate them causally to the phenomenon at hand. Thirdly, the notion of an 'age difference' between a child learner and an adult learner collapses at least three types of development:

(1) *Biological development.* It includes all physiological changes of central and peripheral organs which are somehow involved in language, that is, of some parts of the brain, but also of ears and articulatory organs.

(2) *Social development.* A child born in a Chinese-speaking environment does not just learn Chinese as a mother tongue; in doing so, he or she becomes at the same time a member of a particular social group, with particular norms, particular convictions, particular forms of social behaviour, in brief: learning a first language means at the same time to gain a particular social identity. The adult second language learner, for example a Moroccan foreign worker coming to Holland, has such a social identity when he starts to learn Dutch. For the child to learn a language does not just mean to become a 'zoon logon echon' but also a 'zoon politikon' whereas this is not the case for the adult learner. It is open to which extent this developmental difference affects language acquisition but it is surely a factor which has to be taken into account.

(3) *Cognitive development.* It is open, and a matter of much dispute, to which extent linguistic development depends on cognitive development, and vice versa (Behrens, 1993). But there are some salient examples which show that the interaction is strong. In English, as in all Indoeuropean languages, the finite verb is marked for tense, that is, with each sentence, the speaker is simply forced to express a temporal marking such as past, present, or future – whether he wants this or not. This requires not only mastery of a particular morphology on the verb but also a particular conceptualisation of time which varies, within limits, from culture to culture. Therefore, children must not only learn a set of language-specific linguistic means, such as the inflectional morphology of the verb; they also have to elaborate

---

* What we do not know, of course, is how perfect the pronunciation of these scholars was. But at any time in its history, the pronunciation of Latin exhibited a rich variation. Note, incidentally, that we are speaking here of classroom acquisition, and the argument does not show that 'full mastery' can be attained outside the classroom. But it suffices to show that there are no absolute biological obstacles.

a usually quite complex concept of time which underlies the use of the language-specific expressions. It is complex because it not only involves temporal relations such as *before, after, simultaneous* but also the handling of 'deixis' and other forms of context dependency. Time, as expressed by natural languages, is not absolute but varies with one or even sometimes two changing 'reference points'. A similar argument can be made for many other cognitive domains normally reflected in language, such as the expression of space, of possession, of modality. The adult learner, by contrast, already has such a cognitive system, and many ways are imaginable in which this fact may affect his acquisition of a second language.

In short, a child's acquisition of his or her mother tongue and the adult's acquisition of a second language in social context share a number of features, but they also differ in many respects, and if we want to understand these processes and how they vary with age, we must take a closer look at the various determining factors. In the next section, I shall sketch, in very global terms, what these factors are and how they vary. In section 3, we present some empirical findings which exemplify the LA age effect and, in section 4, we will discuss how these differences can be explained. Given the state of our knowledge in this field, the discussion can hardly be more than a series of speculations of what may be the case, rather than solid conclusions of what is the case. The chapter closes with a look at the possibility that there is a specific 'language module' in our brain which is responsible for first language acquisition but no longer available after a certain age and thus causes the LA age effect.

2. A GLOBAL MODEL

Imagine that you are a 22 year-old Moroccan hired to work in a Dutch factory in the city of Tilburg. You do not know a single word of Dutch, in fact, or any other language than your home dialect and, upon arrival, it turns out that the job does not exist. For some reason, you do not want, or are not able to return but decide to stay in Tilburg, and you are lucky enough to find some temporary occupation. In such a situation, you had better learn the language. What are the factors that make the start of this acquisitional process possible?

First, there must be a reason for the learner to solve this complex and tedious task of learning the language, a kind of motivation or, as I shall say, a *propensity*. Such a propensity must also be present in other types of language acquisition, in particular in FLA, albeit perhaps of a very different nature. The learner need not be aware of the nature of his/her propensity, and in the case of FLA, he/she surely is not. Clearly, different types of propensity may lead to very different acquisition processes, and hence, this factor is another possible cause of the observed differences in the final outcome.

Secondly, the learner must possess – still possess – the capacity to acquire a language and to make appropriate use of the acquired knowledge for communicative purposes. In the psycholinguistic literature, this capacity is often called the *language processor*. It encompasses a number of very hetero-geneous, but well-coordinated subfaculties, such as:

    (1) the ability to discriminate speech sounds and to produce them correctly;

    (2) the ability to decompose sound chains into smaller units and to relate these units to particular things or events in the social environment, that is, to identify lexical units;

    (3) the ability to remember these sound-meaning relationships and to combine them appropriately to larger units (phrases or sentences),

and so on. It is an interesting question whether these abilities are 'domain-specific', that is, whether they are only observed in the acquisition and processing of linguistic knowledge, or whether they are just a special application of more general mental and biological capacities. Whereas this latter view seems more parsimonious, an influential school in linguistics, generative grammar, advocates the former view – the language processor is a special, domain-specific component in the human mind, the 'language module'. We shall return to this question in section 5.

These two conditions, propensity and language processor, do not suffice, however. Should you avoid any contact with the Dutch community, or should they refrain from talking to you, it is not very likely that you will much progress with your acquisition of Dutch. A further, obvious condition is therefore *access* to the language to be learned (the *target language*), and here that means access to specimens of sound waves structured according to the regularities of the target language, and used appropriately in context for communicative purposes.*

Each of these three components is indispensable for language acquisition; each of them may vary considerably. The propensity may be very different for child and adult. In the adult's case, it varies with the learner's particular communicative needs and life plans, it is also very different for language in the classroom and outside the classroom. The language processor may undergo considerable changes with age, some of which have been mentioned already. These include biological changes in the brain, but also deteriorating capacities of audition or muscular control of the articulatory organs, or simply expanding knowledge which make some things easier and others more difficult. Access may vary both in amount and type. In the child's and in the

---

* It is crucial that the input does not only consist of the sound waves that hit the learner's ear. It is impossible to analyse these sound waves – to decompose them, to combine them with meaning, etc. – unless they are embedded in all sorts of accompanying information from the situational context. If you just listen to radio programs in Chinese, you will simply not learn it (except some of its phonological features), because all of this parallel nonlinguistic information is missing.

foreign worker's case, it is given by sound waves and accompanying information; in the classroom case, an essential part – if not the largest part – consists of a metalinguistic description of the target language. If we want to understand why some types of language acquisition differ substantially from others, we must carefully determine the particular constellation of these three factors.

Suppose now all three components are given; then the process of language acquisition will begin. It will last for many years, and its course will be characterised by a certain *structure* – the many phonological, syntactical, morphological, lexical properties of the target language, Dutch in this case, will be acquired in a certain order. This order, and hence the structure of the acquisitional process, may vary considerably, depending on factors such as frequency of occurrence, communicative importance of certain forms and constructions, the ease with which they are perceptually or cognitively processed, and perhaps others.

What also varies is the *speed* of the acquisitional process; it depends on factors such as the strength of the propensity, the excellence of the language processor (there are gifted and less gifted learners), the amount and perhaps type of access, and the like. Speed may also change during the acquisition process, for the very reason that the three factors access, propensity and language processor change. After some time, the most vital communicative needs are perhaps satisfied, and hence, the tempo slows down; then, for some change in the social conditions, it might speed up again. In any event, the process ceases at some point: the learner has reached a certain *end state*. This end state is normally not absolute: little changes may still occur, for example some new words may be learned. But basically, the acquisitional process has come to a close. As was said above, in FLA, this point is normally reached when the learner's language does not significantly differ from that of his or her social environment, whereas in SLA, it normally ends much earlier. The question naturally arises whether the premature end of SLA is the only substantial difference between FLA and SLA, or whether we observe a similar variation also in *structure* and in *speed*. We shall now discuss all three cases in more detail.

3. THE LA AGE EFFECT: WHERE ARE THE DIFFERENCES?

Speed: a common myth

There is hardly any comparative research on the speed of language acquisition. Therefore, the question as to potential differences between FLA and SLA in this respect is largely a matter of speculation. What can be said, however, is that a common view held by the layman and by numerous linguists is false – the view that first language acquisition is an amazingly rapid process, given the complexity of the task. We all are usually surprised and pleased to see this sudden explosion in the linguistic skills of children between about one and three years of age, especially if it is our own children. But this impression is somewhat misleading. Even though a child at school age is normally very fluent in his or her language, closer inspection shows that many important structural features are not mastered before nine or 10.* This means that the entire process of FLA extends over at least 10 years; counted by the hours of exposure to the target language and the possibility using it in social context, this is much more time of access than is given to the average second language learner. Hence, the common notion that FLA is much faster than SLA is somewhat doubtful, to say the least. If there are strong differences between FLA and SLA, speed is not the likeliest place to look.

End state: the selectivity of fossilisation

The mere fact that SLA normally ends far before complete mastery is beyond any doubt. But this 'fossilisation' does not affect all aspects of linguistic knowledge in the same way. Mastering a language requires, among others, knowledge of:

(1) *phonological rules*, segmental (correct sound structure) as well as suprasegmental (correct intonation and stress patterns);
(2) *morphological rules*, in particular inflection of nouns and verbs;
(3) *syntactical rules*, such as word order, phrase structure, government relations, etc.
(4) *lexical items* (vocabulary) and their correct use.

Fossilisation affects these components to a different extent. There are no really reliable comparisons of lexical richness between children and adults after the same exposure to the target language. It appears, however, that adults normally have no problem in learning a lexical item whenever there is need; there is, apparently, no substantial fossilisation in the growing vocabulary (cf. Broeder et al., 1988).

The extreme opposite is phonology; even on a very advanced level of syntax or vocabulary, the adult learner is typically identified as such by his or her 'foreign accent'. The point is strikingly illustrated by cases such as the Polish-born writer Joseph Conrad, whose mastery in written English was far beyond that of the normal English speaker of his time but who never acquired an authentic English pronunciation.

Fossilisation also strongly affects morphology; in fact, many second language learners stop at a level where the words are strung together without

---

* An excellent survey of what children in various languages have learned at a certain age is found in Slobin's voluminous *The Cross-linguistic Study of Language Acquisition* (Slobin, 1986); the contributions in Fletcher and Garman (1984) give a concise picture of the various domains of first language acquisition.

any sign of inflection. This has consequences for the syntactical organisation of their utterances as well. We shall return to this phenomenon in the next section.

This selectivity of fossilisation is well attested. How can it be explained? It is apparently incompatible with the notion that the language processor as a whole deteriorates. Hence, we either assume that the language processor is selectively affected by aging processes – not just for phonology but even for special parts of phonology – or else we assume that there are other factors which contribute substantially to fossilisation. Such reasons could be, for example:

(1) The learner simply no longer notices the difference between his own production and that of his social environment, especially for sound features which are not distinctive (for example the degree of aspiration which distinguishes French and English unvoiced consonants, or the varying diphthongisation of English and German long vowels: the German word *rot* when spoken with a diphthongised 'o' is easily understood – it just 'sounds English'.

(2) The learner is aware of his imperfection but 'intuitively feels' that it is unnecessary to improve his pronunciation any further, because he understands and is understood by others; in other words, his communicative needs are satisfied, and any further approach to the target would seem an unnecessary 'mimicking' of his social environment.

(3) Taking this feeling one step further, the learner may even feel the need – perhaps without being aware of it – to maintain a minimal distance from his social environment, that is, to keep at least some part of his previous social identity. Children, obviously, do not have this fear when learning their mother tongue because they have no social identity to loose. They have to develop a social identity.

Clearly, these possibilities do not speak against the idea that the different end state in FLA and SLA is influenced by biological aging of the brain or of the peripheral organs. But they should make us aware that other factors might be involved; we shall return to this point in section 4.

The structure of acquisition: the basic variety

Both the child and the adult learner must derive the particular structural regularities of the target language from an analysis of the input – the sound waves used for communicative purposes in communicative contexts. To some extent, their input differs in structure; the caretakers' language is sometimes very idiosyncratic, and so may be, albeit in a different way, the language of the natives when talking to what they take to be a foreigner. But as a rule, the language to which the learner is exposed exhibits all of the normal characteristics of the target language. In particular, its morphology and syntax are normal. Nevertheless, the way in which morphology and syntax are learned typically shows some salient differences in SLA and FLA – irrespective of speed and end state. In a nutshell, the difference is this: children pick up morphology very rapidly, both regular and irregular forms; they tend to make a few overgeneralisations (*swimmed* instead of *swam*), but those are rapidly corrected. Adult learners, by contrast, often develop no morphology at all. If they do, then only after having passed through a 'learner variety', which is very fluent and efficient but lacks any morphology and exhibits a number of very specific syntactic regularities – a type of language which we shall call here the 'Basic Variety'.

The existence of such a pidgin-like interim language has been observed very early in the first systematic empirical investigations of adult SFA outside the classroom (Heidelberger Forschungsprojekt, 1975; Schumann, 1978, von Stutterheim, 1986). More recent cross-linguistic work has uncovered a number of its structural properties (Klein and Perdue, 1992; Perdue, 1993). In what follows we shall discuss one component of the basic variety – the expression of temporality.* In all Indoeuropean and in most other languages, temporality is systematically expressed by two verbal categories, tense and aspect. Their precise encoding varies, and hence has to be learned by analysis of the input. But the main device is always the inflectional morphology of the (simple or compound) verb. In some languages, such as Polish, Spanish and French, this system is very complex; in others, as in German or Dutch, it is relatively simple. But no matter how simple or complex, children normally have no problems in learning the various morphological forms (see the survey in Weist, 1984). This does not necessarily mean that children rapidly know how to express temporality. For a very long time, they may have problems with the underlying time concepts, such as the various tense and aspect differentiations – just as they often have odd ideas about *yesterday*, *later*, and *tomorrow*. In a word: children easily pick up the forms that they hear, but they may have problems in using them appropriately for *conveying temporal information*.

The way in which adult learners approach the problem of expressing temporality is fundamentally different. Whatever the learner's first language and the target language may be the acquisitional process always centers around a learner variety with very distinct features – the 'basic variety'. It is characterised by the following four properties:

    (1) Utterances typically consist of uninflected verbs, their arguments and, optionally, adverbials. There is no case marking, and, except in rote forms, there are no finite constructions. In contrast to 'pre-basic varieties', the way in which the words are put together follows a

---

* The findings briefly summarised here result from a larger cross-linguistic project on the second language acquisition of adult immigrant workers. Forty speakers were observed and recorded over a period of about three years; source language-target language pairs were Punjabi-English and Italian-English, Italian-German and Turkish-German, Turkish-Dutch and Moroccan-Dutch, Moroccan-French and Spanish-French, Spanish-Swedish and Finnish-Swedish. Analysis included a number of aspects, such as syntax, lexicon, the expression of time and space, feedback processes, and others. More detailed accounts are found in Perdue (1993), Klein and Perdue (1992) and, specifically on the acquisition of temporality, in Dietrich, Klein & Noyau (1995).

number of clear organisational principles which are neither those of the source language nor those of the target language.

(2) Lexical verbs show up in a 'base form', and there is normally no copula. Most learners of English use the bare stem as their base form, but also V-*ing* occurs. Learners of other languages may use the infinitive (German, French) or even a generalised inflected form (as often in Swedish). Turkish learners of Dutch, for example, use the infinitive, Moroccan learners of Dutch use the bare stem.

(3) There is a steadily increasing repertoire of temporal adverbials. Minimally, this repertoire includes: (a) the calendaric type adverbials such as *Sunday, in the evening*; (b) anaphoric adverbials which allow the speaker to express the relation AFTER such as *then, after*, and also typically an adverbial which expresses the relation BEFORE; (c) some deictic adverbials such as *yesterday, now*; (d) a few frequency adverbials, notably *always, often, two times*, etc.; (e) a few durational adverb-ials, normally as bare nouns, such as *two hours*, etc. Temporal adverbials such as *again, still, already* do not belong to the standard repertoire of the basic variety.

(4) There are some boundary markers, which mark the beginning and the end of some situation, as in constructions like *work finish*, 'after working is/was/will be over.'

The basic variety does not allow for tense or aspect marking. Compared to the rich expressive tools for temporality in fully developed languages, this seems to impose strong restrictions on what can be said. This impression, however, is premature. At this stage, learners are often extremely good story tellers, and telling a story requires the expression of all sorts of temporal information. Their guitar, so to speak, has only one string, but they play it masterly. How is this possible?

What the basic variety allows is the specification of some time span X, its position on the time line, its duration and (if iterated) its frequency. The event, process or state to be situated in time is then simply linked to this time span X. All the speaker has to do now, is to shift X, if there is need. More systematically, the functioning of the basic variety is described by the following three principles:

(1) At the beginning of the discourse, a time span $TAss_1$ is fixed. $TAss_1$ is not the time at which the event, state, process obtains – this time we shall call 'time of the situation ' (TSit) – but the 'time of assertion'; this is the span about which an assertion is made by the utterance in question.* $TAss_1$ can be introduced in three ways:

(a) by explicit introduction on the informant's part; this is usually done by a temporal adverbial in initial position;

---

* We assume that tense expresses the relation of TAss to the time at which the utterance is made, and aspect expresses the relation between TAss and TSit (Klein, 1994).

(b) by explicit introduction on the interviewer's part (e.g., *what happened last Sunday?*);

(c) by implicitly taking the 'default topic time' – the time of utterance; in this case, nothing is explicitly marked.

TAss$_1$ is not only the assertion time of the first utterance. It also serves as a point of departure for all subsequent assertion times in the text.

(2) If TAss$_i$ is given, then TAss$_{i+1}$ is either maintained or changed. If it is maintained, nothing is marked. If it is changed, there are two possibilities:

(a) the shifted assertion time is explicitly marked by an adverbial in initial position;

(b) the new assertion time follows from a principle of text organisation. For narratives, this is the classical principle of chronological order 'Unless marked otherwise, the order of mention corresponds to the order of events'. In other words, TAss$_{i+1}$ is some interval more or less right-adjacent to TAss$_i$.

This principle does not obtain in all text types. It is only characteristic of narratives and other texts with a similar temporal overall organisation – texts which answer a question like *What happened next?* Even in those texts, it only applies to 'foreground sequences', that is, those parts which represent the plot line. In other text types, such as descriptions or arguments, the principle of chronological order does not apply, nor does it hold for side structures in narratives, that is, those sequences, which give background information, evaluations, comments, and so on. For those cases, change of TAss must be marked by adverbials.

Principles I and II provide the temporal scaffold of a sequence of utterances – the time spans about which something is said. The 'time of situation' is then given by a third principle:

(3) The relation of TSit to TAss in the basic variety is always 'more or less simultaneous'. TAss can be contained in TSit, or TSit can be contained in TAss, or TAss and TSit are contained in each other. In other words, the basic variety allows no aspectual differentiation by formal means.

This system is very simple, compared to what we find in all source and target languages, but extremely versatile. It allows an easy expression of when what happens, or is the case, provided (a) there are enough adverbials, and (b) it is cleverly managed. Therefore, one way to improve the learner's expressive power is simply to enrich his vocabulary, especially by adding temporal adverbials, and *to learn how to make optimal use of it*. Precisely this is done by very many adult second language learners. In the project mentioned in the footnote on page 253, about one-third of the 40 learners whose acquisition was investigated do exactly this: they do not go beyond the basic variety, but they steadily improve it in these two respects – more words, better practice. The other two-thirds move towards the target language, and some of them actually come very close to it, although no one really attains native-like proficiency.

Summary of LA age effects

As was said above, the state of acquisition research does not provide us with a really comprehensive picture of the differences between FLA and SLA in social context; in particular, we hardly know anything about the potential variation in speed between the child learner and the adult learner. Still, we can sum up some salient LA age effects regarding end state and structure. These are:

(1) Adult SLA learners normally stop at a level where their language is more or less far from the target variety – the language of the social environment in which they learn. This is hardly ever observed for children and, where it occurs, it is considered to be pathological.

(2) This difference in end state is not observed for children who learn a second language: if there is sufficient access, they normally do not fossilise.

(3) The adult's fossilisation is highly selective:
   (a) adults regularly have problems with phonological features of the target language – distinctive as well as non-distinctive segmental properties, but also, and particularly so, with prosody ('foreign accent').
   (b) Fossilisation affects not so very much the acquisition of lexical items; adults can easily learn all the words they need for their communicative purposes. If there are differences in this regard, then they are minor.

(4) Less known but no less salient are differences in the *structure* of acquisition, rather than in final attainment. We have illustrated this with the way in which child and adult learners learn the means to express temporality. This is, of course, only one of the various cognitive domains which are regularly expressed in language, but it is a particularly important one in that in all Indoeuropean languages, temporal marking is obligatory for most sentences: the finite verb automatically carries temporal information. In a nutshell, the main differences are:
   (a) children have no problems with the various morphological forms, even when these are extremely complex; they soon reproduce exactly the precise verb forms of their social environment;
   (b) they often have problems with the exact meaning of these forms, that is, with the underlying time concepts encoded by the various forms. Their language *sounds* like the language of their social environment, but it does not always express the same *contents*.

(c) Adults invariably pass through a particular language form, the basic variety, which lacks any morphology, hence the usual devices to express tense and aspect. In many ways, the basic variety resembles a pidgin and, in fact, it is plausible that this is the way in which pidgins originate – they are fossilised basic varieties.

(d) Communicatively, the basic variety is very efficient – at least as for the expression of temporality: if there is enough vocabulary, and if it is cleverly managed, then virtually everything that is needed can be expressed. Therefore, going beyond the basic variety does not so very much increase the expressive potential – it only makes the language more look like the language of the social environment.

These findings are selective and preliminary. They leave little doubt, however, that there are some salient differences between the child's first language acquisition and the adult's second language acquisition. What causes these differences? There are a number of possibilities which we shall now discuss in some detail.

4. LA AGE EFFECTS: WHAT ACCOUNTS FOR THE DIFFERENCES?

As was said in section 2, essentially three components are involved in language acquisition: access, language processor, propensity. Each of them may vary with age and hence be responsible for the observed differences. They will not be discussed in turn.

Access

Essentially, child and adult have the same kind of access to the language to be learned – sound waves, and the accompanying information in which these sound waves are functionally used. This rules out access as a main causal factor. But this general statement must be relativised in some respects:

(1) Children may have the same but simply *more* access to the target language. This is probably true but can hardly account for the differences (except for the fact perhaps that some rarely used words are not learned by the adult, for the very simple reason that they do not occur in the input). Phonological features are very recurrent, and after three years, the adult learner must have heard all of them 10,000 times. Still, he does not pick them up whereas the child does.

(2) Adults often have additional access, for example to the written language. But it is hard to see how this additional input should lead to the particular differences in structure and end state. If anything, one would predict that it facilitates acquisition, for example because it can be of some help in the identification of words.

(3) Both children and adults are sometimes exposed to a particular simplified version of the language – 'motherese' and 'foreigner talk'. But motherese is only used by some caretakers, notably old aunts, for quite a limited time, and it is uncontroversial in language acquisition research that children learn up to perfection with and without motherese. Foreigner talk, on the other hand, is relatively rare, compared to the huge amount of 'normal input' to which the adult learner has access (Roche, 1989).

Summing up, it does not seem that differences in access play a significant role in the explanation of the LA age effect.

Language processor

The language processor is the individual's capacity to acquire and to use a language appropriately for communicative purposes. This capacity is species-specific, it is innate, it changes over the lifespan. The way in which it operates at a particular time depends on two factors: on certain biological determinants, and on the knowledge available at that time.

The biological component of the language processor includes several peripheral organs (the articulatory apparatus ranging from the larynx to the lips as well as the aural tract), and some parts of the central nervous system – those that are responsible for perception, memory and various higher cognitive functions (for example the ability to generalise from individual cases and to withdraw from false generalisations). A precise classification and characterisation of the various cognitive capacities involved in language acquisition and language processing is a difficult issue, far beyond the scope of the present chapter. There is no doubt, however, that the ones just mentioned belong to them. The other component of the human language processor is much more dynamic: it is the more or less rich knowledge which the human mind has stored at a given point in time. This 'available knowledge' includes

(1) all sorts of factual knowledge, which is not directly related to a particular language – knowledge about persons, objects, the courses of events, and so on;

(2) partial knowledge about the target language – the first language in FLA, the second language in SLA; the process of acquiring a language is always step by step, and whatever is known at a particular point in time about the language to be learned is exploited to further this process;

(3) knowledge about other languages, notably knowledge of the first language in SLA.

This knowledge constantly changes during the lifespan, to a higher or lesser degree, and for very different reasons, and any of these changes could be responsible for the differences described in the last part of section 3 above.

In examining their relative impact, it should be kept in mind that the relevant watershed is around puberty. Five year-olds normally never fossilise; young adults of, say, 20, hardly ever attain full mastery.

Beginning with the peripheral capacities, it is well-known that audition deteriorates with age. But heavy-metal rock fans aside, it is doubtful whether these changes are so dramatic at the age of 20 as to affect the perception of a new sound system. In fact, there is clear evidence to show the opposite. In a series of studies, Neufeld (1979) has shown that American college students at age 20 are able to learn the phonology of languages such as Quechua, Japanese or Eskimo to the extent that native speakers of these languages cannot distinguish these learners from native speakers. The subjects of these studies were systematically and intensively taught, and similar findings are normally not observed outside the classroom (nor are they normally observed inside the classroom). Hence, these findings do not directly bear on the LA effects from the last part of section 3, since these relate to SLA outside the classroom. But they demonstrate one point: at that age of 20, there are no absolute biological constraints to the acquisition of phonology. This applies analogously to the articulatory organs. It is well known, again, that complex and fine-tuned motor control becomes increasingly difficult with age. But it is doubtful whether the relevant threshold has been passed at age 20. Still, we cannot exclude that these peripheral changes contribute to the fact that the acquisition of phonology *normally* fossilises in the adult's case, but it seems unlikely that they fully explain this fact.

Turning now to the central components of the language processor, we know of a number of cortical changes over the lifespan which, in principle, could be held responsible for the selective LA effects from the last part of section 3. In fact, the probably best-known explanation of the deteriorating language learning capacity, Lenneberg's 'critical period theory', argues along these lines (cf. section 1). But any such account, attractive as it is, faces three major problems. First, the major cortical changes over the lifespan do not typically occur during the age period considered here. Secondly, there is no evidence that central capacities such as memory, concept formation, or the various reasoning abilities which may be involved in language learning significantly deteriorate from say five years of age to 20 years of age. Thirdly, as we look more closely at the characteristic differences described in the last part of section 3, it becomes clear that they are not primarily related to these central capacities. Vocabulary learning, for example, is largely a memory problem. Phonology does not require much memory. Adult learners, however, except at a much more advanced age, have no substantial problems with lexical learning; they have problems with phonology. Apparently, those parts of linguistic knowledge which require 'higher cognitive abilities' are much less affected than more peripheral properties, such as accurate pronunciation, authentic prosody, correct morphological forms, and the like.

There is the possibility that in addition to the domain-neutral central capacities of the language processor, which have been mentioned and which are in fact indispensable, there is also a domain-specific 'language module' somewhere in our cortex. Then, cortical changes in just this component from before to after puberty could be responsible for the observed differences. The assumption that there is such a component is not very parsimonious but cannot be excluded *a priori*. We shall return to this assumption in section 5 below.

Summing up, it appears that age-related changes in the biological components of our language processor may contribute to the LA age effect; but at present, there is little evidence that this contribution is substantial. Future research in the neurobiology of the changing brain might force us to reevaluate the impact of this contribution (see, for example, the still speculative but highly interesting considerations to this effect by Pulvermüller and Schumann, 1994).

The other, much more dynamic component of the language processor is the knowledge available at a given time in the acquisitional process; this knowledge is constantly changing, and in fact, language acquisition *is* part of this knowledge change. There are two crucial differences here between FLA and SLA learners. First, the adult's general knowledge is normally much richer. It is hard to see, however, how this should hamper the acquisition of another language (although experience of life shows that excessive knowledge can be detrimental in many ways). Secondly, in SLA, the available knowledge includes knowledge of (at least) one other language. This may have positive and negative effects, which were extensively studied under the label of (positive and negative) 'transfer' (see, for example, Kellerman, 1986).

Unfortunately, most of this research deals with language acquisition in the classroom, and therefore is not directly comparable. Still, one general finding seems beyond doubt: the fossilised language even of the advanced adult learner typically shows distinct traces of the first language – ranging from the wrong choice of gender to the 'French, German, Swedish foreign accent' which we all know from everyday experience. In this sense, the difference of available knowledge might indeed be a major reason for the LA age effect.

But there are three problems with this explanation. First, the mere fact that knowledge of the first language somehow *influences* the precise form, for example the pronunciation, of the learner's performance in the second language does not necessarily mean that it is an *obstacle* or even blocks its acquisition. It could simply mean that the learner 'works' with his old pronunciation until the new pronunciation is acquired. Somehow, he or she must articulate the words, so why not in the old way – for a while. The problem is that in the adult's case, this 'while' lasts forever, and this is what has to be explained. Secondly, while some of the differences from the last part of section 3 (p. 256) can be traced back to first language influence, this is not so for others. The 'basic variety' described in the penultimate part of section 3 (p. 257) is found in many source language-target language pairs, for example

Turkish-Dutch, Moroccan-Dutch, Spanish-French, Italian-English. None of the source languages is even remotely structured like the basic variety, hence, the particular form of the Basic Variety cannot be due to the influence of, in these cases, the structure of Turkish, Moroccan, Spanish, or Italian.

Thirdly, children at the age of, say, six or seven have already acquired most – though not all – of their first language. In particular, their phonology acquisition is usually completed. Hence, when learning a second language at that age, they should be subject to the same influences. But they are not. Normally, children at that age have no problem picking up a second language when transplanted into a new social environment in which this language is spoken.

The conclusion seems clear: the fact that there is already a language stored in the brain may affect, and in fact does selectively affect, the acquisition of another language. Hence, just as with changes in the 'hardware component' of the language processor, differences in its 'software component' may contribute to the LA age effect in one way or another, but they cannot fully explain it.

Propensity

This leaves us, somewhat unexpectedly, with a last causal factor: the different motivations that push a learner forward in the acquisition of the mother tongue and in the acquisition of a second language. It seems that the Moroccan worker coming to Holland at the age of 22 is driven by other forces to learn Dutch than the child born in a Dutch family by Dutch parents and with Dutch siblings and peers. One might say that the adult's motive is: '*understand others and make yourself understood for concrete purposes*', whereas the child's motive is: '*become – with little differences – like the others*'. These two motives are not mutually exclusive. It is impossible to understand and to be understood without becoming to some extent like the others, and vice versa, becoming like the others includes the capacity to understand and to be understood. But the priorities are set in very different ways. If someone with a strong French accent asks you in the street: *Station where?*, then you will most likely understand him. But at the same time, you will immediately identify him as an outsider, as someone who does not belong to your social group. For the child, language acquisition is more than building up knowledge about phonological, syntactical or lexical rules: it is but one aspect in becoming a social being with all the convictions, norms and habits of a particular social group. To this end, it is not enough to get the intended meaning across. It is vital to reproduce exactly the form of the language. The form *He leaved yesterday* is no less understandable than *He left yesterday*. But the social environment only uses the second form and stigmatises the first. In fact, the least redundant way to express this very meaning would be to say *He leave yesterday*, since the information 'past', as expressed by the irregular tense form or the ending *-ed*, only duplicates in less specific form what is more precisely said by the adverbial _yesterday_. Therefore, if the task were only to express the intended meaning, the basic variety form _he leave yesterday_ is _optimally adapted to the communicative needs_. But it deviates from the established way of expressing this meaning in the particular social community. Lexical items are indispensable, if certain meanings are to be expressed, if certain communicative needs are to be realised; but their exact pronunciation is not mandatory to this end. We typically find fossilisation in phonology, or some parts of it, but not in the lexicon. Depending on whether you primarily want to realise some clear, limited, well-defined communicative needs, or whether you want to become a nonsalient, nonstigmatised member of a social group, structure and end state of your acquisitional process are pushed into quite different directions. This, I believe, explains most of the pecularities of the LA age effect. It does not, however, exclude the fact that the other factors discussed above – access and the various components of the language processor – contribute to this effect as well. But judging from the limited evidence we have, this contribution seems to be comparatively small.

5. CONCLUSION

In this final section, I will not sum up what has been said so far but briefly address one remaining issue, that is the possibility that there is a special 'language module' in our cortex whose change over the lifespan might be responsible for the LA age effect.

In FLA as well as in SLA, whatever is acquired, is acquired step after step by successive analysis of sound stream and accompanying information in the communicative setting. But one might ask whether indeed all components in the mature speaker's linguistic knowledge are acquired in this way. At least part of the final knowledge of the mature speaker could be there by birth. This is indeed assumed by acquisition researchers who work in the 'generative paradigm' (Chomsky, 1985). It leads to an interesting, because simple, theory of language acquisition. Essential parts of the speaker's linguistic knowledge are innate, and only some open slots, so to speak, must be filled by input analysis. This general idea has been worked out in some detail in the so-called 'parameter setting approach' (Weissenborn, Goodluck and Roeper, 1992). In this view, there is a 'peripheral part' of linguistic knowledge, which has to be learned by input analysis, and a 'core part', which is innate but contains by birth some 'open parameters' with a limited number of options. All the child has to do is to choose one of the options, and this is done by input analysis. This view assigns a very minor role to the access, and it does not consider the potential role of different types of propensity. This innate part with the open parameters is called 'universal grammar', and it is assumed that universal grammar is a domain-specific cognitive ability, which interacts with, but is in principle separated from, other mental abilities, such as memory, concept formation, or deductive reasoning. If we now assume (a) that there is not only such an innate 'universal grammar' but also (b) that, for biological reasons, it is only 'available' for some time – say roughly up to puberty – then this could explain the LA age effect (see, for example, the papers in Anderson, 1990). Both assumptions, though, are not particularly plausible.

Consider first the idea that not only the language capacity but also a significant part of the individual's linguistic knowledge is innate, or, as we may say, genetically transmitted. Clearly, this can apply only to those components of linguistic knowledge which are common to *all* languages. No one is born to learn just Tzeltal or Kiksht, every new-born can learn any language, even German. Hence, whatever distinguishes Tzeltal from English, for example, must be learned by input analysis. This includes:

(1) the entire vocabulary (except the expression Coca Cola);
(2) the entire morphology;
(3) the entire syntax to the extent to which it is covered in descriptive grammars;
(4) most (if not all) of phonology.

It includes, in other words, practically everything. This does not necessarily exclude the possibility that, on some abstract level, there are also some universal properties. But if this is the case, then it remains to be shown that these universal properties go in any way beyond the constraints on perception, motor control and cognition which are characteristic of the human mind in general. At present, there is not enough empirical evidence to settle this issue. But clearly, a theory which only operates with general, not domain-specific constraints on the human mind rather than with a specific 'language module', characterised by domain-specific mental principles, is more general. Hence, it is preferable – so long as there is no convincing evidence to the contrary. Secondly, if there is such an innate 'language module', then why should it be no longer active after a certain period? It is true that some functions of the human body are limited to a particular age range. The various processes around puberty illustrate the point. But in all of these cases, there is palpable biological evidence – changes in cell structure, hormone production and the like. No such evidence has been given so far for the 'language module'. This does not exclude that such evidence may be found in future research. But at present, any explanation of the LA age affects in terms of a 'language module' and its changing availability resembles the explanation of life and death by the existence and the fading of the *vis vitalis*. Still, it may be correct.

REFERENCES

Anderson, R. (ed.) (1990) Special Issue of *Studies in Second Language Acquisition*, **12**.

Behrens, H. (1993) Temporal reference in German child language. Doctoral Dissertation, University of Amsterdam.

Birdsong, D. (1992) Ultimate attainment in second language acquisition. *Language*, **68**, 706–55.

Broeder, P., Extra, G. van Hoor, R., Strömqvist, S. & Voionmaa, C. (1988) *Processes in the Developing Lexicon*. Final Report. Strasbourg: European Science Foundation.

Chomsky, N. (1985) *Knowledge of Language*. New York: Prager.

Dietrich, R., Klein, W. & Noyau, C. (1995) *The Acquisition of Temporality in a Second Language*. Amsterdam: Benjamins.

Fletcher, P. & Garman, P. (eds.) (1984) *First Language Acquisition*. Cambridge: Cambridge University Press.

Heidelberger Forschungsprojekt 'Pidgin-Deutsch' (1975) *Sprache und Kommunikation ausländischer Arbeiter*. Kronberg: Scriptor.

Kellerman, E. (ed.) (1986) *Crosslinguistic Influence in Second Language Acquisition*. London: Pergamon.

Klein, W. & Perdue, E. (1992) *Utterance Structure*. Amsterdam: Benjamins.

Klein, W. (1994) *Time in Language*. London: Routledge.

Lamendella, J. (1977) General principles of neurofunctional organization and their manifestation in primary and non-primary language acquisition. *Language Learning*, **27**, 155–96.

Lenneberg, E. H. (1967) *Biological Foundations of Language*. New York: John Wiley.

Long, M. (1990) Maturational constraints on language development. *Studies in Second Language Acquisition*, **12**, 251–85.

Neufeld, E. (1979) Towards a theory of language learning ability. *Language Learning*, **29**, 227–41.

Perdue, C. (ed.) (1993) *Adult Second Language Acquisition*. Cambridge: Cambridge University Press.

Pulvermüller, F. & Schumann, J. (1994) Neurobiological mechanisms of language acquisition. *Language Learning*, **44**, 681–734.

Roche, J. (1989) *Xenolekte*. Berlin: de Gruyter.

Schumann, J. (1978). *The Pidginization Process*. Rowley: Newbury House.

Slobin, D. (ed.) (1986) *The Crosslinguistic Study of Language Acquisition*. Hillsdale, NJ: Erlbaum.

von Stutterheim, Ch. (1986) *Temporalität in der Zweitsprache*. Berlin: de Gruyter.

Weist, R. M. (1984) Tense and aspect. In Fletcher, P. & Garman, M., (eds.) *Language Acquisition*. Cambridge: Cambridge University Press, pp. 356–74.

Weissenborn, J., Goodluck, H. & Roeper, T. (eds.) (1992) *Theoretical Issues in Language Acquisition*. Hillsdale, NJ: Erlbaum.

13 Commentary **Advances in cognitive neuroscience**

ANTONIO R. DAMASIO AND HANNA DAMASIO

The understanding of human cognition and behavior has been limited by a number of practical and theoretical shortcomings. Foremost among the former has been the difficulty in obtaining, in the living human, contemporaneous neural and cognitive-behavioral measurements. Foremost among the latter have been the conceptualization of brain and mind as separate from the body, and of the mind as a software program that might be run on a hardware implement called the brain. In this brief discussion we outline some recent developments and suggest that these shortcomings are being overtaken.

TECHNICAL DEVELOPMENTS

The principal method developments in the broad field of inquiry known as cognitive neuroscience include the advent of new experimental techniques to evaluate separate components of cognitive processes, and the advent or refinement of new techniques to study human brain structure and function *in vivo*. The most significant progress has perhaps occurred in relation to the latter, as we note below.

Lesion studies

One of the means to gain knowledge about the human brain and mind has been the time honored lesion method. The early success of this approach, however, which coincided with the first decades of what is now known as neuroscience, was followed by the realization that lesion studies depended far too much on single and sometimes nonreplicable observations, and that those observations were often made outside of an experimental framework. Moreover, the correlation between abnormal behavior or cognition, on the one hand, and abnormal brain structure, on the other, did not coincide in time, patient autopsies often being obtained many years after particular clinical observations were made.

All of these problems can be obviated now. The availability of patient registries permits the study of several individuals with similar neuropsychological manifestations and similar lesions, individually or as a group. Normal as well as brain lesioned controls can also be studied and compared to target patients so that the effects of factors such as education, age and gender, can be teased apart. Abnormal cognitive or behavioral profiles can be immediately correlated with contemporaneous neuroanatomical facts, obtained *in vivo* by means of neuroimaging technologies. Those include X-ray computerized tomography and magnetic resonance imaging.

The advances in neuroanatomical analysis are decisive because they permit the use of circumscribed lesions as probes to the performance of hypothetical neural systems. In other words, given a large-scale neural system constituted by multiple components in specific cortical regions or subcortical nuclei, it is possible to hypothesize the putative cognitive-behavioral functions of the whole system, and of its parts, and to make predictions about the system's behavior in conditions under which a lesion destroys one of the system's components. Lesion probes are thus a direct window into brain function (Damasio & Damasio, 1989).

One reason why magnetic resonance imaging has made such an impact in this field has to do with its excellent anatomical resolution which permits the reliable detection of structural damage when lesions are as small as only a few cubic millimeters. Another reason is that new techniques now permit the reconstruction of the living human brain in three dimensions. By bringing such reconstructions on-line in computer workstations, and segmenting, slicing and quantifying those images, it is possible to carry out neuroanatomical analyses with a degree of detail no different and sometimes superior to that available in a conventional macroscopic evaluation using post-mortem tissue (Damasio, H. & Frank, 1992; Damasio, H., 1995).

The new age of lesion studies making use of the above developments has produced a number of new findings in investigations of the visual system, memory, language, emotion and reasoning. In the paragraphs below we outline some of these results.

Some advances based on lesion studies

The modern study of patients with brain lesions has confirmed the idea that the visual system is organized in parallel fashion and is functionally regionalized, an idea that also gained support from neurophysiological studies in extrastriate cortices (see Zeki, 1993 for review). For instance, the ability to perceive color depends on a sector of visual association cortices located, in the human, in the region below the calcarine fissure (Damasio et al., 1980; Rizzo et al., 1993). The anatomical correlations obtained with patients with achromatopsia dovetailed with neurophysiological studies in color processing carried out in the macaque monkey (Hubel & Livingstone 1987; Livingstone & Hubel 1987; Zeki 1993). Related studies also made clear that the ability to perceive movement was dissociable from other aspects of visual perception (Zihl, Von Cramon & Mai 1983).

The process of visual recognition, namely, that of recognizing human faces and objects has also gained immensely from lesion studies (Damasio, A. R. et al., 1990; Damasio et al., 1990; Zeki 1993). On this topic, the key development is the determination that not only extrastriate but extravisual areas are part of the system that supports the visual recognition.

On the topic of memory, lesion studies have contributed no less remarkably, ever since the study of patient HM helped decisively the understanding of the neural basis of memory and learning. The contribution of lesion studies has become especially marked as different systems in medial and nonmedial temporal lobe, basal forebrain and frontal cortices, and sensory motor cortices, have been related to different aspects of learning and memory, such as the acquisition or recall of factual knowledge or skills (Squire et al., 1990; Goldman-Rakic, Funahashi & Bruce, 1990; Damasio, Tranel & Damasio 1989; Tranel 1994).

The contribution of lesion studies to the understanding of the neural basis of language has perhaps been the most impressive. Several brain areas in addition to the areas that have been traditionally related to language have now been described, within the left hemisphere, in both anterotemporal and dorsolateral frontal regions. Those areas contain language-related systems too. They are engaged in such tasks as the retrieval of word-forms which denote entities, or the retrieval of word forms that denote actions or states of entities (Damasio, 1992; Damasio & Damasio, 1992; Damasio & Tranel, 1993). Lesion studies are also helping elucidate the basis for the neural processing of sign language (Bellugi, Poizner & Klima, 1989; Anderson et al., 1992).

Last but not least, the understanding of the processes of emotion, feeling and reasoning, is also benefiting from lesion studies. There is evidence, in fact, that emotion/feeling, on the one hand, and reasoning and decision making, on the other, are closely interconnected and depend on neural systems which include both cortical and subcortical structures within (a) the brain core (e.g., hypothalamus, brain stem, basal forebrain), (b) the limbic system, and (c) both prefrontal and somatosensory cortices (Damasio, A. 1994; 1995a).

Functional studies

Until recently the only effective functional correlates of cognitive processes were electrophysiological. Important information has been obtained with those methods which have the clear advantage of preserving the temporal dimension of cognitive phenomena. Unfortunately, the spatial localization of the origin of those electrophysiologic manifestations has been a major challenge. The recent combination of electroencephalographic and magneto-encephalographic technologies, however, promises to overcome the traditional limitations and offers important new information on temporal and spatial information of neural activity (Givens et al., 1981).

A novel approach to human brain function is positron emission tomography, usually known as PET, the current heir to the radio-nuclide scans of previous decades of nuclear medicine. PET uses the detection of dual photons, emitted from the same site but in opposite directions, to help determine changes in cerebral blood flow within the specific brain regions from which the photons arise. Given the presumed relation between regional cerebral blood flow and regional brain metabolism, the technique permits the measurement of functional changes induced by cognitive tasks, and thus permits us to make inferences about the link between certain cognitive operations, on the one hand, and the components of neural systems which appear to be functionally modified by those cognitive operations, on the other (see Raichle 1990 for review).

Compared to electrophysiological techniques, PET has some advantages in spatial resolution but is far less accurate in the temporal aspect. A variety of new modes of analyses, however, promises to optimize the anatomical definition considerably such that the loss in temporal resolution may be an acceptable trade off (Damasio, H. et al., 1993; Grabowski et al., 1995a, 1995b).

Yet another technical development in dynamic imaging pertains to functional magnetic resonance scanning or fMR, the companion to the structural MR we discussed above. It is too early to make a comprehensive assessment of this new technique, although it would not be surprising if it will eventually become the functional imaging approach of choice. The technique preserves the fine anatomical resolution of its structural predecessor and adds a dynamic element within that fine anatomical resolution. There are many technical problems to be solved before further progress is possible, but none of these appear insurmountable.

By and large, functional imaging studies have helped confirm a large number of observations obtained with lesion studies in humans, or with neurophysiological studies in experimental animals. This is true for studies in visual and auditory perception, memory, attention and language. On occasion, the detail obtained with the PET result far surpasses the knowledge available from either the lesion studies, or obtainable from experimental studies in animals. An example is the determination of the probable site of area V5 in the human (Watson et al., 1993). This area, also known as MT, is presumed to contribute importantly to the perception of movement. A recent study performed with fMR strengthens that notion (Tootell et al., 1995, see also Damasio, 1995b).

As dynamic imaging techniques become more reliable and as means of data analysis become more sophisticated, it is apparent that a variety of hypotheses which could not be approached with lesion studies will be investigated fruitfully.

THEORETICAL DEVELOPMENTS

Organismic and developmental perspectives

For most of the twentieth century the investigations of brain and mind have not been directly influenced either by a comprehensive biological perspective or by a social science perspective. A discussion as to why this has been so is outside the scope of this text, although two reasons may be mentioned with some confidence. The first concerns the special nature of both neural phenomena and psychological phenomena. We believe it generated the need for a number of autonomous approaches and techniques which disengaged neuroscience and cognitive science from biology and from the social sciences. The second reason concerns the powerful influence of the computer metaphor in the conceptualizations of brain and mind. The lack of a biological framework, namely a framework informed by evolutionary biology, and the inclination to model neural and cognitive phenomena in computational terms, have obscured the connection between brain and 'body-proper', and prevented the view of both neural and cognitive phenomena in terms of the organism and the environment to which they relate. We believe, on the contrary, that the body, as represented in the brain, may constitute the indispensable frame of reference for the neural processes that we experience as the mind; that our very organism rather than some absolute external reality is used as the ground reference for the constructions we make of the world around us and for the construction of the ever-present sense of subjectivity that is part and parcel of our experiences. We also believe that the mind exists in and for an integrated organism; that our minds would not be the way they are if it were not for the interplay of body and brain during evolution, during individual development, and at the current moment.

The following statements, for which there is ample supporting evidence, summarize what we have in mind; (1) the human brain and the rest of the body constitute an indissociable organism, integrated by means of mutually interactive biochemical and neural regulatory circuits (including endocrine, immune, and autonomic neural components); (2) the organism interacts with the environment as an ensemble: the interaction is neither of the body alone nor of the brain alone. We propose, on this basis, that the physiological operations that we call mind are derived from the structural and functional ensemble rather than from the brain alone. Mental phenomena, seen in this light, can be fully understood only in the context of an organism's continuous interaction within an environment (see Magnusson 1988; Damasio, A. 1994).

Levels of neural organization and the emergence of new functions

Another important theoretical problem concerns the issue of levels of neural organization, the interrelation among such neural levels and, ultimately, the role that knowledge about the lower levels can play in our understanding of the levels at the top, or vice-versa. Consider the following example.

The neural processes subserving short-term and long-term memory appear to have distinct molecular machinery. Long-term memory requires the activation of particular genes whose expression determines a set of specific molecular activities (Alberini et al., 1994). It is possible then that all processes of long-term memory rely on this same basic mechanism regardless of the content of the material being committed to long-term memory. On the other hand, it should be clear that knowledge about the *molecular* underpinnings of long-term memory is not sufficient to explain the underpinnings for *different* types of long-term memory. In other words, knowing about the molecular basis of long-term memory is necessary to provide a comprehensive account of any one memory held in the long-term, but is not sufficient to explain how separate memories are made for unique faces or nonunique objects, for unique melodies or nonunique noises. In order to explain why and how the brain is structured such that it can support those different memories in different systems, we must know about the organization and function of circuits, both small and large scale.

The nature of memory records

Another important theoretical problem concerns the conceptualization of memory, namely, the nature of the records created by the process of learning. On the cognitive side of the problem, the idea that memories of entities or events are not facsimile reproductions held in explicit form is gaining hold. This idea was first advanced by the psychologist Frederic Bartlett (1964) but was largely ignored in neuroscientific thinking. Edelman, among others, has made it a central aspect of his conceptualization of mind (Edelman, 1992).

On the neural side of the problem, a number of important issues are under discussion concerning the mechanism through which records are acquired and retrieved (see Edelman on the role of selection and instruction in learning; and see Damasio & Damasio, 1994).

Future advances in cognitive neuroscience are likely to depend as much on the type of technical progress outlined at the beginning of this text as on the sort of theoretical attitude changes discussed in the latter paragraphs. The understanding of a presumably simple function such as vision, or of a complex function such as social behavior, can only benefit from an evolutionary perspective, an individual lifespan perspective, and a whole organism perspective. It does not appear that the investigation of the purposes and goals of such functions, simple or complex, will succeed without taking into account those three broader perspectives.

Likewise, it must be realized that general biological, neurobiological, psychological, and social phenomena are not only interrelated but have different levels of structural and functional complexity. What happens at molecular levels of organization cannot possibly predict the full scope of what happens at the level of large-scale neural systems, or at the level of social collectives. Conversely, investigations within the latter level will never be able, independently, to elucidate the nature of structures and functions at cellular or subcellular levels. Concerted, integrative, and multilevel approaches are the only viable avenues towards the understanding of the complex nature of being.

REFERENCES

Alberini, C. M., Ghirardi, M., Metz, R. & Kandel, E. R. (1994) C/EBP is an immediate-early gene required for the consolidation of long-term facilitation in aplysia. *Cell*, **76**, 1099–14.

Andersen, S. W., Damasio, H., Damasio, A. R., Klima, E., Bellugi, U. & Brandt, J. P. (1992) Acquisition of signs from American Sign Language in hearing individuals following left hemisphere damage and aphasia. *Neuropsychologia*, **4**, 329–40.

Bartlett, F. C. (1964) *Remembering: A Study in Experimental and Social Psychology.* Cambridge: Cambridge University Press.

Bellugi, U., Poizner, H. & Klima, E. S. (1989) Language, modality, and the brain. *Trends in Neurosciences*, **12**, 380–8.

Damasio, A. (1995a) Toward a neurobiology of emotion and feeling: operational concepts and hypotheses. *The Neuroscientist*, **1**, 19–25.

Damasio, A. R. (1992) Aphasia. *New England Journal of Medicine*, **326**, 531–9.

Damasio, A. R. (1994) *Descartes' Error: Emotion, Reason and the Human Brain.* New York: Grosset/Putnam.

Damasio, A. R. (1995b) Knowing how, knowing where. *Nature*, **375**, 106–7.

Damasio, A. R. & Damasio, H. (1992) Brain and Language, *Scientific American*, **267**, 89–95.

Damasio, A. R. & Damasio, H. (1994) Cortical systems for retrieval of concrete knowledge: the convergence zone framework. In Koch, C. (ed.) *Large-Scale Neuronal Theories of the Brain.* Cambridge, Mass.: MIT Press, pp. 61–74.

Damasio, A. R., Damasio, H., Tranel, D. & Brandt, J. P. (1990) Neural regionalization of knowledge access: preliminary evidence. *Symposia on Quantitative Biology, Vol. 55.* New York: Cold Spring Harbor Laboratory Press, pp. 1039–47.

Damasio, A. R. & Tranel, D. (1993) Nouns and verbs are retrieved with differently distributed neural systems. *Proceedings of the National Academy of Sciences of the USA*, **90**, 4957–60.

Damasio, A. R., Tranel, D. & Damasio, H. (1989) Amnesia caused by herpes simplex encephalitis, infarctions in basal forebrain, Alzheimer's disease, and anoxia. In Boller, F. & Grafman, J. (eds.) *Handbook of Neuropsychology, Vol. 3.* Amsterdam: Elsevier, pp. 317–32.

Damasio, A., Tranel, D. & Damasio, H. (1990) Face agnosia and the neural substrates of memory. *Annual Review of Neuroscience*, **13**, 89–109.

Damasio, A. R., Yamada, T., Damasio, H., Corbett, J. & McKee, J. (1980) Central achromatopsia: behavioral, anatomic and physiologic aspects. *Neurology*, **30**, 1064–71.

Damasio, H. (1995) *Human Brain Anatomy in Computerized Images*. New York: Oxford University Press.

Damasio, H. & Domasio, A. (1989) *Lesion Analysis in Neuropsychology*. New York: Oxford University Press.

Damasio, H. & Frank, R. (1992) Three-dimensional *in vivo* mapping of brain lesions in humans. *Archives of Neurology*, **49**, 137–43.

Damasio, H., Grabowski, T. J., Frank, R., Knosp, B., Hichwa, R. D., Watkins, G. L. & Ponto, L. L. B. (1993) PET-Brainvox, a technique for neuroanatomical analysis of positron emission tomography images. *Proceedings of the PET 93 Akita: Quantification of Brain Function*. Amsterdam: Elsevier, pp. 465–73.

Edelman, G. M. (1992) *Bright Air Brilliant Fire*. Basic Books, New York.

Givens, A. S., Doyle, J. G., Gutillo, B. A., Schaffer, R. E., Tannehill, R. S., Ghannam, J. H., Gilcrease, V. A. & Yeager, C. L. (1981) Electrical potentials in human brain during cognition: new method reveals dynamic patterns of correlation. *Science*, **213**, 918–22.

Goldman-Rakic, P., Funahashi, S. & Bruce, G. J. (1990) Neocortical memory circuits. *Cold Spring Symposium on Quantitative Biology, Vol. 55*. New York: Cold Spring Harbor Laboratory Press, pp. 1025–38.

Grabowski, T. J., Damasio, H., Frank, R., Brown, C. K., Bolos-Ponto, L. L., Watkins, G. L. & Hichwa, R. D. (1995a) Neuroanatomical analysis of functional brain images: validation with retinotopic mapping. *Human Brain Mapping*, **2**, 134–48.

Grabowski, T. J., Damasio, H., Frank, R., Hichwa, R. D., Boles-Ponto, L. L. & Watkins, G. L. (1995b). A new technique for PET slice orientation and MRI-PET coregistration. *Human Brain Mapping*, **2**, 123–33.

Hubel, D. H. & Livingstone, M. S. (1987) Segregation of form, color, and stereopsis in primate area 18. *The Journal of Neuroscience*, **7**, 3378–415.

Livingstone, M. S. & Hubel, D. H. (1987) Psychophysical evidence for separate channels for the perception of form, color, movement, and depth. *The Journal of Neuroscience*, **7**, 3416–68.

Magnusson, D. (1988) *Individual Development in an Interactional Perspective: A Longitudinal Study*. Hillsdale, NJ: Erlbaum.

Raichle, M. E. (1990) Anatomical exploration of mind: studies with modern imaging techniques. *Cold Spring Symposium on Quantitative Biology, Vol. 55*. New York: Cold Spring Harbor Laboratory Press, pp. 983–94.

Rizzo, M., Smith, V., Pokorny, J. & Damasio, A. R. (1993) Color perception profiles in central achromatopsia. *Neurology*, **43**, 995–1001.

Squire, L., Zola-Morgan, S., Cave, C. B., Haist, F., Musen, G. & Suzuki, W. A. (1990) Memory: organization of brain systems and cognition. *Cold Spring Symposium on Quantitative Biology, Vol. 55*. New York: Cold Spring Harbor Laboratory Press, pp. 1007–23.

Tootell, R. B., Reppas, J. B., Anders, M. D., Look, R. B., Sereno, M. I., Malach, R., Brady, T. J. & Rosen, B. R. (1995) Visual motion aftereffect in human cortical area MT revealed by functional magnetic resonance imaging. *Nature*, **375**, 139–41.

Tranel, D., Damasio, A. R., Damasio, H. & Brandt, J. P. (1994) Sensorimotor skill learning in amnesia: additional evidence for the neural basis of nondeclarative memory. *Learning and Memory*, **1**, 165–79.

Watson, J. D. G., Myers, R., Frackowiak, R. S. J., Hajnal, J. V., Woods, R. P., Mazziotta, J. C., Shipp, S. & Zeki, S. (1993) Area V5 of the human brain: evidence from a combined study using positron emission tomography and magnetic resonance imaging. *Cerebral Cortex*, **3**, 79–94.

Zeki, S. (1992) The visual image in mind and brain. *Scientific American*, **267**, 68–76.

Zeki, S. (1993) *A Vision of the Brain*, London: Blackwell.

Zihl, J., Von Cramon, D. & Mai, N. (1983) Selective disturbance of movement vision after bilateral brain damage. *Brain*, **106**, 313–40.

PART IV
BIOLOGY AND SOCIALIZATION

The ability of the human species to develop complex social structures is un-paralleled, and is an explanation for its ecological primacy. The development of sociality is a characteristic of normal childhood when the biological imperatives of the individual become subordinate to social structure. Deviances (e.g. aggressiveness) have both been interpreted in terms of biologic factors, or early childhood experiences (broken homes, drug abuse). A large body of literature suggests certain critical periods during development, including the prenatal period and adolescence, which are crucial for sexual assertion and social competence.

Contributors to Part IV were asked to review a large area of research. The field is so broad, however, that only certain aspects could be covered.

The topic for Cairns in Chapter 14 is the socialization process. The theme is discussed in the framework of a general biosocial view on individual development. Two empirical studies concerned with the role of timing in developmental processes and with the socialization of aggression and violence, respectively, are presented. In a concluding section, Cairns argues for a holistic, sociogenetic model for social behavior, implying that it should be viewed simultaneously in terms of ontogenesis (the development of the individual) and phylogenesis (the development of the species).

Two contributions address the organizational role of steroid hormones for behavior. As pointed out, the central nervous system not only reacts differently to female or male sex steroids, but certain brain nuclei also show morphological differences in between sexes. Morphologic deviations may have a bearing on the development of homosexual orientation although, as pointed out in Chapter 16 by Gorski, this is controversial. Both Gorski and Goy (Chapter 16) report on the influence of early steroid manipulation on sexual orientation and other behaviors. There is, however, almost complete ignorance regarding the effects of sex steroids during puberty either in experimental animals or humans. During this period these hormones are probably important formative principles for adult human behavior.

In his commentary, Karli (Chapter 17) discusses the main theme of this section from a neurobiologist's perspective. He does this with reference to what he describes as an integrated, holistic bio-psycho-social approach of aggressive behavior. Of particular interest is his discussion of the mediating role of affective processes in the development of social behavior or rather a lack of social behavior (withdrawal, aggressiveness).

14 Socialization and sociogenesis

ROBERT B. CAIRNS

Unraveling the secrets of socialization is one of the major challenges that faces contemporary biological and behavioral science. Violence and aggression – from inner-city gangs to national wars of ethnic separation – threaten to disintegrate societies and reduce human genetic diversity. Other issues of socialization, albeit less dramatic and slower-acting, also possess the capacity to modify the course of human evolution. In this regard, changes in the structure of families have been coincident with trends to reduce the parental commitments and societal responsibilities for children. These phenomena suggest that the complexities and biological consequences of social behavior have been seriously underestimated, and that research on these issues deserves high priority in the science.

It has been proposed that such social phenomena can be clarified by viewing them from a new framework that has emerged from recent human and nonhuman studies on social development (Magnusson & Cairns, 1995). These fields seem closer now than they ever have been to achieving an integrative account of social development across the lifespan. One goal of this chapter therefore is to examine the foundation for this work and how the study of socialization has been pursued in biology and psychology. A second and related goal is to outline how the common ground of development can support an integrative, cross-disciplinary framework for the study of social phenomena.

DEVELOPMENT, EVOLUTION AND SOCIAL BEHAVIORS

Since the publication of Darwin's *The Expression of the Emotions in Man and Animals*, social behaviors have presented an enigma for the biological sciences. Darwin (1873) demonstrated that social and emotional behaviors have distinctive adaptive properties in ontogeny and evolution, and they should not be ignored by biology. The problem has been to figure out how to integrate social and biological processes into a single bio-social theoretical model, or to determine whether a single model was possible.

Sociobiology and the development of social behavior in animals

The complexities of social development have led some theorists to question whether its proximal determinants are beyond the reach of biological science. As an alternative, Wilson (1975) proposed that 'sociobiology' should investigate the roots of social behaviors by study of the evolution of social structures in populations rather than the development of interactions in individuals. Hence the rubric 'sociobiology' was derived by joining 'sociology' and 'biology'. This strategy was designed to leap-frog the complexities of psychology and ontogeny and thereby eliminate the 'developmental noise' of psychological changes in immature lives. This pragmatic strategy abandoned the search for proximal biological and behavioral processes in order to focus upon ultimate genetic and evolutionary mechanisms. Regularities observed in social structures permitted inferences about immanent biosocial motives in individuals, including such issues as whether there were genes for prosocial and aggressive behaviors.

More broadly, Hamilton's (1964) concept of inclusive genetic fitness permitted a revision of the Darwinian model to explain why animals could be cooperative and altruistic. When coupled with Maynard Smith's (1982) game-theory analysis of evolutionarily stable strategies, it provided a persuasive account of why organisms were not destroyed by the escalation of mutual competition.

How well have sociobiological proposals aged? Despite controversy, sociobiology gained immediate and broad influence across the biological and social sciences (Cairns, 1977). It provided a useful theoretical model for introducing the concepts of kin selection into anthropological, sociological and economic analyses (e.g. Alexander & Noonan, 1979; Becker, 1993). Sociobiology continues to be a dominant model in behavioral zoology (e.g. Alcock, 1993). Wilson's (1975) specific proposal that ontogenetic change should be dismissed as 'noise' has been a minor point in a larger model, but it has continued to influence concepts and methods.

Counter to this view, T. C. Schneirla (1966), Z.-Y. Kuo (1967), and others argued that recognition of the complexity of social development is the first step toward understanding its elegant coherence and integration. This perspective emphasized the importance of developmental history in the study of behavior. Rather than eliminate developmental observations and experimental analyses, they should be expanded to permit a better integration of information. Kuo expressed 'the firm conviction that the study of behavior today needs a new orientation, a wider and broader horizon' (Kuo, 1967). He continued:

the study of behavior is a synthetic science. It includes comparative anatomy, comparative embryology, comparative physiology (in the biophysical and biochemical sense), experimental morphology, and the qualitative and quantitative analysis of the dynamic relationship between the organism and the external physical and social environment.

(Kuo, 1967, p. 25, author's emphasis)

This developmental perspective has now become the dominant model in modern comparative psychology (Schneirla, 1966; Aronson et al., 1970). The chapters in the present volume by Gottlieb (Chapter 5; also Gottlieb, 1992) and Goy (Chapter 15) provide further illustrations of this integrative model.

Parallel themes emerged in ethology, which has been defined as the subdiscipline of biology concerned with the biological bases of behavior (Lorenz, 1965; Tinbergen, 1972). Ethological methods initially focused on the development of unrestrained behavior of species in the natural environment. This focus inevitably identified the centrality of social behaviors and development in evolutionary adaptations (Lorenz, 1965). Ethologists have provided compelling demonstrations that the evolutionarily meaningful social behaviors could be productively explored through direct observations.

Modern ethology – as represented in Hinde (1970), Bateson (1979, 1991), and Immelmann et al. (1981) – has extended these themes across disciplines, species and methodologies, increasing the overlap between concepts and findings of comparative psychology and ethology (Hinde, 1970). Bateson's Chapter 1 provides a summary of progress in contemporary ethology (for more comprehensive accounts, see Hinde, 1970; Bateson, 1991; Immelmann et al., 1981).

Socialization in childhood and adolescence

The term 'socialization' has typically referred to the social development of human beings, specifically the process of 'making fit for society' (OED, 1972). As in studies of animal behavior, two broad orientations have emerged: one emphasizes proximal determinants, and the other, ultimate genetic determinants. But the research literatures in human social behavior have evolved in separate pathways from those in animal behavior. This is seen in the kinds of proximal determinants emphasized and the sorts of evidence cited for genetic regulation. Despite seemingly common concerns, the literatures have spoken different languages.

Social learning investigations concerned with socialization have focused on how behaviors and beliefs are transmitted from one generation to the next, and how children become similar to their parents in actions and attitudes (Bandura, 1977; Bandura & Walters, 1963; Sears, Maccoby & Levin, 1957). But the proximal concepts employed to explain the transmission and similarities – such as 'social reinforcement', 'imitation', and 'modeling' – focused attention on learning processes rather than biological ones. The idea that children were active agents in this process was explicit in the early works on socialization (e.g. Sears, 1951; Sears et al., 1953) but few methods were available to expand on this theoretical insight; instead, research focused attention on the parental activities as antecedents, and the child social behaviors as consequences.

The development of procedures and models for tracking the interactions between children and parents and how they influence each other provided a major advance for the area (e.g. Patterson, 1982). Bell & Harper (1977) discussed the implications of the findings that children affect their parents as well as vice-versa. It was then but a small step for Scarr (Scarr & McCartney, 1983; Scarr & Kidd, 1983) and others to argue that the genetic background shared by parents and offspring provided a parsimonious account for behavioral similarities across generations. On this view, resemblances reflected the operation of heritable characteristics, so that the 'clouds of correlations' typically observed in studies of the relationship between child-rearing practices and child outcomes were epiphenomenal (Scarr, 1986).

Convergence across disciplines

Given this brief overview, one might conclude that even though studies of human socialization and biosocial studies of animals proceeded along separate routes, they generated parallel controversies. That is generally correct, but two major points of convergence should be underscored. One has been the recognition by investigators in both humans and animals that the study of development could be key to understanding how internal and external influences are integrated (e.g. Bronfenbrenner, 1979; Cairns, 1979; Magnusson, 1988; Sameroff, 1983). Bronfenbrenner (1944), for example, early recognized the need for an integrative analysis of social development, proposing that

the proper evaluation of social status and structure requires the envisagement both of the individual and the group as developing organic units. Piecemeal analysis, fixed in time and space, of isolated aspects is insufficient and even misleading, for the elements of social status and structure are interdependent, organized into complex patterns, and subject both to random and lawful variation.

(Bronfenbrenner, 1944; 75)

Beyond this insight, there have been severe limits on the research methods available to investigators who aspire to investigate human socialization by integrated, multi-level research designs. This is less a handicap for research with nonhuman animals. Animal behaviorists can simultaneously conduct field observations, experimental manipulations, genetic and neurobiological modifications, and longitudinal observations under controlled circumstances. By 1980, investigations conducted in ethology and developmental psychobiology had provided relatively comprehensive accounts of particular domains of social development in several mammalian species over the lifespan.

That brings us to the second major point of convergence. Over the past two decades, there has been a significant dove-tailing of research strategies and findings from human and nonhuman studies on specific domains of social development such as attachment and aggression. Several longitudinal investigations have now been completed on social behavior from birth or childhood to maturity (e.g. Block, 1971; Eron et al., 1971; Magnusson & Bergman, 1990; Rutter, 1989). The findings from this work have significantly expanded the depth and generality of our information on the nature of human social adaptation. They have also promoted the re-introduction of biological measures and concepts into the study of human socialization and an integrative account of social development across the lifespan.

A DEVELOPMENTAL FRAMEWORK

Building upon these advances in research and theory, Magnusson & Cairns (1995) recently summarized a set of propositions relevant to the study of behavior from the common ground of development. The propositions were revised in collaboration with colleagues at Stockholm University and the Carolina Consortium on Human Development (Cairns, Elder & Costello, 1995). For this chapter, I have modified six of the proposals in order to heighten their focus on social development. These are listed below, along with some comments on implications.

An individual develops and functions socially as an integrated organism. Maturational, experiential and cultural contributions are fused in ontogeny. Single aspects do not develop and function in isolation, and they should not be divorced from the totality in analysis.

This organismic proposition lies at the heart of a systemic developmental approach to social behavior and socialization. The kernel idea is that individuals develop and function socially in an integrated fashion. By extension, social behaviors are seen as essential components of evolutionary change and developmental adaptations.

The organismic proposition has been adopted by virtually all investigators of animal behavior (King, 1977; Bertalanffy, 1962), but not by students of human social behavior, despite Bronfenbrenner's (1944) early insights on the matter. In this regard, human socialization researchers have traditionally given only modest attention to organismic, biosocial factors in accounts of social development. One objection has been that the organismic proposition is not wrong so much as it is a truism beyond scientific analysis (Buss & Plomin, 1984; Hansen, 1968).

There are other, more substantial, methodological reasons that underlie the reluctance of socialization researchers to embrace an integrative developmental orientation. If adopted, the orientation would challenge the hegemony of some research designs, measurements, and analyses that are standard for the area (Cairns, 1986; Wohlwill, 1973). Consider, for example, that the effects of age have been eliminated by design or otherwise controlled in traditional socialization research. The rationale was that the effects must be controlled in order to identify the contributions of other theoretically relevant differences (say, in families, peers, or schools). Once the effects of age on social development have been eliminated methodologically, it becomes easier to ignore them theoretically. Moreover, the procedures implicated by the organismic proposition – multi-method, multi-agent information over time – tend to overwhelm existing statistical analytic models.

An individual develops and functions in a dynamic, continuous and reciprocal process of interaction with his or her environment, including relations with other individuals, groups and the subculture.

Social actions organize the space between the organism and its physical and social environment. According to this proposition, social actions must be flexible, responsive, constructive, and rapidly acting in order to serve their distinctive functions in adaptation. Even in simple dyadic exchanges, one's actions must simultaneously achieve within person-organization and between-person social behavior organization. Dynamic social processes, although enormously complicated in themselves, must be effectively synchronized with parallel processes in two or more individuals.

What makes the 'miracle' of social exchange possible and even common-place in everyday life? The available evidence is consistent with an immanent, inherent bias for social interactions from infancy through maturity. Cases of autism – where reciprocal processes fail to become established in the first year of life – occur infrequently, with an incidence rate of $3 : 10,000$. The rarity of the pathology underscores the universality of the social bias in normal human infancy (Rutter & Schopler, 1978). It should be noted that the proposal of an inherent social bias cannot 'explain' the ubiquity of social reciprocity. However, it can become the starting point for a developmental analysis.

What is adaptive in social behavior jointly depends upon the constraints of the social/physical ecology and the characteristics of the individual. Of singular import is the fact that social interactions permit the organism to rapidly change or restructure the effective environment. Relative to most major morphological and physiological modifications, social accommodations are rapid and reversible. They are able to promote changes in the biological organization as well as vice versa. In this basic sense, social actions may be viewed as a leading edge of biological adaptation. If social accommodations work and prove functional in development and in microevolution, they may be buttressed by enduring changes in the biological equipment of the individual (Cairns, Gariépy & Hood, 1990).

A final implication is that social interactions cannot be static and maintain their distinctive functions in adaptation. This follows from the proposition that the malleable properties of social actions confer upon them distinct advantages for rapid biological and social adaptation that cannot be otherwise duplicated. These properties also ensure that social patterns must remain open to sources of variance that extend beyond the biological states of the organism. The irony is that virtually all socialization constructs – from aggression and attachment to self-concept and intelligence – traditionally have been considered to be stable properties of the individual. Such reification of social interactions is inconsistent with their dynamic properties.

Novel patterns of social functioning arise during individual ontogeny.

Tracing backward from adulthood to childhood and infancy reveals few novelties in individual functioning. But it is easier to look backwards than forwards. Retrospection is always more organized and predictable than anticipation. When one tracks development forward – from infancy to childhood and maturity and senescence – the story has novelties and twists. In a lifetime, each individual has the capacity to develop truly novel patterns of action and thinking that are as distinctive as the individual's DNA configuration.

Such novelties may grow out of the reorganization of existing patterns, or the creation of entirely new ones. The conditions of development help determine the nature, form and function of these behavioral adaptations. In this view, social development is bidirectional and constructive throughout the lifespan. The individual is continuously adaptive and active throughout the course of development, not merely in its early stages.

Differences in the rate of development may produce major differences in the organization and configuration of social functions. The developmental rate of individual components may be accelerated or delayed relative to other features.

Individual development reflects a mosaic of ontogenetic trajectories. Sexual maturation is a case in point. Acceleration in the age of menarche in humans has been associated with various outcomes, most of which have been viewed as negative for girls and positive for boys (Simmons & Blyth, 1987; Stattin & Magnusson, 1990). This biological trajectory must be interpreted in conjunction with societal changes in age-related expectations for behavior. Beyond maturational influences on developmental timing, early entry into school (by chance or by geography) has been associated with accelerated cognitive development in children. The advantages are enduring, and they extend beyond scholastic achievement to include advances in basic information processing and intellectual test performance (Morrison, Griffith & Frazier, 1993). The more days a child spends in school, the higher the child's IQ (Ceci, 1990).

Shifting to demonstrations in animal behavior, changes in the developmental timing of social behaviors could be a major force in social evolution, a point that Mason (1979) and I have argued elsewhere (Cairns, 1976, 1979). This proposition follows de Beer's (1958) more general proposal that variations in ontogenetic timing – or alterations in the rate of maturation of key organismic features – could provide essential mechanisms for evolutionary change. On this score, Gould (1977: 408) wrote, 'I predict that this debate [on the role of heterochrony] will define the major issue in evolutionary biology for the 1980s.'

That decade has come and gone, and the predicted centrality of heterochrony did not materialize. Instead, genetic diversity emerged as a burning issue for evolutionary biology in the 1980s. Although Gould's timing was off, his point on the centrality of development was certainly correct. A primary thesis of this chapter is that the common ground of development is key for establishing a rapprochement between biological and psychological approaches to human social behaviors.

Patterns of social functioning develop like dynamic systems. They are capable of reorganization because windows of change exist throughout development, not only in the early stages of life. Social patterns thus cannot be described in terms of hierarchical organization, nor can they be reduced to simpler experiential antecedents or more elementary biological units.

According to this proposition, it is an illusion to view social functioning as regulated hierarchically over the lifespan. It makes little difference whether the hierarchy is presumed to be built upon genetic reductionism, learning processes, or poor early social experiences. The problem with such hierarchical conceptions is that they draw attention away from the organization and reorganization of social patterns that occur throughout ontogeny. According to this proposition, social behaviors may be reorganized throughout the lifespan, not only at conception or birth, and not only by genes or early experience. Periods of organization, features of the individual and the social environment can be synchronized in ways that enhance individual social functioning in the present context.

One thesis that follows from the present framework is that social behaviors cannot be fixed, whether by genes or by early experience, and maintain their distinctive functions in social accommodation and social adaptation. The social systems must be capable of reorganization at critical points if they are to be effective.

Conservation in social development is supported by correlated constraints from without and from within the individual. The upshot is that social and cognitive organization in development tends to be continuous and conservative despite fluidity and change.

For developmentalists, fluidity and change are expected to dominate in ontogeny. The problem for a developmental perspective is to explain stability. Nevertheless, most social behaviors which have been studied longitudinally show reasonably high levels of stability. Aggressive behaviors constitute a case in point. Olweus (1979) concluded that individual differences in aggressive behaviors are virtually as stable as individual differences in intelligence.

The dilemma may be resolved when it is recognized that the antecedents and outcomes of social behavior occur together in 'packages', not as separate or independent variables. Longitudinal studies confirm that there are correlations between individual, family, social, educational and economic constraints (e.g. Cairns & Cairns, 1994; Magnusson, 1988). Cairns & Cairns (1994) observed that multiple changes occurred in the lives of each of the 695 persons they followed from childhood to adulthood. Some of the modifications led to new pathways of living, but most of the changes were ephemeral and persons resumed old habits and ways of living. These investigators comment:

Why did some shifts in trajectory become more enduring while most did not? The answer seems to lie not simply in the person, but in whether the changes were supported by other forces in the person's life. This brings us back to the folly of divorcing a single trend or shift in behaviors from the broader contexts in which they are embedded. Developmental theorists, from Magnusson (1988) to Bronfenbrenner (1979) argue for the necessity of considering regulatory constraints across levels, from individual to dyad to social network to society. Furthermore, our data indicate that biases which operate at one level are usually correlated with those that operate at other levels. These systems collaborate rather than compete, and they funnel behavior in the direction best suited for the context in which development occurs.

(Cairns & Cairns, 1994: 233)

This line of reasoning is not limited to studies of human socialization. A parallel set of conclusions has been reached from investigations in behavioral genetics (Plomin, DeFries & Loughlin, 1977) and developmental psycho-biology (Cairns et al., 1990). On logical grounds, this pattern of correlated constraints is precisely the outcome that should be expected if there is significant bidirectionality in structure-function relationships. There are strong implications for how one should approach socialization research and analysis. If biological, contextural and personal characteristics are inextricably woven over time, one can get lost in attempting to untangle the threads of effects. This proposition leads to methods of analysis which permit descriptions of persons in terms of configurations of characteristics, not single variables taken alone (Magnusson & Bergman, 1990).

TWO EMPIRICAL ILLUSTRATIONS

Coming of age

One example of the utility of the developmental propositions involves the linkage between social development and the timing of pubertal maturation. Developmental timing has long been a focus in both psychological and biological investigations (Turkewitz & Devenny, 1993; de Beer, 1958; Gould, 1977). One of the more active areas in the study of developmental timing in humans involves investigations of variations in the onset of puberty. Is the very early onset of puberty an advantage or a handicap? A consensus of research findings indicates that very early pubertal maturation is associated with negative social outcomes for girls. Depending upon the investigation, very early maturing girls are seen as less capable academically, less socially skilled, and more deviant in their behavior than late maturing girls. The picture is not clear for males, however, and there is some evidence to suggest that the relations are reversed among boys. Why the apparent advantage of neoteny – delayed sexual maturation – for girls, and why is the picture not the same for both genders?

The work of Magnusson, Stattin, and their colleagues offers an answer to this puzzle of socialization (e.g. Magnusson, 1988; Stattin & Magnusson, 1990). In a comprehensive study of over 1000 representative Swedish subjects from childhood through maturity, they assessed not only pubertal maturation but other, potentially related characteristics of girls. These investigators reasoned that the biological effects of maturation must be mediated through social processes in order to have an effect upon adaptation. Specifically, they proposed that early maturing females would appear to be physically older than same-age peers, and girls would tend to hang around with persons who matched their physical age rather than their chronological age. Such differential association could, in turn, accelerate their social and sexual behaviors. In contrast, 'on-time' and late-maturing girls would be less likely to adopt the behaviors and values that were in advance of their age.

Evidence from three longitudinal investigations supports the proposal on the social mediation of the effects of pubertal timing (Magnusson, 1988; Caspi & Moffitt, 1991; Simmons & Blyth, 1987). Consistent with the social mediation proposal, Magnusson and his colleagues have discovered that very early maturing girls (i.e. those who achieved menarche at 10–11 years of age) tended to show a strong bias in their social affiliations (e.g. Magnusson, 1988; Stattin & Magnusson, 1990). At age 13, they differed from less physiologically mature females in that they joined groups of peers – both females and males – who were older than themselves. Their social and sexual behavior patterns were more characteristic of their older peers than other, physically immature members of their cohort. In terms of alcohol consumption and sexual behavior, both the early maturing females and the other boys with whom they associated differed markedly from the rest of the sample.

Magnusson (1988) hypothesized that the rate of biological maturation does not act upon behavior directly; rather, its effects are mediated by a differential selection of older deviant friends and the values they endorse. When subsequent assessments were made at age 16, virtually all girls had attained menarche. Furthermore, the behavioral differences between the early and later maturing girls had also been eliminated by mid-adolescence. Drinking patterns and sexual activities at age 16, as well as other measures of social behavior, were no longer related to maturation rate. It appears that the 'advanced' standards for the early maturing girls at age 13 had become the norm for the entire sample by age 16. Although the differences in social behavior were eliminated in follow-up, differences in school achievement proved to be residual. When early–late comparisons were made among the women in their late 20s, the very-early maturing women had married earlier, had more children, and did not attend the university.

Very early onset of sexual maturity did not directly produce deviance in the Swedish sample. To the contrary, a key mediational variable appears to be social affiliations that were promoted by the pace at which normal biological changes occur. When other girls reached menarche at the normative age, there was no difference in female deviance as a function of the rate of maturation. The behavioral differences have been eliminated, in part, by similarities in levels of sexual maturation that have been mediated by similarities in social interchange. Nor is it the case that early biological maturation is the only route that leads to differential association and deviance. It merely provides a biasing condition.

Essential features of these findings have been replicated in other settings and with other samples. For instance, Caspi & Moffitt (1991) find the same early maturation-deviance phenomenon in the longitudinal study of a sample of New Zealand girls. The effect was obtained, however, only if the girls were enrolled in a coeducational school. Caspi and Moffitt argue that the opportunities for deviance by differential association were greater in the coeducational setting than in all-girl schools.

This work signals a new way of thinking about the relationships between biological characteristics, on the one hand, and social adaptations, on the other. The idea that there is a straight line between biology and behaviour is rejected. Rather, biological influences must be filtered through a social system which has values and pathways of its own. The sequence also implies that different societies could have different pathways for the same biological influence.

On the latter point, it should be emphasized that the proposal does not assume that a single depiction should suffice for how biological states, social organization, and behaviors are fitted together. To the contrary, it points to the need to understand both the development of the components and the mediation of relations in the biobehavioral system. Modest change in one key parameter of the system presumably could drastically modify the outcomes produced. In this regard, work on the social organization of adolescents has shown that affiliation is based upon several factors, only one of which is the sexual maturation level of the members. In societies, for example, where there is great ethnic and social diversity, the effects of early sexual maturation on deviance and on social affiliation might be expected to be significantly modified (Cairns & Cairns, 1994). The larger point is that biosocial processes should be understood in social context.

The socialization of violence and aggression

Violence is one of the great threats to the integrity of modern society. Assaultive youth are not merely perpetrators, they are victims themselves. In both males and females, high levels of childhood aggression are associated with early school dropout, teenage parenthood, high levels of substance abuse and criminal arrests.

A challenge of socialization research and its applications for society is to identify ways to change the course of the behavior. A number of robust single-variable antecedents to the occurrence of high aggressive behavior have been firmly established through longitudinal and experimental study. These include coercive parenting, lack of mentoring or monitoring by committed adults, affiliation with aggressive peers, residence in poverty and/or the inner-city, differences in serotonergic or dopaminergic neurotransmitter activity, being intoxicated, or having at least one parent who is criminal (Cairns & Cairns, 1994; Farrington, 1986; Farrington & West 1990; Magnusson, 1988; Patterson, Reid & Dishion, 1992). The empirical effects are robust, and virtually every reasonable hypothesis has won support when focus is given to a single variable analysis. The multidetermined nature of aggressive patterns has ensured a cornucopia of significant results. Yet efforts to change aggressive and antisocial behaviors in adolescents have achieved only modest success (Cairns & Cairns, 1994).

Recent longitudinal studies have been informative in addressing the paradox between ontogenetic change and the stability of aggressive behaviors. If social acts occur at the interface between the individuals and their environments, and are dynamically responsive to events from within and without, why is there conservatism rather than plasticity? In the case of aggressive behaviors, there are correlated constraints within the individual, in the interactions, and in the society. Accordingly, attempts to modify aggressive behavior must simultaneously address the multiple levels of its support, including internal states as well as the powerful effects of peer group influence in deviant behaviors (e.g. Giordano, Cernkovich & Pugh, 1986; Neckerman, 1992). In practice, intervention fails because of the sheer difficulty in disrupting the correlation between supportive internal and external factors. Even if they are disrupted temporarily, there will be pressure to reorganize the behavior once the intervention constraint is removed.

In this regard, Cairns and Cairns (1994) concluded from their longitudinal investigation that:

> Virtually all teenagers in our time are at risk. The web of events that help regulate their lives become increasingly interwoven over time. To be effective, lifelines that are extended must be kept in place long enough to become opportunities for a lifetime. The fresh and hopeful news is that new opportunities recur and they are not limited to windows that appear early in life.   (Cairns & Cairns, 1994: 273)

These findings from the study of humans are consistent with the evidence from nonhumans, except animal research also permits precise analysis of biological contributions to aggressive behavior. In this regard, genetic influences on the social behaviors of nonhuman mammals have been shown to be ubiquitous, powerful, and readily detected. In all systems that have been investigated to date, robust differences in social behavior have been rapidly established by selective breeding. This includes aggressive and violent behaviors. Fuller and Thompson (1960) offered this claim in their pioneering volume *Behavior Genetics*, and it has yet to be disputed by data.

Demonstrations that aggressive behaviors are influenced by genes constitute only part of the story and, arguably, not the most important part (Scott, 1977). Findings from the development of lines of mice that have been selectively bred for aggression have helped complete the picture (e.g. Cairns, et al., 1990; Gariépy, Lewis & Cairns, in press; Lagerspetz & Lagerspetz, 1975). These studies show that:

(1) Genetic effects for aggressive and violent behaviors are highly malleable over the course of development. Demonstrable genetic effects on aggressive behavior in animals can be accentuated, reversed, or canceled out over the lifespan of individuals. These ontogenetic effects can be produced by modifying the individual's rearing conditions, manipulating social interactions, changing the context of interaction, and aging.

(2) Genetic influences on aggressive behavior are more dynamic, more easily achieved, and more open to rapid manipulation than has been recognized in current models of social evolution and behavior genetics. Specifically, virtually non-overlapping distributions of individuals that differ with respect to aggression can be produced within 1–3 generations of selective breeding. These behavioral changes are not accompanied by obvious morphological and hormone differences, though reliable differences in neurobiology have been consistently identified (e.g. Gariépy et al., in press).

(3) Developmental timing has a significant impact upon the nature and magnitude of the genetic effects observed in the organization of aggressive and violent behaviors. The identification of these effects of developmental timing appear to be critical in identifying the windows of vulnerability to behavior change and the possible implications for intervention strategies in males and females.

These empirical results are consistent with the view that social behaviors – including aggressive and violent actions – are dynamic and adaptive features of organisms. Accordingly, social behaviors constitute a leading edge of biological change. They are among the first features to be influenced by genetic selection and by environmental experience. In this regard, Fuller (1967: 1647) observed that 'behavior most modifiable by variation in experience may also be particularly sensitive to genetic variation'. Although most properties of social systems may be closed to rapid ontogenetic and microevolutionary change, some elements in their organization appear to remain open in both time frames. The recent empirical literature brings attention to the correlation between biological constraints within and environmental constraints without, and how they become integrated over time in the individual and in the species (Cairns et al., 1990; Maynard Smith et al., 1985).

Social actions have distinctive properties in adaptation because they organize the space between the organism and the environment, and thereby promote rapid, selective and novel adaptations. Once the action is effective, or ineffective, it can provide the scaffold for further changes in morphological and physiological activity (Bateson, 1991; Cairns, 1979; Hinde, 1970).

CLOSING COMMENTS

Socialization research historically has been pulled by two opposing forces. One competitor in the tug-of-war has been society's need to ensure the meaningfulness of research and to promote solutions to pressing social issues. It tends to consider the niceties of measurement and research design as trivial pursuits. The other tension can be traced to the need for science to ensure rigor in measurement and precision in analysis, and it tends to view the reduction of complex phenomena to their individual parts as inevitable. Neither side can be a winner in this competition. One can claim relevance, but employ only the veneer of science and thereby lose its critical core and methodological strengths. The other can claim precision and rigor, but overlook the problem of integration and thereby obscure the meaning and function of the phenomena that it aspires to explain.

It has been assumed that biological and behavioral science can clarify the principles of social development by a careful study of individual ontogenies and the natural history of the species. That is, social behaviors should be viewed simultaneously in terms of ontogenesis (the development of the individual) and phylogenesis (the development of the species). Socio-genesis is the proposal that there is a developmental fusion of these sources of variance in social behavior. It emphasizes the essential bidirectionality of processes within the individual and those in the social environment. Accordingly, multiple levels of analysis are required, and the study of social behavior is necessarily a synthetic science.

The propositions outlined in this chapter provide a foundation for a theory and not a theory itself. In its present state, the developmental framework is appropriately viewed as an orientation rather than a tightly bolted structure. The unfinished business has a lot to do with the distinctive properties of human beings and how these are organized over time.

What are these distinctive properties of human social patterns? They include the capacity to think and reflect upon one's actions and one's potential futures. Humans hold the ability to learn rapidly, to communicate ideas symbolically, and to reconstruct memories from the past that are in line with the constraints and needs of the present. These constructions often occur outside the individual's own awareness yet serve basic needs to protect the person's own sense of well-being. These capacities are also combined in development to permit us to be awestruck by beauty, and burdened by guilt.

Nor are one's views of oneself immutable from childhood to maturity. There appears to be as much variability in the individual's own concept of self as there is in the concepts that others share about her/him. One beguiling finding of longitudinal study is that concepts from the self and sources external to the self often show only modest overlap (Cairns & Cairns, 1994). Personal beliefs and values are not necessarily mirrors of an individual's own life. Rather, each of us may exist in a hall of mirrors created by our own projections and by projections of others. Despite one's personal beliefs to the contrary, conceptions of oneself are not static. Like other features of social behavior and social cognition, self-concepts are dynamic and adaptive.

Yet there is relative stability of the self and social behavior, despite changes within and without the individual. In social perceptions as in social behaviors, the stability arises because of the correlated constraints of living. Consider, for instance, the role of peer social networks in maintaining one's sense of oneself. Groups are remarkably fluid for most individuals throughout childhood and youth, yet their effects on social behavior and social cognition seem to be relatively stable. How can there be stability in the midst of change? The empirical answer is that even though faces change, individuals tend to gravitate toward others who are similar to their previous friends and companions (Cairns & Cairns, 1994; Neckerman, 1992). Even social networks can serve as correlated constraints that help maintain continuity in social behaviors.

The sociogenetic model stands in sharp opposition to static conceptions of human behavior. Nevertheless, the dualism remains alive and well in the 1990s. The acceptance of the nature–nurture dualism occurs despite the wealth of evidence that renders untenable its basic assumptions on behavior causation (compare, for instance, Ceci, 1990, with Herrnstein & Murray, 1994). Why the strong attraction in the public and in the science to ideas that run counter to empirical evidence? One must suspect that the criteria for these judgment and interpretations resides in the beliefs of society rather than the hard-won findings of empirical research.

A heavy burden rests upon any area that aspires to understand the distinctive properties of social behavior in humans. The task demands high standards of research, multilevel longitudinal and cross-generational studies, critical evaluations of available findings, and a commitment to understanding the integration of social processes as well as their parts.

Despite these tensions and the sheer complexity of social phenomena, there have been fundamental advances in research and understanding over the past two decades. The primary sources are (i) animal research, which has promoted the synthesis of ethology and comparative psychology on the common ground of development, and (ii) human research, which has provided longitudinal and cross-generational accounts of human beings over formative periods of the life span. Taken together, the findings expand markedly the depth and generality of our information on the nature of social adaptation. The upshot is that developmental science can now offer a coherent and integrative account of human socialization.

ACKNOWLEDGEMENTS

The work reported in this chapter was supported by funds from the National Institute of Mental Health (R01 MH45532 and P50 MH26834). I thank Beverley D. Cairns and David Magnusson for their comments on this chapter, and their contributions to much of the research that is cited. Requests for reprints should be sent to Robert B. Cairns, Center for Developmental Science, CB#8115, University of North Carolina at Chapel Hill, Chapel Hill, NC 27514-8115.

REFERENCES

Alcock, J. (1993) *Animal behavior: An Evolutionary Approach*. Sunderland, Mass.: Sinauer Associates.

Alexander, R. D. & Noonan, K. M. (1979) Concealment ovulation, paternal care, and human social evolution. In Chagnon, N. A. & Irons, W. (eds.) *Evolutionary Biology and Human Social Behavior: An Anthropological Perspective* (pp. 436–53). North Scituate, Mass: Duxbury.

Aronson, L. R., Tobach, E., Lehrman, D. S. & Rosenblatt, J. S. (eds.), (1970) *Development and Evolution of Behavior: Essays in Memory of T. C. Schneirla*. San Francisco, Calif.: Freeman.

Bandura, A. (1977) *Social Learning Theory*. Englewood Cliffs, NJ: Prentice-Hall.

Bandura, A. & Walters, R. H. (1963) *Social Learning and Personality Development*. New York: Holt, Rinehart & Winston.

Bateson, P. P. G. (1979) How do sensitive periods arise and what are they good for? *Animal Behavior*, **27**, 470–86.

Bateson, P. P. G. (1991) *The Development and Integration of Behaviour: Essays in Honour of Robert Hinde*. Cambridge: Cambridge University Press.

Becker, G. S. (1993) *Human Capital: A Theoretical and Empirical Analysis, with Special Reference to Education* 3rd edn. Chicago, Ill.: The University of Chicago Press.

Bell, R. Q. & Harper, L. V. (1977) *Child Effects on Adults*. Hillsdale, NJ: Erlbaum.

Bertalanffy, L. V. (1962) *Modern Theories of Development: An Introduction to Theoretical Biology*. New York: Harper & Brothers. (First published in 1933.)

Block, J. (1971) *Lives Through Time*. Berkeley, Calif.: Bancroft Press.

Bronfenbrenner, U. (1944) A constant frame of reference for sociometric research: Part II. Experiment and inference. *Sociometry*, **7**, 40–75.

Bronfenbrenner, U. (1979) *The Ecology of Human Development: Experiments by Nature and Design*. Cambridge, Mass.: Harvard University Press.

Buss, A. H. & Plomin, R. (1984) *Temperament: Early Developing Personality Traits*. Hillsdale, NJ: Erlbaum.

Cairns, R. B. (1976) The ontogeny and phylogeny of social behavior. In Hahn, M. E. & Simmel, E. C. (eds.) *Evolution and Communicative Behavior*. New York: Academic Press, pp. 115–39.

Cairns, R. B. (1977) Sociobiology: a new synthesis or an old cleavage? (Review of *Sociobiology: A New Synthesis*, by E. O. Wilson.) *Contemporary Psychology*, **22**, 1–3.

Cairns, R. B. (1979) *Social Development: The Origins and Plasticity of Social Interchanges*. San Francisco, Calif.: Freeman.

Cairns, R. B. (1986) Phenomena lost: issues in the study of development. In Valsiner, J. (ed.) *The Individual Subject and Scientific Psychology*. New York: Plenum Press, pp. 97–112.

Cairns, R. B. & Cairns, B. D. (1994) *Lifelines and Risks: Pathways of Youth in Our Time*. New York: Cambridge University Press aid.

Cairns, R. B., Elder, G. H., Jr. & Costello, E. J. (eds.) (1995) *Developmental Science*. New York: Cambridge University Press.

Cairns, R. B., Gariépy, J.-L. & Hood, K. E. (1990) Development, microevolution, and social behavior. *Psychological Review*, **97**, 49–65.

Caspi, A. & Moffitt, T. (1991) Puberty and deviance in girls. Symposium paper read at the Biennial Meeting of the Society for Research in Child Development, Seattle, April, 1991.

Ceci, S. J. (1990) *On Intelligence … More or Less: A Bio-ecological Treatise on Intellectual Development*. Englewood Cliffs, NJ: Prentice-Hall.

Darwin, C. (1873) *The Expression of the Emotions in Man and Animals*. New York: D. Appleton.

de Beer, G. (1958) *Embryos and Ancestors*, 3rd edn. London: Oxford University Press.

Eron, L. D., Walder, L. O. & Lefkowitz, M. M. (1971) *Learning of Aggression in Children*. Boston, Mass.: Little, Brown.

Farrington, D. P. (1986) Stepping stones to adult criminal careers. In Olweus, D., Block, J. & Radke-Yarrow, M. (eds.) *Development of Antisocial and Prosocial Behavior: Research, Theories and Issues*. New York: Academic, pp. 359–84.

Farrington, D. P. & West, D. J. (1990) The Cambridge study in delinquent development: a long-term follow-up of 411 London males. In Kerner, H.-J. & Kaiser, G. (eds.) *Criminality: Personality, Behavior and Life History*. Berlin: Springer-Verlag.

Fuller, J. L. (1967) Experimental deprivation and later behavior. *Science*, **158**, 1645–52.

Fuller, J. L. & Thompson, W. R. (1960) *Behavior Genetics*. New York: John Wiley.

Galton, F. (1871) *Hereditary Genius: An Inquiry into its Laws and Consequences*, rev. edn. New York: D. Appleton.

Gariépy, J.-L., Lewis, M. H. & Cairns, R. B. (in press). In Stoff, D. & Cairns, R. B. (eds.) *Aggression and Violence: Genetic, Neurobiological, and Biosocial Perspectives*. Hillsdale, NJ: Erlbaum.

Giordano, P. C., Cernkovich, S. A. & Pugh, M. D. (1986) Friendship and delinquency. *American Journal of Sociology*, **91**, 1170–201.

Gottlieb, G. (1992) *Individual Development and Evolution: The Genesis of Novel Behavior*. New York: Oxford University Press.

Gould, S. J. (1977) *Ontogeny and Phylogeny*. Cambridge, Mass.: Harvard University Press.

Hamilton, W. D. (1964) The genetical evolution of social behavior. *Journal of Theoretical Biology*, **7**, 1–52.

Hansen, E. W. (1968) Behavior as a continuous process. (Review of Z.-Y. Kuo, *The Dynamics of Behavior Development: An Epigenetic View*.) *Science*, **160**, 58–9.

Herrnstein, R. J. & Murray, C. (1994) *The Bell Curve: Intelligence and Class Structure in American Life*. New York: Free Press.

Hinde, R. A. (1970) *Animal behaviour: a synthesis of ethology and comparative psychology*. New York, McGraw-Hill.

Immelmann, K., Barlow, G., Petrinovich, L. & Main, M. (eds.) (1981) *Behavioral Development: The Bielefeld Interdisciplinary Project*. Cambridge & New York: Cambridge University Press.

King, J. A. (1977) Behavioral comparisons and evolution. In Oliverio, A. (ed.) *Genetics, Environment and Intelligence*. Amsterdam: Elsevier/North Holland, pp. 23–36.

Kuo, Z.-Y. (1967) *The Dynamics of Behavioral Development: An Epigenetic View*. New York: Random House.

Lagerspetz, K. M. J. & Lagerspetz, K. Y. H. (1975) The expression of the genes of aggressiveness in mice: the effect of androgen on aggression and sexual behavior in females. *Aggressive Behavior*, **1**, 291–6.

Lorenz, K. Z. (1965) *Evolution and the Modification of Behavior*. Chicago, Ill.: University of Chicago Press.

Lorenz, K. Z. (1966) *On Aggression*. New York: Harcourt, Brace & World.

Magnusson, D. (1988) *Individual Development from an Interactional Perspective. Vol. 1.* In Magnusson, D. (ed.) *Paths Through Life: A Longitudinal Research Program*. Hillsdale, NJ: Erlbaum.

Magnusson, D. & Bergman, L. R. (1990) A pattern approach to the study of pathways from childhood to adulthood. In Robins, L. N. & Rutter, M. (eds.) *Straight and Devious Pathways from Childhood to Adulthood*. Cambridge, UK: Cambridge University Press, pp. 101–15.

Magnusson, D. & Cairns, R. B. (1995) Developmental science: an integrated framework. In Cairns, R. B., Elder, G. H., Jr. & Costello, E. J. (eds.) *Developmental Science*. New York: Cambridge University Press.

Mason, W. A. (1979) Ontogeny of social behavior. In Marler, P. & Vandenbergh, J. G. (eds.) *Social Behavior and Communication*. New York: Plenum Press, pp. 1–28.

Maynard Smith, J. (1982) *Evolution and the Theory of Games*. Cambridge; New York: Cambridge University Press.

Maynard Smith, J., Burian, R., Kauffman, S., Alberch, P., Campbell, J., Goodwin, B., Lande, R., Raup, D. & Wolpert, L. (1985) Developmental constraints and evolution. *The Quarterly Review of Biology*, **60**, 265–87.

Morrison, F. J., Griffith, E. M. & Frazier, J. A. (1993) Two steps from the start: Individual differences in early literacy. Paper presented at biennial meeting of the Society for Research in Child Development, New Orleans, LA, March.

Neckerman, H. J. (1992) A longitudinal investigation of the stability and fluidity of social networks and peer relationships of children and adolescents. Unpublished doctoral dissertation. University of North Carolina at Chapel Hill. Chapel Hill, North Carolina.

Olweus, D. (1979) Stability of aggressive reaction patterns in males: A review. *Psychological Bulletin*, **86**, 852–75.

OED (Oxford English Dictionary) (1972) Oxford: Oxford University Press.

Patterson, G. R. (1982) *Coercive Family Process*. Eugene, Oreg.: Castalia.

Patterson, G. R., Reid, J. B. & Dishion, T. J. (1992) *Antisocial Boys.* Eugene, Oreg.: Castalia.

Plomin, R., DeFries, J. C. & Loehlin, J. C. (1977) Genotype-environment interaction and correlation in the analysis of human behavior. *Psychological Bulletin,* **84**, 309–22.

Rutter, M. (1989) (ed.) *Studies of Psychosocial Risk: The Power of Longitudinal Data.* Cambridge: Cambridge University Press.

Rutter, M. & Schopler, E. (1978) *Autism: a Reappraisal of Concepts and Treatment.* New York: Plenum Press.

Sameroff, A. J. (1983) Developmental systems: contexts and evolution. In Mussen, P. H. (gen. ed.) & Kessen, W., (vol. ed.) *Handbook of Child Psychology, Vol. 1, History, Theory and Methods.* New York: John Wiley, pp. 237–94.

Scarr, S. (1986) Cultural lenses on mothers and children. In Friedrich-Cofer, L. (ed.) *Human Nature and Public Policy: Scientific Views of Women, Children and Families.* New York: Praeger, pp. 202–38.

Scarr, S. & Kidd, K. K. (1983) Developmental behavior genetics. In Mussen, P. H. (ed.) *Handbook of Child Psychology. Vol. 2,* 4th edn. New York: John Wiley, pp. 345–434.

Scarr, S. & McCartney, K. (1983) How people make their own environments: A theory of genotype-environment effects. *Child Development,* **54**, 426–33.

Schneirla, T. C. (1966) Behavioral development and comparative psychology. *Quarterly Review of Biology,* **41**, 283–302.

Scott, J. P. (1977) Social genetics. *Behavior Genetics,* **7**, 327–46.

Sears, R. R. (1951) A theoretical framework for personality and social behavior. *American Psychologist,* **6**, 476–83.

Sears, R. R., Maccoby, E. E. & Levin, H. (1957) *Patterns of Child Rearing.* Evanston: Row, Peterson.

Sears, R. R., Whiting, J. W. M., Nowlis, V. & Sears, P. S. (1953) Some child-rearing antecedents of aggressive and dependency in young children. *Genetic Psychology Monographs,* **47**, 135–234.

Simmons, R. C. & Blyth, D. A. (1987) *Moving into Adolescence: The Impact of Pubertal Change and School Context.* New York: Aldine.

Stattin, H. & Magnusson, D. (1990) Pubertal-maturation in female development. In Magnusson, D. (ed.) *Paths Through Life, Vol. 2.* Hillsdale, NJ: Erlbaum.

Tinbergen, N. (1972) *The Animal in its World. Explorations of an Ethologist.* London: Allen & Unwin.

Turkewitz, G. & Devenny, D. A. (1993) (eds.) *Developmental Time and Timing.* Hillsdale, NJ: Erlbaum.

Wilson, E. O. (1975) *Sociobiology: The New Synthesis.* Cambridge, Mass.: Harvard University Press.

Wohlwill, J. (1973) *The Study of Behavioral Development.* New York: Academic.

15 Patterns of juvenile behavior following early hormonal interventions

ROBERT W. GOY

In the past 35 years an extensive animal literature has been developed on the masculinization of behavior of genotypic females by administration of exogenous androgen at early stages of development. In addition, a less voluminous but no less convincing literature has been provided on feminization of the behavioral traits of the genotypic male by induction of androgen deficiency during the same early developmental stages that are critical to the masculinization of females. Both of these kinds of studies have striking parallels in human clinical syndromes. The literature on human female pseudohermaphroditism induced by congenital adrenal hyperplasia bears close comparison to the experimental treatment of female animals with androgen before birth (Ehrhardt & Baker, 1974). The experimental work on androgen deficiency in male animals is provided with a number of human parallels in the excellent papers of Wilson (1987, 1991). The similarities in behavior of androgenized female humans and androgen-deficient male humans have been highlighted recently (Money, Schwartz & Lewis, 1984). For comprehensive discussion of the experimental animal research the readers are referred to the following reviews (Ward & Ward, 1985; Baum, 1987; Hutchison & Hutchison, 1990). Most of this work has focused on the development of patterns of adult sexual behavior, and much less attention has been paid to the development of juvenile behavior patterns that are known to be sexually dimorphic. Yet the distinction is of considerable theoretical importance, because juvenile behaviors that are sexually dimorphic are expressed in the absence of concurrent gonadal hormones. The secretions of the gonads do not appear in the blood stream in biologically significant concentrations during the juvenile period between infancy and puberty. In contrast, adult sexual behavior is most typically not expressed in mammals until the gonads are actively producing biologically effective amounts of hormones. Thus, sexual behaviors have hormonal requirements which must be met both during early stages of development and again during adolescence and adultload, whereas juvenile behaviors require only appropriate hormonal stimulation at early stages before the behavior has ever been expressed. Thus the study of the differentiation of juvenile behaviors is not attributable to, and is not confounded by, the altered sensitivity of the neural substrate to the hormones which is one of the principal effects of the actions of the hormones on the fetus.

Sexually differentiated juvenile behaviors serve as basic validation of behaviorally significant hormonal actions on the embryonic, fetal or larval brain, and their presence in a wide number of mammals justifies the study of biochemical interactions between hormones and fetal neural tissues. Before such biochemical-neural studies can be undertaken, however, evidence has to be provided on the kinds of hormones that are effective in altering behavior as well as the times in early development when the hormone must be active. The present work was undertaken in order to make some contribution to the development of this essential background of information. It was hoped that the information sought would be provided at least in part by studies that varied the amount of hormone, the type of hormone, and the timing of administration of hormone. In addition, the work was planned to make use of the rhesus monkey, a nonhuman primate biologically more similar to man than the common laboratory rodents and a species known to require social experience for the normal development of sexual behavior.

SUBJECTS, METHODS AND TREATMENTS

The studies described in this chapter were conducted over a period of nearly 15 years. They contain the findings obtained from longitudinal studies of social and protosexual behavior displayed by more than 300 rhesus monkeys. Each subject used in this report was studied in a specific and highly similar social context. The experimental subjects were all genotypic females that were either potentially or manifestly virilized by injecting testosterone proportionate into pregnant females. Each treatment began and ended on arbitrarily determined days of gestation so that an array of various treatments could be assessed for their behavioral consequences. Most of the treatments involved injection of 10 mg/day of the androgen. In this report, however, variation in daily dosage did not significantly alter the effects on behavior over the range of dosages used. For that reason results from all dosages are used in this report in which the primary concern is the detection of effects related to the duration rather than to the daily dosage of the treatment. Accordingly, some few subjects injected with 15 mg/day, 12.5 mg/day and even as little as 5 mg/day have been included. These irregular cases are distributed among two of the treatments shown in Figure 15.1 which presents a schematic summary of the various treatments analyzed for this report. The figure displays codes for the various treatments in the vertical left-hand column. In each code the first number indicates the duration of the treatment in days, and the number following the slash indicates the gestational age of the fetus on the day of the first injection of androgen. Readers should note that treatments are arranged in order of beginning age (youngest ages at the top of the figure) and duration of treatment. The longest treatment (H80/40)

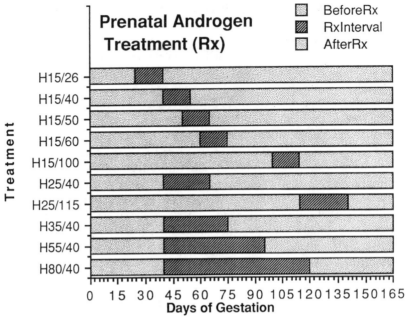

Figure 15.1. Summary of testosterone propionate treatments given to pregnant females for purposes of masculinizing the behavioral characteristics of their female offspring. The lightly filled bar represents the duration of pregnancy, on average, and the darkly filled bar is the period within pregnancy when the androgen was injected daily. The different treatments, listed on the left, are designated with an H followed by four or five digits. The first two digits indicate the total duration of the treatment in days, and the remaining digits after the slash indicate the day of gestation when the treatment was initiated.

consists of only three subjects, one treated with 12.5 mg/day and two treated with 5 mg/day. The single subject that received 15 mg/day was treated for 55 days and is included in the group of subjects treated from day 40 through day 94 (H55/40). These irregular treatments were used early on in the course of these studies but were discontinued, either because the higher doses appeared to produce abortion or because the lower dose was associated with microphallus. This association between the low dose and microphallus is worth some emphasis, because this same treatment was also associated with some of the most extensive virilizations of infant and juvenile behavioral development. At birth each subject was assigned randomly to a group containing its own mother and three to five other mothers and their infants. The criterion for assignment to a social group was the birth date of the infant, and assignments were made so that youngest and oldest infants in a group did not differ by more than one month, usually by not more than two weeks. In addition, an attempt was made to constitute groups so that each subject of experimental interest was raised with two normal male and two normal female peers. Since the final determination of group size depended upon the calendar of births, this latter aim could not always be met.

It is important for the social development of monkeys that a large amount of continuous social experience be provided (Goy and Wallen, 1979) and this cannot be accomplished if the animals are only allowed one half hour each day to play with their peers. Accordingly, during all periods of time when the animals were not being housed singly for the purpose of observation, they were housed in large cages with the members of their unique social group.

Following establishment of the social group, infants and their mothers were left undisturbed in a large housing unit which permitted easy observation of all resident animals. They were observed for one-half hour per day for 150 successive days between the postnatal ages of 3 and 12 months. This nine-month period represents a developmental stage when the infant rhesus is gradually gaining increasing independence from the mother, and during which time its social and protosexual interactions with peers and adult females are being elaborated and consolidated.

When infants reached 12 to 13 months of age they were weaned from their mothers by removing each infant to an individual cage. All infants in the same social group were weaned on the same day. Two weeks later the infants were reunited for a half-hour period of observation, and such reunions and observations were repeated daily for 50 successive days over the ensuing three months. The 50-day periods of observation were repeated annually when the infants were 24 and 36 months of age. Behavioral data were obtained during these specified periods of observation only, and for each infant a record was made of its social behavior with the same peers during the first, second, third, and fourth years of life. The obtained data can be analyzed in terms of successive 50-day blocks (three such blocks in the first year of life and one such in each of the second, third and fourth years); or the data from all blocks can be summed to permit assessment of the tendency to display the behavior over a protracted period of development. The behavior of the androgenized females during this first year of life has been described quite extensively in previous reports (Goy, 1978; 1981; Goy & Robinson, 1982; Goy & Kemnitz, 1983), so in the present report, except as described in the results, the emphasis has been on measures of behavior that sum the data across the entire period of observational studies.

Results

Effects of prenatal testosterone on genitalia of female offspring

The most complete genital transformations were associated with those treatments beginning on the 40th day of gestation. In all such cases the vaginal orifice of the female fetus was completely obliterated and replaced by a scrotal raphe. The embryonic genital tubercle was transformed into a phallus which either showed hypospadius (when the treatment lasted for only 15 days, H15/40) or which showed a complete penile urethra when the treatment lasted for 25 days or more. Treatments lasting more than 25 days (H35/40, H55/40 and H80/40) caused a continuous enlargement and growth of the phallus whenever the daily dosage of androgen equalled at least 10 mg/day. Treatments begun after day 100, or those ending before gestational day 40, did not obliterate the vaginal orifice or cause the formation of a true phallus. The only genital consequence of these treatments was a slight clitoral hypertrophy which, though evident at birth, became less obvious during the first year of life. More extensive descriptions of genital anatomy following prenatal exposure to androgen have been published elsewhere (Goy, Uno & Sholl, 1989).

Behavior of mothers

Aside from the long periods of time spent nursing and grooming their infants, the behavior of each mother toward her own infant was characterized by a nearly complete absence of any aggression. Mild threats were displayed not infrequently, but these were not displayed differentially toward males, females or the androgenized females.

According to our experience with more than 80 groups of monkeys housed in this way, only genital grooming or genital exploration and sexual presentation by the mother has been shown to be displayed differentially toward infants according to their gender. All adult females in the group display these behaviors to infant partners, although the infant's own mother is the principal actor in this behavioral relationship.

The relationship between genital grooming by the infant's own mother and hormonal treatment prior to birth is shown in Table 15.1. The reader's attention is directed to the finding that this behavior of adult females is quite well limited to infants that showed virilization of the external genitalia. While it is clear that adult females are interested in the genitalia of infants of both sexes as well as of the experimental females, those females that were androgenized for the longest periods of time prenatally, and that accordingly showed the greatest degree of genital virilization, received the highest frequencies of genital explorations.

Whether in response to or as a result of this attention from the adult females, or due to other factors altogether, male and female infants behaved differently toward the mothers in their group (other mothers as well as their own). This sex-related behavior is particularly conspicuously manifested in the mounting of mothers by the infants. As the results in Figure 15.2 illustrate, mounting by infants was augmented above that shown by normal females in all females androgenized starting between days 40 and 60 of gestation. The increase in mounting occurred regardless of whether the phallus was complete or

Table 15.1. *Relation between type of prenatal treatment with androgen and the number of genital explorations received from adult females during the first year of life*

Type of treatment	N[a]	Mean	SD	SE
Female[b]	116	0.6412	1.7010	0.1486
H1526	5	0.2000	0.4472	0.2000
H1540	7	5.1429	7.1047	2.6853
H1550	3	4.3333	4.1633	2.4037
H1560	5	2.2000	2.1679	0.9695
H15100	6	1.1667	1.6021	0.6540
H2540	7	1.2857	1.1127	0.4206
H25115	7	0.4286	0.7868	0.2974
H3540	4	0.7500	0.9574	0.4787
H5540	8	6.0000	3.7417	1.3229
H8040	3	17.6667	7.7675	4.4845
Cmale[c]	19	7.5789	6.8257	1.5659
Male	118	12.9169	24.5531	2.2603
RxMale[d]	27	10.7407	14.0318	2.7004

Notes: [a] The number of animals per treatment group. The numbers shown here are those used throughout the presentation of results.
[b] No prenatal exposure to exogenous androgen.
[c] Males castrated within three months of birth.
[d] Males exposed to exogenous androgen during prenatal life.

hypospadic, as long as the vaginal orifice was obliterated. In short, mounting the mothers was augmented to varying degrees in those subjects that showed genital virilization regardless of the duration of androgenization. Moreover, castration of genetic males shortly after birth reduced the frequency of the behavior below that shown by intact males. This finding supports the notion that the important time for androgenic action is prior to birth and not at the time the behavior is actually being displayed.

The results for the infant mounting response are by no means perfectly concordant with those for amount of genital stimulation received, but there is enough agreement to suggest that the behavior of mothers might influence the infant's expression of dimorphic patterns of social response. This statement is not intended to imply that the specific behavior of exploration of infant genitalia is the cause of the restriction of infant mounting of mothers largely to infant males and females with the most virilized genitalia. In fact it could be some other maternal behavior altogether which has not been recorded and which is highly subtle in nature. The genital exploration response is used here merely to indicate that mothers and other adult females are aware, and fairly keenly so, of the infant's gender, and respond quite differently to the two normal

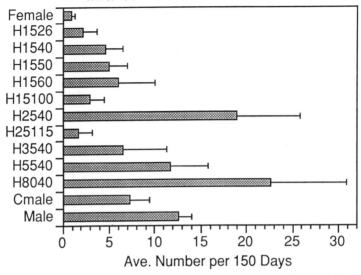

Figure 15.2. The relation between type of prenatal treatment (sex type) and the number of times each infant mounted its own mother during the first year of life (run 1 = 150 successive days). In this and subsequent figures the slash mark separating duration from start of treatment has been eliminated.

sexes as well as to the array of experimentally produced sexual phenotypes.

The large effects of specific prenatal treatments on the behavior of female offspring is clearly attributable to the circumstance that the exposure to the androgen was accomplished prior to birth. The circumstance that all exposures of fetuses to androgen were accomplished by injecting the hormone into the pregnant female afforded the opportunity to see if this procedure affected the male-like mounting behavior of the mothers. Mothers of virilized offspring were exposed to the same levels of androgen as the offspring themselves, but these injections had no effect on the frequency with which the treated mothers mounted other mothers in their social group (Figure 15.3). Data shown in the figure were obtained only on about one-third of the subjects used in all of the studies done, but the numbers are adequate to demonstrate the lack of any effect of the androgen. In this analysis, treatments were grouped according to their duration (long, medium, or short), and no relationship was found for this classification. Moreover, there was no difference in the mounting behavior of females that gave birth to male offspring and those that gave birth to normal female offspring. Since fetal males have higher levels of endogenous androgens than fetal females, the possibility exists these higher concentrations might gain access to maternal tissues and might thereby influence the behavior of the mother.

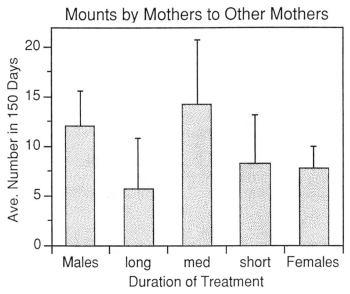

Figure 15.3. The relation between maternal exposure to androgens (during pregnancy) and the number of mounts displayed to other adult females in the group. In this figure, the mothers from different treatment groups have been grouped into those receiving treatments of short, medium and long duration.

Effects of prenatal testosterone on juvenile female behavior

Prenatal treatments also had marked effects on play and mounting of juvenile females. The total amount of play shown by each sexual phenotype during the four years of observation is shown in Figure 15.4. The data include play shown to both male and female partners by each sexual type, and inspection of the figure reveals that when treatments started prior to gestational day 100, a duration of 35 days was required for augmentation of rough play. In constrast, females exposed to androgen after day 100 of gestation showed elevated frequencies of rough play across the four-year span when the duration of exposure was as short as only 15 days (group 15100). When treatments beginning after day 100 lasted as long as 25 days (group 25115), then the augmentation of rough play was even more pronounced.

Mounting of peers was also affected by the prenatal testosterone treatments. The total number of mounts shown by each sex type ranged from a mean of approximately 10 for normal females to more than 160 mounts for females exposed for 80 days prior to birth (Figure 15.5). The interesting feature of these results is the clear evidence that mounting behavior is only elevated when females are exposed to androgen for at least 25 days regardless of when

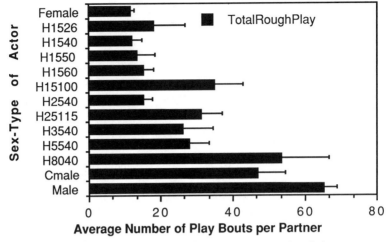

Figure 15.4. The relation between type of treatment (sex type) and the average total number of bouts of rough play shown during the first four years of life.

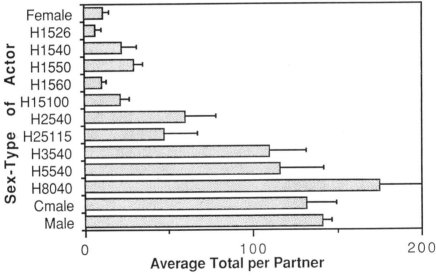

Figure 15.5. The relation between type of treatment (sex type) and the total number of mounts shown during the first four years of life.

the exposure is initiated. No exposure that lasted for only 15 days had the consequence of increasing the amount of mounting activity above that shown by normal, untreated females. Importantly, however, the augmentation of mounting did not require the formation of a phallus (group 25115), nor did the induction of a phallus ensure that mounting would be augmented (groups 1540, 1550, 1560).

Effects of the prenatal treatments on social dominance were also measurable.

Dominance was determined by constructing the hierarchy of submissiveness that developed for each group during each year of life. During each run all occurrences of the grimacing facial expression, a signal of deference, by one animal to another were recorded. Such data were used to construct a matrix showing who grimaced to whom. It is typical in such matrices that one animal in the group fails to display the grimace to any other group member. Such an individual is assigned a social dominance Rank = 1, to indicate its lack of deference to any other group member. At the other extreme an animal can be identified that grimaces to all group members. Such an animal, which defers to all partners, is assigned a Rank = 5 or 6 depending upon the number of group members.

Social dominance was not affected by any treatment of 25 days duration or shorter. When durations of treatments were 35 days or longer, however, average rank became strikingly similar to the average rank of normal intact males. Moreover, castration of males during the first three months of life does not 'feminize' the social dominance of the male. Thus this psychological trait of the individual appears to be strongly influenced by the individual's history of androgen exposure prior to birth. It is important to emphasize that social dominance rank *per se* does not effect the changes in masculine behavior observed among the testosteronized females. If social rank were the critical factor influencing rough play and mounting, then females given treatments 2540 and 25115 would not differ from normal females (Figure 15.6).

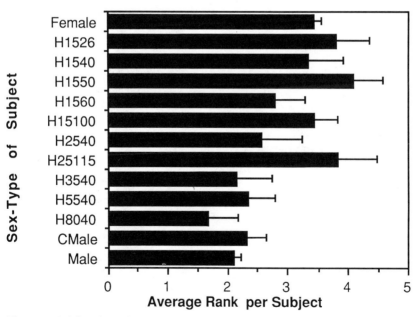

Figure 15.6. The relation between treatment (sex type) and average social rank across all runs. Animals highest in social dominance were assigned a rank of 1.00, and those lowest were assigned a rank of 5 or 6, depending on group size.

Since the pioneering work of Harlow et al. (1966) investigators of rhesus social behavior have studied the play activities of juveniles, but except for Loy & Loy (1976) not much attention has been paid to how they distribute their play in accord with the sex of their partners. Figure 15.7 shows how frequently the different sex types display rough play with male and female partners respectively. The amount of play shown is the average sum of all 50-day periods. Close inspection of the figure reveals that all sex types display the behavior more often with male than with female partners.

The consistently higher frequency of rough play with male than with female partners differs from findings for human children in which males prefer male and females prefer female partners (Hines & Kaufman, 1994). They also found that girls with congenital adrenal hyperplasia (CAH) preferred male over female partners for play. The condition of CAH might be expected to have behavioral effects closely paralleling those produced by the experimental treatments given in the present study. However, it should be noted in Figure 15.7 that males play with males at least five times more often than with females, whereas females only do so about twice as often. If one applies some criterion such as playing at least three times as often with males as with females, then the present findings do resemble those for CAH girls. Inspection of Figure 15.7 shows that according to this criterion only treatments 5540 and 8040 masculinized the partner preference for play.

The hormonal requirements for differentiating a preference for mounting a partner of a particular sex are different from those for elevating the frequency

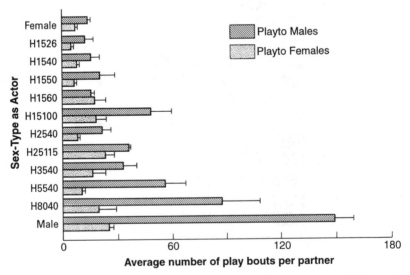

Figure 15.7. The relation between types of treatment and the manner in which juvenile play is distributed between male and female partners.

of mounting. In order to illustrate the preference for a partner of a particular sex the data were separated for mounting of male partners and mounting of female partners. These subtotals were extracted for each 50-day block of observations (each block constituting a separate run). Then the following formula was applied to the data:

$$\text{Preference ratio} = \frac{\text{No. mounts to females} - \text{No. mounts to males}}{\text{No. mounts to females} + \text{No. mounts to males} + 1.0}$$

The preference ratio varies in value from a maximum of $+1.00$ (a complete preference for mounting female partners) to a minimum value of -1.00 (a complete preference for mounting male partners). A value equal to 0.00 indicates neutrality or no preference.

Inspection of Figure 15.8 reveals that males, whether castrated (CMale) or intact (Male-I and Male-NI), manifest a fairly strong preference by run 3 for mounting partners that are also male. This preference continues and even increases during run 4 for CMales and males that are intact but not yet manifesting behavioral signs of puberty (Male-NI). Intact males that manifest behavioral puberty by displaying intromissions with their female peers (Male-I), reverse this trend and manifest a strong preference for mounting female partners during run 4. In comparison to males, normal females prefer

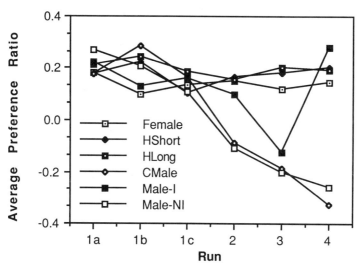

Figure 15.8. The relation between type of treatment and the development of preference for mounting either male or female partners. In this figure prenatal treatments have been grouped into those of long (HLong) or short (HShort) duration. In addition, normal intact males have been divided into two groups, those showing behavioral puberty during Run 4 (Male-I) and those not yet showing signs of behavioral puberty (Male-NI). A positive preference ratio (see text) indicates the female partners were mounted more often than male partners, and a negative ratio indicate the opposite.

Table 15.2. *Play and mounting by rhesus monkeys prenatally exposed to testosterone (T) or dihydrotestosterone (DHT)*

Type of prenatal treatment	Number of mounts[a]	Number of bouts of play[a]
Females (none)	11.3 (3.0)	11.7 (1.0)
DHT-females	81.7 (17.7)	13.9 (2.9)
T-females	132.8 (25.5)	34.9 (6.2)
Males (none)	140.7 (5.8)	65.2 (3.7

Note: [a] Mean and (standard error of the mean) of the total frequency per partner across all four years of observations.

to mount other females rather than males throughout all the runs, and this same behavioral preference is also expressed by females treated prenatally with testosterone regardless of the duration of treatment. To illustrate this latter point, the females exposed to androgen for only 15 days have been grouped together as 'HShort', and those exposed for 25 days or more have been grouped together as 'HLong'. Neither long nor short intervals of treatment during gestation altered the developmental pattern of preference for mounting female partners (Figure 15.8). Thus in regard to this behavioral preference even those females most extensively virilized with prenatal testosterone did not duplicate the developmental pattern of genotypic males.

Effects of other hormonal agents

Testosterone is not the only steroid that influences the development of sex-related behaviors in rhesus. Some work completed in my laboratory with dihydrotestosterone propionate injected for 55 or 80 days into pregnant females from the 40th day of gestation reveals virilizing effects on the behavior of female offspring. The results obtained with dihydrotestosterone can be compared directly with those obtained using testosterone since identical durations of hormonal treatment were given. As shown in Table 15.2, both androgens produced very similar effects on mounting behavior, but dihydro-testosterone, unlike testosterone, failed to masculinize the rough play behavior of treated females. Dihydrotestosterone was effective, however, in elevating the dominance status of treated females and in masculinizing their external genitalia. This point is quite significant, since it demonstrates clearly that a very masculine appearance is not sufficient to promote the display of rough play with peers. In short, rough play is probably not a result of peers' misperceptions of the androgenized females as males.

Data have been obtained more recently in a collaborative study with Bertrand Deputte on the effects of a nonsteroidal estrogen, diethylstilbestrol dipropionate (DES) given from day 40 of gestation to term (about day 165). Using this totally synthetic hormone in a dosage of 100 micrograms per day (a much lower quantity than was employed with the androgens), a modest degree of behavioral masculinization was obtained for both rough play and mounting of peers. Of course, this treatment failed to virilize the external genitalia, which remained totally feminine, and, correspondingly, the infant's relationship to its mother was also distinctly feminine. This is supported by the findings that (1) mothers did not explore the genitalia of estrogenized female offspring, and (2) the estrogenized females did not mount their mothers.

Summary and discussion

Perhaps the most conspicuous feature of the results described above is the almost complete independence of the development of the traits studied. All of the traits (i.e. mounting the mother, mounting peers, preference for a partner of a particular sex, rough play with peers, and genital structure itself) are normally expressed fully in an integrated, manner by the genotypic male monkey. However, the current findings suggest that each trait is organized according to a unique principle. The establishment of male genital structures requires the action of classical androgens, testosterone and dihydrotestosterone. Moreover, the organization of the genital tissues follows a strict principle of androgenic action during a specifiable critical period.

The development of a male type of affective relationship with the mother (involving the expression of mounting the mother) appears to depend upon differentiation of male-type genitalia, since, in the absence of such structures, the display of this behavior is quite uncommon. Because of the requirement of genital masculinization, mounting the mother can appear to depend upon neural differentiation by androgen during a critical period. But a closer look indicates that the mounting behavior of the infant is likely to be coupled to behaviors displayed by the mother. These maternal behaviors (genital grooming and presenting among others) may serve the function of bringing a distinct gender identity to the mother–infant relationship. The full behavioral consequences for the developing infant are not known, but the gender identity of the mother–infant relationship seems irrelevant to the manner in which the infant behaves toward its peers. That is, female infants can be induced to show rough play and mounting of peers when exposed to testosterone during the last third of prenatal life, even though this same treatment fails to masculinize the genitalia and fails to masculinize the mother–infant relationship.

The principle governing the organization of rough play and mounting of peers does not involve a clearly defined critical period before birth. Instead, the experimental organization of these behavioral systems in females requires protracted exposure to appropriate hormones, and a clear relationship exists between the duration of exposure to the steroid before birth and the frequency of display of these responses at later developmental ages. Although mounting and play with peers follow similar principles of quantitative regulation by prenatal hormones, different hormonal mechanisms govern their development. This is shown by their differential expression when dihydrotestosterone rather than testosterone was used as the prenatal masculinizing substance.

Students familiar with the literature on early androgenic hormonal interventions may regard these results as confirming what has been widely and often demonstrated in rodents. Changes in rodent play activities and in the tendency to mount have been widely demonstrated following the treatment of genetic female rats with androgens or estradiol, a principal brain metabolite of androgen. Moreover, effects of early deficiency of androgen in the male have been shown by experiments involving early castration, by administration of antiandrogen, by studies on inherited androgen insensitivity (Beach & Buehler, 1977), and by a unique method of reducing endogenous androgens with maternal stress (Ward & Weisz, 1980; Ward and Ward, 1985). Even the fact that different behavioral systems can be independently affected by hormonal manipulations has been shown previously (Davis, Chaptal, & McEwen, 1979). The protracted period of embryonic and fetal development of the rhesus, however, has made it possible to reveal details of the differentiation process that could not otherwise be made apparent. What has been particularly striking in the results of the work with rhesus is the great variety of behavioral and anatomical modifications that can be induced and with which the animal can come to terms (so to speak) and live amicably in a group of normal social peers. The variety and number of sexual phenotypes determined by hormones before birth far exceeds the easily discernible five types that Fausto-Sterling (1993) so eloquently pleads for. Animals can be produced very nearly at will that display any combination of the behavioral traits that are normally expressed as sexual dimorphisms in the population. Thus animals that show a typically feminine relationship with their mothers can have at the same time a completely different relationship with peers in which a male-type gender role is expressed. Or, animals can be produced that show an ambiguous gender role in which little or no play is shown with their peers, but, at the same time high frequencies of mounting their peers and their mother exist.

The hormone present before birth does not induce new kinds of behavior qualitatively; it merely acts in some way to either decrease or increase the frequency of display of particular behaviors. In monkeys, the prenatal treatments clearly and definitely operate along the quantitative dimension of the behavior. Both mounting and play behavior can be augmented slightly, extensively, or not at all. No explanation can be given for this high degree of control that the hormone prior to birth exercises over the development of behavior. It is as though the hormone acts upon a substrate of a motivational core specific for each behavior, encoding it with a proscription for quantitative limits on the expression of the behavior. Or, the hormone acts in some way to establish predispositions to behave in certain ways. Under either arrangement it seems possible and likely that the quantitative expression is regulated by experience. Viewed in this way, the final control over the quantitative aspects of the behavior lies in the interaction between early endocrine variables and later social experience. Such an interaction between hormonal history and social experience can be seen clearly in the establishment of social dominance rank. The very definition of dominance rank as well as its quantitation depend upon the way that peers behave toward the animal being ranked. Without the behavioral expression of deference by peers, there is no dominance measurable.

There are substantial parallels between this view of hormonal and experiential interaction for juvenile behavior and similar interactions in the determination of adult male sexual behavior. Ward & Reed (1985) have demonstrated in rats that prenatal maternal stress and social experience of male offspring together influence the pattern of adult male sexual behavior. But the interaction of endocrine history with later experience is probably of special relevance to the rhesus monkey in which, along with other Anthropoidea including apes and human beings, complex early experience variables play a greater role in determining the patterning of sexual and sex-related social behavior than they do in lower mammals. Harlow (Harlow et al., 1966) regarded experiential and endocrinological variables to be of equal importance and noted that each is essential to the development and full expression of reproduction. Harlow definitely and unreservedly assigned primacy to infant and juvenile play behavior as experiences crucial to the determination of reproductive behavior patterns. He espoused the position that sex-differences in play gave rise to sex-differences in reproductive behavior. An even greater emphasis was given to the importance of early experience by Nissen (cf. Nissen cited by Young, 1961) who, in his work with chimpanzees, opined that sexual behavior was derived from social play by chance occurrences of responses closely approximating those appropriate to reproduction. The reason why some but not other randomly occurring responses are selected and organized into a repertoire of reproductive responses is not provided in the speculations of Nissen. A conscientious effort to describe the influence of early experience is found in work by Money & Ehrhardt (1972). His studies of human beings born with ambiguous or discordant genitalia largely ignore specific gender role behaviors, however, and instead concentrate on a core gender identity which is thought to be determined by parental influences. The patterning of later sex-related behavior is presumed to be largely determined by the kind of core gender identity that has been established.

The concern for possible experiential variables in the patterning of primate sexual and sex-related behaviors is a traditional view which may be facing a serious challenge in contemporary work. The recent discovery that brain structures may be altered by hormones prior to birth in human beings (Swaab & Fliers, 1985; Allen et al., 1989; Le Vay, 1991) as in other animals (Nottebohm & Arnold, 1976; Gorski et al., 1980; Tobet, Zahniser & Baum, 1986) has given renewed impetus to the notion that biological determination of sexuality may not require the participation of experience. Moreover, evidence has been found for a site on the sex chromosome in a region designated Xq28 (Hamer et al., 1993) that may contain a gene for homosexuality in human males. In addition, there has been renewed interest in accumulating data on human twins to demonstrate the heritability of homosexuality (Whitman, Diamond & Martin, 1993). Although no hormonal variable prior to birth has been implicated in the etiology of homosexuality in human beings, a model for endocrine determination of homosexuality has been proposed (Dorner, 1988). Dorner's endocrine hypothesis and the more recent genetic studies on men and women illustrate the current trend away from social and experiential variables and toward more direct biological mechanisms. On the one hand, the link between a gene and a specific neuronal structure may not be overly obscure, but on the other hand, the link between a specifc neuronal structure and a specific behavioral disposition remains formidably unclear. One direction for the future clearly points to describing such links in a reductionistic manner, and especially the links between neuronal anatomy, biochemistry and the regulation of the expression of behavior. As a beginning effort in this direction it is important to point out the work on hormones, brain mechanisms and learning being conducted in several laboratories (Clark & Goldman-Rakic, 1989; Bachevalier & Hagger, 1991; Hagger & Bachevalier, 1991). These outstanding efforts have shown better than any others that hormonal influences are not restricted to subcortical brain mechanisms, but, at least in primates, also affect the emergence of cortically controlled functions.

ACKNOWLEDGMENTS

This work was supported by funds from the National Institutes of Health by grants RR00167 and MH21312 from the Division of Research Resources and the National Institute of Mental Health respectively. Their support is gratefully acknowledged.

REFERENCES

Allen, L. S., Hines, M., Shryne, J. E. & Gorski, R. (1989) Two sexually dimorphic cell groups in the human brain. *Journal of Neuroscience,* **9,** 497–506.

Bachevalier, J. & Hagger, C. (1991) Sex differences in the development of learning abilities in primates. *Psychoneuroendocrinology,* **16,** 177–88.

Baum, M. J. (1987) Hormonal control of sex differences in the brain and behavior of mammals. In Crews, D. (ed.) *Psychobiology of Reproductive Behavior.* Englewood Cliffs, NJ: Prentice–Hall, pp. 232–57.

Beach, F. A. & Buehler, M. G. (1977) Male rats with inherited insensitivity to androgen show reduced sexual behavior. *Endocrinology,* **100,** 197–200.

Clark, A. S. & Goldman-Rakic, P. S. (1989) Gondonal hormones influence the emergence of cortical function in nonhuman primates. *Behavioral Neuroscience,* **103,** 1287–95.

Davis, P. G., Chaptal, C. V. & McEwen, B. S. (1979) Independence of the differentiation of masculine and feminine sexual behavior in rats. *Hormones and Behavior*, **12**, 12–19.

D'Occhio, M. J. & Ford, J. J. (1988) Sexual differentiation and adult sexual behavior in cattle, sheep and swine: the role of gonadal hormones. In Money, J. & Musaph, H. (eds.) *Handbook of Sexology, Vol. 6*. Copenhagen: Elsevier Science, pp. 209–30.

Dorner, G. (1988) Neuroendocrine response to estrogen and brain differentiation in heterosexuals, homosexuals and transsexuals. *Archives of Sexual Behavior*, **17**, 57–75.

Ehrhardt, A. A. & Baker, S. W. (1974) Fetal androgens, human central nervous system differentiation, and behavior sex differences. In Friedman, R. C., Richart, R. M. & van de Wiele, R. L. (eds.) *Sex Differences in Behavior*. New York: John Wiley, pp. 33–52.

Fausto-Sterling, A. (1993) The five sexes. *The Sciences*, pp. 20–4.

Gorski, R. A., Harlan, R. E., Jacobsen, C. D., Shryne, J. E. & Southam, A. M. (1980) Evidence for the existence of a sexually dimorphic nucleus in the preoptic area of the rat. *Journal of Comparative Neurology*, **193**, 529–39.

Goy, R. W. (1978) Development of play and mounting in female rhesus virilized prenatally with esters in testosterone or dihydrotestosterone. In Chivers, D. J. & Herbert, J. (eds.) *Recent Advances in Primatology, Vol. 1*. London: Academic Press, pp. 449–62.

Goy, R. W. (1981) The differentiation of male social traits in female rhesus monkeys by prenatal treatment with androgens: variations in types of androgens, duration and timing of treatments. In Novy, M. J. & Resko, J. A. (eds.) *Fetal Endocrinology*. New York: Academic Press, pp. 319–40.

Goy, R. W. & Kemnitz, J. W. (1983). Early, persistent and delayed effects of virilizing substances delivered transplacentally to female rhesus fetuses. In Zbinden, G. Cuomo, V., Racagni, G. & Weiss, B. (eds.) *Application of Behavioral Pharmacology in Toxicology*. New York: Raven Press, pp. 303–14.

Goy, R. W. & Robinson, J. A. (1982) Prenatal exposure of rhesus monkeys to potent androgens: morphological, behavioral, and physiological consequences. *Banbury Report II. Environmental Factors in Human Growth and Development*. New York: Cold Spring Harbor Laboratory, pp. 355–78.

Goy, R. W. & Wallen, K. (1979) Experiential variables influencing play, foot-clasp mounting, and adult sexual competence in male rhesus monkeys. *Psychoneuroendocrinology*, **4**, 1–12.

Goy, R. W., Uno, H. & Sholl, S. A. (1989) Psychological and anatomical consequences of prenatal exposure to androgens in female rhesus. In Mori, T. & Nagasawa, H. (eds.) *Toxicity of Hormones in Prenatal Life*. Boca Raton, Fl.: CRC Press, pp. 127–42.

Hagger, C. & Bachevalier, J. (1991) Visual habit formation in rhesus monkeys (Macaca mulatta): reversal of sex difference following neonatal manipulations of androgens. *Behavioral Brain Research*, **45**, 57–64.

Hamer, D. H., Hu, S., Magnusson, V. L., Hu, N. & Pattatucci, A. M. L. (1993). A linkage between DNA markers on the Xchromosome and male sexual orientation. *Science*, **261**, 321–7.

Harlow, H. F., Joslyn, W. D., Senko, M. G. & Dopp, A. (1966) Behavioral aspects of reproduction in primates. *Journal of Animal Science*, **25** (Suppl.), 49–67.

Hines, M. & Kaufman, F. R. (1994) Androgen and the development of sex-typical behavior: rough and tumble play and sex of preferred playmates in children with congenital adrenal hyperplasian (CAM). *Child Development*, **65**, 1042–53.

Hutchison, J. B. & Hutchison, R. E. (1990) Sexual development at the neurochromal level: the role of androgens. In Feierman, J. R. (ed.) *Pedophilia: Biosocial Dimensions.* New York: Springer–Verlag, pp. 510–43.

Le Vay, S. (1991) A difference in hypothalamic structure between heterosexual and homosexual men. *Science*, **253**, 1034–7.

Loy, J. & Loy, K. (1974) Behavior of an all-juvenile group of rhesus monkeys. *American Journal of Physical Anthropology*, **40**, 83–96.

Money, J. & Ehrhardt, A. A. (1972) *Man and Woman, Boy and Girl.* Baltimore, Md: Johns Hopkins University Press.

Money, J., Schwartz, M. & Lewis, V. (1984) Adult erotosexual status and fetal hormonal masculinization and demasculinization; 46XX congenital virilizing adrenal hyperplasia and 46XY androgen-insensitivity syndrome compared. *Psychoneuroendocrinology*, **9**, 405–14.

Nottebohm, F. & Arnold, A. P. (1976) Sexual dimorphism in vocal control areas of the songbird brain. *Science,* **194**, pp. 211–3.

Swaab, D. F. & Fliers, E. (1985) A sexually dimorphic nucleus in the human brain. *Science,* **228**, 1112–15.

Tobet, S., Zahniser, D. J. & Baum, M. J. (1986) Sexual dimorphism in the preoptic/anterior hypothalamic area of ferrets: effects of adult exposure to sex steroids. *Brain Research,* **364**, 249–57.

Ward, I. and Reed, J. (1985) Prenatal stress and prepubertal social rearing conditions interact to determine sexual behavior in male rats. *Behavioral Neuroscience,* **99**, 301–9.

Ward, I. & Ward, B. (1985) Sexual behavior differentiation. In Adler, N., Pfaff, D. & Goy, R. W. (eds.) *Handbook of Behavioral Neurobiology.* New York, Plenum: 77–98.

Ward, I. & Weisz, J. (1980) Maternal stress alters plasma testosterone in fetal males. *Science,* **207**, 328–9.

Whitman, F. L., Diamond, M. & Martin, J. (1993) Homosexual orientation in twins: a report on 61 pairs and three triplet sets. *Archives of Sexual Behavior,* **22**, 187–206.

Wilson, J. D. (1987) Disorders of androgen action. *Clinical Research,* **35**, 1–12.

Wilson, J. D. (1991) Syndromes of androgen resistance. *Biology of Reproduction,* **46**, 168–73.

Young, W. C. (1961) The hormones and mating behavior. In Young, W. C. (ed.) *Sex and Internal Secretions.* Baltimore, Md: Williams and Wilkins, 1173–239.

16 Gonadal hormones and the organization of brain structure and function

ROGER A. GORSKI

INTRODUCTION

In the development of any individual, genomic and phenotypic sex are of fundamental and lasting importance. Although every adult is essentially familiar with sex differences in the genitalia and other physical attributes and the changes which occur during a lifetime (e.g. maturation at puberty, reproductive senescence), the fact that sex differences in brain function and structure also exist is perhaps less well appreciated. Nevertheless, both are quite well established and current research in this area is focused on attempts to link structural sex differences to specific brain functions; the elucidation of how these differences develop; the identification of sex differences in human cognitive function, and most recently, the identification of structural sex differences that correlate with sexual orientation.

The results of research on animals support the fundamental concept of the sexual differentiation of the brain: the mammalian brain is inherently feminine, or perhaps incompletely developed, and the structural and functional features characteristic of the brain of the male of a given species are imposed on this 'feminine' brain by the actions of hormones secreted by the testes during a critical period(s) of development. There is overwhelming evidence, even in human beings, that the basic 'blueprint' of the reproductive system is feminine and that exposure to testicular hormones or their metabolites prevents the development of Mullerian duct derivatives (i.e. the oviducts, uterus and the deepest part of the vagina), and promotes the development of Wolffian duct derivatives (i.e. the ductus deferens [vas], epididymus and seminal vesicles), as well as induces the formation of the male genitalia. (The genitalia of men and women arise from a common anlage, and individuals of either genetic sex possess both the Mullerian and Wolffian ducts during development.) Note that in accord with the feminine blueprint, genetically male (XY) human beings with normal testicular function but completely lacking functional androgen receptors because of a mutation in the androgen receptor gene and therefore, the ability to respond to this hormone, possess female external genitalia and after puberty, marked breast development (the Androgen Insensitivity Syndrome).

The role of the brain in the control of behavior is obvious but it also controls gonadal development and function and in many species the critical reproductive event of ovulation. In a very real sense, the brain is an integral component of the reproductive system and it should not be surprising that parts of the brain also undergo the process of sexual differentiation. What may be surprising is that components of brain structure and function which appear to have little to do with reproduction, at least at our current level of understanding, also display sex differences that may well be determined by the hormonal environment developmentally.

Implicit in the concept of the sexual differentiation of the brain is that changes in brain structure and functional potential induced by gonadal hormones during development are *permanent*. Because of this, much of the research in this area has involved laboratory animals. It is clearly unethical to manipulate deliberately the hormonal environment of developing human fetuses or infants in a way that could well produce permanent changes, the full extent and significance of which remain unknown. Thus, in human beings it is possible to identify sex differences in brain structure and function although direct experimental evidence linking these to hormone action cannot be obtained.

SEXUAL DIFFERENTIATION OF THE BRAIN

Before considering the extent of this process and how it may apply to our species, it is useful to describe briefly the experimental approach that has established the concept of the sexual differentiation of the brain by focusing on just two functional sexual dimorphisms revealed from studies of the laboratory rat: the neural control of the cyclic release of the hormones responsible for ovulation and that of reproductive behavior.

In the female rat, there is a cyclic neural mechanism presumably located within the hypothalamus which, under specific conditions, can lead to a marked surge in the release of the hypothalamic and pituitary hormones that induce ovulation. Under physiological conditions this system is activated (or disinhibited) only on the afternoon of proestrus when plasma estradiol (E_2) levels reach their peak. That E_2 is the trigger has been demonstrated by injecting ovariectomized rats with E_2 and measuring a temporally-defined surge increase in plasma hormone levels. This response is called 'E_2-induced positive feedback'. Adult male rats, even if castrated and given an ovarian graft do not ovulate, nor do they show E_2-induced positive feedback if injected with exogenous ovarian steroids. This is basically an all-or-none sex difference, the male simply does not exhibit E_2-induced positive feedback.

In terms of reproductive behavior the sex dimorphism in rats is not as complete. One behavioral response of the sexually receptive female rat is that she assumes the lordosis posture when mounted. After ovariectomy which eliminates sexual behavior in rats, sexual receptivity can be restored by the injection of ovarian hormones and the receptive female will display lordosis almost every time that she is mounted. Male rats, when castrated as adults and treated with the same regime of ovarian hormones, will display the lordosis posture when mounted but *only occasionally*; males show statistically significantly lower levels of lordosis responding than do females. In terms of masculine behavioral patterns the sex dimorphism in rats is even less marked because the intact female will occasionally mount other animals, but again the male and female differ significantly in terms of the frequency of such behaviors as mounting, intromission and ejaculation when tested under the same hormonal conditions.

Could these sex differences in rat brain function reflect genomic sex differences in the brain? The answer appears to be 'No' based on the results of the following experimental approach: the injection of exogenous steroids or the removal of the endogenous source of these hormones (the gonads) during early postnatal life. The injection of testosterone propionate (TP) in moderate doses to five-day-old males rats has no effect on the neuroendocrine characteristics of these males when adult. However, if the five-day-old female rat is given a single injection of at least 30 μg TP, she becomes anovulatory and permanently sterile and exhibits enhanced masculine but depressed feminine sexual behavior.

Whenever exogenous hormones are administered to an animal, there is the risk that the observed response is a pharmacological artifact. However, the effects of gonadectomy neonatally argue strongly against this possibility. Gonadectomy of the neonatal female rat does not appear to change her adult neuroendocrine characteristics, she exhibits E_2-induced positive feedback and high levels of lordosis responding when given ovarian hormone replacement therapy in adulthood. Remarkably, however, if the male rat is castrated within the first few days of postnatal life, when adult this genetic male displays E_2-induced positive feedback and will support corpora lutea formation in ovarian grafts. Moreover, they will display levels of lordosis responding equivalent to those of the female, but reduced masculine behavior. Thus, after castration neonatally the adult genetic male rat exhibits feminine neuroendocrine characteristics; the effects of injecting TP into females appears to reflect what endogenous testicular hormones do in the male. As the field has progressed it has become useful to distinguish four different components of the process of the sexual differentiation of the brain: *masculinization* – the promotion of male characteristics such as mounting; *demasculinization* – the suppression of the development of male characteristics; *feminization* – the promotion of female characteristics such as E_2-induced positive feedback or lordosis; and *defeminization* – the suppression of the development of female characteristics. Most importantly, these may well be independent processes with different hormonal sensitivities, different temporal patterns and presumably different neural regulatory sites.

The process of the sexual differentiation of the brain is very pervasive in terms of brain function and probably applies to most species which reproduce bisexually, although in certain animals, temperature or social factors determine physiological and behavioral sex (see Crews, 1993). Although one might now also predict the existence of hormone-dependent structural sex differences in the brain, just a few years ago this seemed only remotely possible. Not only was the brain considered 'hard-wired', but as indicated above, male rats can exhibit lordosis and females do mount other females, observations which suggest that the neural circuitry which subserves these sexually dimorphic behaviors are actually present in both sexes. It seemed logical that the most important variable was the hormonal sensitivity of these neural circuits (i.e. could they be activated readily by physiological levels of gonadal hormones), or the existence of functionally specific inhibitory systems as has been proposed for lordosis behavior (Kondo et al., 1990). Although these views may indeed be correct for certain functions, structural sex differences clearly exist and presumably subserve at least some sexually dimorphic functions.

Three landmark studies paved the way for the modern search for sex differences in brain structure. In 1973, Raisman & Field reported the existence of an ultrastructural sex difference in the preoptic area (POA) of the rat hypothalamus, and they also demonstrated that it was hormone dependent and followed the 'rules of sexual differentiation'. In 1976, Nottebohm & Arnold published their findings that in the canary and zebra finch, there are marked sex differences in the nuclear organization of regions of the brain involved in the male-specific production of song. The author's laboratory then discovered a marked sex difference in the POA of the rat which we ultimately labelled the sexually dimorphic nucleus of the preoptic area (SDN-POA; Gorski et al., 1980). The SDN-POA is 3–7 times larger in volume in the male than in the female (Figure 16.1). Since neuronal density within the SDN-POA is apparently equivalent in both males and females, the volume difference implies that more neurons comprise the SDN-POA of the male than of the female. Is it possible that gonadal hormones in some way influence, even determine, the number of neurons which comprise this specific brain structure?

The results of initial studies were inconclusive. The volume of the SDN-POA in the neonatally castrated male when adult is significantly smaller than that of the control male, but still significantly larger than that of the female. In addition, a single injection of TP given to neonatal female rats, although at doses well above those needed to masculinize and defeminize brain function, leads to an increase in SDN-POA volume, but not to the size of that of the normal male. Over time, three explanations of these findings were considered possible: a surge in testosterone (T) levels in male rats at parturition could be important for SDN-POA development; perhaps there is a genomic contribution to the sex difference in SDN-POA volume; perhaps something occurs prenatally in the male but not in the female.

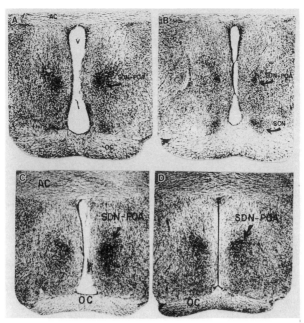

Figure 16.1. Representative photomicrographs at the same magnification through the sexually dimorphic nucleus of the preoptic area (SDN-POA) of adult rats. The animals were chosen for illustration because their individual SDN-POA volumes closely approximated the means for the following groups: (A) male, (B) female, (C) and (D) genetic females exposed perinatally (embryonic day 16 through postnatal day 10) to testosterone propionate (C) or diethylstilbestrol (D) which treatments sex-reversed SDN-POA volume. Abbreviations: AC, anterior commissure; OC, optic chiasm; V, third ventricle. Modified from Döhler et al. (1984a) and reprinted with permission from Gorski (1987).

From the results of several studies, it can be concluded that the surge of T at parturition does not appear to influence SDN-POA volume (Handa et al., 1985), but there is a surge of T in the plasma around embryonic day 18 in the male which is critical (Weisz & Ward, 1973), and finally, daily exposure to TP via injections to the mother from embryonic day 16 until parturition and then directly into the rat pups for the first 10 days of postnatal life, completely sex-reverses SDN-POA volume in the female (Figure 16.1). The latter result cannot rule out a possible contribution of genomic factors but does indicate that experimental hormone exposure *alone* can produce a male-like SDN-POA in the genetic female. The conclusion from these studies is that the functional potential of the rat brain and components of its very structure are sexually dimorphic in the adult because of the action of testicular hormones during a critical phase of development.

Functional sex differences in the brain

It has already been described how male and female rats differ in the neural control of the cyclic release of LH and of reproductive behavior. This has been known for many years since the search for sex differences in brain function has been ongoing for more than three decades. Because of this the literature in this area is very extensive and citations to the known facts will not be provided. For specific references the reader is referred to several reviews (Goy & McEwen, 1980; Kelly, 1988; Döhler, 1991; Gorski, 1991; vom Saal, Montano & Wang, 1992).

Sex differences in brain function and their sexual differentiation in mammals are not limited to behaviors that are obviously related to reproduction and include taste preference, the regulation of food intake and body weight, territorial marking and aggressive, defensive (Blanchard et al., 1991), learning, open field, parenting, play and social behaviors, reliance on visuospatial cues in a maze-learning paradigm (Williams & Meck, 1991). However, a given functional parameter of the brain that is sexually dimorphic in one species is not necessarily sexually dimorphic in all species. An important example of this is E_2-induced positive feedback. Although this is a marked all or none sex difference in rats, this is not true for non-human primates nor for human beings. Male rhesus monkeys can exhibit E_2-induced positive feedback and support ovulation in ovarian grafts. Also, women with the syndrome of congenital adrenal hyperplasia, who are markedly virilized by androgens of adrenal origin, still ovulate. These observations caution against broad generalizations across different species.

Another characteristic of different mammalian species is how mature they are at birth. In some species (e.g. the guinea pig and rhesus monkey) sexual differentiation of the brain is predominantly, if not completely, determined before birth. In the rat it is clearly a perinatal process. It must also be remembered that the various components of the process of sexual differentiation (e.g. masculinization, defeminization) may well be independent of each other.

A critical question is whether there are substantial sex differences in the functional potential of the human brain. Sex differences in human brain function do exist, but most of these are statistical; there is considerable overlap. Thus, any pair of male and female individuals may display a sex difference opposite to the general statistical trend and many men and women would not differ at all. However, in certain cases (e.g. exceptional ability in mathematical reasoning where boys outnumber girls by almost 13 : 1, Benbow & Benbow, 1984), the sex difference is marked. Sex differences in cognitive abilities also appear to be test or task specific and are not observed in all purported tests of the same general skill, although it may be that different tests of one cognitive skill (e.g. visual-spatial ability) actually require different neural processing.

Since there is a very extensive literature in this area, the reader is referred to a number of reviews or recent reports (Eccles, 1987; Macoby, 1987; O'Boyle, Alexander & Benbow, 1991; Watson & Kimura, 1991). In general, males perform better on tasks that test visual-spatial ability and mathematical reasoning while females perform better on those tasks that test verbal ability. Moreover, there appear to be significant sex differences in terms of the lateralization of brain function and an important relationship to handedness. However, no single functional brain characteristic can accurately predict one's sex, let alone one's gender.

Another difference between the sex dimorphisms in human brain function and those in laboratory animals is the basic lack of information about the causes of the former. It is likely that in addition to the specificity of any given test of cognitive function, genomic factors, social, educational and economical status and other experimental factors play a role, but what about hormones? There are relatively few studies which report differences in cognitive function that may be dependent on gonadal hormones (see Gouchie & Kimura, 1991).

Structural sex differences in the non-human mammalian brain

The SDN-POA of the rat is one of the most marked and well-studied structural sex dimorphisms in the mammalian brain, but it is clearly not the only one. (Space limitations preclude the listing of all relevant references here, and the interested reader should see Gorski, 1991 for other citations to the literature.) In addition to the SDN-POA the following are larger in the male rat: accessory olfactory bulb, bed nucleus of the olfactory tract (Collado et al., 1990), bed nucleus of the stria terminalis (BNST; Hines, Allen & Gorski, 1992a), medial amygdaloid nucleus (Mizukami, Nishizuka & Arai, 1983; Hines et al., 1992a); medial preoptic nucleus, spinal nucleus of the bulbocavernosus, supraoptic nucleus (apparently dependent on body weight; Madeira et al., 1993), and the ventromedial nucleus (Matsumoto & Arai, 1983). In rats the male has a greater number of neurons in some areas of the cerebral cortex (Reid & Juraska, 1992) and the cortex exhibits greater asymmetry (Diamond, 1991). The following nuclei are larger in volume in the female rat: anteroventral periventricular nucleus, the locus coerulus (Guillamón, De Blas & Segovia, 1988), and the parastrial nucleus (del Abril, Segovia & Guillamón, 1990). Structural sex differences in nuclear volume within the preoptic area have also been reported in the ferret, gerbil and guinea pig in which species the BNST is also sexually dimorphic.

In addition, a number of sex differences in neuronal connectivity have been reported. These include in the rat, the arcuate nucleus (Perez, Naftolin & García-Segura, 1990), corpus callosum, hippocampus (Juraska, 1993; Gould, Woolley & McEwen, 1991), lateral septum, medial nucleus of the amygdala, medial preoptic area, SDN-POA, suprachiasmatic nucleus, ventromedial nucleus (Matsumoto & Arai, 1986) and the visual cortex (Muñoz-Cueto, García-Segura & Ruiz-Marcos, 1991). Sex differences in connectivity have also been noted in the medial preoptic area of the hamster and monkey.

This list of structural sex differences should not be interpreted to mean that there are no conflicting reports in the literature. For example, Juraska & Kopcik (1988) did not find a sex difference in the midsagittal size of the corpus callosum (CC) or its posterior component (the splenium), but Berrebi et al., (1988) found that the CC measured somewhat lateral to midline was larger in male rats than in females. Surprisingly, although not sexually dimorphic in size in midline, the splenium of the female rat has significantly more neurons than does that of the male (see Juraska, 1993). This observation emphasizes that structural size, albeit a useful parameter, is a relatively gross measurement. Moreover, experiental factors such as early handling (Berribi et al., 1988) or the quality of the environment (see Diamond, 1991; Juraska, 1993) can modify brain morphology. Interestingly, the mouse, in spite of its assumed relatedness to the rat, does not have as SDN-POA (Young, 1982). Perhaps in the mouse there is a population of neurons which are sexually dimorphic but which cannot be readily distinguished by routine staining procedures.

Structural sex differences in the brains of non-mammalian species such as the quail, lizard, frog and teleost fish have also been reported since the pioneering study of the songbird (Nottebhom & Arnold, 1976). As indicated with respect to the SDN-POA of the rat, the fact that appropriate hormonal exposure developmentally can completely sex-reverse the volume of this nucleus, does not preclude a genomic contribution to the sex dimorphism under more physiological conditions. Thus, the development of the structural sex differences could be due to genomic or hormonal factors or both. The sensitivity of the SDN-POA to hormones could be typical and predictive of other structural sex differences, or less likely, atypical and without predictive value.

Structural sex differences in the human brain

The search for structural sex differences in the human brain presents a number of unique challenges. When studying laboratory animals, one ordinarily chooses the precise time of sacrifice and the brain is essentially immediately fixed by perfusion. In the case of human beings, there will be considerable delay and variance between the time of death and fixation of the brain and then only by immersion into fixative. Since herioc efforts are often used to maintain human life, marked pathology or age-related degenerative processes could affect the structure of the individual brain. Although hospital records can be used to rule out frank neuropathology and conditions such as

Alzheimer's disease, more subtle pathological changes in the brain may not be recognized. Finally, the human brain changes with age. Given a limited source of human material it may not be possible to carefully age match subjects. Finally, age *per se* is not necessarily a good index of the aging process. Two 70 year-old individuals may differ markedly in how they are actually aging, physiologically, behaviorally or physically. In spite of these limitations, structural sex differences in the human brain have been identified, but controversy abounds in this area.

One area of controversy relates to possible sex differences in the CC. Following the initial report of de Lacoste-Utamsing & Holloway (1982), there have been a substantial number of reports failing to confirm their observation which are discussed by Hines (1990) and Allen et al. (1991). Suffice it to say that in addition to the possible inherent variability in this structure, there were methodological differences between the various studies and the potentially important factor of age was not always taken into account. The most recent results of Allen et al., (1991) do not support a sex difference in the size of the CC but do confirm a sex difference in the shape of its splenium. Although a difference in the size or shape of the CC is often suggested to be related to more 'cross-talk' between the left and right hemispheres of the brains of women who are apparently less lateralized in terms of brain function than are men, this certainly has not been established conclusively.

Controversy also exists in terms of possible sex differences in the volume of several hypothalamic nuclei. The existence of a SDN-POA in the human brain which is, as in the rat, larger in volume and in neuronal number in males has been reported (see Hofman & Swaab, 1989). However, Allen et al. (1989) independently evaluated four small hypothalamic nuclei which they named the Interstitial Nucleus of the Anterior Hypothalamus (INAH) One to Four (Figures 16.2, 16.3). It appears that the SDN-POA of the Swaab laboratory is the same nucleus as INAH-1, but Allen et al., (1989) did not find this nucleus to be different in volume between men and women. Not only was the brain tissue analyzed in these two studies from different individuals, but there were also methodological and age differences and it is possible that a component of INAH-1 is, in fact, sexually dimorphic. Allen et al., (1989) did find that INAH-2 and INAH-3 were both significantly larger in volume in the male, but not INAH-1 or INAH-4 (Figure 16.3). Subsequently, LeVay (1991) using methodology similar to that of Allen et al., (1989), also found INAH-1 to be equivalent in volume in men and women. He also confirmed that INAH-4 is not sexually dimorphic while INAH-3 is, but he did not confirm the sex difference in volume of INAH-2 reported by Allen et al., (1989).

Another reported structural sex difference in the human brain is the darkly staining component of the BNST (Allen & Gorski, 1990), which is larger in the male. Finally, the midsagittal surface area of the anterior commissure (Allen & Gorski, 1991) is larger in the female, and the highly variable *massa*

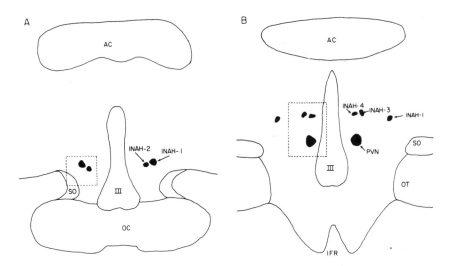

Figure 16.2. Schematic illustration of the general location of interstitial nucleus of the anterior hypothalamus (INAH) one to four, in the human brain. (A) and (B) are approximately 800 μm apart. Details of the area indicated by the area enclosed by the dashed lines in A is illustrated in Figure 16.3 (A) and (B), and that in (B) in Figure 16.3 (C) and (D). Abbreviations: AC, anterior commissure; IFR, infundibular recess; OC, optic chiasm; OT, optic tract; PVN, paraventricular nucleus; SO, supraoptic nucleus; III, third ventricle. (Based on Allen et al., 1989 and reprinted with permission from Gorski, 1988.).

intermedia is present more frequently in the female and when present in both sexes is larger in women (see Allen & Gorski, 1991).

Even if we accept these reports of structural sex differences in the human brain as valid, we are still left with unanswered but fundamental questions. When do the structural sex differences actually develop? Are they determined by the hormonal environment during development? At the time of puberty, during adulthood, or at all? What do they mean functionally? At present, these questions cannot be answered but it must be assumed that over the course of development and then aging, the structure of the human brain changes and that these changes may well have significant functional consequences. In the rat, lesions of the anteroventral periventricular nucleus (AVPV) and its surround appear to disrupt ovulation (see Terasawa & Davis, 1983). Although lesions of the SDN-POA in males do not disrupt their copulatory behavior (Arendash & Gorski, 1983), the results of the electrical stimulation of the SDN-POA strongly suggest that it has a significant role in the regulation of masculine copulatory behavior (Hori & Gorski, unpublished). In the case of the human being, it may well be possible in the future to relate the results obtained with various imaging techniques to putative function (see Hines et al., 1992b).

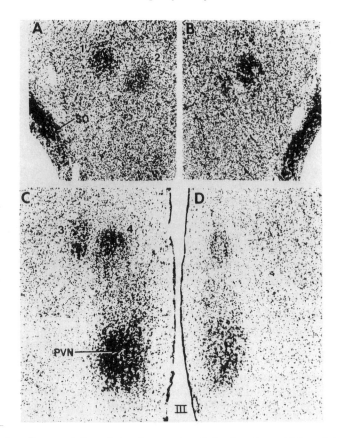

Figure 16.3. Representative photomicrographs of the four interstitial nuclei of the anterior hypothalamus (INAH) in the brain of the human male (A, C) and female (B, D) to illustrate the sex difference in INAH 2 and 3. From these sections it appears that INAH 4 is also sexually dimorphic but this was not true when the volumes from all subjects were averaged. The general location of these photomicrographs is indicated in Figure 16.2. Abbreviations as in Figure 16.2. (From Gorski, 1988, with permission.)

Possible mechanisms responsible for the sexual differentiation of the brain

Given the existence of structural sex differences in the brain, even without an understanding of what they mean functionally, how these differences arise is of critical importance and some progress has been made in this area. Perhaps one of the more surprising observations is that in laboratory animals such as the rat, the actual molecular species of gonadal hormone which acts to masculinize and defeminize the brain is E_2.

This author was the first to show that a single injection of estradiol benzoate would lead to anovulatory sterility in female rats. However, the most reasonable assumption at that time was that this was a pharmacological artifact. The results of subsequent studies, however, strongly suggest that the conversion of T secreted by the testes into E_2 by the enzyme aromatase, is a critical step in the process of sexual differentiation. As illustrated in Figure 16.1 prolonged exposure of the perinatal female rat to the synthetic estrogen, diethylstilbestrol (DES), sex-reverses SDN-POA volume.

The putative role of E_2 offers the possibility that alterations in aromatase activity rather than in testicular activity could affect the process of sexual differentiation. Moreover, there are even more important consequences of this observation, at least at the conceptual level. For example, in the rat, plasma levels of E_2 over the animal's lifetime are actually highest during the first week or so of postnatal life (Weisz & Gunsalus, 1973). If E_2 is the masculinizing hormone it cannot be present in high levels in females during the process of sexual differentiation, but it apparently is.

This inconsistency has not yet been resolved, in fact two essentially opposite hypotheses have been proposed. According to one hypothesis, the *protection* hypothesis, plasma E_2 levels are high postnatally because alpha fetoprotein (AFP), which binds E_2 is present at high levels in the plasma of the postnatal rat. Moreover, AFP is thought to sequester E_2 and prevent it from entering neurons and thus from exerting its masculinizing action. Masculine differentiation of the male's brain occurs, even though AFP has the same role as in the female, because T secreted by the testes is not bound to AFP and can enter neurons where it is aromatized to E_2. However, this elegantly simple hypothesis is challenged by the observations that E_2 is required for neurite outgrowth in explant cultures (see Toran-Allerand, 1984), that anti-estrogen treatment inhibits feminization but does not induce masculinization of brain function (Döhler & Hancke, 1978) and finally, that anti-estrogen treatment postnatally prevents the normal development of the SDN-POA (in terms of its volume) in females as well as in males (Döhler et al., 1984b). Thus, it has been argued that exposure to some E_2 is necessary for the normal development of the female brain while exposure to higher levels leads to the differentiation of the male brain. Particularly in species in which the process of sexual differentiation occurs at least partially postnatally, some mechansim may be required to maintain the high levels of E_2 during pregnancy beyond parturition so that the female brain can develop normally. That mechanism may well be AFP acting as a '*provider*' of E_2.

Thus, there are essentially two hypotheses for the developmental state of the brain of the rat at birth: the brain is inherently feminine or neuter (or perhaps incompletely developed; Figure 16.4). In the first hypothesis AFP serves to protect the genetic female's brain against exposure to E_2, thus allowing it to express its inherently feminine blueprint. In the second hypothesis, the neonatal rat brain is not inherently feminine and AFP provides enough E_2 to permit the normal development of the female brain while the

A ALPHA-FETOPROTEIN PROTECTS THE INHERENTLY FEMALE BRAIN

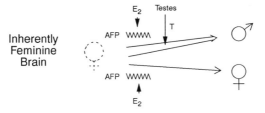

B ALPHA-FETOPROTEIN PROVIDES E$_2$ TO THE DEVELOPING BRAIN

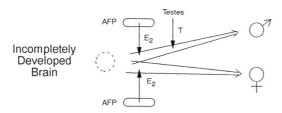

Figure 16.4. A highly schematic diagram of the possible role of alpha fetoprotein (AFP) in the development of the brain in male and female rats. In (A), AFP protects the inherently feminine brain from exposure to estradiol (E$_2$) but not from the action of testicular testosterone (T) after its aromatization. In (B), AFP is proposed to deliver E$_2$ to the developing brain to promote normal development of the female's brain. Again, additional E$_2$ derived from the aromatization of testicular testosterone is assumed to masculinize the male's brain.

additional E$_2$ produced by the aromatization of T secreted in males, leads to masculine differentiation of the brain.

What about animals in which sexual differentiation of the brain occurs prenatally, in the hormonal milieu of pregnancy? Could E$_2$ still be the masculinizing hormone? At least in the guinea pig, exposure to estrogen prenatally does masculinize brain function (Hines et al., 1987). In the human being, one syndrome offers a real challenge to our understanding of the sexual differentiation of the human brain: the androgen insensitivity syndrome. In these genetic male individuals there can be a complete lack of functional androgen receptors, and they develop female external genitalia. As might be predicted by the concept of the sexual differentiation of the brain, these XY women are psychosexually female. Although this would be consistent with their lack of response to T and their sex assignment and rearing as females, their female sexuality actually calls into question the role of E$_2$ in the masculine differentiation of the human brain. Although postpubertal breast development is marked, it is not known whether the levels of E$_2$ derived from the testes directly or from the aromatization of T are high enough prenatally to affect the brain. Until this is established or refuted, the feminine sexuality of XY women with the androgen insensitivity syndrome raises questions about unknown protective mechanisms in human beings similar to the possible role of AFP in the rat, and the role of E_2 in masculine differentiation of the human brain.

Whatever the molecular species of gonadal hormone responsible for the masculine differentiation of the brain, one can still consider putative mechanisms of hormone action. In terms of structural sexual differentiation, the development of three nuclei have been studied: the Spinal Nucleus of the Bulbocavernosus (SNB; Breedlov & Arnold, 1981), the SDN-POA (Gorski et al., 1980) and the AVPV (Bleier, Byne & Siggelow 1982, initially called the medial preoptic nucleus by these authors; Simerly, Swanson & Gorski, 1985a; Bloch & Gorski, 1988). In both the SNB and the SDN-POA, nuclear volume and neuronal number are greater in the male, whereas the AVPV displays the *opposite* sex dimorphism – it is larger in the female.

One mechanism by which gonadal steroids could increase the number of neurons in a given region of the central nervous system (CNS) is by a mitogenic action. However, it currently appears that the stimulation of mitotic activity of neuronal precursor cells is not affected by gonadal hormones (Dodson, Shryne & Gorski, 1988). What probably occurs in both the SNB (Nordeen et al., 1985) and SDN-POA (Dodson & Gorski, 1993) under the influence of gonadal hormones is the prevention of neuronal death. Developmental cell death, possibly apoptosis, is a characteristic of the development of many tissues including the CNS and it is likely that gonadal hormones either promote neuronal survival actively (i.e. by inducing what might be called a 'survival gene mechanism' either directly or through other trophic factors) or prevent apoptosis (possibly by suppressing a 'suicide gene mechanism'). These two hypotheses appear to be amenable to study at the level of molecular techniques.

The AVPV represents something of an enigma since testicular hormones appear to suppress the development of this structure (Simerly et al., 1985b; Ito et al., 1986) and it is not known whether the active hormone is T or E_2. The elucidation of the development of this sexually dimorphic nucleus is quite important because it may well indicate that testicular hormones may both promote and suppress the survival of neurons in different regions of the brain.

One hypothesis of developmental cell death in the CNS is that the survival of neurons depends on their making appropriate synaptic contacts at the appropriate time, thus receiving survival-promoting neurotrophic factors by retrograde transport. If the neurons of the SDN-POA and AVPV happen to compete for a common target area, hormonal stimulation of neurite outgrowth or a direct stimulation of survival in one could lead indirectly to neuronal death in the other. Thus, in the case of the AVPV, we do not know if exposure to testicular hormones causes neuronal death directly or merely stimulates the survival of competitor neurons such as those of the SDN-POA.

It is possible that new insight into the mechanism of action of gonadal hormones will come from the study of chemical agents which interfere with this process. These include the administration of alcohol (Zimmerberg & Reuter, 1989; Ahmed et al., 1991), barbiturates (Arai & Gorski, 1968), cocaine (Raum et al., 1990) and neurotransmitters or their inhibitors (see Döhler, 1991). Maternal stress in the rat also has been reported to lead to the partial demasculinization of sexual behavior (see Ward, 1984) and SDN-POA volume (Anderson, Rhees & Fleming, 1985) in male offspring. In human beings, maternal stress experienced during the Second World War has been correlated with an increased frequency of the birth of homosexual men in Germany (Ellis et al., 1988; see Dörner et al., 1991).

Clinical evidence for the sexual differentiation of the human brain

Since one cannot ethically manipulate the hormonal environment of a human fetus or child experimentally, direct analysis of the possible effects of hormones on the human brain depend on studies of 'experiments of nature', or of those individuals exposed for 'therapeutic' reasons to exogenous hormones. The results of such studies are not particularly consistent and for more details, the reader should consult several reviews (Witelson, 1991; Reinisch & Sanders, 1992a; Hines, 1993).

There are three experiments of nature that are particularly germane to this discussion. Androgen insensitivity, congenital adrenal hyperplasia and 5-alpha-reductase deficiency. The androgen insensitivity syndrome has already been discussed and appears to question the role of E_2 in the masculine differentiation of the human brain, or suggests that there is an unknown protective mechanism that prevents the hormonal masculinization of the female fetus. The results of studies of women with congenital adrenal hyperplasma, who are exposed prenatally to abnormally high levels of adrenal androgens, suggest that these women are shifted towards the masculine direction on a behavioral continuum, that is, they are frequently considered to be tomboyish (see Ehrhardt & Baker, 1974). It has also been reported that they exhibit an increased frequency of lesbianism or bisexuality (Money, Schwartz & Lewis, 1984). Girls with congenital adrenal hyperplasia show male-like toy preference (Berenbaum & Hines, 1992) and after puberty, a possible advantage in spatial ability (Nass & Baker, 1991).

Since it is the metabolite of T produced by the enzyme 5-alpha-reductase (dihydrotestosterone) which masculinizes the human genitalia, males with a deficiency in this enzyme can appear to be females at birth. Imperato-McGinley et al. (1979) found that many individuals with this pathology in the Dominican Republic 'changed' their psychosexual identity from female to male after puberty. Interestingly, in the USA the usual treatment for such individuals is orchidectomy and the continued sex assignment as females. It is not clear that men with this enzymatic deficiency in the Dominican Republic were actually raised unambiguously as girls and/or perhaps reacted *post hoc* to the physical masculinization of their bodies at puberty by assuming a more concordant psychosexual identity. On the other hand, and automatic assignment of such individuals as females and their orchidectomy may be wrong. We must understand the process of the sexual differentiation of the brain more fully so that physicians can avoid making wrong decisions that could cause psychological problems for life.

On occasion, a treatment anticipated to have therapeutic effects may have unexpected and unwanted effects. In an attempt to prevent miscarriage, millions of human fetuses were exposed to the synthetic estrogen, DES, prior to 1972. Unfortunate results of this treatment include clear cell adenocarcinoma of the cervix and vagina and some reproductive dysfunction in men (see Reinisch & Sanders, 1992b). Women exposed prenatally to DES exhibit a male pattern of left/right ear dominance in dichotic listening tests (Hines & Shipley, 1984) and exhibit an increased frequency of lesbianism (Ehrhardt et al., 1985), both perhaps consistent with the general concept of the sexual differentiation of the brain. However, males exposed prenatally to DES exhibit lowered spatial ability and are less lateralized in terms of brain function (Reinisch & Sanders, 1992b). These latter observations are opposite of what one would predict from our current understanding of the role of E_2 in the sexual differentiation of the rat brain.

GONADAL HORMONES AND THE MORPHOLOGY OF THE ADULT BRAIN

The present discussion has emphasized the permanent effects of gonadal hormones on the developing brain. One possible corollary of this concept is that gonadal hormones alter brain structure *only* during the developmental process of sexual differentiation, but this is incorrect. Gonadal hormones have the capacity to alter brain structure, although perhaps only transiently, throughout life.

The most classic example of the morphological plasticity of the adult brain in response to gonadal hormones is the seasonal variation in brain structure observed in songbirds (Nottebohm, 1981). Although it has been suggested that nuclear 'involution' following testicular regression in the non-breeding season may reflect only changes in the histological staining characteristics of some neurons (Gahr, 1990), reactivation of testicular activity during the next breeding season leads to dendritic elongation and the formation of new synapses (see De Voogd, 1991). In the rat, morphological responses to hormonal exposure are clearly not limited to development. Synaptic remodeling appears to occur with the physiological hormonal changes of the estrous cycle (Woolley & McEwen, 1992). The volume of sexually dimorphic nuclei in the gerbil (Commins & Yahr, 1984) and rat (Bloch & Gorski, 1988) can be altered by gonadectomy and hormone treatment, but studies like those of Gahr (1990) performed in the songbird (the results of which question the significance of volume changes) have not been performed in these species.

Another important developmental period when morphological effects might well be expected is at the time of puberty, but this has received little study. In human beings puberty induces marked changes in the physical structure of the body, and also in behavior. Whether the profound changes in hormonal activity at puberty also influence brain structure is not known.

SEXUAL DIFFERENTIATION OF THE BRAIN AND HOMOSEXUALITY

If one were to choose a human behavior to analyze developmentally, it is perhaps unlikely that the choice would be such a private and personal one as sexual orientation, which is often confronted by negative societal pressure. Yet, perhaps because of progress in our understanding of the sexual differentiation of the brain, this topic has been approached recently by several laboratories. Using the rat as the model, it seems clear that the brain is inherently feminine (or as indicated above, perhaps incompletely developed) and that structural and functional characteristics typical of the male are imposed on this feminine blueprint by the action of testicular hormones or their metabolites. In this regard, an understanding of the process of sexual differentiation of the rat brain could be useful for our understanding of the phenomenon of transexualism in which a man, for example, may tell his physician: 'I am a woman, please get me out of this male body.'

When one tries to apply the concept of horomone-dependent sexual differentiation of the brain to homosexuality, an immediate problem arises. Homosexual men consider themselves male and lesbians, female. However, as discussed above, the process of the sexual differentiation of the brain can be divided into four potentially independent processes. A transient alteration in hormonal exposure at a specific time in development might alter one component of sexual differentiation without altering other components or the sexual differentiation of the internal or external genitalia, or adult patterns of hormonal secretion. The literature on homosexuality is replete with examples of men who 'always knew that they were gay', as well as with unsuccessful attempts to alter this behavior. One can ask within the framework of this discussion whether the process of the sexual differentiation of the brain could play any role in the etiology of homosexuality.

To date there are published reports of three structural differences between the brains of homosexual and apparently heterosexual men, but thus far, none involving lesbians. Swaab & Hofman (1990) reported that the suprachiasmatic nucleus (SCN), but not the SDN-POA (presumably INAH-1), is larger in volume and contains more neurons in homosexual men, although men and women do not differ in terms of these parameters (Hofman et al., 1988). One potential difficulty with these studies is that the SCN was visualized and quantified after immunohistochemical staining for vasopressin. It now is clear that neurochemical expression can be state dependent and it is possible that what was measured by this group was influenced by factors other than sexual orientation. Nevertheless, this first report of a putative structural difference correlated with sexual orientation may well be valid.

In the second study, Le Vay (1991) reported that INAH-3 was larger in heterosexual than in homosexual men. As discussed by Le Vay, these results could be confounded by AIDS which clearly can cause neuropathology. He also pointed out that if hospital records did not indicate that a man was homosexual, he was assumed to be heterosexual. Later, Allen & Gorski (1992) reported that the midline surface area of the anterior commissure (AC), which they had earlier shown to be larger in women than in men (Allen & Gorski, 1991), was even larger in homosexual men. In this study, there were adequate numbers of both heterosexual and homosexual men who did not have AIDS to compare the subgroups statistically and no effect of AIDS was noted. As in the LeVay study, men who were not identified on hospital records as homosexual were considered to be heterosexual. If, in either study, homosexual men were erroneously included as heterosexual, that could have made the observed difference between the two groups less marked than they may actually be. As discussed above, dealing with human brain tissue raises problems in terms of variable intervals between death and tissue fixation. Moreover, in these two studies there was considerable variability and great overlap between groups. It is currently impossible to judge, from *any* brain parameter, whether a given individual has a 'male' or 'female' brain or is heterosexual or homosexual.

As is the case for the reports of structural sex differences in the human brain, the results of these studies must be confirmed by independent investigators before they are accepted as fully valid. Again, there is no evidence to relate the structural differences which correlate with sexual orientation to hormone levels or action at a specific point during development, or for that matter, at any time. Based on our understanding of the hormone-dependent process of sexual differentiation of the rat brain, it can be assumed that hormones could have played a role, but this is only a speculative assumption. Moreover, the structure of the brain can be modified by environmental factors (Berrebi et al., 1988; Diamond, 1991; Juraska, 1993). Thus, even if these results are confirmed by others, we will not know which comes first – a difference in brain structure that is related to sexual orientation in some way, perhaps causally, or environmental factors that are related to the homosexual life style which in turn lead to changes in brain structure.

As might be predicted from the variability between the sexes on tests of cognitive function, the influence of sexual orientation, at least on spatial ability, is unclear. Male homosexuals have been reported to perform more poorly than heterosexual men on certain tests of spatial ability but not all, and lesbian women performed as well as heterosexual women except for one test (the water jar test) on which they performed more poorly, rather than better which could be expected if their brains were more 'masculinized' (Gladue et al., 1990). To add even more complexity, it has been reported that both male and female homosexuals have an increased incidence of 'left-handedness', defined as non-consistent right-hand preference (McCormick, Witelson & Kingstone, 1990).

The results of studies at a different level suggest a possible contribution of genetic factors to homosexuality. There have been three approaches to this question: concordance in twins, pedigree analysis and gene linkage. The most recent studies of concordance have included interviews with the subjects and their self-rating on the Kinsey scale and therefore, appear to be the most reliable. It was found that in identical twins, the concordance rate (i.e. the likelihood that if one twin is homosexual the other will be too) ranged from 52–65% for homosexual men (Bailey & Pillard, 1991; Whitman, Diamond & Martin, 1993) and 48–75% for lesbian women (Bailey et al., 1993; Whitman et al., 1993). The concordance rate dropped markedly is non-identical twins. Although these results support a significant genetic contribution to sexual orientation, the fact that about half of the twins with identical genomes were not homosexual indicates that other factors must also be involved.

In 1993, Hamer et al., reported the results of their studies of pedigree analyses of the extended families of 76 homosexual men. These investigators found that in these families there was an increased incidence of homosexuality in maternal uncles and cousins compared to that in their specific control group which suggested a possible involvement of the X chromosome. By gene linkage analysis on blood from 40 pairs of gay brothers (not twins), they found that in the region of the X chromosome known as Xq28, 33 of the 40 pairs of brothers inherited the same alleles of chromosome markers. This region of the X chromosome is large and could be the locus of numerous genes. Although it is possible that this region includes a gene(s) that contributes, or predisposes one, to homosexuality that clearly has not been proven. Note also that seven of the 40 pairs of gay brothers did not share the same alleles in the region of Xq28. Therefore, whatever Xq28 may contain, it does not explain homosexuality *per se*.

The theme of this symposium is the interaction of multiple factors in the development of an individual. The possible factors that contribute to sexual orientation have been presented here not because the results are clear, but rather because they indicate that multiple factors possibly including hormonal, genomic and environmental influences may all play a role in establishing a very fundamental, although presumably multifactorial, aspect of human behavior, that is sexual orientation.

IMPLICATIONS FOR HUMAN SOCIETY

The process of the sexual differentiation of the brain, which has major implications for a given individual, would appear also to have major implications for society. The recent studies on the possible 'biological basis' of sexual orientation have already raised issues concerning the civil rights of homosexuals if their sexual orientation is the consequence of factors beyond their control and not simply a matter of their voluntary decision to follow a different life style. However, sex differences in brain function and brain structure extend well beyond those which appear to be directly related to reproduction. Differences in cognitive abilities could be used to reinforce suppressive societal stereotypes or more appropriately recognized and possibly overcome or minimized by different educational methods or perhaps, simply by encouraging different attitudes among teachers. An understanding of the nature and possibly the hormonal basis of sex differences in the human brain will not immediately eliminate cultural prejudices against one sex or group or other, but with the passage of time and further experimental evidence, perhaps this will eventually occur.

CONCLUSION

Human development is extremely complex and subject to the influences of many factors. The concept of the sexual differentiation of the brain suggests that fundamental and pervasive sex differences in brain function and structure exist and may be determined prenatally in human beings. These differences perhaps should be taken into account in terms of educational, psychiatric and even medical practices. Although the concept of the sexual differentiation of the brain is very well documented in laboratory animals, its role in human development still remains obscure. However, we cannot escape the fact that we are mammals, although very complex mammals, and therefore, we cannot escape the modification of our brains by the hormone environment during certain, presumably critical, periods of development. As human beings, we have developed the ability to overcome many of the laws of nature, but it is not likely that sexual differentiation of the brain is one of them.

REFERENCES

Ahmed, I. I., Shryne, J. E., Gorski, R. A., Branch, B. J. & Taylor, A. N. (1991) Prenatal ethanol and the prepubertal sexually dimorphic nucleus of the preoptic area. *Physiology and Behaviour*, **49**, 427–32.

Allen, L. S. & Gorski, R. A. (1990) A sex difference in the bed nucleus of the stria terminalis of the human brain. *Journal of Comparative Neurology*, **302**, 697–706.

Allen, L. S. & Gorski, R. A. (1991) Sexual dimorphism of the anterior commissure and massa intermedia of the human brain. *Journal of Comparative Neurology*, **312**, 97–104.

Allen, L. S. & Gorski, R. A. (1992) Sexual orientation and the size of the anterior commissure in the human brain. *Proceedings of the National Academy of Sciences of the USA*, **89**, 7199–202.

Allen, L. S., Hines, M., Shryne, J. E. & Gorski, R. A. (1989) Two sexually dimorphic cell groups in the human brain. *Journal of Neuroscience*, **9**, 497–506.

Allen, L. S., Richey, M. F., Chai, Y. M. & Gorski, R. A. (1991) Sex differences in the corpus callosum of the living human being. *Journal of Neuroscience*, **11**, 933–42.

Anderson, D. K., Rhees, R. W. & Fleming, D. E. (1985) Effects of prenatal stress on differentiation of the sexually dimorphic nucleus of the preoptic area (SDN-POA) of the brain. *Brain Research*, **322**, 113–18.

Arai, Y. & Gorski, R. A. (1968) Protection against the neural organizing effect of exogenous androgen in the neonatal female rat. *Endocrinology*, **82**, 1005–9.

Arendash, G. W. & Gorski, R. A. (1983) Effects of discrete lesions of the sexually dimorphic nucleus of the preoptic area or other medial preoptic regions on the sexual behavior of male rats. *Brain Research Bulletin*, **10**, 147–54.

Bailey, J. M. & Pillard, R. C. (1991) A genetic study of male sexual orientation. *Archives of General Psychiatry*, **48**, 1089–96.

Bailey, J. M., Pillard, R. C., Neale, M. C. & Agyei, Y. (1993) Heritable factors influence sexual orientation in women. *Archives of General Psychiatry*, **50**, 217–23.

Benbow, C. P. & Benbow, R. M. (1984) Biological correlates of high mathematical reasoning ability. In De Vries, G. J. H., De Bruin, J. P. C., Uylings, H. B. M. & Corner, M. A. (eds.) *Progess in Brain Research, 61 Sex Differences in the Brain*, pp. 468–90. Amsterdam: Elsevier.

Berenbaum, S. A. & Hines, M. (1992) Early androgens are related to childhood sex-typed toy preferences. *Psychological Science*, **3**, 203–6.

Berrebi, A. S., Fitch, R. H., Ralphe, D. L., Denenberg, J. O., Friedrich, U. L., Jr. & Denenberg, U. H. (1988) Corpus callosum: region-specific effects of sex, early experience and age. *Brain Research*, **438**, 216–24.

Blanchard, D. C., Shepherd, J. K., De Padua Carobrez, A. & Blanchard, R. J. (1991) Sex effects in defensive behaviour: baseline differences and drug interactions. *Neuroscience and Biobehavioral Reviews*, **15**, 461–8.

Bleier, R., Byne, W. & Siggelow, I. (1982) Cytoarchitectonic sexual analysis of the SDN-POA of the medial preoptic and anterior hypothalamic areas in guinea pig, rat, hamster and mouse. *Journal of Comparative Neurology*, **212**, 118–30.

Bloch, G. J. & Gorski, R. A. (1988) Estrogen/progesterone treatment in adulthood affects the size of several components of the medial preoptic area in the male rat. *Journal of Comparative Neurology*, **275**, 613–22.

Breedlove, S. M. & Arnold, A. P. (1981) Sexually dimorphic motor nucleus in the rat lumbar spinal cord: response to adult hormone manipulation, absence in androgen-insensitive rats. *Brain Research*, **225**, 297–307.

Collado, P., Guillamón, A., Valencia, A. & Segovia, S. (1990) Sexual dimorphism in the bed nucleus of the accessory olfactory tract in the rat. *Developmental Brain Research*, **56**, 263–8.

Commins, D. & Yahr, P. (1984) Adult testosterone levels influence the morphology of a sexually dimorphic area in the Mongolian gerbil brain. *Journal of Comparative Neurology*, **224**, 132–40.

Crews, D. (1993) The organizational concept and vertebrates without sex chromosomes. *Brain, Behavior & Evolution*, **42**, 202–14.

del Abril, A., Segovia, S. & Guillamón, A. (1990) Sexual dimorphism in the parastrial nucleus of the rat preoptic area. *Developmental Brain Research*, **52**, 11–15.

de Lacoste-Utamsing, C. & Holloway, R. L. (1982) Sexual dimorphism in human corpus callosum. *Science*, **216**, 1431–2.

De Voogd, T. J. (1991) Endocrine modulation of the development and adult function of the avian song system. *Psychoneuroendocrinology*, **16**, 41–66.

Diamond, M. C. (1991) Hormonal effects on the development of cerebral lateralization. *Psychoneuroendocrinology*, **16**, 121–9.

Dodson, R. E. & Gorski, R. A. (1993) Testosterone propionate administration prevents the loss of neurons within the central part of the medial preoptic nucleus. *Journal of Neurobiology*, **24**, 80–8.

Dodson, R. E., Shryne, J. E. & Gorski, R. A. (1988) Hormonal modification of the number of total and late-arising neurons in the central part of the medial preoptic nucleus of the rat. *Journal of Comparative Neurology*, **275**, 623–929.

Döhler, K. D. (1991) Pre- and postnatal influence of hormones and neurotransmitters on sexual differentiation of the mammalian hypothalamus. *International Review of Cytology*, **131**, 1–57.

Döhler, K. D., Coquelin, A., Davis, F., Hines, M., Shryne, J. E. & Gorski, R. A. (1984a) Pre- and postnatal influence of testosterone propionate and diethylstilbestrol on differentiation of the sexually dimorphic nucleus of the preoptic area in male land female rats. *Brain Research*, **302**, 291–5.

Döhler, K. D. & Hancke, J. L. (1978) Thoughts on the mechanism of sexual brain differentiation. In Dörner, G. & Kawakami, M. (eds.) *Hormones and Brain Development*. Amsterdam: Elsevier, pp. 153–7.

Döhler, K. D., Srivastava, S. S., Shryne, J. E., Jarzab, B., Sipos, A. & Gorski, R. A. (1984b) Differentiation of the sexually dimorphic nucleus in the preoptic area of the rat brain is inhibited by postnatal treatment with an estrogen antagonist. *Neuroendocrinology*, **38**, 297–301.

Dörner, G., Poppe, I., Stahl, F., Kolzsch, J. & Uebelhack, R. (1991) Gene- and environment-dependent neuroendocrine etiogenesis of homosexuality and trans-sexualism. *Experimental and Clinical Endocrinology*, **98**, 141–50.

Eccles, J. S. (1987) Gender roles and achievement patterns: an expectancy value perspective. In Reinisch, J. M., Rosenblum, L. A. & Sanders, S. A. (eds.) *Masculinity/Femininity: Basic Perspectives*. New York: Oxford University Press, pp. 240–80.

Ehrhardt, A. A. & Baker, S. W. (1974) Fetal androgens, human central nervous system differentiation, and behavior differences. In Friedman, R. C., Richart, R. M. & van the Weile, R. L. (eds.) *Sex Differences in Behavior*. New York: John Wiley, pp. 33–52.

Ehrhardt, A., Meyer-Bahlburg, H. F. L., Rosen, L. R., Feldman, J. F., Veridiano, N. P., Zimmerman, I. & McEwen, B. S. (1985) Sexual orientation after prenatal exposure to exogenous estrogen. *Archives of Sexual Behavior*, **14**, 57–77.

Ellis, L., Ames, M. A., Peckham, W. & Burke, D. (1988) Sexual orientation of human offspring may be altered by severe maternal stress during pregnancy. *Journal of Sexual Research*, **25**, 152–7.

Gahr, M. (1990) Delineation of a brain nucleus: comparisons of cytochemical, hodological and cytoarchitectural views of the song control nucleus HVC of the adult canary. *Journal of Comparative Neurology*, **294**, 32–6.

Gladue, B. A., Beatty, W. W., Larson, J. & Staton, R. D. (1990) Sexual orientation and spatial ability in men and women. *Psychobiology*, **18**, 101–8.

Gorski, R. A. (1987) Sex differences in the rodent brain: their nature and origin. In Reinisch, J. M., Rosenblum, L. A. & Sanders, S. A. (eds.) *Masculinity/Femininity: Basic Perspectives*. New York: Oxford University Press, pp. 37–67.

Gorski, R. A. (1988) Hormone-induced sex differences in hypothalamic structure. *Bulletin of the Tokyo Metropolitan Institute of Neuroscience*, 16 Suppl., **3**, 67–90.

Gorski, R. A. (1991) Sexual differentiation of the endocrine brain and its control. In Motta, M. (ed.) *Brain Endocrinology*. New York: Raven Press, pp. 71–104.

Gorski, R. A., Harlan, R. E., Jacobsen, C. D., Shryne, J. E. & Southam, A. M. (1980) Evidence for the existence of a sexually dimorphic nucleus in the preoptic area of the rat. *Journal of Comparative Neurology*, **193**, 529–39.

Gouchie, C. & Kimura, D. (1991) The relationship between testosterone levels and cognitive ability patterns. *Psychoneuroendocrinology*, **16**, 323–34.

Gould, E., Woolley, C. S. & McEwen, B. S. (1991) The hippocampal formation: morphological changes induced by thyroid, gonadal and adrenal hormones. *Psychoneuroendocrinology*, **16**, 67–84.

Goy, R. W. & McEwen, B. S. (1980) *Sexual Differentiation of the Brain*, Cambridge, Mass.: MIT Press.

Guillamón, A., De Blas, M. R. & Segovia, S. (1988) Effects of sex steroids on the development of the locus coerulus in the rat. *Developmental Brain Research*, **40**, 306–10.

Hamer, D. H., Hu, S., Magnuson, V. L., Hu, N. & Pattatucci, A. M. L. (1993) A linkage between DNA markers on the X chromosome and male sexual orientation. *Science*, **261**, 321–7.

Handa, R. J., Corbier, P., Shryne, J. E., Schoonmaker, J. N. & Gorski, R. A. (1985) Differential effects of the perinatal steroid environment on three sexually dimorphic parameters of the rat brain. *Biology of Reproduction*, **32**, 855–64.

Hines, M. (1990) Gonadal hormones and human cognitive development. In Balthazart, J. (ed.) *Hormones, Brain and Behavior in Vertebrates. 1. Sexual Differentiation, Neuroanatomical Aspects, Neurotransmitters and Neuropeptides*. Basel: Karger, pp. 51–63.

Hines, M. (1993) Hormonal and neural correlates of sex-typed behavioral development in human beings. In Hang, M. (ed.) *Development of Sex Differences and Similarities in Behavior*. Amsterdam: Kluwer Academic Publishers, pp. 131–49.

Hines, M., Allen, L. S. & Gorski, R. A. (1992a) Sex differences in subregions of the medial nucleus of the amygdala and the bed nucleus of the stria terminalis of the rat. *Brain Research*, **579**, 321–6.

Hines, M., Alsum, P., Roy, M., Gorski, R. A. & Goy, R. W. (1987). Estrogenic contributions to sexual differentiation in the female guinea pig: influences of diethylstilbestrol and tamoxifen on neural, behavioral and ovarian development. *Hormones and Behavior*, **21**, 402–17.

Hines, M. & Shipley, C. (1984) Prenatal exposure to diethylstilbestrol (DES) and the development of sexually dimorphic cognitive abilities and cerebral lateralization. *Development Psychology*, **20**, 81–94.

Hines, M., Chiu, L., McAdams, L. A., Bentler, P. M. & Lipacmon, J. (1992b) Cognition and the corpus callosum: verbal fluency, visuospatial ability, and language lateralization related to midsagittal surface areas of callosal subregions. *Behavioral Neuroscience*, **106**, 3–4.

Hofman, M. A., Fliers, E., Goudsmit, E. & Swaab, D. F. (1988) Morphometric analysis of the suprachiasmic and paraventricular nuclei in the human brain. *Journal of Anatomy*, **160**, 127–43.

Hofman, M. A. & Swaab, D. F. (1989) The sexually dimorphic nucleus of the preoptic area in the human brain: a comparative morphometric study. *Journal of Anatomy*, **164**, 55–71.

Imperato-McGinley, J., Peterson, R. E., Gautier, T. & Sturla, E. (1979) Male pseudohermaphoditism secondary to 5α-reductase deficiency – a model for the role of androgens in both the development of the male phenotype and the evolution of a male gender identity. *Journal of Steroid Biochemistry*, **11**, 637–45.

Ito, S., Murakami, S., Yamanouchi, K. & Arai, Y. (1986) Perinatal androgen exposure decreases the size of the sexually dimorphic medial preoptic nucleus in the rat. *Proceedings of the Japan Academy*, **62**, 408–11.

Juraska, J. M. (1993) Sex differences in the rat cerebral cortex. In Hang, M. (ed.) *Development of Sex Differences and Similarities in Behavior*. Amsterdam: Kluwer Academic Publishers, pp. 377–88.

Juraska, J. M. & Kopcik, J. R. (1988) Sex and environmental influences on the size and ultrastructure of the rat corpus callosum. *Brain Research*, **450**, 1–8.

Kelly, D. B. (1988) Sexually dimorphic behaviors. *Annual Review of Neuroscience*, **11**, 225–51.

Kondo, Y., Shinoda, A., Yamanouchi, K. & Arai, Y. (1990) Role of septum and preoptic area in regulating masculine and feminine sexual behavior in male rats. *Hormones and Behavior*, **24**, 421–34.

LeVay, S. (1991) A difference in hypothalamic structure between heterosexual and homosexual men. *Science*, **253**, 1034–7.

Macoby, E. E. (1987) Varied meanings of 'masculine' and 'feminine'. In Reinisch, J. M., Rosenblum, L. A. & Sanders, S. A. (eds.) *Masculinity/Femininity: Basic Persepectives*. New York: Oxford University Press, pp. 227–39.

Madeira, M. D., Sousa, N., Cadete-Leite, A., Lieberman, A. R. & Paula-Barbosa, M. M. (1993) The supraoptic nucleus of the adult rat hypothelamus displays marked sexual dimorphism which is dependent on body weight. *Neuroscience*, **52**, 497–513.

Matsumoto, A. & Arai, Y. (1983) Sex difference in volume of the ventromedial nucleus of the hypothalamus in the rat. *Endocrinologica Japonica*, **30**, 277–80.

Matsumoto, A. & Arai, Y. (1986) Male-female difference in synaptic organization of the ventromedial nucleus of the hypothalamus in the rat. *Neuroendocrinology*, **42**, 232–6.

McCormick, C. M., Witelson, S. F. & Kingstone, E. (1990) Left-handedness in homosexual men and women: neuroendocrine implications. *Psychoneuroendocrinology*, **15**, 69–76.

Mizukami, S., Nishizuka, M. & Arai, Y. (1983) Sexual difference in nuclear volume and its ontogeny in the rat amygdala. *Experimental Neurology*, **79**, 569–75.

Money, J., Schwartz, M. & Lewis, V. G. (1984) Adult erotosexual status and fetal hormonal masculinization and demasculinization: 46,XX congenital virilizing adrenal hyperplasia and 46,XY androgen-insensitivity syndrome compared. *Psychoneuroendocrinology*, **9**, 405–14.

Muñoz-Cueto, J. A., García-Segura, L. M. & Ruiz-Marcos, A. (1991) Regional sex differences in spine density along the apical shaft of visual cortex pyramids during postnatal development. *Brain Research*, **540**, 41–7.

Nass, R. & Baker, S. (1991) Androgen effects on cognition: congenital adrenal hyperplasia. *Psychoneuroendocrinology*, **16**, 189–201.

Nordeen, E. J., Nordeen, K. W., Sengelaub, D. R. & Arnold, A. P. (1985) Androgens prevent normally occurring cell death in a sexually dimorphic spinal nucleus. *Science*, **229**, 671–3.

Nottebohm, F. (1981) A brain for all seasons: cyclical anatomical changes in song control nuclei of the canary brain. *Science*, **214**, 1368–70.

Nottebohm, F. & Arnold, A. P. (1976) Sexual dimorphism in vocal control areas of the songbird brain. *Science*, **194**, 211–3.

O'Boyle, M. W., Alexander, J. E. & Benbow, C. P. (1991) Enhanced right hemisphere activation in the mathematically precocious: a preliminary EEG investigation. *Brain and Cognition*, **17**, 138–53.

Perez, J., Naftolin, F. & García Segura, L. M. G. (1990) Sexual differentiation of synaptic connectivity and neuronal plasma membrane in the arcuate nucleus of the rat hypothalamus. *Brain Research*, **527**, 116–22.

Raisman, G. & Field, P. M. (1973) Sexual dimorphism in the neuropil of the preoptic area of the rat and its dependence on neonatal androgen. *Brain Research*, **54**, 1–29.

Raum, W. J., McGivern, R. F., Peterson, M. A., Shryne, J. H. & Gorski, R. A. (1990) Prenatal inhibition of hypothalamic sex steroid uptake by cocaine: effects on neurobehavioral sexual differentiation in male rats. *Developmental Brain Research*, **53**, 230–6.

Reid, S. N. M. & Juraska, J. M. (1992) Sex differences in neuron number in the binocular area of the rat visual cortex. *Journal of Comparative Neurology*, **321**, 448–55.

Reinisch, J. M. & Sanders, S. A. (1992a) Prenatal hormonal contributions to sex differences in human cognitive and personality development. In Gerall, A. A., Moltz, H. & Ward, I. L. (eds.) *Handbook of Behavioral Neurobiology 11 Sexual Differentiation*. New York: Plenum Press, pp. 221–43.

Reinisch, J. M. & Sanders, S. A. (1992b) Effects of prenatal exposure to diethyl-stilbestrol (DES) on hemispheric laterality and spatial ability in human males. *Hormones and Behavior*, **26**, 62–75.

Simerly, R. B., Swanson, L. W. & Gorski, R. A. (1985a) The distribution of monoaminergic cells and fibers in a periventricular preoptic nucleus involved in the control of gonadatropin release: immunohistochemical evidence for a dopaminergic sexual dimorphism. *Brain Research*, **330**, 55–64.

Simerly, R. B., Swanson, L. W., Handa, R. J. & Gorski, R. A. (1985b) Influence of perinatal androgen on the sexually dimorphic distribution of tyrosine-hydroxylase immunoreactive cells and fibers in the anteroventral periventricular nucleus of the rat. *Neuroendocrinology*, **40**, 501–10.

Swaab, D. F. & Hofman, M. A. (1990) An enlarged suprachiasmatic nucleus in homosexual men. *Brain Research*, **537**, 141–8.

Terasawa, E. & Davis, G. A. (1983) The LHRH neuronal system in female rats: relation to the medial preoptic nucleus. *Endocrinologica Japonica*, **30**, 405–17.

Toran-Allerand, C. D. (1984) On the genesis of sexual differentiation of the central nervous system: morphogenetic consequences of steroidal exposure and possible role of α-fetoprotein. In De Vries, C. J., DeBruin, J. P. C., Uylings, H. B. M. & Corner, M. A. (eds.) *Progress in Brain Research 61 Sex Differences in the Brain*. Amsterdam: Elsevier, pp. 63–98.

vom Saal, F. S., Montano, M. M. & Wang, M. H. (1992) Sexual differentiation in mammals. In Colborn, T. & Clement, C. (eds.) *Chemically-induced alterations in sexual and functional development: the wildlife/human connection.* Princeton, Princeton Scientific, pp. 17–83.

Ward, I. L. (1984) The prenatal stress syndrome: current status. *Psychoneuroendocrinology*, **9**, 3–11.

Watson, N. V. & Kimura, D. (1991) Nontrivial sex differences in throwing and intercepting: relation to psychometrically-defined spatial functions. *Personality and Individual Differences*, **12**, 375–85.

Weisz, J. & Gunsalus, P. (1973) Estrogen levels in immature female rats: true or spurious-ovarian or adrenal? *Endocrinology*, **93**, 1057–65.

Weisz, J. & Ward, I. L. (1973) Plasma testosterone and progesterone titers of pregnant rats, their male and female fetuses, and neonatal offspring. *Endocrinology*, **106**, 306–16.

Whitman, F. L., Diamond, M. & Martin, J. (1993) Homosexual orientation in twins: a report on 61 pairs and three triplet sets. *Archives of Sexual Behavior*, **22**, 187–206.

Williams, C. L. & Meck, W. H. (1991) The organizational effects of gonadal steroids on sexually dimorphic spatial ability. *Psychoneuroendocrinology*, **16**, 155–76.

Witelson, S. F. (1991) Neural sexual mosaicism: sexual differentiation of the human-temporo-parietal region for functional asymmetry. *Psychoneuroendocrinology*, **16**, 131–53.

Woolley, C. S. & McEwen, B. S. (1992) Estradiol mediates fluctuation in hippocampal synapse density during the estrous cycle in the adult rat. *Journal of Neuroscience*, **12**, 2549–54.

Young, J. K. (1982) A comparison of the hypothalami of rats and mice: lack of a gross sexual dimorphism in the mouse. *Brain Research*, **239**, 233–9.

Zimmerberg, B. & Reutter, J. M. (1989) Sexually dimorphic behavioral and brain symmetries in neonatal rats: effects of prenatal alochol exposure. *Developmental Brain Research*, **46**, 281–90.

17 Commentary **The brain and socialization: a two-way mediation across the life course**

PIERRE KARLI

If *socialization* refers to those processes that render 'social', that make fit for well-adapted social interactions, two basic questions immediately arise: (1) who is to be rendered social, and (2) what are the properties, the constraints and the forces that contribute to organize and energize these social rendering processes? Right from conception, the biological individual is endowed with the potentialities for developing a specific range of means of expression and action that is characteristic for each member of the species. With the aid of the developed equipment and competences the individual becomes able to establish, maintain or modify a series of relationships so as to become a fully-fledged social actor. As he becomes more and more aware of the opportunities and gratifications, strains and conflicts inherent in the operation of his social relationships, as the full meaning of these relationships is made more and more explicit in his internal representations, the social actor will consciously promote his own socialization and possibly contribute to some kind of social change. In other words, there progressively emerge, coexist and closely interact the three facets of any human 'trinity': a biological individual, a social actor and a reflecting and deliberating subject. Each one of these facets carries on a dialogue with an environment of its own: the organism's material environment; the actor's social milieu; the subject's inner world. Each facet shapes – and, in return, is being shaped by – its own dialogue, an evolving set of appropriate, that is adapted and adaptive, interactions. But the three facets with their respective dialogue obviously share one and the same brain, which means that the latter takes on the mediation of a threefold dialogue which evolves across the life course. At any one time, the concrete events of the dialogue depend on both the way in which the brain is functioning and the nature of the information the brain is currently carrying and processing. But in turn these events and their manifold consequences affect brain functioning and information processing. Needless to say, it is extremely difficult to fully grasp the brain's mediating role with our linear discourse, owing to the highly complex and circular character of the processes involved. Only a few salient points can be dealt with here, in particular those that are relevant to the contributions made in this book by Robert Cairns, Robert Goy and Roger Gorski (Chapters 14,

15 and 16) to the understanding of some general or more specific aspects of socialization.

The human brain can be fully understood only if we consider it as a history-produced and history-producing dynamic entity. More concretely, it is pertinent to examine with an integrated bio-psycho-social approach how the brain shapes, and is shaped by the events of an individual life-history. Robert Cairns (Chapter 14) has rightly stressed both the necessity and the difficulty to combine in a constructive way a holistic, system-orientated and time-sensitive developmental model with rigorous analyses by means of relevant and reliable empirical operations. When studying brain-behaviour relationships, we are usually led – for obvious methodological reasons – to cut some thin slice out of the history *elaborated in close interaction* by an individual brain and the dialogue it mediates. It matters, therefore, to be aware of the fact that the experimental conditions together with the statistical analysis of the data they yield may well wipe out historically determined individual differences, and that things must be put back in their more global, historical context.

DIFFERENTIAL EFFECTS OF TIME

As the ontogeny progresses, the work of time changes its nature. In the initial phase of socialization, which is closely linked to the biological maturation of the individual, time essentially serves as a revealing agent. Owing to the interactions with the environment that take place in its course, time progressively reveals (in a way and to an extent that prove more or less close to an optimum) what is already prefigured in a species-specific genetic endowment. This time-dependent revelation concerns those processes and mechanisms that allow the individual to acquire and to mobilize his social competences. The *meaning* of this beginning life-history is hardly more than the mere expression of a programme which all members of the species have in common. Time is not yet being verbalized and it is experienced as something fragile and evanescent. But later on, time will serve more and more as the site of impact of pregnant contingent events and an autobiographic memory starts to build up that will undergo continuous reconstruction and reappropriation through the use of language. From now on, the individual life history generates a meaning of its own that is no longer rigidly preprogrammed, owing to the interpretation and symbolization of the experienced – and partly *chosen* to be experienced – events. Of course, the individual way in which this occurs also conforms to some specific 'programme'. But the nature of this sociocultural programme is quite different from that of the genetic programme, and the autonomy with regard to it is, or at least can be much greater.

When examining the development of the biological individual and that of the social actor, one should keep in mind a simple, but apparently not always self-evident, fact that the very nature of homeostasis, change and causality is not identical in those two instances. The processes and mechanisms which regulate the organism's internal milieu and the required exchange of matter and energy with the environment correspond to basic biological needs: they are brought into play from within and their efficiency is validated through feedback arising also from within. Things are quite different in the case of the relational homeostasis which the social actor strives to build up and preserve. Both the incitements and the validating feedback come from without, from the interactions with others. Of course, the internally arising affective processes, with all their biological determinants, play an important mediating and integrating role which I wish to discuss later.

In the living organism, cell death and cell proliferation, the flow of matter and energy, the complex and changing interplay of the nervous, endocrine and immunological systems, all aim at preserving or restoring the identity and integrity of the biological self. It is the stability of structure and function that is of vital importance. The social actor, on the other hand, needs a fair degree of plasticity if he has to efficiently adapt to the changes that occur in a society as well as in his own social roles and status. Individual *interests* evolve as a relational construct which develops in and through the dialectical relations between the individual's needs and desires and the people thought to be capable of satisfying them (see van der Wilk, 1991). As regards causality, there is a shift, schematically speaking, from genetically determined cause–consequence relationships, which prevail for the biological individual, to historically determined means–end relationships, which reflect and shape the social actor's interactions with others.

BIOLOGICAL AND SOCIAL DETERMINANTS OF SEXUAL BEHAVIOUR

Both Goy and Gorski (Chapters 15 and 16) have concentrated on sexual behaviour, examining its determination in connection with the sexual differentiation of the brain (Gorski) or with early hormonal interventions (Goy). Sexual behaviour happens to correspond, in the human species, to a biologically controlled reproductive process as well as to a culturally coded interindividual relationship. It follows from this dual character that the concrete behaviour is multidetermined and that the determinants involved as well as the effects they induce are likely to interact in a varied and evolving way. Even in non-human mammals, it is not easy to disentangle the various interacting effects induced at successive developmental stages by a single factor such as a gonadal hormone. In the experiments reported by Goy, testosterone propionate was injected into pregnant rhesus monkey females with the aim of analysing the repercussions of such an early hormonal treatment on the morphology and behaviour of juvenile genotypic females. The observations clearly show that a great variety of anatomical and behavioural modifications can be induced by the prenatal testosterone treatment. These modifications are differentially brought about by the commencement, the duration or the end of the treatment and they are differentially combined in a number and variety of sexual phenotypes that greatly exceed the more typical combinations described in the rat.

A further dissociation worth stressing lies in the fact that the testosterone treatment, while *quantitatively* increasing the females' mounting activity, did not *qualitatively* shift the evolution of their preference for a partner of a particular sex so as to duplicate the developmental pattern observed in genotypic males. The latter initially display a fairly strong preference for male partners before reversing their preference at puberty. On the other hand, even the most extensively masculinized females did not show such an initial preference for male partners.

Whenever a determining factor induces several effects, the question arises as to whether a given effect is directly determined or, at least partly, determined through the mediation of any other(s) of the effects induced. If we consider, for instance, the fact that the prenatal testosterone treatment clearly increased both the frequency of genital exploration by mothers and that of the infants' mounts to mothers, one may wonder to what extent and how the masculinized infants' behaviour might be influenced by the way in which the masculinization of their genitalia influences the mothers' behavior. A more important question concerns the relationships between play activities, social dominance and the development of sexual behaviour. Elevated frequencies of *rough play* were observed in those genotypic females that had been exposed to testosterone beyond day 100 of gestation. In the rat, too, *play fighting* in the juvenile period was found to be influenced by plasma testosterone levels in the perinatal period (Ward & Stehm, 1991; Pellis & McKenna, 1992). With a long enough prenatal androgen treatment (35 days or longer), the masculinized females displayed signs of social dominance ranks that proved similar to the ranks of normal intact males. It is very likely that the individual development of sexual behavior is markedly influenced by the outcomes of rough play interactions, by the dominant-subordinate relations that are possibly shaped by the outcome, and also by the way in which these outcomes and relations act back on both the release and the effects of various hormones and neurotransmitters. This may well partly explain the great variety of the behavioral repercussions observed in genotypic females following the prenatal androgen treatment.

Similar questions obviously arise if we now consider the determination of the naturally occurring sex differences in the genitalia, in brain structure and function, and in the overt behaviour (Gorski, Chapter 16). As regards the early 'organizational' effects of gonadal hormones, it appears that they differ according to both the target and the species being considered. In all mammals including man, the differentiation of the inner and outer genitalia is quite rigidly − and therefore reliably − controlled by the hormonal environment. As for sex differences in brain structure and overt behaviour, they are less clearcut and not as dependent on the action of gonadal hormones. In the male rat, the large size of the sexually dimorphic nucleus of the preoptic area (SDN-POA) actually seems to be largely due to the action of testicular hormones during a critical phase of development. But genomic and environmental factors that modulate both the release of, and the sensitivity to, androgenic hormones may also contribute to determine the differential development of this brain structure. Furthermore, in experiments in which the volume of the SDN-POA was significantly decreased in male rats by exposing them to prenatal stress, no difference in SDN-POA volume was observed between those adult rats that did and those that did not exhibit ejaculatory behaviour when tested with oestrous females (Kerchner & Ward, 1992). In other words, even in the rat there is no straightforward relationship between hormone-induced structural characteristics of the brain and overt behaviour displayed later on. In the adult rat, the 'activational' effects of the gonadal hormones preferentially promote mounting behaviour in the male and lordosis behaviour in the female – two behaviour patterns which actually coexist in one and the same animal. But behaviour is also outcome-determined: it is very likely that mounting behaviour is more rewarding and reinforcing for the male and lordosis behaviour more so for the female. In the monkey, sexual behaviour is greatly influenced by social status and social experience to the extent that subordinate males may appear to be 'psychologically castrated' (Keverne, 1993). Behavioural interactions within the social group alter testosterone secretion as well as other neuroendocrine processes, in particular endogenous opiate activity.

Structural sex differences were also identified in the human brain, but the precise nature of the determining factors as well as the way in which the existing differences, possibly, determine behavioural consequences remain unknown. With regard to cognitive abilities, Gorski stresses the fact that the observed sex differences are basically statistical and that they can be test or task specific. Human males with a deficiency in the enzyme 5-alpha-reductase can appear to be females at birth, but owing to differential sociocultural influences they may display either a female or a male psychosexual identity at adulthood. There is no structural or functional characteristic of the human brain that accurately predicts an individual's sex, and sexual orientation is obviously multidetermined (See also Hines, 1993).

On the other hand, when considering the possible action of a single factor such as a gonadal hormone, one must be aware of the fact that it may influence sociosexual behaviour in many diverse ways. For instance, plasma testosterone levels were shown to determine, in part, the individual sensitivity to the aversive character of frustration, threat or provocation, in man and animal alike (Olweus et al., 1980), and in a group of young men several indices of aggressive behavioural characteristics were found to be positively correlated with resting testosterone levels (Gladue, 1991). In both rat (Aron et al., 1993) and monkey (Dixson, 1993), testosterone influences the development of social communication as it controls the production of, and the sensitivity to, significant olfactory cues. But gonadal hormones are also known to act in more general ways on the structure and activity of neural networks by regulating the development and subsequent remodeling of neural circuits, by modulating the effects of various neurotransmitters, and by controlling signal transduction inside the neuron (see Demotes-Mainard, Vernier & Vincent, 1993).

The correct interpretation of the effects of biological variables on behaviour can further be rendered difficult by the fact that these effects may be mediated through social processes rather than resulting from some more direct action on behaviour. Cairns (Chapter 14) clearly exemplifies this kind of indirect determination by showing how the influence exerted by the sexual maturation rate on the behaviour of 13 year-old girls may well be mediated through a strong bias in their social affiliations. One may add that things are even more complex owing to a high degree of circularity. Having duly considered that 'biological influences must be filtered through a social system which has values and pathways of its own', we must also consider that at any given time social influences are filtered through biological systems which have a number of individual features and that most of them somehow depend on prior interactions with the social system.

TOWARDS AN INTEGRATED BIO-PSYCHO-SOCIAL APPROACH OF AGGRESSIVE BEHAVIOUR

In the field of 'aggression research' behavioural neurobiology strove for decades to define categories and labels for the various forms of aggression and to uncover for each one of the thus defined separate entities a cerebral representation in the form of a separate, linearly organized, neural substrate. Quite naturally, the emphasis was put on the search for brain mechanisms that would specifically facilitate or inhibit the activity of one of these distinct 'motivational systems', thereby enhancing or reducing the propensity to *emit* the motivated behaviour in response to the relevant releasing stimuli. But such a biological perspective could not easily be reconciled with the psychological perspectives that were elaborated in the study of human aggression. Moreover, it proved to be an inappropriate conceptual framework within which the data obtained in animal experimentation could be aptly interpreted. Even when using a model as 'simple' as the rat's mouse-killing behaviour (Karli, 1956), it appeared that the cues emanating from the mouse were quite different according to whether we were considering a naive rat, or a rat which had been given an opportunity to become familiarized with the strange species, or else an experienced killer rat. Moreover, one and the same brain manipulation could produce quite different results depending on the rat's prior experience. To give just two examples: a septal lesion that markedly increases the probability of the killing behaviour in the naive, and 'neophobic', rat is without any such effect in rats that were previously familiarized with mice; an electrical stimulation of the periaqueductal grey induces both an aversive emotional state and an instrumental killing behaviour in the previously non-killing animal, while the same stimulation sharply interrupts an ongoing, and appetite motivated, killing behaviour in the experienced killer rat (Karli, 1981). In other words, it is important to consider both the brain structures and mechanisms that underlie the various operations of information processing and the kind of information that is being processed in any particular case. Cairns stresses the fact that 'genetic-neurobiological biases for aggressive behaviour' may be cancelled out or even reversed by the conditions of rearing as well as by the opportunities for social interaction, that is, by variables that may deeply influence the frames of reference used to process the current sensory input.

It certainly proved fruitful to shift our interest from a genetically-determined universal propensity to emit aggressive behaviour towards a historically determined individual relationship to (and way of coping with) a particular situation. More precisely, rather than to go on analysing and assembling the various components of the 'neural substrate' of a given form of behaviour, the major emphasis was put on the way in which a brain perceives an individually determined relationship to a given situation and on the way in which it anticipates, on the basis of prior experience, a method to cope with it by means of using one or another component of its behavioural repertoire (Karli 1987, 1989a, b, 1990, 1991). Neurobiology provides ways to study brain mechanisms which contribute to determine a number of features that characterize an individual and that in turn contribute to determine the probability that in the face of a given situation this individual will resort to an aggressive behaviour as the appropriate strategy. Among the various individual features that can be studied, the following are worth mentioning: the level of overall emotional responsiveness; the more specific sensitivity to the aversive character of threat, provocation, or frustration; the proneness to impulsive responding; the degree of anxiety; the kind of social bonds and emotions; the way of recording, and referring to, the life-history, especially the history of specific and relevant reinforcement. Obviously, such a biological perspective is much more in keeping with studies that aim at clarifying the role played in the generation of human aggression by personality factors such as 'irritability' and 'emotional susceptibility' (Caprara et al., 1983; Caprara & Pastorelli, 1989), 'weak self-control' with a marked dependence on situational cues and internal impulses (Pulkkinen & Hurme, 1984), and cognitive structures ('scripts') for social behaviour, which both determine and result from social interactions with their outcome expectancies (Huesmann & Eron, 1989). The individual life history should be given considerable attention, since it greatly contributes to shape not only the phenotypic expression – in brain structures and processes – of genetically coded information, but also the development, in close interaction with brain maturation, of personalized psychodynamics and cognitive structures. This is in addition to the continuous updating of the internal representations of a specific sociocultural environment with its values, aspirations, models and myths.

If we are to understand the complex determination of human behaviour, we are bound to elaborate and use an integrated biopsychosocial approach of brain-behaviour relationships. When formulating their 'developmental propositions', Magnusson & Cairns (see Cairns, Chapter 14) rightfully warn that since 'an individual develops and functions psychologically as an integrated organism' and since 'single aspects do not develop and function in isolation', the latter should never 'be divorced from the totality in analysis'.

THE MEDIATING AND INTEGRATING ROLE OF AFFECTIVE PROCESSES

In the development and functioning of such a totality as a social actor, an important (but often neglected) mediating and integrating role is played by affective processes. In social perception and social judgements, emotions and moods play a far more important role than in the case of perception and judgements of the objects of the physical world (see Forgas & Bower, 1988). Affective states have informational value so that a subject may well consult his feelings as a salient source of relevant information instead of basing his evaluation 'on a piecemeal analysis of the available facts' (Schwarz & Clore, 1988). In the development of social behaviour, affective processes ensure a two-way mediation between perception and action: it is in particular the association of a historically determined affective significance with the objective parameters of the sensory information that guides the choice of the behavioural strategy deemed appropriate. In return, the affective experience that results from the comparison of the consequences actually derived from the behaviour (with those that had been anticipated) may modify both the significance of the situation and the evaluation of the relevance of the strategy used. In other words, it is largely through the mediation of affective states that an overt social behaviour is often both a partial reactualization of the past and a determinant that contributes to shape the motivations of behaviours to follow.

Within the brain, one may differentiate – somewhat arbitrarily – three interacting levels of integration and organization that are implicated in the generation and action of affective attributes and states (Karli, 1989a, b, c, 1992). A preliminary remark should be made here: in animal experiments, the 'affective' (pleasant or unpleasant, appetitive or aversive) character of attributes and states can only be inferred from their effects on overt behaviour; they are not mere epiphenomena, but intervening variables, *signals* in their own right (see Kentridge & Aggleton, 1990).

(1) At the mesencephalic and diencephalic level, elementary affective attributes are associated with the current sensory information in an immediate and direct way so that the resulting behaviour merely fits in with the present moment and its basic biological meaning.

(2) It is through the bringing into play of a second level, which essentially corresponds to temporal lobe structures, that the behaviour acquires its historical dimension and that it both reflects and dynamically shapes an individual life history. At this level, the amygdala, in connection with other structures, is deeply involved in the control of social behaviour in two closely related ways: in the face of a given situation, an important step lies in the recognition of its full affective significance through reference to the traces laid down by past experiences, which generates some expectancy and guides the choice of the behavioural strategy to be used; in return, the latter significance may be modulated by the structuring, personalizing, effects of the concrete behavioural interaction with the social environment.

(3) At the 'highest' level where the prefrontal cortex is essentially implicated, there occur more complex cognitive and affective elaborations based on a number of internalized and continuously reshaped frames of reference so that the subject's behaviour can be in keeping with a more conscious, well considered, and deliberate personal plan.

At the mesencephalic and diencephalic level, the generation of elementary affective attributes results from the bringing into play of two distinct but interacting neuronal systems, the activation of which has opposing effects: a lateral system underlies appetence, reward and approach while a medial, periventricular, system underlies aversion, flight or defence. Our group has extensively studied the latter neuronal system which can be locally activated either by applying an electrical stimulation or by injecting an excitatory amino acid (Karli, 1987, 1989b, 1991, 1992; Schmitt & Karli, 1989). The basal activity and the responsiveness of this aversion and defence system are controlled by moderating influences that act on it in a permanent or a more episodic manner and that involve, in particular, GABAergic and opioidergic neurotransmissions. Both the processing of sensory information and the animal's overt behaviour can be manipulated by locally acting on one or the other of these neurotransmissions. For instance, an experimentally induced facilitation or blockade of the GABAergic transmission in the rat brings about an emotive biasing of input-output relationships that clearly affects the individual's social interactions. More concretely, a unilateral microinjection, into the periaqueductal grey, of a GABA agonist (which facilitates GABAergic transmission, thereby reinforcing the moderating influence exerted on the induction of aversion and defence) was found to provoke an ipsilateral hyperreactivity, enhanced *approach* responding to ipsilateral tactile stimulation, together with a clear facilitation of *offensive* behaviours. Conversely, unilateral microinjection of a GABA antagonist (with opposite local effects) was found to provoke a contralateral hyperreactivity, enhanced *withdrawal* and *escape* responding to any contralateral tactile stimulation, together with an increased tendency to display *defensive* behaviours. Some of these aversion-moderating influences most probably originate from the more laterally located reward system: escape responding induced by a medial hypothalamic stimulation can be attenuated by simultaneously stimulating the lateral hypothalamic reward system; and the escape-attenuating effects of the lateral hypothalamic stimulation happen to be closely correlated with its rewarding effects as assessed by self-stimulation experiments (Schmitt & Karli, 1984).

Throughout an individual life history, the amygdala is deeply involved in the mediation of the shaping influence of experience, as it has an essential part in the interplay of appetitive and aversive, positively reinforcing and negatively reinforcing, effects. Quite understandably therefore, amygdaloid lesions often deprive behaviour of some of its history-founded, personalized aspects. And if such lesions take place at an early stage of ontogeny, they interfere with the development of well-adapted, outcome-determined social interactions.

In the adult rat, amygdaloid lesions do not in any way prevent energy needs being satisfied by an adequate intake of food. They only modify certain individual attitudes to food: changes of varying degree in feeding habits and preferences as well as deficiencies in the acquisition of a conditioned aversion for a given food were often observed (e.g. Rolls & Rolls, 1973). As regards sexual behaviour, the classic notion of a lesion-induced 'hypersexuality' (in adult males of various species) takes in phenomena that should probably be considered as essentially *qualitative* anomalies of sexual behaviour, in particular the abolition of selective inhibitions that were developed in the course of ontogenesis (see Karli, 1976).

Behaviour determinants linked with the individual's past experience play a particularly important role in socio-affective interactions, and it is not surprising, therefore, that the latter get severely disrupted by amygdaloid lesions. If such lesions are carried out in monkeys living in the wild, it is noted that the animals so operated on are incapable of rejoining their group or a neighbouring one: they can no longer adapt their behaviour to that of their fellow creatures by referring to experience and their resocialization, therefore, becomes impossible (Kling & Brothers, 1992). In the rat, the probability that an aggressive behaviour is displayed in a given situation depends on the latter's affective significance; and the amygdala is implicated any time this significance is being modified by social interactions. This can be exemplified with the following concrete experimental facts. Various brain manipulations were shown to result in an initiation of mouse-killing behaviour only in those rats that had not been given any prior experience with mice, and a bilateral lesion of the medial amygdala was found to abolish this aggression-preventing effect of a prior familiarization with mice (Karli, 1981; Vergnes, 1981). The aversive experience of defeat as well as that of punishment result in a decreased probability that an aggressive strategy be used again. But the behavioural repercussions of defeat were shown to be markedly attenuated by bilateral lesions of the cortico-medial amygdala, whether the latter lesions were carried out before or after the defeat episode (Koolhaas, 1984).

As regards the ontogenetic development of the emotional and social responsiveness, the amygdala – in connection with the prefrontal cortex and the septum – is implicated in a progressive lowering of the degree of reactivity (more concretely, of the degree of behavioural activation induced by endogenous and exogenous stimuli) during the rat's early post-weaning period. When carried out in the infant rat (at the age of 7–8 days), both amygdaloid lesions (Eclancher & Karli, 1979a) and septal lesions (Eclancher & Karli, 1979b) result in a marked hyperreactivity that is still observed in the adult animal. But the amygdala is further involved in a more selective modelling of behaviour through the structuring influence of experience. It is in particular the *social play* activity that contributes to shape the individual's distinctive *behaviour style*, and Panksepp, Siviy & Normansell, (1984), consider that there is 'some predictable continuity between successes on the playing field and the successes of adult life'. Since early amygdaloid lesions not only provoke a lasting hyperreactivity but in addition reduce the frequency and duration of social play, they are bound to hinder the development of well-adapted social interactions. In the monkey, early temporal lobe lesions were shown to severely disrupt the development of socio-affective behaviour: the animals' behaviour is quite rigid and inappropriate, and their social interactions are extremely poor (Thompson, 1981; Bachevalier, 1990).

Whether an affective significance is being recognized or eventually modified on the basis of the behavioural outcome, the generation of the resulting affective state is brought about through functional interactions of the amygdala with the neural substrates of reward and aversion. The way in which a given stimulus is perceived and orientates the behaviour depends on individual characteristics of the latter functional relationships. In the cat, a naturally existing differential predisposition to respond *offensively* or *defensively* to a variety of environmental threats can be experimentally modified by manipulating the synaptic transmission properties between the amygdala and the ventro-medial hypothalamus (Adamec, 1991). The observed behavioural effect may also be due, in addition, to an increased excitability of the periaqueductal grey and to a modulation of the functioning of the benzo-diazepine receptors within the amygdala (Adamec, 1993). More generally, many individual features of socio-affective behaviour most probably result, in part, from the particular way in which a great variety of chemical transmitters and modulators affect the functional properties of amygdaloid neurons.

But the complexity of brain-behaviour relationships does not merely reflect that of brain functioning. It also, and even more so, reflects the circular character of many processes in the interplay of brain and behaviour. This circularity can be exemplified by considering the reciprocal shaping of septal functioning and social interactions. In the young rat, a similar hyperreactivity can be brought about by a septal lesion or by social isolation. Under normal conditions, the maturation of the septum's functional properties interacts with the developing social contacts so as to achieve an appropriate level of responsiveness. In other words, social interactions cannot have their normal impact on this behavioural dimension without the mediation of the septum and, conversely, the septum (in connection with other brain structures) cannot exert its moderating influence without being shaped and driven by social interactions.

As regards humoral factors, it is well-known that a great number of hormones, neurotransmitters and neuromodulators contribute to determine the generation of affective states and the elaboration of their behavioural expression by acting, in particular, on several 'limbic' brain structures (see Karli, 1987, 1989a, b, 1991, 1992). But in return, behavioural interactions and their outcome do affect the current level as well as the subsequent release of – and/or sensitivity to – one or the other of these chemical agents, and such humoral changes contribute to mediate the shaping influence of experience. For instance, the aversive experience of defeat was shown to provoke a lowering of both testosterone levels (rat, monkey) and corticosterone levels (mouse) with the effect of reducing the subsequent probability of aggressive behaviour and increasing that of submissive behaviour. In the adult rat, social isolation has anxiogenic effects that are partially related to a reduced release of serotonin within the brain (Maisonnette, Morato & Brandão, 1993). The exposure to various stressful situations further produces a certain degree of 'anhedonia' (a reduced sensitivity to the 'rewarding' effects of a given stimulation) which seems to be due to a reduced sensitivity of dopaminergic receptors in the nucleus accumbens (Zacharko & Anisman, 1991; Willner, Muscat & Papp, 1992). At each stage of the ontogenetic development, environmental influences may affect the maturation and functioning of a particular system or mechanism likely to be involved in the elaboration of socio-affective behaviour. Since endogenous opiates are known to play an important role in the generation of social emotions and in the processes of interindividual attachment, it suffices to mention here that the functioning of the rat's opiate systems was found to be altered by maternal stress during fetal life (Kinsley, Mann & Bridges, 1992) as well as by repeated maternal deprivation during the neonatal period (Hoersten et al., 1993).

Brain-behaviour relationships should always be examined in a historical, dynamic and synthetic perspective. When considering the 'bottom-up' elaboration of behaviour, any single mechanism acquires its full significance only if, after isolating it for the sake of analysis, we replace it within the relevant pattern of interacting determinants. Conversely, any possibly occurring 'top-down' modulation of the latter mechanism can be explained by the very fact that it is combined with others into a functional whole of higher order the 'emergent' properties of which get expressed in the overt behaviour and may act back on the mode of functioning of some of its constitutive elements.

FINAL COMMENT

A neurobiologist who studies brain-behaviour relationships using, for obvious ethical reasons, some laboratory species, even though he is basically
interested in a deeper understanding of how his own brain mediates the
dialogue(s) he carries on with his environment(s), is necessarily led to face the
question of whether – and what – he can rightfully extrapolate from animal to
man. Since any experimentally obtained piece of evidence takes on its true
and full meaning from interpretation within an appropriate conceptual
framework, such extrapolations are likely to be valid only to the extent that
the individual's developmental history and present mode of functioning are
being addressed by theory and experimental analysis in reconcilable ways
in both animal and man. As emphasized and concretely exemplified above, it
proved pertinent and fruitful for the study of brain-behaviour relationships
in various animal species to progressively switch from a quite atomized, linear
and static perspective over to a more holistic and dynamic one that would
fully recognize the essential integrating and shaping role played by complex
interactions, reciprocity and time. From such a perspective, valid and
promising bridges can be built between behavioural neurobiology and
human psychology, since the latter entered upon a similar evolution.
Some psychologists put forward an explicitly holistic and interactional
view of human individual development and functioning, emphasizing the
complementary notions that the individual develops and functions as an
integrated and integrating totality, that dynamic reciprocal interactions
take an essential part in the organization of any functional level at each
stage of development and that the actual meaning of any partial process basically derives from the role it plays within the developing and
functioning totality (see Magnusson, 1990; Magnusson & Törestad, 1993;
Cairns, Chapter 14).

REFERENCES

Adamec, R. E. (1991) Partial kindling of the ventral hippocampus: identification of
   changes in limbic physiology which accompany changes in feline aggression and
   defense. *Physiology and Behavior*, **49**, 443–53.
Adamec, R. E. (1993) Partial limbic kindling – brain, behavior, and the benzodiazepine
   receptor. *Physiology and Behavior*, **54**, 531–45.
Aron, C., Chateau, D., Chabli, A. & Schaeffer, C. (1993) Inherited and environmental
   determinants of bisexuality in the male rat. In Haug, M., Whalen, R. E., Aron, C.
   & Olsen, K. L. (eds.) *The Development of Sex Differences and Similarities in Behavior.*
   Dordrecht: Kluwer, pp. 1–18.
Bachevalier, J. (1990) Memory loss and the socio-emotional disturbances following neonatal damage of the limbic system in monkeys: an animal model for
   childhood autism. In Tamminga, C. A. & Schulz, S. C. (eds.) *Advances in Psychiatry: Schizophrenia, Vol. 1.* New York: Raven Press, pp. 129–40.

Caprara, G. V. & Pastorelli, C. (1989) Toward a reorientation of research on aggression. *European Journal of Personality*, **3**, 121–38.

Caprara, G. V., Renzi, P., Alcini, P., D'Imperio, G. & Travaglia, G. (1983). Instigation to aggress and escalation of aggression examined from a personological perspective: the role of irritability and emotional susceptibility. *Aggressive Behavior*, **9**, 345–51.

Demotes–Mainard, J., Vernier, Ph. & Vincent, J.-D. (1993) Hormonal control of neural function in the adult brain. *Current Opinion in Neurobiology*, **3**, 989–96.

Dixson, A. F. (1993) Sexual and aggressive behaviour of adult male marmosets (Callithrix jacchus) castrated neonatally, prepubertally, or in adulthood. *Physiology and Behavior*, **54**, 301–7.

Eclancher, F. & Karli, P. (1979a) Effects of early amygdaloid lesions on the development of reactivity in the rat. *Physiology and Behavior*, **22**, 1123–34.

Eclancher, F., & Karli, P. (1979b) Septal damage in infant and adult rats: effects on activity, emotionality, and muricide. *Aggressive Behavior*, **5**, 389–415.

Forgas, J. P., & Bower, G. H. (1988) Affect in social and personal judgements. In Fiedler, K. & Forgas, J. (eds.) *Affect, Cognition and Social Behavior,* Toronto: Hogrefe, pp. 183–208.

Gladue, B. A. (1991) Aggressive behavioural characteristics, hormones, and sexual orientation in men and women. *Aggressive Behavior*, **17**, 313–26.

Hines, M. (1993) Hormonal and neural correlates of sex-typed behavioural development in human beings. In Haug, M., Whalen, R. E., Aron, C. & Olsen, K. L. (eds.) *The Development of Sex Differences and Similarities in Behavior*. Dordrecht: Kluwer, pp. 131–49.

Hoersten, S. von, Dimitrijevic, M., Markovic, B. M. & Jankovic, B. D. (1993) Effect of early experience on behavior and immune response in the rat. *Physiology and Behavior*, **54**, 931–40.

Huesmann, L. R. & Eron, L. D. (1989) Individual differences and the trait of aggression. *European Journal of Personality,* **3**, 95–106.

Karli, P. (1956) The Norway rat's killing-response to the white mouse. An experimental analysis. *Behaviour*, **10**, 81–103.

Karli, P. (1976) Neurophysiologie du comportement. In Kayser, Ch. (ed.) *Physiologie,* 3rd edn, *Vol. 2.* Paris: Flammarion, pp. 1331–454.

Karli, P. (1981) Conceptual and methodological problems associated with the study of brain mechanisms underlying aggressive behaviour. In Brain, P. F. & Benton, D. (eds.) *The Biology of Aggression*. Alphen aan den Rijn: Sijthoff and Noordhoff, pp. 323–61.

Karli, P. (1987) *L'homme agressif.* Paris: Editions Odile Jacob.

Karli, P. (1989a) Is the concept of 'personality' relevant to the study of animal aggression? *European Journal of Personality*, **3**, 139–48.

Karli, P. (1989b) Studies on neurochemistry and behavior. In Blanchard, R. J., Brain, P. F., Blanchard, D. C. & Parmigiani, S. (eds.) *Ethoexperimental Approaches to the Study of Behavior*. Dordrecht: Kluwer, pp. 434–50.

Karli, P. (1989c) Perception, cognition and action: The mediating role of affective states. *Brain Behavior and Evolution,* **33**, 153–6.

Karli, P. (1990) Acteur social et régulation biologique. In *Acteur social et délinquance.* Liège: Pierre Mardaga, pp. 37–54.

Karli, P. (1991) *Animal and Human Aggression.* Oxford: Oxford University Press. (English version of the book published in French in 1987.)

Karli, P. (1992) De la perception à l'action: le rôle médiateur et structurant des états affectifs et des émotions. In Barreau, H. (ed.) *Le Cerveau et l'Esprit*. Paris: CNRS Editions, pp. 85–104.

Kentridge, R. W. & Aggleton, J. P. (1990) Emotion: sensory representation, reinforcement, and the temporal lobe. *Cognition and Emotion*, **4**, 191–208.

Kerchner, M. & Ward, I. L. (1992) SDN-MPOA volume in male rats is decreased by prenatal stress, but is not related to ejaculatory behavior. *Brain Research*, **581**, 244–51.

Keverne, E. B. (1993) Sex differences in primate social behavior. In Haug, M., Whalen, R. E., Aron, C. & Olsen, K. L. (eds.) *The Developments of Sex Differences and Similarities in Behavior*. Dordrecht: Kluwer, pp. 227–40.

Kinsley, C. H., Mann, P. E. & Bridges, R. S. (1992) Diminished luteinizing hormone release in prenatally stressed male rats after exposure to sexually receptive females. *Physiology and Behavior*, **52**, 925–8.

Kling, A. S. & Brothers, L. A. (1992) The amygdala and social behavior. In Aggleton, J. P. (ed.) *The Amygdala*. New York: Wiley–Liss, pp. 353–77.

Koolhaas, J. M. (1984) The corticomedial amygdala and the behavioural change due to defeat. In Bandler, R. (ed.) *Modulation of Sensorimotor Activity during Alterations in Behavioral States*. New York: Alan Liss, pp. 341–9.

Magnusson, D. (1990) Personality development from an interactional perspective. In Pervin, L. A. (ed.) *Handbook of Personality: Theory and Research*. New York: Guilford Press, pp. 193–222.

Magnusson, D. & Törestad, B. (1993). A holistic view of personality: a model revisited. *Annual Review of Psychology*, **44**, 427–52.

Maisonnette, S., Morato, S. & Brandão, M. L. (1993) Role of resocialization and of 5-HT1A receptor activation on the anxiogenic effects induced by isolation in the elevated plus-maze test. *Physiology and Behavior*, **54**, 753–8.

Olweus, D., Mattson, A., Schalling, D. & Lööw, H. (1980). Testosterone, aggression, physical and personality dimensions in normal adolescents. *Psychosomatic Medicine*, **42**, 253–69.

Panksepp, J., Siviy, S. & Normansell, L. (1984) The psychobiology of play: theoretical and methodological perspectives. *Neuroscience and Biobehavioral Reviews*, **8**, 465–92.

Pellis, S. M. & McKenna, M. M. (1992) Intrinsic and extrinsic influences on play fighting in rats: effects of dominance, partner's playfulness, temperament and neonatal exposure to testosterone propionate. *Behavioural Brain Research*, **50**, 135–45.

Pulkkinen, L. & Hurme, H. (1984) Aggression as a predictor of weak self-control. In *Human Action and Personality, Jyväskylä Studies in Education, Psychology and Social Research No. 54*, University of Jyväskylä, Finland, pp. 172–89.

Rolls, E. T. & Rolls, B. J. (1973) Altered food preference after lesions in the basolateral region of the amygdala in the rat. *Journal of Comparative and Physiological Psychology*, **83**, 248–59.

Schmitt, P. & Karli, P. (1984) Interactions between aversive and rewarding effects of hypothalamic stimulations. *Physiology and Behavior*, **32**, 617–27.

Schmitt, P. & Karli, P. (1989) Periventricular structures and the organization of affective states and their behavioural expression. *Brain Behavior and Evolution*, **33**, 162–4.

Schwarz, N. & Clore, G. L. (1988) How do I feel about it? The informative function of affective states. In Fiedler, K. & Forgas, J. (eds.) *Affect, Cognition and Social Behavior*. Toronto: Hogrefe, pp. 44–62.

Thompson, C. I. (1981) Long-term behavioral development of rhesus monkeys after amygdalectomy in infancy. In Ben-Ari, Y. (ed.) *The Amygdaloid Complex*. Amsterdam: Elsevier, pp. 259–70.

Vergnes, M. (1981) Effect of prior familiarization with mice on elicitation of mouse-killing in rats: role of the amygdala. In Ben-Ari, Y. (ed.) *The Amygdaloid Complex*. Amsterdam: Elsevier, pp. 293–304.

Ward, I. L. & Stehm, K. E. (1991) Prenatal stress feminizes juvenile play patterns in male rats. *Physiology and Behavior*, **50**, 601–5.

Wilk, R. van der (1991) Interests and their structural development: theoretical reflections. In Oppenheimer, L. & Valsiner, J. (eds.) *The Origins of Action*. New York: Springer-Verlag, pp. 159–73.

Willner, P., Muscat, R. & Papp, M. (1992) Chronic mild stress-induced anhedonia: a realistic animal model of depression. *Neuroscience and Biobehavioral Reviews*, **16**, 525–34.

Zacharko, R. M. & Anisman, H. (1991). Stressor-induced anhedonia in the mesocorticolimbic system. *Neuroscience and Biobehavioral Reviews*, **15**, 391–405.

PART V

SOCIAL COMPETENCE

The four chapters of this part all reflect a holistic view on individual functioning and development.

In Chapter 18 on biology and culture, Hinde assumes that the old controversy between the role of nature and nurture is laid down (cf. Chapters 2 and 5). After a discussion of stable and labile characteristics, using the development of gender differences as an illustration, Hinde focuses on the development of social relationships, social networks and beliefs and values in the individual development process. In the framework of a holistic view, the basic proposition is that the individual and the environment function and change as a complete integrated system. The characteristic feature of the development of the individual depends on the interplay of factors at all levels of the total system, from basic physiological and psychological processes to proximal and distal factors in the environment. The chapter ends with a summary of the consequences of this view for further research on individual development.

Kagan, in his introduction to Chapter 19, presents a historical background to the definition of the concept of temperament and the discussion of biological and social factors in the developmental processes underlying individual differences in temperament. Attention is drawn to the distinction between a nomothetical versus an idiographic approach to the study of temperament. With reference to his own and other relevant research, Kagan's main topic is the role of biological and social factors behind temperamental differences, in terms of low versus high reactivity, between inhibited and uninhibited children. Inherent biological factors are assumed to lie behind individual differences in reactivity, but the concluding central message is that though genes play a role in the development of temperament, they always share influence with experience, that is, with the environment.

A rapidly emerging field of scientific inquiry is developmental psychopathology. In Chapter 20, Rutter summarizes main issues in that field. The focus is on causation and on principles and mechanisms in the developmental processes underlying various aspects of psychopathological disorders. Relating to a discussion of different concepts of causation, key research issues are identified and appropriate research strategies and tactics are discussed. The author emphasizes the complexity of the processes to be studied which follows from a holistic, integrated view, but also that they are analyzable in terms of main principles and mechanisms.

In the last chapter in this part, Chapter 21, Hamburg takes a broad perspective in a discussion of social behavior. His main concern is means by which we can influence the development of individuals who can contribute to a peaceful world. He underlines the importance of the development of various aspects of prosocial behavior early in life. He discusses the role of the schools in empathy training, in training cooperation and in teaching conflict resolution, and he emphasizes the role of life skills training in adolescence. Attention is drawn to the positive and negative potentialities of television in the development of prosocial and antisocial behavior.

18 The interpenetration of biology and culture

ROBERT A. HINDE

INTRODUCTION

It is easy to seek explanations in terms of polar opposites. Fortunately, the dichotomies between nature and nurture, or innate and learned behaviour, have now been laid to rest – though they occasionally try to rear their ugly heads (Oyama, 1985). Contrasting 'biology' and 'culture' can be useful as an analytical tool, but it can easily lead us back into the same trap. Culture can appear as something laid on from the outside, an addition to the framework which processes of socialisation have constituted from a biological basis. This chapter attempts to avoid that dilemma. Although only certain aspects can be treated here, the full argument could be summarised as follows.

Development depends on processes of reciprocal interaction between embryo, foetus, baby or person and the environment. For most aspects of psychological development, the most important part of the environment is constituted by other persons (e.g. Magnusson, 1990). The interaction involves the individual responding selectively, acting on the environment, assigning meanings, and changing the environment, which in turn may act on the individual. As a result of such interactions, all babies and all persons of a given age/sex class come to resemble each other in certain ways, and to differ in others. Among the characteristics common to all individuals, of special importance are various propensities conducive to the formation of relationships with other persons. The relationships that are formed depend on the characteristics of the individuals involved, including their beliefs and values, and reciprocally affect those individuals, including their beliefs and values. Relationships affect relationships, and thus the influence they exert on the participating individuals depends in part on the social structure – that is, on the dynamic and potentially changing pattern of interdependent relationships and groups. The social structure is influenced by, and influences, the beliefs and values of the individuals involved and their relationships. Thus, to understand development, it is necessary to come to terms with diachronic relationships between physiology, individuals, their interactions, relationships, groups and societies, the physical environment and the sociocultural structure.

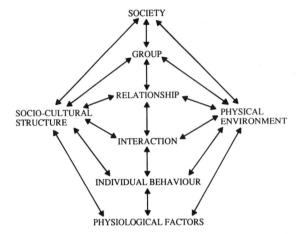

Figure 18.1. The dialectical relations between successive levels of social complexity.

Each of these levels, from individual behaviour to society, involves properties not relevant to the level below and requires new explanatory concepts. For instance, the relationships within a group may be arranged hierarchically, centripetally, and so on, but these are properties not relevant to individual relationships. Moreover, an aggressive interaction between two siblings may be ascribed to desire for possession of a toy, but ongoing aggressiveness in their relationship to sibling rivalry. But more importantly, each level of complexity affects and is affected by those adjacent to it, including the sociocultural structure of beliefs, values, and so on. For example, the course of a relationship depends both on the nature of the constituent interactions and on the group (or family) in which it is embedded. The whole forms a dynamic system such that no part can be fully understood in isolation from the others. This is illustrated in Figure 18.1.

A few key points from this sketch form the subjects of the following sections.

STABLE AND LABILE CHARACTERISTICS

Given that development involves continuous person-environment-person interactions, where can we break into the circle? Fortunately, it is not necessary to start at the very beginning: for the psychologist a convenient starting point is provided by the identification of psychological characteristics which, although variable, are recognisably present in all humans of a specified age and sex. Just as humans have noses, though no two noses are quite alike, so babies have a rooting reflex, mothers respond to a baby's smile, children learn to talk, adults seek for food, and so on, though of course individuals vary in degree on all these characteristics. We can regard such characteristics as the basic biology of human behaviour. This is not to return to the old dichotomy between innate and learned characteristics, but merely to recognise that it is possible to arrange psychological characteristics along a continuum from those that are developmentally stable with respect to environmental influences, and thus appear over virtually the whole range of environments over which life is possible, to those that are developmentally labile with respect to environmental conditions and are thus highly variable between individuals or appear over only a narrow range of conditions. For present purposes we need not concern ourselves with whether a character is ubiquitous because its development is unspecific in its environmental require-ments, or because its requirements are ubiquitously present. To take an animal example, all male chaffinches (*Fringilla coelebs*) have a predisposition to learn the species-characteristic song, but not other songs. This is a characteristic of chaffinches. The behaviour of singing the species-characteristic song is relatively stable because the presence of models to mimic and other necessary conditions are nearly always present in nature. But chaffinches not allowed to hear the normal song sing only a simple version, so the behaviour is not completely stable (Thorpe, 1961).

These relatively developmentally stable characteristics provide a basis for understanding both the similarities between humans across all cultures and all conditions and also, as we shall see, for understanding cultural diversity. They include aspects of perception (e.g. distinguishing figure from ground), motor patterns (e.g. the Moro reflex, the smile), responsiveness to stimuli (e.g. the alarm response of children to loud noises), motivation (e.g. to eat, drink, behave sexually), certain aspects of basic cognitive processes, pre-dispositions to learn, and so on.

Of course each of these developmentally stable characteristics has its own developmental history involving continuing interactions between the organism at each stage and its environment. Each is only *relatively* stable, varying within limits, and it is usually a reasonable assumption that each was evolved by natural selection in the environments in which our species evolved – some having a long history, others being specifically human. With some charac-teristics, such as the baby's response to loss of support, darkness or being alone, the role of natural selection seems clear enough, but in most it is a matter of reasonable conjecture, unlikely ever to be proven (Hinde, 1991).

At the other end of the developmentally stable-labile continuum, some characteristics are critically dependent on the environment. While the pro-pensity of a chaffinch to learn the species-characteristic song, as of a child to learn a language, is a stable characteristic, the actual song as learned is environmentally labile. Again, in the short-term, how an individual behaves is markedly influenced by the relationship context. In young children, observational data indicate that behaviour differs between, for instance, home and school (Hinde & Tobin, 1986). In adults, this is often described as involving the display of different role identities in different social situations

(McCall, 1970). In the longer term, interactions have consequences on the subsequent perceptions and behaviour of the participants: no aspect of what an individual does in interaction with another is independent of the past history of their relationship with each other or indeed with others.

But the diversity and complexity of human life depend on dialectical relations of the type illustrated in Figure 18.1. Let us trace out one example of the way in which biological, social and cultural factors interact – the genesis of gender differences in behaviour. To scotch the controversy almost invariably associated with the issue, it is helpful to consider four independent but interrelated questions. The *direction* of the differences between the behaviour of men and women in close relationships is remarkably similar across cultures, though the extent and patterning of the differences is highly variable. Thus we may first ask why the differences are in the direction in which they are. Why, for instance, are women not more assertive and aggressive than men? Why do relationships seem to matter more to women than to men? Comparisons of anatomy and behaviour between humans, non-human primates and other species strongly suggest that the direction of the differences is the result of natural selection. The sexes differ in reproductive physiology, and must therefore differ in their behavioural strategies if they are each to maximise individual reproductive success (or inclusive fitness). The issues here have been rehearsed often elsewhere, and turn on the characteristics likely to have been favoured in evolution to maximise the reproductive success. These differ between men and women: (a) male reproductive success depends in large measure on the number of females fertilised, so natural selection has operated to promote male competitiveness; (b) females are certain of their parenthood whereas males can be cuckolded, and females must invest more in each offspring than males: offspring survival is therefore more important to females than to males. Moreover, following from that, (c) if male assistance in parenthood is beneficial, the male-female relationship will be more important to the female than to the male (see e.g. Alexander, 1980; Buss, 1994; Hinde, 1984).

We may next ask how the differences develop. In earlier contributions to this volume, Gorski has shown how hormone treatment early in life can cause sex differences in brain structure in animals, and that differences in brain structure occur also in humans; and Goy has described the effects of early hormone treatment on sex differences in behaviour. While it is clear that pre- or perinatal hormones may determine the direction of gender differences, it is likely that postnatal experience plays an important role in their extent and patterning. In monkeys effects of postnatal experience on sex differences have been demonstrated, though they tend to be context dependent. but in humans social experience plays on the biologically influenced predispositions to produce long-term effects (Huston, 1983). The influence of parents, family and peer group have been widely studied, though they operate in different ways in different cultures. The processes include reinforcement, modelling and the internalization of norms. All of these are influenced by the gender stereotypes current in the culture: parents encourage in their children behaviour deemed appropriate for little girls or little boys and, acquiring the stereotypes, children of each sex attempt to behave as that sex is supposed to behave. Moreover, it must be noted, these stereotypes are affected by the way in which individuals actually behave. Thus the ways in which men and women are shown in advertisements reflect the societal stereotypes and both influence and are influenced by the way individuals actually behave.

A further question is why, at least in industrial societies, differences are so great as they are and why the stereotypes so greatly exaggerate and distort reality. A number of processes seem to be involved:

(1) In developing a self-concept, children see themselves as members of some categories and not of others. Of these, perhaps the most important is boy versus girl. As with membership of almost any other social group (Rabbie, 1991), they then tend to exaggerate the difference between their own group and the other, and (at least in the case of boys) to see their own group as superior.

(2) Denigration of the out-group (i.e. the other gender) may enhance an individual's status in his or her own.

(3) Games from which the opposite sex are excluded in children's games may express gender solidarity and help exaggerate the gender differences (Thorne, 1990).

(4) Individuals may enhance their chances of attracting a member of the opposite gender by exaggerating in themselves those characteristics deemed to be attractive to them (Deaux & Major, 1990).

(5) The stereotypes channel the behaviour of individuals, who act in a manner that confirms the stereotype (Rhode, 1990).

There is a further question of why the stereotypes differ between cultures. In any group the complex of values and beliefs, together with the patterning of relationships, must be seen as a structure, with different characteristics influencing each other. We must therefore expect both stereotypes and behavioural propensities to vary with a number of factors such as, for example, the economic possibilities for a woman to support herself and her children, the advantages and disadvantages of polygyny in the prevailing circumstances, and the extent to which residential arrangements make cuckoldry possible. Such issues will be influenced by both ecological and historical factors.

We see, then, that gender differences arise through an ongoing interplay between biological, psychological and sociocultural factors. Gender role development is not a matter merely of biological motivation, nor merely of psychological experience. What an individual experiences is influenced by his or her 'biological' nature, and experience interacts with biologically influential predispositions. Furthermore, the nature of that experience varies according to the nature of the individual's relationships with others, and with the prevailing culture, and affects those relationships and that culture.

BIOLOGY AND WHAT IS 'BEST'

Because the mention of natural selection in the last section may have caused the hackles of some psychologists to rise, it is as well to add that what is biologically natural is not necessarily *ipso facto* best. While it is true that any upset to the balance of developmental processes that has been adjusted by natural selection may bring unforeseen consequences, the issue is not simple. There are several points:

(1) What is biologically best means what is best for survival and reproduction. But what is best in one situation may not be so in another. Natural selection tends to produce alternative strategies of behaviour. For instance Main & Weston (1982) have argued that, if parents are not sensitively responsive, it may be better for infants to adopt an 'avoidant' style, enabling them to maintain contact without being pressing; while if conditions are harsh, it may be better for the infant to be competitive and assertive.

(2) The environment we live in now is not that in which natural selection acted. The principles that operated in development now may be different from those that operated then, and given infant characteristics may lead to different adult ones.

(3) What is biologically best for one partner in a relationship may not be best for both. Thus, it may be in a child's interests to seek more parental care than it is in the parents' biological interests to give (Trivers, 1974).

(4) What is biologically desirable may not be what is culturally desirable. 'Sensitive responsiveness' by a mother may mitigate against her own self-fulfilment according to the cultural norms. One can argue that such norms are 'wrong', but that will not lessen the maternal unhappiness, which may in turn rebound on the child.

(5) By definition, what is culturally best in one culture may not be so in another.

(6) The desideratum of 'psychological health' may depart from those of either biology or culture or both: this is an open issue (Hinde & Stevenson-Hinde, 1990).

PROPENSITIES CONDUCIVE TO THE FORMATION OF RELATIONSHIPS

In the present context, some of the most important of the relatively stable characteristics concern the propensities of infants to interact with, and form relationships with other individuals.

Babies are equipped with reflexes that facilitate finding the nipple and maintaining contact with the mother (Prechtl & Lenard, 1968). They are predisposed to respond to stimuli characteristic of people, in particular to faces and voices. They smile and cry, and parents are attuned to respond. They are predisposed to *interact* with others, and become disturbed if, in a face-to-face dialogue, the behaviour of the other is not related to their own (e.g. Trevarthen, 1979). They rapidly come to distinguish familiar from unfamiliar people, and respond differentially to approving and disapproving tones of voice (Papousek et al., 1991). Soon after the end of the first half year they monitor the expressions of their mothers, seeming to distinguish their emotions, and their behaviour to new situations is influenced by that of their mothers (Klinnert et al., 1983).

Towards the end of the first year, communication becomes increasingly advanced, and they start to use others to facilitate their own ends. Interactive games become common (e.g. Bruner & Sherwood, 1976). In their second year their responsiveness to the emotions of others becomes more finely tuned, and they begin to become aware of what is and is not appropriate in their culture (Kagen, 1981). Recently studies of 2-year-olds in their own homes, interacting with known others, have revealed that children develop powers of social and moral understanding much earlier than had earlier been supposed (Dunn, 1988). Two- and 3-year-olds show considerable understanding of others' feelings and goals, and have acquired considerable knowledge of social rules. They talk about mental states, and show curiosity about the behaviour of others.

These studies, which represent only a small fraction of those available in the literature, carry no implication that these abilities of babies are in any sense 'inborn' or 'innate'. Rather all, with the exception of early reflexes, are probably consequences of processes necessarily arising when a human infant grows up in an appropriate social environment. They are important here for two reasons. First, they show that children rapidly develop propensities to form *relationships* with other individuals, relationships of rapidly increasing complexity which involve quite sophisticated interpersonal perception. Secondly, these processes of socialisation are accompanied by acculturation. Dunn (1988: 183) put it thus:

From their first year, children are active participants in discourse about the social rules of their world. It is through the implicit and explicit messages in this moral discourse that they learn much of the nature of the rules of their particular culture.

Coming from a rather different orientation, Schweder (1990: 1) writes:

... human beings, starting at birth (and perhaps earlier), are highly motivated to seize meanings and resources out of a sociocultural environment that has been arranged to provide them with meanings and resources to seize and use.

... human beings and sociocultural environments interpenetrate each other's identity and cannot be analytically disjoined into independent and dependent variables.

These predispositions of the infant are matched by corresponding ones in the caregiver. Thus maternal behaviour is broadly similar across all cultures.

In its general outlines, the parent–child relationship has characteristics that seem likely to have promoted the biological fitness (i.e. inclusive fitness) of both mother and child in our environment of evolutionary adaptedness (Hinde, 1984). Bowlby (1969, 1973) conceptualised the mechanisms involved by postulating an 'attachment behaviour system' in the infant and a corresponding 'caregiver behaviour system' in the adult. ('Behaviour system' here refers to a software description of the relations between the various types of behaviour conducive to proximity. It is held to operate initially primarily in conditions of stress, and to lead to the formation of a parent–child relationship.)

The process by which early relationships affect subsequent personality are no doubt diverse, but an important role has been ascribed to the 'internal working models' of external reality which, it is postulated, the child acquires. Bowlby suggested that working models of the self and of the principal caregivers are of special significance and form a basis for future behaviour. Such working models tend to be stable, though they also have some flexibility and may be updated as relationships develop and change, and defensive processes may interfere with their formation in situations of mental pain and stress. The concept of the internal working model has recently been linked to object relations theory and to theories of cognitive development (e.g. Bretherton, 1990) and is proving to be a useful tool for understanding the development of social behaviour (Bartholomew, 1993). Interference with the formation of internal working models by defensive mechanisms provides a potential means for the intergenerational transmission of differences in relationship style (Bretherton, 1990).

While those with a psychoanalytical orientation regard the mother–child relationship as the primary influence on personality development, other relationships soon start to play a role. During recent decades attention has focused on the father, siblings, peers and a variety of life events. These matters are beyond the scope of this chapter: a recent review of children's relationships is provided by Dunn (1993).

It must not be forgotten not only that any interaction depends on and has consequences for both partners, but also that many interactions occur in the context of ongoing relationships and, as mentioned above, relationships may have properties in addition to those of their constituent interactions (Hinde, 1979). Thus it may be the global qualities of a relationship that are important for personality development, rather than, or as well as, the component interactions. For example Bowlby (1969, 1973) and Ainsworth et al. (1978) have emphasised the importance of 'maternal sensitivity', as manifested in diverse types of interaction, for the mother–child relationship. Similarly Maccoby & Martin (1983; see also Baumrind, 1971) related children's aggressive behaviour to two dimensions of parental style, namely high versus low control and accepting/responsive versus rejecting/unresponsive. In general, highly aggressive children were likely to have parents high on strong control and low on responsiveness, or low on both. Full understanding of development will therefore require an understanding of the dynamics of relationships. A discussion of current knowledge in this field would take us far afield, and space permits here only the statement that a science of interpersonal relationships requires (a) a solid basis of description; (b) an understanding of the various psychological processes that occur in inter-personal relationships; and (c) an analysis of the manner in which those processes enter into relationships of different sorts (see e.g. Hinde, 1979, 1995; Auhagen & von Salisch, 1993).

THE SOCIAL NETWORK

Relationships seldom occur in isolation. A's relationship with B may be affected by B's relationship with C, even if A and C never meet. This has been studied specifically in the family context.

Thus a number of studies have shown that the nature of the marital relationship is related to that of the parent–child relationship; that the parent–firstborn relationship is related to the parent–secondborn and the sibling relationship (Dunn, 1988); and that conflict may spread through the family (Hinde & Stevenson-Hinde, 1988). In all such cases the effects are likely to be two-way: thus not only may the marital relationship affect the mother–child relationship, but the reverse is also true. A considerable body of evidence is now available to show that mental health continues to depend on relationship support from others throughout life.

Clinically, it is important to recognise that such influences of one relationship on another may involve a number of different processes (Hinde & Stevenson-Hinde, 1988), such as:

(1) A's relationship with B may reduce the time or energy that A has for C.

(2) The psychological support provided by one relationship may provide fuel for the demands of another.

(3) Deficiencies in one relationship may increase the demands made on another.

(4) Competition between A and B for the attentions of C may affect their relationship with each other.

(5) The quality of one relationship may affect the general atmosphere of the group or family.

(6) The nature of one relationship *as perceived* by a participant may affect the future of that and other relationships as much as its actual nature.

(7) Social learning or modelling may occur.

Since the several relationships within a family may affect each other, the family can be regarded as a system of relationships (e.g. Minuchin, 1985). For instance, Byng-Hall & Stevenson-Hinde (1991) have shown that insecurity in attachment relationships may cause individuals to attempt to 'capture' an attachment figure, to turn to an inappropriate attachment figure, to respond inappropriately to attachment behaviour, and/or to expect loss comparable to that already experienced.

Furthermore the family must be seen as a psychological group (cf. Rabbie, 1991) and acquires properties of its own. Each family, for instance, may develop its own system of norms and values. While some like to ascribe properties of homeostasis or progressive change to the family as a whole, it seems preferable to seek for the underlying processes in individuals or in dyadic relationships.

A number of workers have attempted to demonstrate effects of relationships on relationships across generations in the context of transmission of parenting. For instance Caspi & Elder (1988) used data across four generations indicating the following sequence: personal instability leads to marital conflict, which leads to nonoptimal parenting which leads to a difficult child and thus to personal instability in the next generation. Problems recurring across generations may of course be due to the sharing of genetic factors, or to the sharing of similar social and physical circumstances, and not necessarily or directly to continuity in parenting attitudes or styles. As a result van IJzendoorn (1992) suggests that many cross-sectional studies are inadequate to demonstrate conclusively intergenerational transmission of parenting styles. Furthermore, the supposed effects are in any case usually small. However, IJzendoorn is apparently optimistic about the application of the Adult Attachment Interview (Main & Goldwyn, 1984). In studies using this instrument it is not supposed that childhood experiences translate directly into childrearing style, but rather that the current internal representation of the past held by the individual (e.g. Bretherton, 1990) plays a crucial role. Thus parents who had secure relationships with their own parents, and those who did not but have come to terms with their experiences, are likely to have secure relationships with their own children.

PERSONAL AND CULTURAL BELIEFS AND VALUES: THE SOCIOCULTURAL STRUCTURE

How an individual behaves depends in large measure on how he or she perceives the world, including the perception of the self. Here again relationships play a crucial role. Mead (1934) argued that we can evaluate ourselves only through the ways in which we perceive others to respond to us. Lewis & Brooks-Gunn (1979) have emphasised that the self is developed through the consequences of the infant's actions on the world. An important aspect of this is the individual's perception of his or her ability to control the environment (Seligman, 1975). This is probably one area in which the sensitive mothering emphasised by Bowlby and Ainsworth plays an important role.

In addition to the self-concept, the individual acquires notions of how the world functions – norms of behaviour, values, beliefs and knowledge of the institutions of the society and the rights and duties associated with the roles in those institutions. Some of these beliefs and values may be idiosyncratic, but most are acquired from and shared with at least some others, especially others with whom there is a close relationship. As we have seen, each family may have its own norms, and norms and values may be shared with peers in the workplace or members of a political or religious institution. In addition, individuals may share beliefs with others of their sex or age group, social class, and so on. Finally, some norms, beliefs and values may be shared by most or all members of a society.

It is to the latter that the term 'culture' is usually applied. Briefly, 'culture' refers here to those ways in which human groups or subgroups differ that are communicated between individuals, with special reference to beliefs, values and behaviour. 'Culture' is thus best viewed as existing in the minds (separately or collectively) of the individuals in a group. There is thus a continuum between the culture of a given society and the beliefs and values of the component individuals. It is an unfortunate fact that the former has become the province of sociologists and anthropologists, the latter of social and developmental psychologists: the ways in which beliefs affect behaviour must be basically similar whether they are idiosyncratic or shared by many others.

The culture of a group involves beliefs about the relations between the relationships between the component individuals, that is about the structure of the group. Furthermore, norms or beliefs relevant to one situation may influence and be influenced by those relevant to another. It is thus convenient to refer to the 'sociocultural structure', though there is no implication that in some instances the structure may not be dictated by the (e.g. authoritarian) views of one individual. The term 'structure' is important because not only do relationships affect relationships, but individuals seek for some coherence in their beliefs and values.

An individual's beliefs and values are acquired through the processes of socialisation/acculturation in the group in which she or he lives. But it is important to remember that the group culture is not a given, but a consequence of the activity of individuals. Thus views about divorce both reflect and influence the stability of marriages. This is an aspect of the series of dialectical relations between the several levels of social complexity shown in Figure 18.1 and the sociocultural structure. Physiological mechanisms (including the brain), individuals, interactions, relationships, groups, societies and the sociocultural structure itself are not to be seen as fixed entities, but as continuously created through the agency of these dialectics.

BELIEFS, VALUES AND DEVELOPMENT

Kohn (1969) suggested that the goals and values that parents have for their children are influenced by their social situation, including social class, that these goals and values influence their parental style, and this in turn affects child outcomes. A number of studies have shown relations between parenting styles and beliefs and child performance. For instance, as we have seen, Baumrind (1971) found that children whose parents have an authoritarian style (i.e. high control and low responsiveness) tend to show more problematic behaviour than those with authoritative parents (i.e. moderate control and moderate/high responsiveness). Okagaki & Sternberg (1993) found that the children of parents with strong beliefs about conformity tended to do less well in school.

That parents from different cultural backgrounds do in fact differ in their views about parenting and child development has been shown in a number of studies (e.g. Bornstein, 1991; Okagaki & Sternberg, 1993). However, studies involving direct comparisons across cultures face a number of problems. The major one is that of ensuring representativeness and comparability of samples. Since societies (e.g. countries) are themselves culturally heterogeneous, studies claiming to compare country X with country Y may in fact be using non-representative groups in one or the other. Furthermore, a given concept may have different meanings in different cultures. Thus Fujinaga (cited Okagaki & Sternberg, 1993) found that both Japanese and American middle-class mothers value independence in their children, but for the former this means the ability to engage in interdependent relationships and for the latter it means self-assertiveness.

Both the difficulty of heterogeneity within a society and that of the suitability of methods are illustrated by a meta-analysis of studies of 'attachment'. Ainsworth et al. (1978), studying the relations of 1 year olds to their mothers, recognised three patterns of mother–child relationship – avoidant (A), secure (B) and ambivalent (C) attachment. Subsequently, a fourth disorganised (D) category has been recognised (Main & Solomon, 1986), and the scheme has been somewhat elaborated for older children. IJzendoorn & Kroonenberg (1988) carried out a meta-analysis of 32 studies from eight different countries. This showed that, in a number of instances, samples from one country resembled those from other countries in the relative frequencies of A, B & C patterns more than they did each other. While the authors term this 'intracultural variation', it could perhaps better be seen as indicating the diversity of cultures within a society. However, it was also clear that A classifications were more prevalent in Western European countries and C classifications in Israel and Japan. Other studies have shown marked differences in the frequencies of the different patterns between samples differing in socioeconomic status or maternal mental health.

Yet another problem in cross-cultural work stems from the very complexity of cultural differences. Any two cultures differ along so many dimensions that it is extremely difficult to ascribe a difference in behaviour, development or capacity to any particular aspect of the culture – indeed, it is nearly always a mistake to do. The shortcomings of global characteristics of cultural factors has been illustrated by Liddell (in press) in a discussion of the complexity of the influences associated with the first year of schooling and with urbanisation in third world children.

In spite of problems such as these, a considerable number of cross-cultural studies have been carried out, classic examples being those organised by Whiting & Whiting (1975) of child-rearing in six cultures. Recently, considerable interest has been shown in the similarities and differences between the processes of socialisation and education in Europe and America on the one hand and Japan on the other. Early studies focusing on maternal style and infant activity produced rather contradictory data and gave rise to a prolonged discussion as to whether the differences were primarily genetic or cultural. Bornstein and colleagues (e.g. Bornstein, 1993), in more detailed studies, found both consistencies and differences in mother–child interaction across cultures. Not only some direct measures of infant or mother behavior, such as maternal responsiveness to infant distress or non-distress vocalizations, but also some aspects of the relations between maternal and infant behaviour, showed little cross-cultural variation. For instance, in most cultures mothers who often encouraged their infants' social-interactive behaviour had infants who orientated to them and interacted with them often, and mothers who called their infants' attention to external objects had infants who oriented more to objects in the environment. However, while American mothers induced their infants to attend to the environment more than Japanese mothers, Japanese mothers induced their infants to attend to themselves more than American mothers. Fernald & Morikawa (1993) similarly found that American mothers labelled objects more than did Japanese mothers, while Japanese mothers used objects to engage infants in social routines more than American mothers did. Again in comparisons of maternal speech between Argentina, France, Japan and the USA, Bornstein and colleagues (Bornstein, 1993; Tamis-LeMonda et al., 1992) showed that in all four countries there was substantial similarity in the types and frequency of the functional classes of speech addressed to infants. Both affect- and information-salient speech increased from five to 13 months in amount, but the proportion of the former fell. There were, however, differences in the amount of affect-salient speech (greater in Japan) and in information-salient speech (greater in the Western cultures), and further differences between cultures in the subcategories of information-salient speech. While these studies are in harmony with the popular conception that American mothers encourage more social forms of stimulation while Japanese mothers encourage closeness, it also emphasises some of the difficulties in understanding the processes involved in cross-cultural differences. At 13 months, American toddlers were more advanced in productive and receptive vocabularies, but less advanced in symbolic play, than their Japanese counterparts, and these differences also were correlated with differences in maternal style (Tamis-LeMonda et al., 1992).

A somewhat different approach involves investigating the precursors of a particular characteristic in several societies. For instance, the emphasis in many

Asian cultures on group harmony, cooperation with, and the prosocial behaviour towards, in-group members, contrasts with the emphasis on individualism in many Western countries, and especially the USA (Triandis, 1991). The Asian characteristics seem to be the result of purposeful efforts to train children from their early years to demonstrate prosocial behaviour. This early training may have long-term sequelae in superior academic success, the children being attentive and responsive to their teachers and helpful to each other, and subsequently in commercial success (Stevenson, 1991). Goody (1991) emphasises that the bases of prosocial behaviour may differ markedly between different small-scale societies. She distinguishes two modes. In the 'anxious mode' human social relations and the world are culturally defined as dangerous, so that the child must learn shyness and fearfulness (Urku, Semai). There may also be an insecure relationship with the mother leading to an insecure personality. In the 'secure mode', prosocial behaviour is learned through shaping and modelling within a strongly supportive setting, and developed in interdependence with other children in mixed age peer groups (Mbuti, Birifor, Fore).

CONCLUSION

We have seen how infants are born with a repertoire of behaviour patterns, propensities and potentialities for learning. We have hinted at, and other contributions to this conference have spelled out, how these give rise to the characteristics of the adult. Especially important are propensities to develop interpersonal relationships. These relationships with others play a crucial role – relationships whose nature depends on and influences the nature of the participating individuals. Moreover, those relationships, and the groups within which they are embedded, influence and are influenced by each other and by the beliefs, values, and so on of individuals, many of which are shared between individuals and form the sociocultural structure of the society.

In conclusion, then, we may underline three lessons for the future. We must cease to expect one-way causal relations, and expect action and reaction throughout development. We must not confine our studies to one level of analysis, but seek to find relations between them, combining analysis with synthesis. This will require us to cross and re-cross the divisions between developmental, personality, experimental and social psychology and anthropology.

REFERENCES

Ainsworth, M. D. S., Blehar, R. C., Waters, E. & Wall, S. (1978) *Patterns of Attachment: a Psychological Study of the Strange Situation.* New Jersey: Erlbaum.

Alexander, R. D. (1980) *Darwinism and Human Affairs.* London: Pitman.

Auhagen, A.-E. & von Salisch, M. (1993) *Zwischenmenschiche Beziehungen.* Göttingen: Hogrefe.

Bartholomew, K. (1993) From childhood to adult relationships: attachment theory and research. In Duck, S. (ed.) *Learning about Relationships*. Newby Park, Calif.: Sage, pp. 30–62.

Baumrind, D. (1971) Current patterns of parental authority. *Developmental Psychology Monographs*, **4**, (1,Pt 2).

Bornstein, M. H. (ed.) (1991) *Cultural Approaches to Parenting*. Hillsdale, NJ: Erlbaum.

Bornstein, M. H. (1993) Cross-cultural perspectives on parenting. In Eelen, P., d'Ydewalle, G. & Bertelson, P. (eds.) *Psychology at the XXV International Congress*. Hove: Erlbaum.

Bowlby, J. (1969, 1973) *Attachment and Loss. I. Attachment, II. Separation*. London: Hogarth.

Bretherton, I. (1990) Communication patterns, informal working models and the intergenerational transmission of attachment relationships. *Infant Mental Health Journal*, **11**, 237–52.

Bruner, J. S. & Sherwood, V. (1976) Peekaboo and the learning of rule structures. In Bruner, J. S., Jolly, A. & Sylva, K. (eds.) *Play: its Role in Development and Evolution*. New York: Basic Books, pp. 277–85.

Buss, D. (1994) *The Evolution of Desire*. New York: Basic Books.

Byng-Hall, J. & Stevenson-Hinde, J. (1991) Attachment relationships within a family system. *Infant Mental Health Journal*, **12**, 187–200.

Caspi, A. & Elder, G. H. Jr. (1988) Emergent family patterns: the intergenerational construction of problem behaviour and relationships. In Hinde, R. A. & Stevenson-Hinde, J. (eds.) *Relationship within Families: Mutual Influences*. New York: Oxford University Press, pp. 218–40.

Deaux, K. & Major, B. (1990) A socio-psychological model of gender. In Rhode, D. L. (ed.) *Theoretical Perspectives on Sexual Difference*. New Haven, Conn.: Yale University Press, pp. 89–99.

Dunn, J. (1988) *The Beginnings of Social Understanding*. Oxford: Blackwell.

Dunn, J. (1993) *Young Children's Close Relationships*. London: Sage.

Fernald, A. & Morikawa, H. (1993) Common themes and cultural variations in Japanese and American mothers' speech to infants. *Child Development*, **64**, 637–56.

Goody, E. (1991) The learning of prosocial behaviour in small-scale egalitarian societies. In Hinde, R. A. & Groebel, J. (eds.) *Cooperation and Prosocial Behaviour*. Cambridge: Cambridge University Press, pp. 106–28.

Hinde, R. A. (1979) *Towards Understanding Relationships*. London: Academic Press.

Hinde, R. A. (1984) Why do the sexes behave differently in close relationships? *Journal of Social and Personal Relationships*, **1**, 471–501.

Hinde, R. A. (1991) A biologist looks at anthropology. *Man*, **26**, 583–608.

Hinde, R. A. (1995) A suggested structure for a science of relationships. *Personal Relationships*, **2**, 1–15.

Hinde, R. A. & Stevenson-Hinde, J. (eds.) (1988) *Relationships within Families: Mutual Influences*. New York: Oxford University Press, pp. 365–85.

Hinde, R. A. & Stevenson-Hinde, J. (1990) Attachment: biological, cultural and individual desiderata. *Human Development*, **33**, 62–72.

Hinde, R. A. & Tobin, C. (1986) Temperament at home and behaviour in preschool. In Kohnstamm, G. A. (ed.) *Temperament Discussed*. Lisse: Swets & Zeitlinger, pp. 123–32.

Huston, A. C. (1983) Sex-typing. In Hetherington, E. M. (ed.) *Mussen: Handbook of Child Psychology, Vol. 4*, 4th edn. New York: John Wiley, pp. 387–468.

IJzendoorn, M. H. (1992) Intergenerational transmission of parenting. *Developmental Review*, **12**, 76–99.

IJzendoorn, M. H. & Kroonenberg, P. M. (1988) Cross-cultural patterns of attachment: a meta-analysis of the strange situation. *Child Development*, **59**, 147–56.

Kagan, J. (1981) *The Second Year*. Cambridge, Mass.: Harvard University Press.

Klinnert, M. D., Campos, J. J., Sorce, J. F., Emde, R. N. & Svejda, M. (1983) Emotions as behaviour regulators: social referencing in infancy. In Plutchik, R. & Kellerman, H. (eds.) *Emotion: Theory, Research and Experience. Vol. 2*. New York: Academic Press, pp. 57–86.

Kohn, M. L. (1969) *Class and Conformity: A Study in Values*. Homewood, Ill.: Dorsey.

Lewis, M. & Brooks-Gunn, J. (1979) *Social Cognition and the Acquisition of Self*. New York: Plenum Press.

Liddell, C. (in press) Diversities of Childhood in Developing Countries. In Eisenberg, L. & Desjarlais, R. (eds.) *Culture and Medicine*. Cambridge, Mass.: Harvard Medical School.

Maccoby, E. E. & Martin, J. A. (1983) Socialisation in the context of the family: parent–child interaction. In Hetherington, M. (ed.) *Mussen: Handbook of Child Psychology, Vol. IV*. New York: John Wiley, pp. 1–103.

Magnusson, D. (1990) Personality development from an interactional perspective. In Pervin, L. A. (ed.) *Handbook of Personality: Theory and Research*. New York: Guildford Press.

Main, M. & Goldwyn, R. (1984) Predicting rejection of her infant from mother's representation of her own experience. *Child Abuse and Neglect*, **8**, 203–17.

Main, M. & Solomon, J. (1986) Discovery of an insecure-disorganized/disoriented attachment pattern. In Brazelton, T. B. & Yogman, M. (eds.) *Affective Development in Infancy*. Norwood, NJ.: Ablex.

Main, M. & Weston, D. R. (1982) Avoidance of the attachment figure in infancy. In Parkes, C. M. & Stevenson-Hinde, J. (eds.) *The Place of Attachment in Human Behaviour*. London: Tavistock, pp. 31–59.

McCall, M. (1970) Boundary rules in relationships and encounters. In McCall, G. J., McCall, M., Denzin, N. K., Suttles, G. D. & Kurth, S. B. (eds.) *Social Relationships*. Chicago, Ill.: Aldine, pp. 3–34.

Mead, G. H. (1934) *Mind, Self and Society*. Chicago, Ill.: University of Chicago Press.

Minuchin, P. (1985) Families and individual development: Provocations from the field of family therapy. *Child Development*, **56**, 289–302.

Okagaki, L. & Sternberg, R. J. (1993) Parental beliefs and children's school performance. *Child Development*, **64**, 36–56.

Oyama, S. (1985) *The Ontogeny of Information*. Cambridge: Cambridge University Press.

Papousek, H., Papousek, M., Suomi, S. J. & Rahn, C. W. (1991) Preverbal communication and attachment: comparative views. In Gewirtz, J. & Kurtines, W. M. (eds.) *Intersections with Attachment*. Hillsdale, NJ.: Erlbaum, pp. 97–122.

Prechtl, H. F. R. & Lenard, M. G. (1968) *Verhaltens physiologie des Neugebornen*. *Fortschritte der Paedologie*. Berlin: Springer-Verlag.

Rabbie, J. M. (1991) Determinants of instrumental intra-group cooperation. In Hinde, R. A. & Groebel, J. (eds.) *Cooperation and Prosocial Behaviour*. Cambridge: Cambridge University Press, pp. 238–62.

Rhode, D. L. (1990) Definitions of difference. In Rhode, D. L. (ed.) *Theoretical Perspectives on Sexual Difference*. New Haven, Conn.: Yale University Press, pp. 197–212.

Schweder, R. A. (1990) Cultural psychology – what is it? In Stigler, J. W., Schweder, R. A. & Herdt, G. (eds.) *Cultural Psychology*. Cambridge: Cambridge University Press, pp. 1–46.

Seligman, M. E. P. (1975) *Helplessness: On Depression, Development and Death*. San Francisco, Calif.: Freeman Cooper.

Stevenson, H. W. (1991) The development of prosocial behaviour in large-scale collective societies: China and Japan. In Hinde, R. A. & Groebel, J. (eds.) *Cooperation and Prosocial Behaviour*. Cambridge: Cambridge University Press, pp. 89–105.

Tamis-LeMonda, C. S., Bornstein, M. H., Cypress, L., Toda, S. & Ogino, M. (1992) Language and play at one year: a comparison of toddlers and mothers in the United States and Japan. *International Journal of Behavioural Development*, **15**, 19–42.

Thorne, B. (1990) Children and gender: constructions of difference. In Rhode, D. L. (ed.) *Theoretical Perspectives on Sexual Difference*. New Haven, Conn.: Yale University Press, pp. 109–13.

Thorpe, W. H. (1961) *Bird Song*. Cambridge: Cambridge University Press.

Trevarthen, C. (1979) Communication and cooperation in early infancy. In Bullowa, M. (ed.) *Before Speech: The Beginning of Interpersonal Communication*. Cambridge: Cambridge University Press, pp. 321–48.

Triandis, H. C. (1991) Cross-cultural differences in assertiveness/competition vs. group loyalty/cooperation. In Hinde, R. A. & Groebel, J. (eds.) *Cooperation and Prosocial Behaviour*. Cambridge: Cambridge University Press, pp. 78–88.

Trivers, R. L. (1974) Parent-offspring conflict. *American Zoologist*, **14**, 249–64.

Whiting, B. B. & Whiting, J. W. M. (1975) *Children of Six Cultures*. Cambridge, Mass.: Harvard University Press.

19 Temperamental contributions to the development of social behavior

JEROME KAGAN

HISTORY OF THE CONCEPT OF TEMPERAMENT

The belief that some of the variation in human behavior is a result of inherent biological processes is an old idea. The ancient Greeks assumed, without a detailed appreciation of genetics or physiology, that the balance among the four humors of yellow and black bile, blood and phlegm created an opposition, within each person, of two complementary qualities of warm-cool and dry-moist. The balance in these two qualities produced an inner state that was responsible for observed variation in rationality, emotionality and behavior. Galen elaborated these Hippocratic ideas and named four fundamental personality types that were derivative of these qualities: melancholic, sanguine, choleric and phlegmatic (Siegel, 1968).

These ideas remained popular until the end of the nineteenth century when a sharp contrast between temperament and character emerged. Temperament referred to an inherited predisposition to particular emotional states while character referred to the expression of those predispositions in behaviors that were a joint function of both life history and the individual's biology (Roback, 1931). Jung supported this distinction in the twin notions of a private anima and public persona. The idea that certain body types represented partial signs of a person's temperament (Lombroso, 1911; Kretschemer, 1925) was especially popular in the last part of the nineteenth century and the early decades of this century. The Nazis were threatening Europe when William Sheldon (1940) published his data on the relation of body type to personality. The suggestion that inherited physical qualities, some of which were characteristic of ethnic groups, were linked to personality was too close to Hitler's version of the Aryan type. Hence, this research, along with a powerful eugenics movement in the United States, stopped suddenly.

Freud was a critical figure in the history of temperamental ideas for he substituted the concept of libido for Galen's four humors and made the balance among the motives of the id, thoughts of the ego, and the feelings of the superego the primary determinant of behavior. Although Freud's early writings awarded influence to temperament as well as to experience, the contribution of temperament faded in his later essays when he undermined the sharp boundary between an anxious, somewhat shy introvert who was not yet ready to see a physician and a phobic patient by arguing that both profiles were influenced by early social encounters. Freud muted the differences between the small proportion of adults with serious psychopathology and everyone else by arguing that both the terror of leaving home and worry about next month's debts could be derivatives of the same conflict (Freud, 1948). Thus, psychoanalytic ideas turned minds away from a temperamental category of person who was especially vulnerable to acquiring a symptom to a category of environment that produced symptoms. The adjective 'fearful' became a continuous dimension on which any person could be placed.

These ideas arrived in America when segments of the society were trying to quiet a group of scientists who claimed that the recent European immigrants were genetically less fit than those who had arrived in the seventeenth and eighteenth centuries. Because Freudian, and later behavioristic, principles minimized the significance of temperament, both sets of concepts were accepted with minimal resistance.

There are several reasons why temperamental concepts have returned after over 50 years of exile. First, scientists have documented the fact that closely related animal strains raised under identical laboratory conditions behave differently in response to the same intrusion; some of these behavioral tendencies can be bred in a remarkably small number of generations (Corey, 1978; Scott & Fuller, 1965). Secondly, recent progress in neuroscience has contributed to the community's receptivity to temperamental ideas. The brain contains over 150 different chemicals which, along with their receptors, influence the excitability of specific sites in the central nervous system. Individuals inherit different concentrations of these chemicals along with their receptors; hence, one can begin to imagine how a person might be especially vulnerable to depression, anxiety, or hyperactivity. Finally, the work of Thomas & Chess (1977) on infant temperaments motivated a number of developmental scientists to probe these ideas.

DEFINITIONS OF TERMS

There is legitimate disagreement surrounding the most useful sense and referential meanings of temperament, even though most scientists agree that temperament refers to stable emotional and behavioral reactions that appear early in life and are influenced, in part, by genetic factors. The most popular view, a derivative of the Thomas–Chess conception, emphasizes infant behaviors that are stable and functionally relevant for adaptation, especially those involving interactions with others (Thomas & Chess, 1977). It is assumed, further, that each characteristic is likely to be a continuous dimension. Because the nine Thomas–Chess temperamental dimensions were inferred from parental descriptions of infants, this functional perspective has been associated with a particular referential meaning; namely, replies to questionnaires by parents or other adults familiar with the child (Rothbart, 1989).

A less popular view of temperament, which has a shorter history and slightly different sense and referential meanings, is closer to the philosophical assumptions of scientists who describe strain differences in animal behavior. The sense meaning of temperament in this perspective emphasizes the inherited physiological foundations of a class of observed behaviors that is stable over time. This view minimizes, although not completely, the adaptive quality of the temperamental profile. I intend no pejorative evaluation in this contrast between a functional and a descriptive empirical strategy.

A descriptive perspective usually relies on behavioral observations rather than questionnaires to supply the primary referential meaning of temperament. Choice of this strategy is obvious when animals are the targets of research. However, because the correlations between direct observations of children and parental descriptions of what appear to be the same behaviors are modest, the theoretical meaning of a temperamental quality when observed behavior is the referent may not be the same as the meaning when parental report is the source of evidence. The agreement between parents and observers is low for most temperamental qualities – the correlations between the two are rarely above 0.4 and are often much lower (Seifer et al., 1994). The reasons for the poor agreement include parental distortions of their children's characteristics due to lack of objectivity and contrast effects, as well as variation among parents in the interpretations of the sentences presented on the questionnaires. Finally, some scientists invent temperamental constructs that involve physiological characteristics that parents are unable to observe.

Thus, conclusions about the stability and future consequences of a temperamental quality can be different when the data are derived from the two different sources, even though both perspectives define a temperamental quality as an inherited predisposition favoring particular emotions and responses that is moderately stable from infancy forward. Each set of conclusions is valid, but we should not automatically treat the two as equivalent. A reasonable analogy is the fact that the meanings of sentences about interspecific relations in phylogeny are not identical when bones rather than biochemistry supply the relevant evidence.

CONTINUA OR CATEGORIES

An important issue requiring discussion is the choice between a conception of a temperamental characteristic as a continuous behavioral dimension or as a qualitative category. Scientists who view temperament from a functional perspective prefer to treat temperamental concepts as continuous. For example, Thomas & Chess described the approach-withdrawal dimension as if all infants could be placed on a continuum with respect to the tendency to withdraw or to approach unfamiliar objects or events. Kagan and his colleagues believe that young children who are extreme in their avoidance of unfamiliar events are qualitatively different from those who consistently approach the same events (Kagan, Reznick & Snidman, 1988). Although temperature and volume can be measured continually, ice, liquid and steam are qualitatively different phenomena that emerge when particular values on these variables are actualized.

Recent research tends to favor the notion that some temperamental characteristics should be treated as qualitative categories. For example, patients with the profiles that psychiatrists call panic, obsessive-compulsive and social phobia show qualitatively different patterns of autonomic response in heart, muscle, arterial vessels and skin (Hoehn-Saric & McLeod, 1988). Further, analyses of psychological and physiological data that treat the sample of adults as composed of smaller qualitatively distinct groups arrived at a more coherent understanding than analyses that treated the corpus of data as comprising continuous dimensions of personality or autonomic arousal (Myrtek, 1984). The evidence supports David Magnusson (1988, 1992) who has argued that categories of people, not continuous variables, are stable and each category changes in a lawful way over time. David Lykken and his colleagues (1992) also argue for the usefulness of categories. Some personality constellations are the result of a combination of genes located on several different chromosomes that form a special configuration. When only one of the genes is missing a totally different phenotype is produced, not just a less extreme version of the one that defines the original profile. Meehl (1992) has made an equally persuasive argument for the theoretical utility of categories of people in the study of personality and mental illness.

INHIBITED AND UNINHIBITED CHILDREN

Psychologists study a variety of social behaviors in children, including shyness, sociability, aggression, conformity, dominance, nurturance, dependence and affiliation. Unfortunately, investigations of temperamental characteristics have not devoted equivalent effort to each of these behavioral classes. Because the most extensive body of evidence refers to shy and sociable behavior much of this chapter focuses on these two characteristics and what has been learned about the influence of temperament on their development. It is possible that when an equivalent level of progress has been attained for other behavioral categories, the theoretical structure of some of them will resemble the one to be described for inhibited and uninhibited temperaments. We view the two profiles as qualitative, defined by behavioral observations, influenced by genetic factors and leading to distinctly different psychological outcomes with growth.

One-third of 1 to 2 year-old children who are extremely fearful or avoidant in unfamiliar situations and shy with unfamiliar people, compared to those who are sociable and relatively bold, preserve these characteristics through late childhood and adolescence (Kagan et al., 1988). The stability correlations over periods of five or six years are between 0.3 and 0.5. It is important to appreciate that a consistent tendency to be shy or sociable in a 7 year-old is heterogeneous as to its origin. Some shy or sociable chldren (or adults) are born with a temperamental predisposition while others are not. The former group will show characteristics that the latter does not display; for example, temperamentally shy children are likely to show signs of sympathetic reactivity while those who acquired their shy profile are less likely to do so. One central, defining feature of the categories of inhibited and uninhibited temperaments is the 1 year-old's initial reaction to unfamiliar people, places and events. The inhibited 1 year-old child is typically subdued, quiet and avoidant to most unfamiliar events while the unihibited child usually approaches the same unfamiliar situations. If the unfamiliar event is a person, the child is called shy; the uninhibited child is called sociable. However, if the unfamiliar event is a physical challenge, the inhibited child is called avoidant and the uninhibited child is called bold. When the unfamiliar event is a high risk opportunity, the inhibited person is called cautious and the uninhibited one impulsive. However, with growth, some inhibited children learn to overcome their shyness with strangers but may retain a timid, fearful profile to unfamiliar nonsocial events. Hence, only some shy school-age children possess an inhibited temperament and some temperamentally inhibited children are not shy but display excessive timidity and caution. Thus, shy behavior and possession of an inhibited temperament are not synonyms in older children because a temperamentally inhibited child need not display all of the early features of the category. The predicate 'ability to fly' seems an apt analogy. Flying is characteristic of most birds, but not all birds fly and some animals that fly (like bats) are not birds. A similar stance must be taken with reference to shy behavior and an inhibited temperament (or sociable behavior and an uninhibited temperament) in older children.

Infant reactivity

Two distinct profiles of reactivity to stimulation seen in 4 month-old infants are predictive of the inhibited and uninhibited profiles in the second year (Kagan, 1994; Kagan & Snidman, 1991). These profiles can be understood by assuming that some infants are born with a low and some with a high threshold of excitability in the amygdala and its projections to ventral striatum, lateral hypothalamus, cingulate and downstream sympathetic targets. It is assumed that infants with low thresholds in both the basolateral and central areas of the amygdala and their projections will show high levels of motor activity, muscle spasticity and prolonged irritability to a standardized laboratory battery composed of visual, auditory and olfactory stimulation. These easily aroused, distressed infants, which make up about 20% of unselected, healthy Caucasian populations, are called high reactive. A complementary group of infants who show low levels of motor arousal and minimal irritability to the same stimulus events are assumed to have high amygdalar thresholds to stimulation. These infants, called low reactive, comprise about 40% of the same volunteer populations. The remaining infants show either high motor arousal and low irritability or low motor arousal with high irritability.

The concepts high and low reactive are related to Rothbart's (1989) theoretical ideas. Rothbart regards ease of arousal to stimulation, which she calls reactivity, and the ability to modulate that arousal, called self-regulation, as the two fundamental temperaments of the first year of life. Reactivity, for Rothbart, refers to the ease with which motor activity, crying, vocalization, smiling and automatic and endocrine responses are provoked by stimulation. Self-regulation refers to the processes that modulate reactivity, like attention, approach, withdrawal, attack and self-soothing.

Strelau (1983) places Rothbart's two temperamental categories in the brain by positing the two central nervous system processes of excitability and inhibition – an idea derived from Pavlov's writings. The reactive infant is presumed to have an excitable brain. The infant who regulates arousal well and does not move into a distressed or excessively excited state is presumed to have a strong inhibitory system.

Longitudinal study

We selected, from over 450 infants tested at 4 months of age, 73 high reactives and 147 low reactives and evaluated them at 14 and 21 months in a laboratory battery consisting of a variety of unfamiliar procedures. The incentives for the display of inhibited or uninhibited behavior included intrusion into their personal space (placing electrodes on their body or a blood pressure cuff on their arm), exposure to unfamiliar objects (robots, toy animals, papier mâché puppets), and encounters with unfamiliar people who behaved in an atypical way or wore a novel costume. A child who cried to any one of these events or did not approach an unfamiliar object when requested to do so was called fearful for that episode.

Figure 19.1 reveals that the high reactive infants were significantly more fearful at 14 months than low reactive infants ($F = 36.3$, $p < 0.0001$). Most of these children were evaluated again in a similar battery when they were 21 months old. About 40% of the high reactive infants were highly fearful (four or more fears) at both 14 and 21 months of age, while less than 10% showed minimal fear (zero or one fear) at the two ages. By contrast, about 40% of the low reactive infants were minimally fearful at the same two ages and less than 10% showed high fear (see Figure 19.2). Three-fourths of the children who were consistently high or low fear had been classified as either high or low reactive when they were 4 months old. Moreover, high reactive infants became dour and serious as they grew while low reactives became joyful and spontaneous. One can see the origins of

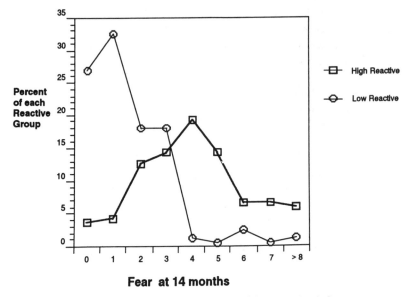

Fear at 14 months

Figure 19.1. Fear scores at 14 months for high and low reactive infants.

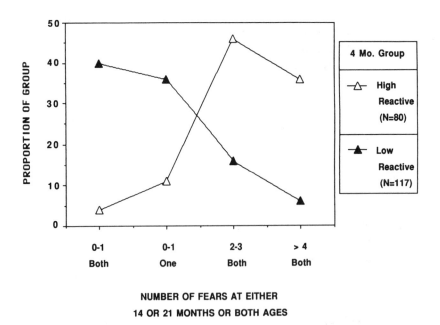

Figure 19.2. Relation of reactivity at 4 months to fear at 14 and 21 months.

Galen's melancholic and sanguine temperamental types before a child is 2 years old.

These two temperamental groups differ in facial skeleton in ways that would not have been surprising to some nineteenth-century observers and which imply the categorical nature of these two temperaments. Infants with very narrow facial skeletons at 14 months (ratio of width of the face at the bizygomatic to the height of the face) were more often high reactive at 4 months and showed high fear and infrequent smiling in the second year (Arcus & Kagan, in press). Children with broad faces were more often low reactive minimally fearful, and showed frequent smiling (see Figure 19.3). The 10 children with the narrowest faces (ratio <0.46) were significantly more fearful at 14 and 21 months than were the 10 children with the broadest faces (ratio >0.65).

As might be expected, the inhibited children with narrower faces are also more likely to have an ectomorphic body build. The fact that facial skeleton is a significant correlate of two temperamental groups argues for the influence of a set of genes that affects features as diverse as the growth of facial bone, ease of arousal in infancy, smiling and fear of unfamiliar events. It is of interest that inbred mouse strains, like A/Jax, that are susceptible to inhibition of palatal shelf growth following pharmacological doses of glucocorticoids, are more fearful in an open field than strains, like C57BL/6, that are far less susceptible to the influence of this molecule on facial bone (Walker & Fraser, 1956; Thompson, 1953).

A group of 95 children from the large cohort of over 450 children have been evaluated in our laboratory at $4\frac{1}{2}$ years of age. The study is ongoing;

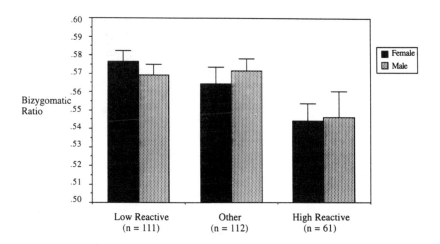

Four Month Classification

Figure 19.3. Ratio of facial width to length at 14 months in low reactive, high reactive, and other infants.

therefore, the analysis is preliminary. The children who had been high reactive infants displayed less frequent spontaneous comments and smiling, compared with those who had been low reactive, during a one hour interview with an unfamiliar female examiner (see Asendorpf, 1990). One-half of the high reactive children uttered fewer than 40 spontaneous comments and smiled less than 15 times. By contrast, over one-half of the low reactives uttered more than 40 spontaneous comments and smiled more than 15 times. Some low reactives smiled more than 50 times during the testing session. Spontaneous talking and smiling with an unfamiliar adult are two extremely sensitive signs of inhibited and uninhibited children. These responses differentiate the two groups in late childhood and adolescence.

Further, the children who had been low reactive were less intimidated by the adult female examiner. In one of the episodes the examiner asked the child to perform some actions that would normally be punished by parents. For example, the examiner opened a photo album containing pictures of herself, took out a large color photograph and as she handed it to the child said, 'This is my favorite picture; tear up my favorite picture'. Many more low than high reactives either asked her why they should perform that act or refused to do so. The refusal was not accompanied by signs of fear; rather, their behavior seemed to reflect the fact that low reactives were less fearful of not conforming to the requests of this authority figure. The high reactives seemed afraid to disobey the examiner and sheepishly tore a small corner from the photograph.

In addition, the high reactive infants showed greater interference in a variation of the Stroop procedure in which the child was required to name the color of a series of 27 pictures. One-third of the pictures, each one displayed on a screen, had a threatening symbolic quality (snake, knife, gun, witch), one-third were symbolic of happy states (ice cream, birthday cake, Mickey Mouse), and one-third were neutral in affective content. The children who had been high reactive, compared with low reactive, infants showed significantly longer response latencies to name the colors of the threatening compared to the positive pictures. Ohman (in press) notes that stimuli like snakes and angry faces have a biologically prepared potency to elicit a brief fear state in adults. These two pictures – an angry face and a snake – often produced long latencies among the $4\frac{1}{2}$ year-old children.

Heritability

Inhibited and uninhibited behaviors appear to be heritable. Matheny (1990), who has been studying identical and fraternal twins at the University of Louisville, reports that identical twins are more similar in their display of inhibited behavior than are fraternal twins; the heritability coefficient is about 0.5. The Institute of Behavioral Genetics at the University of Colorado is conducting a longitudinal study of a large number of same sex twin pairs who were first observed at 14 and 20 months and are being followed through late childhood. The heritability coefficients for inhibited and uninhibited behavior, based on observations in the laboratory in the second year, were between 0.5 and 0.6. The heritability estimates were higher (0.7 to 0.9) when the sample was restricted to the children who were extremely inhibited or uninhibited (i.e. greater than one standard deviation from the mean score for all children) (Robinson et al., 1993).

Physiological correlates of reactivity and inhibition

If future research affirms that inhibited and uninhibited children differ in the thresholds of excitability in the amygdala and its projections to motor and autonomic centers, then high reactive and inhibited children should show evidence of greater sympathetic reactivity than low reactive, uninhibited children. The data support that prediction for older inhibited children show greater pupillary dilation, greater cardiac acceleration, and larger changes in blood pressure to appropriate stressors than do uninhibited children (Kagan et al., 1988).

More impressive is the fact that more high than low reactive infants have higher fetal heart rates (over 140 bpm) a few weeks before birth than do low reactive infants. High reactive infants also showed higher two-week sleeping heart rates while being held erect, but not when held supine. This result, supported by power spectral analyses of the infants' sleeping heart rates, suggests that high reactive infants have greater sympathetic reactivity to challenge (Snidman et al., 1995).

Asymmetry and inhibition

Richard Davidson has been studying asymmetries in cerebral activation in frontal areas using desynchronization of alpha frequencies (6 to 12 Hz) as the index of activation (Davidson et al., 1990). Inhibited, compared with uninhibited, children show greater activation in the right compared with the left frontal area (Davidson et al., 1991). Moreover, high reactive infants show greater activation of the right frontal area, during both the first and second year, while low reactive infants show greater activation in the left frontal area (Fox, personal communication). It is of interest that the right archistriatum of chicks is more involved in fearful reactions to novelty than the left (Bradshaw & Rogers, 1993) and that kindling of the right amygdala in rats leads to greater avoidance in an elevated maze than does kindling of the left amygdala (Adamec & Morgan, 1994).

We have been studying bilateral asymmetry of skin temperature on the forehead. Skin temperature is controlled by the degree of sympathetically mediated vasoconstriction in the arterioles of the forehead. Because the sympathetic nervous system, unlike the skeletal motor system, does not cross, children with a more active right hemisphere might show greater constriction of vessels on the right side while those with greater left hemisphere activation, which is more common, should show greater constriction on the left side. Two year-old girls who had a cooler temperature on the right compared with the left forehead were significantly more inhibited than those with a cooler left forehead. Further, 2 year-old children, of both sexes, who had a cooler left compared with right forehead smiled more frequently and had a lower heart rate during the laboratory battery.

A profile that combined low reactivity and a low heart rate at four months with low fear, frequent smiling, and a cooler left forehead in the second year was characteristic of a very small group of boys who were exuberant, sociable, and full of vitality. This small, select group supports Magnusson's (1992) suggestion to search for categories of people, each defined by a distinct profile of characteristics, and Lykken's concept of emergenesis. The fact that less than 10% of this sample of over 450 infants displayed this combination has implications for current practices in research. Most laboratory studies of children or adults contain fewer than 40 unselected volunteers. If some temperamental categories, perhaps hyperactivity or attention deficit disorder, comprise less than 5–10% of the population, samples as small as 40 will contain only three or four subjects with these profiles. Investigators are unlikely to detect them because the correlations among the defining variables in a large sample of unselected subjects are low.

IMPLICATIONS

It appears that infants inherit two independent qualities: ease of arousal to stimulation, which is one of Rothbart's temperamental concepts, and the quality of the affective state that follows the heightened arousal. Motor activity and perhaps vocalization to auditory and visual stimulation in young infants seem to reflect ease of arousal. Smiling or distress reflects the valence of the state that follows the increased arousal. High reactive infants are easily aroused and, in addition, usually move into a state of distress following their heightened arousal. Low reactive infants, by contrast, do not become aroused easily. On those occasions when they do, about 20% assume a state investigators might call happy or joyful. Many of these children have very low and highly variable heart rates. We estimate that about 20% of infants show both ease of arousal and a distressed state while about 30% show ease of arousal and a joyful state.

Peter Lang and his colleagues also believe that ease and valence of arousal are separate adult characteristics (Lang et al., 1993). It may not be a coincidence that 16% of an adult sample in one of Lang's investigations showed a combination of both high sympathetic reactivity and minimal smiling – two salient characteristics of inhibited chilren, who comprise 20% of volunteer samples. By contrast, 33% of Lang's adults displayed low sympathetic reactivity and frequent smiling; a proportion remarkably close to our estimate of 35–40% for low reactive, uninhibited children.

Relevance for moral affects

These two temperamental categories may have implications for individual variation in morality. Kochanska (1991) first determined which of 58, 1 to 3 year-old middle-class children were inhibited and which uninhibited and observed their mothers to determine if they reasoned with their child when they made requests or simply demanded obedience by relying on their authority. When these children were 8 to 10 years old, they completed a set of stories and described the feelings of the protagonists. The children who had been inhibited six years earlier and, in addition, had mothers who used reasoning in their discipline told more stories indicative of a relatively strict conscience. Among the children who were uninhibited, maternal discipline style was unrelated to strictness of conscience.

Mothers of inhibited children report that their children are unusually sensitive to punishment and are intimidated by adult authority. It is possible that uninhibited children experience a diluted fear of adult punishment and, therefore, feel a less urgent need to conform to all family and community standards. If these children grow up in homes that do not punish antisocial behavior and interact with peers who invite such behavior, they may be at risk for conduct disorder. Obviously, if they grow up in homes in which asocial behavior is punished, there is little danger that they will become delinquent adolescents. Thus, David Magnusson (1988) is probably correct when he suggests that some boys are temperamentally vulnerable to a delinquent career. However, it is not that some children inherit genes for criminal behavior; rather, their biology probably affects their vulnerability to experiencing fear to the violations of ethical standards.

Anxiety disorders and introversion

It is likely that inhibited and uninhibited temperaments make a modest contribution to the later syndromes psychiatrists call anxiety disorders. Stability of inhibited behavior is more common in girls than in boys and extreme anxiety, phobias and panic attacks are more frequent among adult women than adult men. The heritability of generalized anxiety disorder or phobias (between 0.4 and 0.6) is close to the heritability of inhibited behavior. However, most inhibited children will not become adults with a profile that will fit one of the psychiatric categories. Prediction of a shy, restrained, introverted adult personality from early inhibition is much more likely.

Temperament and individual development

The inheritance of an initial temperamental quality, for example, an inhibited or an uninhibited disposition, leads to different phenotypic displays over the life course. The 4 month-old infant who is an inhibited type displays vigorous motor activity and extreme distress to stimulation. During the second and third years, the same child is likely to be shy with strangers and fearful in unfamiliar situations. By adolescence, however, many inhibited children are no longer excessively shy or timid, but still retain a dour emotional appearance, high muscle tension, and a preference for activities that are solitary. One of the most inhibited boys in our longitudinal sample told an interviewer, when he was a young adolescent, that he wanted to be an astrophysicist because he likes to work alone. Thus, as Jung anticipated, adults who were inhibited children are more likely to become introverts rather than extroverts.

The inhibited child is likely to carry a special vulnerability to uncertainty and anxiety throughout the lifespan. If life conditions are minimally stressful this individual may not appear to others to be very different from most in the society. However, should an unusual stress occur, for example, an earthquake, the possibility of unemployment, or uncertainty over promotion, the inhibited adult is more likely to react with signs of anxiety than the uninhibited individual facing the same situation. It is a demonstrated fact that only a proportion of adults react to a trauma with an extreme affective reaction. Thus, each temperamental category is linked to an envelope of outcomes; the one that is actualized will depend on the specific life experiences encountered.

Ethnicity and temperament

Finally, there is the possibility that the prevalence of some temperamental categories may differ among the world's ethnic groups. Reproductively isolated populations across the world possess different frequencies of particular genes. For example, northern Europeans, compared with Asians, have a higher incidence of the gene associated with a Rh negative blood type – 15% versus 1% (Cavalli-Sforza, 1991). Asians, however, have a higher frequency of one of the genes that is linked to a vulnerability to bladder cancer and lack an enzyme needed to metabolize alcohol, as well as one needed to tolerate the lactose present in milk (Lin et al., 1993; McCracken, 1971).

Over 25 years ago, Freedman & Freedman (1969) reported that newborn Asian-American infants, compared with European-American infants, were calmer, less emotionally labile, and more easily consoled when distressed. Chinese-American infants living in Boston were less active and far less vocal to visual and auditory events during the first year than Caucasian infants of the same social class living in the same neighborhoods (Kagan, Kearsley & Zelazo, 1978). Bronson (1972) also found that Caucasian infants showed higher reactivity than infants of Asian pedigree and Weisz and colleagues have reported similar personality differences between American and Thai adolescents (Weisz et al., 1988).

Table 19.1. *Means and standard deviations for five responses in American, Irish and Chinese 4 month-old infants*

Variable	American n = 247	Irish n = 106	Chinese n = 80
Motor activity	48.6 (31.9) 0–194	36.7 (26.2) 0–116	11.2 (1.3) 0–57
Cry (sec.)	7.0 (14.7) 0–89	2.9 (11.0) 0–98	1.1 (0.5) 0–32
Fret (% trials)	10.0 (12.3) 0–70	6.0 (8.9) 0–46	1.9 (5.2) 0–22
Vocalize (% trials)	31.4 (15.9) 0–78	31.1 (16.8) 0–67	8.1 (1.0) 0–54
Smile (% trials)	4.1 (6.0) 0–38	2.6 (4.2) 0–30	3.6 (0.6) 0–24

Note: Data are M(SD) with the range of values printed below.

We compared the four-month behavior of our Boston infants with 106 infants living in Dublin, born to parents who were born in Ireland, and 80 Beijing infants living with parents born in the People's Republic of China. The Caucasian infants, from both Dublin and Boston, had much higher levels of motor activity, irritability and vocalization to visual, auditory and olfactory stimulation than did the Chinese infants – a factor of four for motor and a factor of five for crying. Thus, significantly more Caucasian than Chinese infants were high reactive (Kagan et al., 1994) (see Table 19.1).

FINAL REFLECTIONS

Although genes make a contribution to infant reactivity and inhibited and uninhibited child profiles, genetic factors are not omnipotent and always share power with experience. Over one-third of high reactive infants were not exceptionally fearful in the second year; a small number were fearless. Home observations on 50 of the high reactive infants indicated that a mother's actions with the child affected the probability that a high reactive infant would become inhibited. A nurturing parent who consistently protected her high reactive infant from all minor stresses made it more, rather than less, difficult for that child to control an initial urge to retreat from strangers and unfamiliar events. Equally accepting mothers who made mundane age appropriate demands for cleanliness and conformity helped their high reactive infants tame their fearfulness. We expect that there will be interactions with experiences for all temperamental categories.

Because not all high reactive infants become inhibited, we propose that the terms inhibited type and uninhibited type refer to the two contrasting hypothetical genotypes that are inferred from features displayed in the first few months of life, especially high or low reactivity. The concept inhibited refers to the actualization of a shy, timid, fearful profile in the second year in children who are an inhibited type; the term uninhibited refers to the appearance of a bold, sociable, outgoing behavior in 2 year-old children who are an uninhibited type. We believe that analogous constructs will be useful for all temperamental categories.

We stress behavioral over physiological features in defining the temperamental categories because each of the peripheral biological signs we quantified was only modestly correlated with the behavioral characteristics. The biological measurements are analogous to seasonal migration as a defining characteristic for birds. Finally, we require a name for the inhibited or uninhibited child who later loses most of the defining behavioral characteristics of their category. We suggest that the terms formerly inhibited or formerly uninhibited name these children.

Because the theoretical meaning of the term inhibited involves a biological, behavioral and emotional profile, the behavior and affect displayed in a specific situation should not be regarded as conceptually separate from the biology that mediates the psychological profile. The idea of an inhibited child – and this conclusion may apply to all temperaments – combines both features.

The independence of an entity (for example, a child) from its functions was a major node of disagreement between Whitehead and Russell. Russell believed that the two ideas were independent, while Whitehead insisted they were a unity. Consider the statement, 'Lions stalk gazelles'. Russell would have argued that the predicate 'stalk' was applicable to a variety of animals and could be treated as an independent function. Whitehead would have claimed that lions stalk in a very particular way, different from that of hyenas; hence, the original idea should not be parsed into one class of agents and another class of actions. I side with Whitehead, as do all who believe that the motives, emotional mood, and posture of an agent who 'kisses' another are different if the agent is a 3 year-old child, a lover, or a grandfather. The predicate 'habituate' provides another example, for that term does not have the same meaning in the following four statements: infants habituate to repetitions of a stimulus, children habituate to unfamiliar settings, neurons habituate to electrical stimulation, and couples habituate to each other in the first year of marriage. The social behavior of inhibited children in unfamiliar situations is not exactly like the behavior of those who acquired their shy, timid demeanor through experience alone. The former group smiles less often and has greater muscle tension. Thus, it is unwise to treat the predicate 'is shy with others' as an independent function that is separable from the agent and the context of behavior. Thus, we must take into account the biology and history of a child, in addition to contemporary behavior. Scientists differ in the degree to which they impose an analytic or a holistic strategy on a phenomenon. Most human social behavior benefits from a holistic strategy because the context, as well as the cognitive structures, emotions and temperament of the agent, contribute to the behavior. None can be ignored. Hans Krebs, the biochemist with a metabolic cycle named after him, explained at age 70 why he, rather than Carl Martius, a leading chemist at the time, discovered the citric acid cycle 35 years earlier.

My guess is that it was a matter of scientific outlook ... Martius regarded himself ... as a theoretical organic chemist interested in reaction mechanisms. The degradation of citrate was for him a chemical and not a biological problem ... My outlook was that of a biologist trying to elucidate chemical events in living cells. I was accustomed to correlating reactions in living matter with the activities of the cell as a whole.

(Holmes, 1993: 426)

When a scientific domain is immature and underlying mechanisms are unknown, investigators have no choice but to invent categories that are defined primarily by similarity in surface characteristics. In the eighteenth century, animals that appeared different were placed in separate phyla, families, or species. But the evolutionary classifications of animals are reshuffled when new knowledge about origins is acquired. Nature is permissive with respect to the language we choose to name the forms in her garden of delights. She only insists that we respect the integrity of the objects that we move back and forth between our verbal inventions.

ACKNOWLEDGMENT

This research was supported in part by the John D. and Catherine T. MacArthur Foundation.

REFERENCES

Adamec, R. E. & Morgan, H. D. (1994) The effect of kindling of different nuclei in the left and right amygdala on anxiety in the rat. *Physiology and Behavior*, **55**, 1–12.

Arcus, D. & Kagan, J. (in press) Craniofacial variation and temperament in the first two years. *Child Development*.

Asendorpf, J. B. (1990) Development of inhibition during childhood. *Developmental Psychology*, **26**, 721–30.

Bradshaw, J. L. & Rogers, L. J. (1993) *The Evolution of Lateral Asymmetries, Language, Tool Use, and Intellect*. New York: Academic Press.

Bronson, G. W. (1972) Infants' reactions to unfamiliar persons and objects. *Monograph of the Society for Research in Child Development*, **37**, 1–81.

Cavalli-Sforza, L. L. (1991) Genes, people, and language. *Scientific American*, **265**, 104–11.

Corey, D. T. (1978) The detectors of exploration and neophobia. *Neuroscience and Biobehavioral Reviews*, **2**, 232–53.

Davidson, R. J., Ekman, P., Saron, C. D., Senulis, J. A. & Friesen, W. V. (1990) Approach-withdrawal and cerebral asymmetry. *Journal of Personality and Social Psychology*, **58**, 330–41.

Davidson, R. J., Finmann, R., Straus, A. & Kagan, J. (1991) Childhood temperament and frontal lobe activity. Unpublished manuscript.

Freedman, D. G. & Freedman, N. (1969) Behavioral differences between Chinese-American and American newborns. *Nature*, **224**, 1227.

Freud, S. (1948) *Inhibition and Symptoms*. London: Hogarth. (Originally published in German 1926.)

Hoehn-Saric, R. & McLeod, D. R. (1988) The peripheral sympathetic nervous system. *Psychiatric Clinics of North America*, **11**, 375–86.

Holmes, F. L. (1993) *Hans Krebs. Vol. 2*. New York: Oxford.

Kagan, J. (1994) *Galen's Prophecy*. New York: Basic Books.

Kagan, J., Arcus, D., Snidman, N., Wang, Y., Hendler, J. & Greene, S. (1994) Reactivity in infants. *Developmental Psychology*, **30**, 342–5.

Kagan, J., Kearsley, R. B. & Zelazo, P. R. (1978) *Infancy*. Cambridge: Harvard University Press.

Kagan, J., Reznick, J. S. & Snidman, N. (1988) Biological bases of childhood shyness. *Science*, **240**, 167–71.

Kagan, J. & Snidman, N. (1991) Infant predictors of inhibited profiles. *Psychological Science*, **2**, 40–4.

Kochanska, G. (1991) Socialization and temperament in the development of guilt and conscience. *Child Development*, **62**, 1379–92.

Kretschmer, E. (1925) *Physique and Character*, 2nd edn. Translated by Sprott, W. J. H. New York: Harcourt Brace.

Lang, P. J., Greenwald, M. K., Bradley, M. M. & Hamm, A. O. (1993) Looking at pictures: affective facial, visual and behavioral reactions. *Psychophysiology*, **30**, 261–73.

Lin, H. J., Han, C. Y., Lin, B. K. & Hardy, S. (1993) Slow acetylated mutations in the human polymorphic-acetyltransferease gene in the 786 Asians, Blacks, Hispanics and Whites. *American Journal of Human Genetics*, **52**, 827–34.

Lombroso, C. (1911) *Crime and Its Causes*. Boston: Little Brown.

Lykken, D. T., McGue, M., Tellegen, A. & Bouchard, P. J. (1992) Emergenesis. *American Psychologist*, **47**, 1565–77.

Magnusson, D. (1988) *Individual Development from an Interactive Perspective*. Hillsdale, NJ: Erlbaum.

Magnusson, D. (1992) Back to the phenomena. *European Journal of Personality*, **6**, 1–14.

Matheny, A. (1990) Developmental behavior genetics: the Louisville Study. In Hahn, M. E., Hewitt, J. K., Henderson, N. D. & Benno, R. H. (eds.) *Developmental Behavior Genetics: Neural, Biometrical, and Evolutionary Approaches*. New York: Oxford University Press, pp. 25–38.

McCracken, R. (1971) Lactose deficiency. *Current Anthropology*, **12**, 479–517.

Meehl, P. E. (1992) Factors, taxa traits, and types. *Journal of Personality*, **60**, 117–74.

Myrtek, M. (1984) *Constitutional Psychophysiology*. New York: Academic Press.

Ohman, A. (in press) Preferential preattentive processing of threat in anxiety. In Rapee, R. M. (ed.) *Current Controversies in the Anxiety Disorders*. New York: Guilford.

Roback, A. (1931) *The Psychology of Character*, 2nd edn. New York: Harcourt Brace.

Robinson, J. L., Kagan, J., Reznick, J. S. & Corley, R. (1993) The heritability of inhibited and uninhibited behavior. *Developmental Psychology*, **28**, 1030–7.

Rothbart, M. K. (1989) Temperament in Childhood. In Kohnstamm, G. A., Bates, J. E. & Rothbart, M. K. (eds.) *Temperament in Childhood*. Chichester: John Wiley, pp. 59–76.

Scott, J. P. & Fuller, J. (1965) *Genetics of the Social Behavior of the Dog*. Chicago: University of Chicago Press.

Seifer, R., Sameroff, A. J., Barrett, L. C. & Krafchuk, E. (1994) Infant temperament measured by multiple observations and mother report. *Child Development*, **65**, 1478–90.

Sheldon, W. H. (1940) *The Varieties of Human Physique*. New York: Harper.

Siegel, R. E. (1968) *Galen's System of Physiology and Medicine*. Basel: Karger.

Snidman, N., Kagan, J., Riordan, L. & Shannon, D. (1995) Cardiac function and behavioral reactivity in infancy. *Psychophysiology*, **32**, 199–207.

Strelau, J. (1983) *Temperament, Personality, and Activity*. New York: Academic Press.

Thomas, A. & Chess, S. (1977) *Temperament and Development*. New York: Brunner Mazel.

Thompson, W. R. (1953) The inheritance of behaviors: behavioral differences in 15 mouse strains. *Canadian Journal of Psychology*, **7**, 145–55.

Walker, B. E. & Fraser, F. C. (1956) Closure of the secondary palate in three strains of mice. *Journal of Embryology and Experimental Morphology*, **4**, 185–96.

Weisz, J. R., Suwanlert, S., Chaiyasit, W., Weiss, B., Walter, B. R. & Anderson, W. W. (1988) Thai and American perspectives on over and under controlled child behavior problems. *Journal of Consulting and Clinical Psychology*, **56**, 601–9.

20 Developmental psychopathology as an organizing research construct

MICHAEL RUTTER

For most of their history, the research fields of child development and of child psychiatry have remained rather separate. The approach of developmental psychopathology came into being during the 1970s and 1980s: because clinicians came to appreciate the importance of developmental issues in psychopathology; because developmentalists came to recognize the need to study the origins and course of individual patterns of behavioural maladaptation; and because of the accumulating evidence that a combination of developmental and clinical research strategies was particularly helpful in tackling many developmental questions. Developmental psychopathology does not constitute a theory, or even a body of knowledge, but rather it comprises a set of research strategies and tactics that capitalize on developmental variations, and on psychopathological variations, to ask questions about mechanisms and processes involved in the origins and course of psychopathology, about individual differences in responses to developmental challenges and transitions, and about individual differences in psychological development. A particular research design feature has involved the use of abnormal situations or abnormal cases as a means to pull apart variables that ordinarily go together. This has been evident, for example, in studies of autistic children, of *idiots savants*, and of deaf and blind children (see Rutter, 1993).

Because of the prime focus on understanding the causal mechanisms, there has been a need to find ways of applying experimental principles outside the laboratory (Rutter, 1994). The necessity of using epidemiological methods arises because so few of the risk variables are of a kind that are open to experimental manipulation in the laboratory. Nevertheless, it has proved possible to apply the same principles when using epidemiological and longitudinal data in real-life situations. The same need has led to research approaches that may disaggregate age into its separate components. Age indexes a wide variety of features including different types of biological maturation and also different types of experiences. If the changes associated with increasing chronological age are to be understood, it is necessary to determine which aspect of age is involved in the causal processes. A further feature that is inherent in the focus on causal mechanisms is the central concern to integrate neurobiological, psychological and sociocultural perspectives.

This chapter seeks to provide a 'flavour' of some of the most characteristic methods of study employed in developmental psychopathology, to note the range of different concepts of causation that have to be considered, to outline some of the key overarching research issues that dominate this field of enquiry, and in doing so to provide a few examples of some of the principles that have emerged from research in the field of developmental psychopathology (see Rutter, 1993; Rutter & Rutter, 1993; Rutter & Hay, 1994 for bibliography).

SOME RESEARCH STRATEGIES AND TACTICS

Use of longitudinal data

The first key research design feature concerns the emphasis on the use of longitudinal data (Rutter, 1994). Farrington (1988) pointed out the major advantage, when tackling causal questions, of moving from a focus on between group differences to a focus on changes within the individual over time as they relate to the experience of specified risk and protective factors. Many advantages accrue but five warrant special mention. First, the existence of longitudinal data, provided they are available before the risk experience under investigation, allow determination of whether or not there were psychopathological differences between exposed and non-exposed groups *before* risk exposure. That has proved to be an important consideration with respect to several risk factors. For example Block, Block & Gjerde (1986) showed that, to some extent, the psychopathological risks associated with parental divorce were already evident in the children before the divorce took place. Cherlin et al. (1991) have confirmed this finding in two further large data sets. The strong implication is that, although family break-up as such may add to the risks, the main risk must lie in features associated with the divorce rather than divorce as an isolated event. Much the same applies to the psychopathological risks associated with children being taken into group foster care. Children admitted into care because of family breakdown or a failure in parenting are indeed at an increased psychopathological risk but, as with divorce, the risks stem from associated factors rather than from the act of being taken from the parental home into group foster care. Findings of this sort have been crucially important in providing a redirection of focus on the possible risk processes that may be operating in these circumstances.

Secondly, the availability of longitudinal data allows concentration on what happens to children who appear psychologically normal at the outset but who then encounter the risk experience that is being considered. If such children develop psychopathology anew following the risk experience, this provides a strong pointer to the likelihood that change reflects some causal mechanism associated with the experience. Thus, Richman, Stevenson & Graham (1982) in their longitudinal epidemiological study of children followed from the age of 3 to the age of 8 showed that the experience of family discord was accompanied by adverse within-individual psychopathological change in children exposed to these family risk circumstances.

Thirdly, longitudinal data allow use of the test of reversal. That is, they may be employed to determine whether there are the predicted reductions in psychopathology that are supposed to follow the loss, or at least major reduction in, the specified risk factor. Thus, the finding that psychological distress goes down when unemployed people are successful in obtaining paid work, combined with the finding that there is an increase in distress when people lose their job does much to support the causal inference. Similarly, the evidence of cognitive recovery following children's rescue from grossly depriving circumstances or following head injury adds to the strength of the causal inference.

Fourthly, there are substantial gains associated with the possibility of focusing on within-individual change during the course of exposure to the experience under study. For example, Mortimore et al. (1988) were able to demonstrate the major effects of variations in the quality of schooling by studying changes in scholastic achievement over the course of the elementary school years in children attending different schools within London. School effects, when studied in this way, were substantially greater than those evident in studies considering only the end point. That is because family influences (both genetic and experiential) had already led to major individual differences at the time of starting school. Schools could not have effects before the children began to attend them. Findings such as these have led to a reevaluation of the importance of school effects.

Fifthly, longitudinal data are important in determining whether risk effects persist over time in ways that are independent of social context. For example, numerous studies have shown the strong associations between reading difficulties and conduct disturbances in childhood. Moreover, numerous studies have also shown the strong persistence of conduct disorders from childhood into adult life and the persistence of reading difficulties. One might suppose, therefore, that individuals with serious reading difficulties in childhood would have a major increase in psychopathological disorders in adult life. Rather surprisingly, the longitudinal study undertaken by Maughan et al. (in press) has shown that, at least with an inner city sample, the increase in disorder in adulthood is quite trivial. The finding is important because it suggests that the risk may not be a function of the basic neuropsychological deficit that is commonly supposed to be important but rather a function of the combination of scholastic difficulties and the demands imposed by the education system. Once people have left school, their reading difficulties continue but it seems that the psychopathological risks associated with them may well diminish. Of course, the finding needs to be replicated in other samples but it indicates the additional research leverage provided by long-term longitudinal data.

'Natural experiments'

The essence of a laboratory experiment consists of waggling one variable, while holding everything else constant, in order to determine if it causes another variable to move. Its strengths lie in the ability to separate the effects of different variables by manipulating only one at a time, by the power to determine whether the effects follow a consistent and predictable temporal relationship, and by the ability to determine whether the effects are found consistently across a range of circumstances that vary in all sorts of features except the one under direct study. These derive from the control provided by the laboratory situation and by the planned changes introduced by deliberate manipulation of variables. The challenge for epidemiologists and developmentalists is to find parallels that mimic these controls as closely as possible but do so in the natural environment.

Genetic designs that use circumstances separating nature and nurture provide the best known of these experiments of nature. Both twins and adoptees provide circumstances that separate genetic and nongenetic effects in ways that provide great research leverage. There are quite a few different variants of these designs (for example, identical twins separated at birth, the offspring of identical and of nonidentical twins, etc.), and each has a rather different pattern of strengths and limitations. Together, however, they provide a most powerful means of differentiating genetic and nongenetic effects and, within the latter, between shared and nonshared effects. Traditionally, they have been mainly used to quantify the strength of genetic effects. But that is of very limited interest in its own right. Rather, the strength of these genetic designs lies in their power to test hypotheses about causal mechanisms both genetic and nongenetic. Thus, it is only with genetically sensitive designs that environmental risk hypotheses can be put to the test in a satisfactory manner. Also, contrasting hypotheses about genetic mechanisms may also be examined. For example, does the genetic component in the risk for alcoholism lie in individual differences in susceptibility to alcohol, in a risk-taking tendency or in vulnerability to a disease state?

Twinning provides other experimental opportunities that are independent of genetic considerations. For example, it has been found that, as a group, twins tend to lag behind singletons in the acquisition of language and of verbal skills more generally. This difference provides the opportunity to examine influences on language development. The tactic consists of determining whether the environmental features that differentiate twins and singletons also account for variations in language development within twin samples, within singleton samples, and thereby account for the group differences between twins and singletons. The two chief contenders as possible causal influences in this connection concern obstetric complications on the one hand and differences in postnatal family interaction on the other hand.

Naturally occurring sample variations offer another opportunity to separate variables, provided that the variations arise for reasons unconnected with the postulated risk mechanism. For example, Cahan & Cohen (1989) used this method to differentiate the effects of chronological age from the effects of schooling on different aspects of cognitive performance. They noted that if the organization of the educational system required that children enter school at a fixed time (e.g. in September), a contrasting of variations by age within a school year and variations by duration of schooling, by comparing one school year with the next one, provided just the experimental separation necessary. The findings showed that both chronological age and education were influential but that for most cognitive outcomes, the effects of the latter were somewhat stronger.

The very substantial individual variation in the age at which children reach puberty provides a comparable opportunity to separate the effects of puberty from chronological age. For example, Angold & Rutter (1992) showed that the rise in depressive syndromes over the course of adolescence was more strongly associated with age than with pubertal status. By contrast, the rise in eating disorders during the same age period is probably more a function of puberty (or rather the weight changes associated with puberty) than of age per se. The same disjunction between age and puberty has been used most effectively to examine the behavioural consequences of girls reaching the menarche unusually early. Stattin & Magnusson (1990) found that early maturing girls showed a rise in norm breaking behaviour and also a tendency to drop out of schooling compared with girls reaching puberty later. However, they went on to demonstrate that this effect was a function of the tendency for many, but not all, unusually early maturing girls to associate with older peers. Caspi et al. (1993) replicated the finding in a New Zealand longitudinal study.

A further quasi-experimental opportunity is provided by circumstances involving a change in risk factor. This is a satisfactory research strategy, however, only when there are longitudinal data (or failing those, satisfactory retrospective data) that can allow documentation of a change in psychological functioning that follows the risk or protective experience. For example, West (1982) was able to show that when boys move from inner London to somewhere outside the Metropolis this was accompanied by a significant reduction in their delinquent activities as measured by both self report and crime records. It has still to be determined which aspects of the move were responsible for this beneficial alteration in behaviour. The causal explanation could lie in factors as diverse as a change in peer group, altered crime opportunities, and changed patterns of family interaction. Nevertheless, the data are convincing in showing that the move is highly likely to index some influential causal process.

The dispersal of children to a wide range of secondary schools at the time that they leave primary school has been used similarly to investigate the effects of the quality of schooling experience. In this case, the experiment was constrained by the fact that the distribution of children to secondary schools was far from random. Accordingly, there was the need to take into account differences prior to secondary school admission and to adjust for them accordingly in the statistical analysis. Inevitably, that means that there has to be heavy reliance on the measurement of possibly relevant confounding variables. That is a common problem in research outside the laboratory but it is one in which the combination of careful measurement of relevant variables, the analysis of changes over time, and replication across widely differing samples provides a strong means of examining causal hypotheses with some rigour. As already noted, the 'rescue' of children from severely depriving circumstances provides another experimental opportunity (as does the experience of head injury).

Contrasting patterns of correlates

The third key strategy involves the use of competing patterns of correlates in order to separate variables. The essential first step in this tactic is the specification of some postulated mediating mechanism. That is crucial in order to move from risk indicators to causal risk processes. For example, at one time 'broken homes' were considered as an important risk factor for child and adult psychopathology. The contrasting of the effects of parental death and parental divorce or separation have provided one of the first means of testing the competing hypothesized mechanisms of parental loss and family discord. The finding that with both child outcomes and adult outcomes, the ill effects of parental divorce or separation far outweighed those of parental death provided a strong pointer to the likelihood that the mechanism involved some aspect of discord rather than some aspect of loss. Of course, in many circumstances, it is crucial to go beyond a simple comparison of risks. Thus, for example, Fergusson, Horwood & Lynskey (1992) found that the overall psychopathological risks associated with family discord and those associated with family separations, changes and disruptions were approximately the same. The crucial next step consisted of comparing the effects of one after controlling for the other. The results showed that there was a substantial dose-response relationship between the degree of family discord and the risks to the children, after controlling for family changes, whereas there was no dose-response relationship between the number of changes and the risk to the child once discord had been taken into account. Again, the findings pointed to the probability that the risk mechanism involved some aspect of discord.

The examples just given all involved analyses within a single sample. However, in most circumstances it is better if one can compare subgroups that differ in their pattern of correlates or, better still, take entirely different samples that do so. For example, Vorria (1991) compared the psychological functioning of children reared in group homes according to whether they had been admitted because they had been orphaned or because of parental poverty as compared with those admitted because of family discord or a breakdown in parenting. The finding that ill effects were mainly found in the latter group suggested either that the main risk mechanism lay in the experiences before coming into the institution or, alternatively, that institutional ill effects were mainly evident in those who were vulnerable by virtue of prior experiences or genetic susceptibility. In much the same way, Rutter & Quinton (1984) and Quinton et al. (1993) examined the effects of parental mental disorder and an institutional upbringing respectively by using contrasts with general population samples. In both cases, the findings indicated that the main risks were associated with experiences evident in all samples but which occurred more often in association with parental mental disorder or an institutional upbringing. The implication is that the two risk factors mainly operated because they predisposed to other risk factors rather than because they constituted a major risk in themselves (although there was evidence that to some extent that was also the case).

DIFFERENT CONCEPTS OF CAUSATION

There is a general tendency with respect to psychopathology to think of causation only in terms of the 'who' question of individual differences. That is, causation is conceptualized in terms of the factors that result in 'A' showing a high level of aggression and 'B' showing a low level or 'X' exhibiting a depressive disorder and 'Y' not doing so. That is indeed an important causal question but it is very far from the only one that needs to be posed.

Dimensions and categories

Perhaps the first feature that characterizes the distinctiveness of a developmental psychopathology approach to causation is a concern with the contrasting of dimensions and categories. Traditionally, psychologists have tended to adopt a dimensional perspective in which clinical disorders are viewed as the extreme negative end of a continuum. By contrast, psychiatrists tend to think of disorders as qualitatively distinct from normality, rather than as an end of a continuum. Developmental psychopathology accepts neither assumption but, instead, puts the issue of continuities and discontinuities across the span of behavioural variation as a key issue to be investigated. The answer may differ according to the facet that is the object of attention. For example, it is clear that IQ functions as a dimension across the whole of its range (including the span covered by severe mental retardation) insofar as predictions to educational success or occupational level of concern. On the other hand, it is equally clear that, with respect to aetiology, there is a sharp discontinuity between severe retardation and the normal range of intelligence. Thus, major chromosome anomalies (such as those associated with Down's syndrome and fragile X syndrome) account for much of severe retardation whereas they play an absolutely trivial role in variations within the normal range. When genetic factors are likely to play a substantial role, genetic research strategies may well be useful in tackling the question of continuities and discontinuities, However, the general need is not for a genetic design as such but rather for research strategies that can determine whether the causes of variations within the normal range are the same as, or different from, those applying in relation to clinical disorders.

In that connection, however, it is essential to appreciate that disorders are very rarely defined only in terms of an extreme on a single behavioural trait. Magnusson & Bergman (1988, 1990) showed this clearly in their findings from the Stockholm longitudinal study. In their sample of males as a whole, aggression in childhood was a significant predictor of adult criminality (as it had been found to be in numerous other studies). When the findings were examined more closely, however, criminality in adult life was largely accounted for by individuals who in childhood had shown a combination of aggression, hyperactivity, poor peer relations, and other problem behaviours. When this multi-problem group was removed from the sample, aggression ceased to predict adult criminality. The implication is that it may often be necessary to examine constellations of behaviour that characterize individuals rather than separate individual traits as they apply across the population at large. In the same kind of way, Moffitt (1993) and Patterson, Capaldi & Bank (1991) have suggested the need to differentiate between early onset antisocial behaviour (which is often associated with hyperactivity and poor peer relations as indicated above) and adolescent onset antisocial behaviour. The former tends to be quite persistent into adult life whereas the latter is often a transient phenomenon. Antisocial behaviour has been taken here as an example but exactly similar issues apply to features such as depression, alcoholism, drug taking, eating disorders and anxiety. In each case there is a clinical disorder that has a similarity with something that is widely distributed in the population. The question is whether it represents the same phenomenon or something rather different. Causal processes would be much better understood if we knew more about continuities and discontinuities across the span of behavioural variation.

Persistence of psychopathology

There are many examples of psychopathological traits that show quite high persistence over long periods. That is clearly the case, for example, with antisocial behaviour. Until relatively recently there has been a tendency to assume that it was only change or discontinuity that required an explanation, with persistence or lack of change being the biological norm. Clearly, however, that must be a false assumption. The whole process of development is concerned with change. The mature adult is radically different from the new-born infant in a host of different ways. There has, of course, long been an interest in the developmental processes involved in this maturational change but there is no reason to suppose that individual differences should be expected to remain stable over the two decades of physical growth. Accordingly, it is necessary to examine the factors predisposing to stability as those involved in change. For example, Quinton et al. (1993) showed that the high persistence of antisocial behaviour was, to a substantial extent, dependent on the operation of a chain of influences over time – including family relationships, the characteristics of the peer group, and the choice of marriage partner. To a surprising extent, the persistence of antisocial behaviour was contingent on these intervening links in the chain. That is not to say that there are not important intrinsic factors that play a part in this process (with genetic factors possibly more important in the continuation of antisocial behaviour than in its occurrence initially), but indirect effects stemming from external influences appear rather more important than has sometimes been supposed. The answer, obviously, is likely to vary with the type of psychopathology being considered. Thus, genetic factors seem to predominate with respect to autism. Childhood depression shows a very strong, diagnosis-specific increase in risk for the recurrence of affective disorder in adult life but the relative importance of genetic and nongenetic factors in this case remains quite uncertain. Kessler et al. (1992) have suggested that factors involved in the initiation of depression and those involved in its persistence or recurrence may well not be synonymous. The crucial point is that there is as much need to investigate causes of persistence or nonpersistence as with individual differences in occurrence of psychopathology. In that connection, there is a particular interest in so-called turning point effects in which there is a change of psychological trajectory in individuals who are part of a group in which persistence is much more usual. Findings have been striking in showing that even experiences in adult life may be associated with such changes in trajectory. For example, both Quinton et al. (1993) and Sampson & Laub (1993) showed that a harmonious marriage was accompanied by a marked reduction in the persistence of antisocial behaviour in individuals exhibiting conduct disturbances or delinquency in childhood.

Change in level

A further causal question concerns differences in the overall level of a trait, rather than individual differences in its manifestation. Thus, although a predisposition to antisocial behaviour shows substantial consistency over time, nevertheless there is a marked tendency for antisocial behaviour to diminish in early adult life. Curiously, this desistance from antisocial behaviour has been very little investigated until recently. We have very little idea as to whether this is a function of some biological change or rather a consequence of altered social circumstances. For obvious reasons, it is important to determine which is the case. That change in level concerns something that affects individuals in the course of their development over time. In addition, we need to consider changes in level as they apply to whole populations over time. For example, the evidence is consistent in showing that in all Western countries there has been a massive increase in crime over the last 50 years. A careful examination of the evidence indicates that this change is, to a very large extent, a real one and not just an artefact of police practices, crime definition, or methods of recording. It is by no means self-evident that the causes of this major increase in antisocial behaviour will turn out to be the same as those leading to individual differences in the propensity to crime as they apply at any one time period. The investigation of this causal question follows much the same principles but certain adaptations in research strategy are needed (Rutter & Smith, 1995).

Situational effects

There are many aspects of psychopathology in which it is important to draw a distinction between a propensity to behave in a particular way and the actualization of that potential in the form of manifest behaviour. There is a substantial literature showing the importance of situational influences on delinquent behaviour. Such situational influences are quite varied in the ways in which they operate. Thus, some concern variations in opportunities for crime; some concern variations in degrees of community surveillance; some involve differences in peer group norms; some involve changes in the person's own state (as induced by drugs or alcohol); and some may reflect variations in attitude or incentive (as through the effects of unemployment). It will be appreciated that the term 'situation' has been used in rather a broad sense here. The point, however, is that it is seriously misleading to regard behavioural propensities as something that are a fixed part of an individual's makeup. There are individual differences in propensity but their actualization varies considerably according to transient changes in the individual and alterations in the circumstances in which the individuals find themselves.

Person-environment interactions

It is a universal finding that individuals vary greatly in their susceptibility to all manner of risk experiences. It has to be said that we know relatively little about such interactions in relation to psychological attributes. That is largely because such interactions have usually been looked for in terms of statistical interaction effects in multivariate analyses of total population genetic designs and have considered gene-environment interactions in terms of unspecified genetic risks and unspecified environmental risks, rather than specific hypotheses about particular types of interactions. The well-documented person-environment interactions in the fields of biology and medicine almost all concern circumstances that apply only to subgroups (often quite small subgroups) of the population and they apply to quite specific environmental features. For example, the genetically determined intolerance of many Asiatic people to alcohol is an instance of this kind; moreover it is one that appears to play a significant role in the relative protection against alcoholism. Also the same feature may be a risk factor for some outcomes and yet a protective one against others. Thus, physiological and behavioural hyper-reactivity seems likely to be a risk factor for anxiety disorders but a protective factor against antisocial disorders. Individual differences of many kinds do play an important role in shaping psychological development but, although some of the effects are direct, rather more are influenced by social context.

Person characteristics are by no means confined to 'constitutional' factors of one kind or another. One of the most important developmental questions concerns the ways in which experiences at one age may influence people's reactions to environmental circumstances at a later age. Also, long-standing social circumstances may affect the ways in which people respond to acute events. We know relatively little about such effects but there are indications that they are operative. For example, there is some suggestion that children who have been exposed to chronic psychosocial adversities are more likely to respond negatively to recurrent hospital admission than those from a more favoured family environment and children who have had experiences of happy separations may be more resistant to the negative effects of hospital admission. Also, there is an increased risk of marital breakdown with the second marriages of individuals whose first marriage was in the teenage years. It is not clear whether this reflects the characteristics of people who make teenage marriages or rather the effects of an early marriage breakdown. But, either way, it does represent some kind of person-environment interaction.

Person-environment correlations

Too much psychosocial risk research has seemed to operate on the assumption that psychosocial risks are randomly distributed in the population and that it is not necessary to ask questions about their origin. It is clear, however, that that is a quite mistaken assumption. From Robins' (1966) classic follow-up study of child guidance clinic patients onwards, it has been very evident that individuals vary greatly in their environmental risk exposure. Her data showed that individuals who exhibited antisocial behaviour in childhood had a much increased rate in adult life of unemployment, repeated marital breakdown, social isolation, and dependency on welfare. More recently, Quinton et al. (1993) have shown a very substantial tendency for antisocial individuals to marry or cohabit with partners who are themselves antisocial in one way or another. Champion, Goodall & Rutter, 1995) in their 20 year follow-up study of individuals first investigated at age 10 found that those with emotional or behavioural disturbance in childhood were twice as likely to experience severely negative stress events and chronic adversities in adult life. The precise mechanisms involved in the ways in which people shape and select their environments remain ill understood as yet but it is clear that causal questions need to be posed about the origins of individual differences in environmental risk exposure as well as in the psychological effects of such exposure.

Mediating mechanisms

Finally, causal mechanisms need to be considered in terms of those that are involved in the carry forward of risk sequelae. Thus, it is not enough to determine which aspects of child abuse or neglect constitute the most important component of the risk. We have also got to go on to enquire *how* such risk experiences get translated into behavioural propensities, such as those evident in antisocial behaviour. It is only very recently that investigators have begun to tackle this crucially important, but quite difficult, causal question. One example is provided by the longitudinal study undertaken by Dodge, Bates & Pettit (1990) of children exposed to abuse (mostly of mild degrees). Their results suggest that cognitive processing of the experience may constitute one of the mediating mechanisms. Those children exposed to abuse who developed a hostile attributional style were the ones most likely to exhibit aggressive behaviour.

SOME KEY RESEARCH ISSUES

Choice of variables

Surprisingly little attention has been paid, until recently, to the choice of variables in developmental research. Several rather different issues are involved. First, much too much research has been based on single measure, single informant, variables. Not surprisingly, weak associations and inconsistent relationships have tended to be the pattern. Not only is there a very considerable problem of error if there is reliance on a single data source at a single time of measurement, but also there is a failure to take into account the systematic biases in perception, context and reporting that are an inevitable part of measurement by questionnaire or interview. It is clear that there is much to be gained by the use of multiple informants and multiple measurements and, especially, in their combination through latent construct statistical approaches of one sort or another. This has been evident, for example, in the ways in which the Christchurch longitudinal study data have been used to examine pervasive conduct disturbance and in the separation of hyperactivity, inattention and conduct problems (Fergusson & Horwood, 1993). But, the issue is not just one of data sources and multiple measures, it is also a question of conceptualization of the characteristics to be examined.

For example, numerous studies have shown that as observed and as reported, there is a huge overlap between hyperactivity and conduct disturbance. Nevertheless, these features have a rather different pattern of correlations with other variables and a different course of development. Similarly, there appear to be important differences between conduct disorders that begin in early childhood and those that do not start until adolescence. Somewhat similarly, major depressive disorders that begin in childhood function somewhat differently from those beginning in adolescence or early adult life. It is not enough just to take characteristics as they derive out of factor analyses and the like. Rather, the need is to differentiate behaviours according to differing patterns of correlations and course.

A key issue in this connection concerns the need in many cases to focus on constellations of behaviour. Mention has already been made of the important Magnusson & Bergman (1988, 1990) findings that, so far as adult criminality is concerned, the main predictive value lies in a combination of problem behaviours in childhood, rather than any one of these considered in isolation. Much the same applies to the childhood precursors of schizophrenia.

Magnusson & Bergman (1988, 1990) have dealt with this issue in terms of the distinction between person-orientated and variable-orientated approaches. That is one useful way of viewing things but perhaps it is preferable to make several different sorts of distinctions. First, there is that between single behavioural traits and constellations of behaviour. Secondly, there is the distinction between traits (either single characteristics or constellation of characteristics) considered in isolation and characteristics considered in relation to their context. That is, although some variables have strong predictable effects regardless of context (for example that between IQ and educational attainment), many have effects that vary by context. Insofar as that is the case, the distinction is not so much between traits and persons as between behaviours (simple or complex) and person-environment interplay. It is not, of course, that interaction effects should be assumed. Rather, the need is to separate those where interactions are important and those where they are not. For example, the meaning of illegitimacy has changed radically over the last generation. Fifty years ago it tended to imply, in most of Western culture, unwanted babies born to single mothers living without the support of a partner. Nowadays, by sharp contrast, 'illegitimate' babies are frequently born following planned pregnancies in couples living together but not legally married. So-called illegitimacy rates have risen astronomically over the last 50 years but the meaning of illegitimacy is quite different now to what it was half a century ago. By contrast, psychological risks associated with divorce have remained much the same over the same time period in spite of the fact that divorce has become very much more common. The need is to examine the extent to which the effects of particular experiences are, or are not, context dependent. Empirical findings will show that some are and some are not. Research needs to tell us which is which.

Dimensions within categories

The importance of examining continuities and discontinuities between dimensions and categories in the field of psychopathology has been noted already. This is a major issue with respect to all the common forms of psychopathology that have parallels between diagnosed disorders (such as major depressive disorders or anorexia nervosa) and apparently comparable continuously distributed behavioural dimensions. To date, there are very few examples where we have good data that would enable us to determine the extent and pattern of continuities and discontinuities across the span of behavioural variation. But, it is not an issue that is by any means confined to psychopathology where there is an obvious 'normal' parallel. Much the same applies to qualitatively distinct conditions such as schizophrenia or autism. In both cases, the disorder is characterized by symptoms that are qualitatively distinct from normality. Yet it is clear from genetic evidence that the phenotype extends beyond the traditional diagnosis to include variations in personality functioning of a more frequent kind. Also, in both cases, the twin and family data suggest strongly that the genetic component involves several genes, and not just one. The possibility remains, therefore, that although the disorder as traditionally diagnosed is qualitatively distinct, the liability to that condition may be reflected in some continuously distributed feature. The internal medicine parallels here would be conditions such as hypertension and epilepsy where the severe disorder is obviously qualitatively different but yet where the liability seems to be continuously distributed to an important extent.

Comorbidity

Epidemiological and clinical studies in child psychiatry have all shown the very high frequency of various patterns of comorbidity. Some of these doubtless reflect artifacts deriving from the wrong specification of diagnoses and others stem from the use of categories when dimensions might be more appropriate. Nevertheless, even after due allowance has been made for the likely operation of artifacts of this and other kinds, it seems that the co-occurrence of supposedly separate forms of psychopathology is surprisingly common. The question is what mechanisms does this comorbidity reflect? Obviously, there will not be a single answer to this but the need is to use the existence of comorbidity as a means of investigating a causal mechanism, rather than dismissing it as just a nuisance variable to be taken into account in some fashion. For example, why is there such a strong association between hyperactivity and conduct disorders? It cannot be that they are just two alternative manifestations of the same trait because longitudinal data show that, although early hyperactivity much increases the risk for later conduct disturbance, the converse does not apply. Similarly, why do reading difficulties in childhood predispose to conduct disorders begin-ning before adolescence, but not psychopathology beginning after adoles-cence or occurring in adult life? Why does conduct disorder in childhood predispose to some forms of, mostly minor, depressive disorders in adulthood but apparently reduce the risk for major depressive disorders in adult life?

Heterotypic continuity

Most longitudinal studies have focused on the examination of continuities over time in the occurrence of behaviours that are manifest in the same way at all ages. Thus, there is a large literature on continuities in aggression and similar, albeit smaller, literatures on other aspects of psychopathology. For many behaviours, this is a perfectly appropriate way of considering develop-mental patterns. Nevertheless, it is also clear that some behaviours change in their manifestations over time, although the basic underlying construct remains the same. For example, the childhood precursors of adult schizo-phrenia are not to be found in delusions, hallucinations, and thought disorder but rather in attentional deficits, neurodevelopmental impairments and social abnormalities. More recently, evidence has begun to accumulate that the adult outcome of childhood conduct disturbance extends much more broadly than criminality and antisocial personality disorder. Especially in females, the continuity may lie in other forms of personality disturbance and in a predisposition to episodic affective disorders. There is, moreover, a growing body of evidence that infant attention and habituation measures constitute the precursors of intelligence as measured in later childhood (although there are some contradictory data). It should not necessarily be assumed that the finding that a behaviour of one kind predicts a behaviour of another kind at a later age means heterotypic continuity. An alternative explanation would be that the first behaviour creates a risk factor for the second behaviour although their meaning is quite different. Thus, in the field of internal medicine, obesity creates a risk for later osteoarthritis and for diabetes; yet there is abundant evidence that obesity, osteoarthritis and diabetes represent quite different conditions. Just as it must not be assumed that continuity will be reflected in unchanging behaviour manifest in the same way at all ages, it must not be assumed that just because there are correlations over time between two different sorts of behaviour, that this represents differing manifestations of the same underlying construct. The need is to design studies to determine just what the mechanisms might be.

Indirect chain mechanisms

Longitudinal studies have thrown up numerous examples of indirect chain mechanisms underlying continuities over time, even in the case of quite strong continuities. At one time, research interest focused on the extent to which there were enduring long-term effects of early adverse experiences that were independent of later circumstances. It has come to be appreciated in more recent times that that is actually the wrong way of posing the question. The reason is that the long-term sequelae are so often dependent upon setting in motion a chain of events in which no one cog in the chain has inevitable permanent sequelae but in which the sum of all the chain elements may be very substantial continuity over time. The reality of such indirect chain effects is no longer in doubt and the need now is to analyse what happens at each stepping stone on the path or each link in the chain so that we may understand how continuity and discontinuity arise. Among other things, this means that it is necessary to treat experiences as both independent variables (in terms of effects on what happens afterwards) and dependent variables in terms of their having arisen as a result of prior characteristics or experiences.

The 'accentuation principle'

Psychosocial risk researchers have tended to think of stress experiences as things that bring about change. In one sense, that is correct. The evidence is consistent that seriously adverse negative events (both acute and chronic) serve as important precipitants of psychopathological disorders of different kinds. What is misleading, however, is the supposition that when considered developmentally this results in overall changes in pattern of characteristics. For the most part, it does not. Elder & Caspi (1988) have coined the term 'accentuation principle' to describe the very common finding that negative experiences tend to accentuate previously existing characteristics, rather than change their direction. Thus, for example, girls who reach the menarche unusually early show a rise in norm-breaking behaviour but this rise is most apparent in girls who had already shown more norm-breaking behaviour than average before the onset of menstruation. As the evidence reviewed by Caspi & Moffitt (1993) indicates, this is a common state of affairs. For the most part, challenging or stressful experiences enhance or exaggerate characteristics that were already present rather than make people into something rather different from what they were before. The finding is an important one because it emphasizes the role of experiences in promoting stability and continuity.

Effects of experiences brought about by the individuals themselves

One important methodological advance in the field of life events research was the measurement of the extent to which life events were dependent or independent of illness behaviour. The separation was important in order to provide a rigorous test of the hypothesis that the life events precipitated psychiatric disorder. It has sometimes led, however, to the wrongheaded assumption that events that are brought about by people's own actions cannot have subsequent effects on their behaviour. That is far from the case. There is no necessary logical connection between the causes of a risk factor and the mode of its operation. That is obvious, for example, with respect to smoking cigarettes. People choose to smoke (for reasons associated with personality variables, opportunities, habit and social pressures) but the risks for lung cancer and for coronary artery disease are mediated by an entirely different set of mechanisms. The same need to differentiate between factors involved in the origins of a risk factor and factors involved in the mediation of the risks for disorder applies in the field of psychopathology. There is good evidence that events brought about by people's own actions do actually have substantial effects on their subsequent behaviour. For example, Rowe, Woulbroun & Gulley (1994) have reviewed the evidence on peer group effects. Analysis of data from studies with measures at the beginning and end of an academic year show that the choice of peers is indeed a matter of personal selection in large part but also that, having chosen to enter a particular peer group, the characteristics of that group serve to shape people's subsequent behaviour. Sampson & Laub (1993), in their reanalysis of the Gluecks' longitudinal study of delinquents, showed that incarceration for antisocial behaviour made it more likely that antisocial acts would continue. The details in the analysis indicated that the effect was not a direct one; rather, the risk for persistence of antisocial behaviour arose because incarceration made it so much more difficult for people to find employment when they were released. In the same sort of way, alcoholism predisposed to the continuation of antisocial behaviour. Obviously, it is essential to undertake rigorous analyses that eliminate the possibility that the effects are simply a function of unmeasured aspects of the underlying construct. Nevertheless, there are statistical techniques for doing just that and findings are convincing that there are real effects from circumstances brought about by people's own behaviour.

'Turning point' effects

Much the same applies to circumstances that lead to a change in people's behaviour – a change that sometimes involves an alteration in life trajectory from maladaptation to adaptation, or the reverse. For example, mention has already been made of the finding from both the Gluecks' longitudinal data and the British longitudinal studies that a harmonious marriage has a substantial effect in leading individuals who had shown previous conduct disturbance to desist from antisocial behaviour and to achieve normal, or near normal, levels of overall social functioning. When viewed in general population terms, such turning point effects account for little of the variance. What is striking, however, is that the effects are quite large when considered at the individual level. The disparity arises from the fact that individuals who are at risk rarely find themselves in circumstances that represent a disjunction from their previous social experiences and which, therefore, are likely to provide the opportunity for a change in life trajectory. Nevertheless, for the subsample who do experience such advantageous circumstances, the beneficial effects can be quite major.

CONCLUSIONS

The bringing together of developmental and clinical research perspectives, in the way that is characterized by developmental psychopathology, has led to some important changes in conceptualizations of both developmental processes and of the genesis of psychopathological disorders. In some respects, the findings have led to an increase in complexity of the issues that have to be considered. Nevertheless, the research approach has provided a set of strategies and tactics that provide good opportunities for the delineation of causal mechanisms. The patterns may be complex but they are analysable and research findings have already gone some way towards the delineation of some of the developmental principles that need to be considered. The same approaches have also provided a means of integrating biological, psychological and social-cultural influences and, as such, developmental psychopathology constitutes a most useful organizing research construct.

REFERENCES

Angold, A. &. Rutter, M. (1992) Effects of age and pubertal status on depression in a large clinical sample. *Development and Psychopathology,* **4**, 5–28.

Block, J. H., Block, J. & Gjerde, P. F. (1986) The personality of children prior to divorce: a prospective study. *Child Development,* **57**, 827–40.

Cahan, S. & Cohen, N. (1989) Age versus schooling effects on intelligence development. *Child Development,* **60**, 1239–49.

Caspi, A., Lynam, D., Moffitt, T. E. & Silva, P. A. (1993) Unraveling girls' delinquency: Biological, dispositional, and contextual contributions to adolescent misbehavior. *Developmental Psychology*, **29**, 19–30.

Caspi, A. & Moffitt, T. E. (1993) When do individual differences matter? A paradoxical theory of personality coherence. *Psychological Inquiry,* **4**, 247–71.

Champion, L. A., Goodall, G. M. & Rutter, M. (1995) Behavioural problems in childhood and stressors in early adult life. I. A twenty year follow-up of London school children. *Psychological Medicine.* **25**, 231–46.

Cherlin, A. J., Furstenberg Jr., F. F., Chase-Lansdale, P. L., Kiernan, K. E., Robins, P. K., Morrison, D. R. & Teitler, J. O. (1991) Longitudinal studies of effects of divorce on children in Great Britain and the United States. *Science,* **252**, 1386–9.

Dodge, K. A., Bates, J. E. & Pettit, G. S. (1990) Mechanisms in the cycle of violence. *Science,* **250**, 1678–83.

Elder, Jr., G. H. & Caspi, A. (1988) Human development and social change: An emerging perspective on the life course. In Bolger, N., Caspi, A., Downey, G. & Moorhouse, M. (eds.) *Persons in Context: Developmental Processes.* Cambridge: Cambridge University Press, pp. 77–113.

Farrington, D. P. (1988) Studying changes within individuals: the causes of offending. In Rutter, M. (ed.) *Studies of Psychosocial Risk: The Power of Longitudinal Data.* Cambridge: Cambridge University Press, pp. 158–83.

Fergusson, D. M. & Horwood, L. J. (1993) The structure, stability, and correlations of the trait components of conduct disorder, attention deficit, and anxiety, withdrawal reports. *Journal of Child Psychology and Psychiatry,* **34**, 749–66.

Fergusson, D. M., Horwood, L. J. & Lynskey, M. T. (1992) Family change, parental discord and early offending. *Journal of Child Psychology and Psychiatry,* **33**, 1059–75.

Kessler, R. C., Kendler, K. S., Heath, A. C., Neale, M. C. & Eaves, L. J. (1992) Social support, depressed mood, and adjustment to stress: A genetic epidemiologic investigation. *Journal of Personality and Social Psychology,* **62**, 257–72.

Magnusson, D. & Bergman, L. R. (1988) Individual and variable-based approaches to longitudinal research on early risk factors. In Rutter, M. (ed.) *Studies of Psychosocial Risk: The Power of Longitudinal Data.* Cambridge: Cambridge University Press, pp. 45–61.

Magnusson, D. & Bergman, L. R. (1990) A pattern approach to the study of pathways from childhood to adulthood. In Robins, L. & Rutter, M. (eds.) *Straight and Devious Pathways From Childhood to Adulthood.* Cambridge: Cambridge University Press, pp. 101–15.

Maughan, B., Pickles, A., Rutter, M. & Hagell, A. (in press) Reading problems and antisocial behaviour. *Journal of Child Psychology and Psychiatry.*

Moffitt, T. E. (1993) Adolescence-limited and life-course persistent antisocial behavior: A developmental taxonomy. *Psychological Review,* **100**, 674–701.

Mortimore, P., Sammons, P., Stoll, L., Lewis, D. & Ecob, R. (1988) *School Matters: The Junior Years.* Wells, Somerset: Open Books.

Patterson, G. R., Capaldi, D. & Bank, L. (1991) An early starter model for predicting delinquency. In Pepler, D. J. & Rubin, K. H. (eds.) *The Development and Treatment of Childhood Aggression.* Hillsdale, NJ: Erlbaum, pp. 139–68.

Quinton, D., Pickles, A., Maughan, B. & Rutter, M. (1993). Partners, peers, and pathways: Assortative pairing and continuities in conduct disorder. *Development and Psychopathology,* **5**, 763–83.

Richman, N., Stevenson, J. & Graham, P. (1982) *Pre-School to School: A Behavioral Study.* London: Academic Press.

Robins, L. (1966) *Deviant Children Grown Up.* Baltimore, Md: Williams and Wilkins.

Rowe, D. C., Woulbroun, J. & Gulley, B. L. (1994) Peers and friends as nonshared environmental influences. In Hetherington, E. M., Reiss, D. & Plomin, R. (eds.) *Separate Social Worlds of Siblings.* Hillsdale, NJ: Erlbaum, pp. 159–73.

Rutter, M. (1993) Developmental psychopathology as a research perspective. In Magnusson, D. & Casaer, P. (eds.) *Longitudinal Research on Individual Development.* Cambridge: Cambridge University Press, pp. 127–51.

Rutter, M. (1994) Beyond longitudinal data: Causes, consequences, changes and continuity. *Journal of Consulting and Clinical Psychology.* **62**, 928–940.

Rutter, M. & Hay, D. (eds.) (1994) *Development Through Life: A Handbook for Clinicians.* Oxford: Blackwell Scientific.

Rutter, M. & Quinton, D. (1984) Parental psychiatric disorder: Effects on children. *Psychological Medicine,* **14**, 853–80.

Rutter, M. & Rutter, M. (1993) *Developing Minds: Challenge and Continuity Across the Lifespan.* Harmondsworth: Penguin; New York: Basic Books.

Rutter, M. &. Smith, D. J. (1995) *Psychological Disorders in Young People: Time Trends and Their Causes*. Chichester: John Wiley.

Sampson, R. J. & Laub, J. H. (1993) *Crime in the Making: Pathways and Turning Points Through Life*. Cambridge, Mass.: Harvard University Press.

Stattin, H. & Magnusson, D. (1990) *Pubertal Maturation in Female Development*. Hillsdale, NJ: Erlbaum.

Vorria, P. (1991) Children Growing up in Greek Institutions: Their Behaviour and Relationships at School and in the Institution. PhD Thesis in Education, University of London, Institute of Education.

West, D. (1982) *Delinquency: Its Roots, Careers and Prospects*. London: Heinemann.

21 Commentary **Social competence and human conflict**

DAVID HAMBURG

It is a privilege to read the chapters in this part of the book by three masters of the scientific study of behavior. They provide a comprehensive overview of major areas of inquiry and give many insights. For example, Kagan's Chapter 19 reflects his career-long interest in integrating biological and psychological perspectives in the development of behavior. This is a perspective of fundamental importance in the scientific study of behavior.

One of Hinde's observations (in Chapter 18) stimulates a long-standing interest of mine that deals with the theme of this book: social competence. Indeed the problem I wish to address may well be the most serious, widely prevalent social incompetence of our time – that is, incompetence in reaching mutual accommodation among human groups in a highly diverse, deeply interdependent world – saturated with very destructive weapons beyond any prior experience. How can child and adolescent development be shaped in ways likely to foster our learning to live together amicably – at last?

Hinde's chapter noted,

In developing a self-concept, children see themselves as members of some categories and not of others . . . As with membership of almost any . . . social group, they then tend to exaggerate the difference between their own group and the other, and to see their own group as superior . . . denigration of the out group . . . may enhance an individual's status in his own.

THE UNPRECEDENTED CHALLENGE OF OUR TIME

In a brief moment of evolutionary time – since the industrial revolution and mainly in the twentieth century – we humans have thrust ourselves headlong into a world of enormous complexity, vast scale, unprecedented rates of change, technical and social transformation, brilliant new horizons and weaponry of destructive power beyond previous imagination. Our power for better and worse suddenly dwarfs everything that went before in millions of years of human evolution. This power is rich in promise for the human future if we can at last come to master the pervasive tendency toward conflict in our species.

An underlying orientation of great importance here is the ubiquitous human tendency toward egocentrism and ethnocentrism. We find it easy to put ourselves at the center of the universe, attaching a strong positive value to ourselves and our group, while attaching a negative value to many other people and their groups. It is prudent to assume that human beings are all, to some extent, egocentric and ethnocentric. But these tendencies, under certain conditions, can lead to violent conflict.

The world is now, as it has been for a long time, awash in a sea of ethnocentrism, prejudice and violent conflict. The worldwide historical record is full of hateful and destructive indulgences based on religious, racial, ethnic and other distinctions. What is new is the destructive power of our weaponry: not only nuclear but chemical, biological and conventional – that is, pervasive proliferation. The worldwide spread of technical capability, the miniaturization of weapons, the widely broadcast justifications for violence, and the upsurge of fanatical behavior are occurring in ways that can readily provide the stuff of very deadly conflicts in every nook and cranny of the earth. To be blunt, we have as a species a rapidly growing capacity to make life everywhere absolutely miserable.

No longer have we the luxury to indulge in harsh prejudice and in ethnocentric extremes. The consequences are simply too devastating – and getting more so with each passing year. These are anachronisms grounded in our ancient past. There may be 'tough-minded' people who believe that this is the human condition and that we must make the most of it. But technology has passed them by. The destructive capacity of modern weapons – large and small – has made the 'tough-minded' view unrealistic, if not today, then tomorrow. If we cannot learn to accommodate each other respectfully – within nations and across nations – we will destroy each other at such a rate that humanity will soon have little to cherish, assuming there is any humanity left on earth.

THE HUMAN GROUP, ADAPTATION, AND DEADLY CONFLICT

There are powerful links between human groups, survival and social competence. The basic facts have implications for conflict resolution and mutual accommodation. There is a very long evolutionary background of human groups. Monkeys and apes typically live in groups whose internal structure is based upon intense and persistent attachments between individuals. They have long-term, complex relationships that are crucial for their survival and reproduction. Hunter-gatherers, the earliest form of human societies, typically live in groups of about 20 to 50 members. Reciprocity is crucial in relationships, both within and between groups. Disapproval enforced by jeopardy to sharing in the future or by the threat of rejection from the group are powerful sanctions that reinforce conformity to group norms. The importance of sharing is conveyed to children from infancy onward.

In the simple societies of human origin over many millennia, a sense of personal worth is built on one's sense of belonging to a valued group; a sense of belonging, in turn, depends on the ability to master the traditional tasks of that society, to engage in social interactions in ways that are mutually supportive. All this is further reinforced by deeply meaningful experiences of participation in group rituals that constitute shared experiences of social identity invested with emotional significance. All of these traditional experiences occur within the context of a small, face-to-face group that provides the security of familiarity, support in times of stress, shared coping strategies, and enduring attachments that sustain hope and adaptation for a lifetime.

The evidence of modern biological, anthropological and historical research indicates that these basic facts of small-scale, traditional life apply to the several million years in which our ancient ancestors organized in hunting and gathering societies, the extended family of agricultural village society that began to appear about 10,000 years ago, and the primary group of the homogeneous neighborhood in pre-industrial towns of historical times.

As times have drastically changed in the past two centuries – especially since the Industrial Revolution – and people have flowed like floodwaters across the earth, they have always sought fervently to maintain social support networks similar in basic functions to the small societies in which our species evolved. Such social support systems facilitate the development of coping strategies that help people make a living, keep distress in bad times within tolerable limits, maintain self-esteem, preserve human relationships, meet requirements of new situations, and prepare for the future.

During the past few decades, fruitful insights have come from experimental research on the psychology of intergroup behavior. Social psychologists as well as anthropologists and sociologists have been interested in the human propensity to distinguish between in-groups and out-groups. Both in field studies and experimental research, the flow of evidence is very impressive. Human beings are readily able to learn in-group favoritism or in-group bias. People are remarkably prone to form partisan distinctions between their own and other groups, to develop sociometric preferences for their own group, to discriminate against other groups, to accept favorable evaluations of the products and performances of the in-group, to accept unfavorable characterizations of other groups that go far beyond the objective evidence or the requirements of the situation. This is true not only of long-standing group commitments, but even in experimental situations where only a brief orientation is given to distinguish a newly formed group. It is difficult to avoid invidious distinctions even when the experimenter wishes to do so.

Overall, it is easy to stimulate a strong sense of 'my people' – the in-group. This easily learned response may have had adaptive functions in human evolution over a very long period. Now our circumstances are much more complex than those in which we evolved, and responses of this sort are far more problematical. It is important to note that these invidious distinctions can readily be exacerbated by political demagogues. As we see so vividly in the twentieth century, such exacerbation can have disastrous consequences.

Let me try to put the long sweep of evolutionary historical evidence in a very concise way. Human societies have a pervasive tendency to make distinctions between in-groups and out-groups in ways that are highly susceptible to harsh interpretations that justify violence. Many different political, social, economic and pseudoscientific ideologies have been utilized in support of these hostile positions. Groups have been specified in many ways: religion, race, language, region, tribe, nation and various political entities. The worldwide historical record is full of hateful and destructive activities based on such invidious distinctions – often associated with deeply felt beliefs about superiority, a sense of jeopardy to group survival, or justification by supernatural powers. All that is an ancient part of the human legacy and now more dangerous than ever before. Yet, there is no need to assume that membership in a supportive group must be hateful, let alone lethal toward others. On the contrary, it is reasonable to assume that we can indeed learn to live together, in spite of very bad habits from the past, and that we must now avidly seek ways to do so.

PREJUDICE AND ETHNOCENTRISM IN CHILD DEVELOPMENT AND EDUCATION

How do we acquire orientations of ethnocentrism, prejudice, dogmatism and a susceptibility to hateful pseudo-solutions? Are there ways to foster more constructive orientations? The nature of parental care, child care, experience with siblings and with peers, exposure to hatred and violence in schools, streets and mass media, and the cumulative effect of frustrating conditions are all important factors. So, also in some places are official propaganda and the religious cultivation of stereotypes.

The extent of prejudice can be affected by home, school and community factors as well as by opportunities to gain familiarity with other groups under constructive circumstances. This is shown in a fine research tradition over several decades reflecting such contributors as Musafer Sherif (Sherif & Sherif, 1966), Gordon Allport (1958) and Morton Deutsch (1973).

Putting together a great deal of laboratory and field research, it appears that the quantitative amount of contact between negatively orientated groups does not have a high degree of relevance to the outcome. Much depends on whether the contact occurs under favorable conditions. If the conditions involve an aura of suspicion, if they are highly competitive, if they are not supported by relevant authorities, or if they occur on the basis of very unequal status, then they are not likely to be helpful, whatever the amount. Indeed such unfavorable conditions can exacerbate old tensions and can reinforce stereotypes.

On the other hand, there is a strong positive effect of friendly contact in the context of equal status, especially if such contact is supported by relevant authorities, is embedded in cooperative activity and fostered by a mutual aid ethic – especially superordinate goals. Under these conditions, the more contact the better. Such contact is associated with improved attitudes between previously suspicious or hostile groups as well as changes of patterns of interaction between them in constructive ways.

Superordinate goals have the potentially powerful effect of unifying disparate groups. They are shared goals that can only be achieved by cooperative effort and therefore override the differences that people bring to the situation. In Sherif's experiments, he readily made strangers at a boys' camp into enemies with isolation and competition, but when he introduced powerful superordinate goals, he was able to transform enemies into friends.

These experiments have been fundamentally replicated since then in work with large numbers of business executives and many different kinds of groups. So the effect is certainly not limited to children and youth. Indeed, the findings have been extended in ways that indicate the beneficial effects of working cooperatively under conditions that lead people to formulate a new, inclusive group that goes beyond the subgroups with which they entered the situation. Such effects are particularly strong when there are tangibly successful outcomes of cooperation – for example, clear rewards from cooperative learning. Schools and community-based youth development organizations could be organized in ways that utilize the principles of research on intergroup relations and conflict resolution.

Indeed, this problem of intergroup relations importantly involves child and adolescent development and presents crucial new opportunities. These lie in finding ways through research and innovation to educate for conflict resolution and mutual accommodation – not only in schools but also in community organizations and the media, both print and non-print. In short, the scientific community can challenge pivotal institutions to consider how the various groups of this global human species can at last learn to live together. Perhaps it is something like learning that the earth is not flat. We may even need a paradigm shift in our outlook toward human groups.

Education in all its forms, from family to schools to mass media, can increasingly convey the facts of a pluralistic and interdependent world, not one that is strange and hateful. Yet today's education worldwide is still considerably enthnocentric. We bring up our children everywhere to be negative toward some other group(s). On the other hand, education everywhere could convey an accurate concept of a single highly inter-dependent, worldwide species – a vast extended family sharing fundamental human similarities and a fragile planet. We ultimately rely for survival on the give-and-take learned in childhood but now extending far beyond childhood games toward adult and even international mutual accommodation.

In point of fact, all research-based knowledge of human conflict, diversity and mutual accommodation is grist for the education mill – via the education system, the media and other modalities. What follows is a sketch of some possibilities for making use of many different educational vehicles for learning to live together.

DEVELOPMENT OF PROSOCIAL BEHAVIOR IN EARLY LIFE

In the context of secure attachment and valued adult models, provided by either a cohesive family or a more extended social support network, certain social norms are established early in life: (1) taking turns; (2) sharing with others; (3) cooperating, especially in learning and problem solving; (4) helping others, especially in times of stress. These norms, though established on a simple basis in the first few years of life, open the way to constructive human relationships that have significance throughout the lifespan. They tend to earn respect, provide gratification, and amplify the effectiveness of anything the individual could do alone. For this reason, early intervention programs need to take account of the factors that influence the development of attachment and prosocial behavior. This is important in parent education, child care centers, and preschool education.

There is research evidence that settings in which the requirements and expectations incorporate prosocial behavior do in fact foster such behavior. For example, children who are responsible for tasks helpful to family maintenance, especially caring for younger siblings, are generally more altruistic than similar children who do not have these prosocial experiences. Both direct family observations and experimental studies have examined the effects of a model on later prosocial or antisocial behavior. In the experimental studies, typically an adult (presumably much like a parent) demonstrates a prosocial act such as sharing toys, coins, or candy that have been won in a game. The sharing is with someone else who is said to be in need though not present in the experimental situation. The adult plays the game and models the sharing before leaving the child to play.

The results are clear. Children exposed to such models, when compared to similar children in control groups, tend to show the behavior manifested by the models whether it be honesty, generosity, helping or rescuing behavior. Given the child's pervasive exposure to parents and teachers, the potential for observational learning in this sphere as in others is very great. Prosocial behavior is particularly significant in adaptation because it is likely to open up new opportunities for the growing child, strengthen human relationships, and contribute to the building of self-esteem.

EMPATHY TRAINING

Empathy is defined as a shared emotional response between observer and stimulus person. It may be expressed as 'putting myself in the shoes of another person'. Empathy training has been carried out in elementary school classrooms. Studies have been done in which experimental groups show positive results when compared with control groups. Evidently, empathy can be taught and can contribute to the formation of prosocial behavior.

TEACHING CONFLICT RESOLUTION IN THE SCHOOLS

Professor Morton Deutsch, of Columbia University, a distinguished scholar in conflict resolution, has delineated programs that schools can use to promote attitudes, values, and knowledge that will help children develop constructive relations throughout their lives (Deutsch, 1973). Such programs include: (1) cooperative learning; (2) conflict resolution training; (3) constructive use of controversy in teaching; and (4) creation of dispute resolution centers. These efforts are most effective if they have a serious curriculum with repeated opportunities to learn and practice cooperative, conflict resolution skills. Students get a realistic understanding of the amount of violence in society and the deadly consequences of such violence. They learn that violence begets violence, that there are healthy and unhealthy ways to express anger, and that non-violent alternatives to dealing with conflict are available and will be useful to them throughout their lives.

COOPERATIVE LEARNING

Research on cooperative learning has burgeoned since the early 1970s. It involves a mutual aid ethic and appreciation for student diversity. In cooperative learning, the traditional classroom of one teacher and many students is reorganized into heterogeneous groups of four or five students who work together to learn a particular subject matter, for example, mathematics.

Research has demonstrated that student achievement is at least as high, and often higher, in cooperative learning activities as in traditional classroom activities. At the same time, cooperative learning methods promote positive interpersonal relations, motivation to learn and self-esteem. These benefits are obtained in middle grade schools and also high schools, for various subject areas, and for a wide range of tasks.

In my view, there are several overlapping yet distinctive concepts of cooperative learning that offer a powerful set of skills and assets for later life: learning to work together; learning that everyone can contribute in some way; learning that everyone is good at something; learning to appreciate diversity in various dimensions; learning complementarity of skills and division of labor: learning a mutual aid ethic.

LIFE SKILLS TRAINING IN EARLY ADOLESCENCE

The Carnegie Council on Adolescent Development's Working Group on Life Skills Training provided in 1990 the factual basis and organizing principles on which such interventions can be based. It also described a variety of exemplary programs.

One category of life skills is assertiveness, which has several components: (1) taking advantage of opportunities, for example, how to use community resources such as health and social service agencies or job training opportunities. (2) Another aspect of assertiveness is resistance to pressure or intimidation, for example, drugs or weapons. How does one stand up to pressure without spoiling relationships or isolating oneself? (3) Yet another aspect of assertiveness is nonviolent conflict resolution, assertiveness to achieve goals in ways that make use of the full range of nonviolent opportunities that exist in the society.

Altogether, social competence is a central area for life skills training. Such skills can be taught not only in schools but in community organizations.

TELEVISION AND PROSOCIAL BEHAVIOR

Research has established causal relationships between children's viewing of aggressive or prosocial behavior on television and their subsequent behavior. Children as young as 2 years old are facile at imitating televised behaviors. Television violence can affect behavior as early as age 3 or 4, and the effect continues in adolescence. In general, the relationship between television violence or prosocial behavior and subsequent viewer behavior holds in a variety of countries. Cross-national studies have included countries diverse as Australia, Finland, Israel, the Netherlands, Poland and the United States.

There is some research evidence that television need not be a school for violence, but can indeed be used in a way that reduces intergroup hostility. The relevant professions need to encourage the constructive use of this powerful tool to promote compassionate understanding, nonviolent problem solving, and decent intergroup relations. Television can portray human diversity while highlighting shared human experiences – including the common humanity of our adversaries, even in times of stress. But so far we have had only glimpses of its potential for reducing intergroup conflict. Television can teach a wide range of skills and behaviors that are important for the social development of children. Television can both entertain and educate simultaneously. These features are vividly illustrated by the program *Sesame Street*.

Professor Gerald Lesser (1989) of Harvard University has recently summarized features of *Sesame Street* that are of interest in this context (Lesser, 1989). The program originated in the United States but appears in 100 other countries. Each program is fitted to the language, culture, and traditions of a particular nation. The atmosphere of respect for differences permeates all of *Seasame Street's* many versions.

Research from a variety of countries is encouraging. For example, the Canadian version of *Sesame Street* shows many sympathetic instances of English and French-speaking children playing together. Research from Canada clearly shows that both English and French-speaking children who see these examples of cross-group friendships are more likely to actually form such friendships than Canadian children who do not see them. The same is true for Dutch, Moroccan, Turkish, and Surinamese children who see *Sesame Street* in Holland. The findings suggest that appealing and constructive examples of social tolerance help young children to learn such behavior.

CONCLUDING COMMENT

Let me close with a crucial question for the human future. Can human groups achieve internal cohesion, self-respect and adaptive effectiveness without promoting hatred and violence? Altogether, we need to strengthen research and education on child development, prejudice, ethnocentrism and conflict resolution. We can generate new knowledge and explore vigorously the application of such knowledge to urgent problems in contemporary society.

Old attitudes, beliefs, emotions, political ideologies and stereotypes from our ancient and recent past will often hinder such efforts, but our motivation for survival is strong and our problem-solving capacities are great.

The intimate, slowly changing world of our nonhuman primate ancestors and of early humans is long gone. So, too, is the small and relatively simple world of more recent ancestors who lived in agrarian societies. Our contemporary world is the crowded, heterogeneous, impersonal, super-armed, rapidly changing environment shaped during the past two centuries. There is little in our very long history as a species to prepare us for this world we have suddenly made. Perhaps we just cannot cope with it – witness Yugoslavia and Rwanda. But we have learned the very hard lesson that the earth is not flat. Maybe it is not too late for a paradigm shift in child development and education that would at long last make it possible for human groups to learn to live together in peace and mutual benefit.

REFERENCES

Allport, G. W. (1958) *The Nature of Prejudice*. New York: Doubleday.

Deutsch, M. (1973) *The Resolution of Conflict*. New Haven, Conn.: Yale University Press.

Groebel, J. & Hinde, R. A. (1989) *Aggression and War: Their Biological and Social Bases*. Cambridge: Cambridge University Press.

Hewstone, M., Stroebe W. & Codol, J. (1988) *Introduction to Social Psychology*. Oxford: Blackwell.

Lesser, G. (1989) Taking children beyond hate. Presented at a conference, 'Beyond Hate', chaired by Elie Wiesel, Boston University, 12 June 1989.

Sherif, M. & Sherif, C. (1966) *Groups in Harmony and Tension: An Integration of Studies on Intergroup Relations*. New York: Octagon.

PART VI
AGING

This part deals with human aging from biological, psychological and social perspectives.

In Chapter 22, Baltes & Graf point out that psychological research on human aging is in its infancy. The challenge of future research is to explore links between psychological and social aspects of aging and to their interaction. He highlights several features of human aging: its multifaceted nature, heterogeneity and plasticity and analyzes that future efforts involve studying the constraint and plasticity of psychological aging, latent potentials of old persons and strategies for compensation for age-related dysfunction.

Hardy in Chapter 23 examines the impact of molecular genetics on the understanding of the causes of dementia and longevity. Molecular genetics has helped us to better understand the causes of Alzheimer's disease (AD) and longevity. Three genes have been shown to be involved in the etiology of AD. These are the amyloid precursor protein gene on chromosome 21, an as yet unidentified gene on chromosome 14 and the apolipoprotein-E gene on chromosome 19. ApoE alleles are associated with longevity. Specifically, apolipoprotein-E2 homozygotes have a fourfold increase in the chance of reaching 100 years and apolipoprotein-E4 homozygotes almost never reach this age. Human molecular genetics offer both opportunities and hazards, and Hardy ponders some of the ethical dilemmas of predictive testing for common late onset causes of mortality and morbidity. These are: does the individual have the right to know his/her own genome? Do the insurers have the right to know their clients' genome? Should the employers have the right to know their employees genome?

In Chapter 24 Morgan & Gordon discuss how molecular changes, observed in aged organisms may arise for a number of reasons. An important goal of research is to identify causal mechanisms responsible for aging. While alterations in protein and RNA synthesis are potential mediators of aging, it is likely there are additional mechanisms. Extra nuclear factors rather than modified transcription or translation capacity appear in many instances to be important in regulating specific genes during aging. Morgan concludes that aging may be the result of an accumulation of diverse alterations lacking molecular determinants but leading to similar physiological changes in many organisms.

In his commentary to this section (Chapter 25) Finch integrates issues raised by the previous authors and, in examining the mechanisms that govern the timing of life, offers a broad perspective on age-associated plasticity. Finch gathers evidence from a variety of studies to support his contention that aging is associated with enormous plasticity, rather than being rigidly programmed. Included among the factors that have an important influence on aging are the prenatal and postnatal hormonal environments and nutrition. While the progressive age-related accumulation of glycated proteins in the brain and other tissues may set some upper limit on plasticity, he suggests that the linkage of hormones and nutrition to age-related diseases provides many targets for intervention.

22 Psychological aspects of aging: facts and frontiers

PAUL B. BALTES AND PETER GRAF

This chapter is arranged into four distinct sections. First, we offer some observations on the history of gerontology focusing especially on the ontogenetic dynamic between growth and decline. Secondly, we present the main elements of psychological lifespan theory and illustrate how psychologists approach the phenomenon of aging at a metatheoretical level. Thirdly, we organize the current evidence on the nature of human aging in the form of three propositions about facts and frontiers. In a concluding section, we offer three integrative perspectives. These illustrate the complexity of aging, and they demonstrate the close interconnections between biology, behavior, and societal conditions, but also the kind of theoretical efforts that might emerge from transdisciplinary dialogue and collaboration.

INTRODUCTORY OBSERVATIONS

Gerontology and old age are 'young'

Human gerontology is still a relatively 'young' member in the family of sciences. Of course one can find precursors of gerontological investigations in biology, medicine, psychology, and the social sciences (see Gruman, 1979 for historical reviews), but only during recent decades has the field of gerontology fully emerged as an intellectual force with a reasonably well-specified agenda of concepts and methods. The handbook edited in 1959 by James Birren (*Handbook of Aging and the Individual: Psychological and Biological Aspects*) was a critical event, especially for social scientists. Since its publication, the quantity of scientific work has expanded at an extraordinary rate, as has the growth of professional specializations and gerontological research organizations.

Gerontology is also 'young' when considered in the larger context of human civilization. From the perspective of culture and civilization, old age as a 'mass phenomenon' had its advent in the twentieth century. Although some individuals reached old age throughout the last millennia, the proportion of individuals that live to old age has increased dramatically in the twentieth century so that old age is no longer an exception in today's industrialized world. In the industrialized world, close to 50% of the population reach the age of 75, resulting in what is often called the 'graying' or aging of the population (Brock, Guralnik & Brody, 1990). This demographic graying of the population is primarily due to an increase in the number of persons reaching old age, however, and it does not reflect an increase in the maximum lifespan. In fact, there is little evidence for any increase in the maximum human lifespan during the last millennia (Fries, 1989).

Because we are in the demographic 'infancy' of old age, we are still in what one might call a 'societal or cultural exploration' phase of old age, a situation high in uncertainty and, possibly, in innovation (Baltes & Mittelstrass, 1992). Contrary to earlier periods of the lifespan, especially infancy and childhood, which have benefited from centuries of cultural attention and investment and thereby achieved a high level of support and stability, there is no long-standing tradition of a broadly based and refined 'culture' of old age (Alterskultur). Thus, what we witness today as old age has not yet settled into a stationary, stable condition. Instead, in the years and decades to come, the facts and processes of old age are likely to undergo rapid change, at least insofar as its cultural forces and behavioral manifestations are concerned.

On the limits of biological theories of aging and the role of culture

One key feature that sets the role of evolution-based biological theories of aging apart from biology-based theoretical conceptions in childhood and adolescence is the age-related decrease in evolutionary selection pressure (see Finch, Chapter 25). Aging is a process located primarily in the phase of life where reproduction- and parenting-related evolutionary selection effects are of lesser significance. This does not mean that evolution-based genetic factors are less important in old age; instead, it signifies that the genetic factors of aging are less well selected and, therefore, are likely to contain a larger proportion of dysfunctional (deleterious) genes. This is the reason why it is occasionally argued that 'biology is not a good friend of old age'.

The other side of the same coin is that cultural factors are of crucial importance for the evolutionary development of old age. These factors are part of another stream of 'inheritance', the cultural-social one with its own special features of transmission and dissipation (Durham, 1990). How these two streams of genetic and cultural inheritance interact is a central piece of the intellectual story of theories of aging (Baltes & Mittelstrass, 1992), and in this chapter we will offer several illustrations on the psychological level of analysis.

Toward multidimensional (multidirectional) and dynamic conceptions of aging

Current views of and expectations about aging are influenced by general societal beliefs and stereotypes; in part because gerontology is still a young field of study, it lacks a broad theoretical and empirical foundation, and especially because its domain includes each one of us personally. Survey research shows that personal and societal expectations about old age are generally negative, with most people regarding old age as a period of decline and increased frailty. Instead of looking forward to old age, we enter this life stage with an increasing preference for being younger (see Figure 22.1; see also Figure 22.9). Unfortunately, these same negative expectations and stereotypes about aging are also likely to shape the conceptual and empirical orientations of scientists and scholars, and thus, it is not surprising that much of the early psychological research on aging was akin to counting 'the wrinkles of old age.'

Negative expectations about old age can also be found in classical definitions of aging that originated in the biological and life sciences (Shock, 1977). Biology defines aging as that period or interval in the life course when biological systems lose their efficacy and functioning, that is, when the range of adaptivity or adaptive fitness decreases and the organism becomes thus less effective and more vulnerable. Even though there may be solid methodological and theoretical reasons for this kind of limited definition of aging, its disadvantage is that it reifies a decline and deficit conception of aging, thereby perhaps preventing us from discovering whatever potential for growth that remains.

In the behavioral and social sciences, and in modern gerontology, this biological, unidimensional view of aging and old age is slowly being cast off and replaced with more multifaceted and dynamic and less fixed conceptions (Birren & Bengtson, 1988; Gerok & Brandstädter, 1992; Rowe & Kahn, 1987). Old age and aging are now no longer viewed as reflecting a

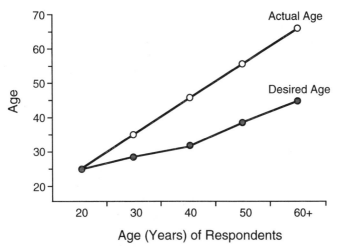

Figure 22.1. Results of a representative study (USA) on the topic 'If you could maintain a certain age, which age would it be?' Unpublished data from Research Network on Midlife Development (Director: O. G. Brim) of the John D. and Catherine T. MacArthur Foundation.

unidimensional process of decline, nor are they considered as immutable and impervious to intervention. In recognition of the spirit of this change in perspective, we uphold the image of the Roman god Janus whose special expertise was the ability to see at the same time in two or more directions. Recent behavioral-science research has been especially effective in showing that old age is indeed a period of life with more than one face.

Deficits as catalysts for progress (innovation)?

Yet a different perspective on aging emerges when we consider the dynamic link between deficits and innovation. The core question highlighted by this link is whether deficits – the symptoms that guide our general expectations about old age and aging – necessarily foreclose the possibility of development in the sense of progress and 'growth.' At least since the publication of 'Limits of Growth' by the Club of Rome, there is an increasing awareness that more is not always better and that progress is possible even in the context of limitations and constraints (see also Baltes, 1987).

A number of theoretical arguments has been made, especially in the cultural sciences, that it is exactly the condition of a limitation or a loss which generates new forms of mastery and innovation. And under the influence of cultural-anthropological traditions, some contemporary behavioral scientists now maintain that suboptimal biological states or imperfections are catalysts or primary motivators for the evolution of culture and for the advanced states achieved in human ontogeny. In this line of thinking, the human organism is by nature a 'being of deficits' (Mängelwesen). Furthermore, it is suggested that individual and social culture have developed or emerged in part to deal specifically with biological deficits. Because of the fact that old age is accompanied by 'radical deficit,' the graying of the population may also give rise to major cultural changes (advances) in knowledge, technology, and social norms. Moreover, this deficits-breed-growth view may account not only for cultural evolution, but also for selection pressures during individual ontogeny (Marsiske et al., 1995). It is possible that when individuals reach states of increased vulnerability in old age, they invest more and more heavily in efforts that are explicitly geared toward regulating and compensating for age-associated biological deficits, thereby generating a broad range of novel behaviors.

In our view, one of the essential problems of human aging is indeed the search for an effective and reality-based mastery of the dynamics between growth and decline, or between expansion and contraction (Baltes, 1987, 1993). On the one hand, the biology of old age is characterized by a progressive weakening of the human body. On the other hand, it is the special strength of human culture and individual behavior that it can generate conditions that promote psychological progress despite or even because of such increasing biological limitations. Throughout this chapter, we will make an effort to elaborate this point.

DEVELOPMENT AND AGING: METATHEORETICAL OBSERVATIONS FROM LIFESPAN THEORY

Because of the complexities associated with ontogenetic processes, but also because of the meaning of the words 'development' and 'aging' in psychology, there has been much discussion – at a metatheoretical level – of what constitutes development, what constitutes aging, the degree to which there are separate processes, and the extent to which development and aging are simultaneous as opposed to sequential-interactive components of the life course. Discussion of these issues was heavily influenced by the emergence of lifespan psychology (Thomae, 1979).

Table 22.1 summarizes a few of the central assumptions and principles of lifespan theory in psychology (Baltes, 1987). Each of the assumptions/principles is relevant, of course, to research concerned with earlier periods of life, and their understanding and investigation may be even more advanced in other sciences (e.g. developmental biology) than in psychology. We feature these assumptions/principles in this chapter in order to highlight their critical importance and the fact that they form a coherent gestalt or unifying perspective that guides the efforts of lifespan researchers. This kind of perspective seems especially important for gerontological research, in part, because it furnishes the investigator with a strong mental schema that serves to counterbalance the pervasive societal 'everyday' stereotype of aging as a negative and largely fixed process of decline.

The first and perhaps most important principle is that development is a *life-long process*, and moreover, that each state of aging is not only the result of age-specific but also of lifespan precursor conditions. A second assumption is that in contrast to traditional developmental 'child' psychology which focuses on development as a positive change in the structure and function of behavior (adaptive capacity or growth), a lifespan view of development emphasizes the *multidirectionality* of development. Embedded in the idea of multidirectionality is the assumption that throughout life there are positive and negative changes in adaptive capacity, both within specific functions as well as in the profile of all available behaviors. The domain of intelligence can be used to illustrate these changes. Throughout adulthood and in old age, some categories of intelligence show long-term stability or even growth, whereas others reveal declines that begin fairly early in adulthood.

The idea of multidirectionality is pushed to its extreme by the *gain-loss dynamic* and the related argument that development is always a combination of gains and losses. The strong claim is that there is no such thing as a pure gain in adaptive capacity with ontogeny, just as there is no pure loss (Baltes, 1987). As argued also in developmental biology (e.g. Edelman, 1987; Chapter 9), psychologists now explore whether the very process of ontogenetic development as 'specialized adaptation' always involves negative features and outcomes. Among the losses concurrent with gains are, for instance, the

Table 22.1. *Family of theoretical propositions characteristic of lifespan developmental psychology*

Concepts	Propositions
Development as selection and adaptation	Development can be defined as a life-long adaptive process. Some adaptive processes are cumulative, others discontinuous. Adaptivity is local, specific, and time-bound.
Development as gain/loss	Throughout life, development consists of the joint occurrence of gain (growth) and loss (decline). The process of development is multidirectional.
Historical and evolutionary embeddedness	Ontogenetic development varies substantially in accordance with historical-cultural conditions. Because of the relative recency of a 'culture' of old age and of lesser 'evolutionary-genetic' selection pressure on later life, old age is less 'optimized' than earlier age periods.
Contextualism as paradigm	Development can be understood as the outcome of the interactions (dialectics) among three systems of biological and environmental influences: age-graded, history-graded and nonnormative. The mechanisms involved can be characterized in terms of the metatheoretical principles associated with contextualism.
Successful development as selective optimization with compensation	On a general level of analysis, 'successful' development can be conceived of as resulting from the collaborative interaction involving three components: selection, optimization, and compensation. The ontogenetic pressure for this dynamic increases with age.

(Modified after Baltes, 1987.)

exclusion of alternative pathways of development or the allocation of resources that under certain conditions could be relevant in the mastery of other aspects of life. In the psychology of learning and cognition, another example is 'negative' transfer. An everyday example is children's relative loss of fantasy as they acquire the skill of formal 'decontextualized' logic, or their increased difficulty in acquiring a second language (see Klein, Chapter 12). As to old age, its negative features may reflect the costs of investments into earlier developmental 'acquisitions.' As a consequence, late-life structures and functions are constrained by the costs of early life outputs.

The search for gains and losses in adaptive capacity across the lifespan has been paralleled by the rapid growth of investigations into the *range and limits of plasticity* of mind and behavior (Baltes, 1987). Research into age-related changes in plasticity (intra-individual variability) is motivated, first, by a search for the 'latent potential' of structure and function in old age, and second, by questions about the fundamental component processes associated with such concepts as 'norm of reaction,' 'developmental reserve' or 'competence' (Salthouse, 1991). A better understanding of latent potential is critical for ferreting out those aspects of the current cultural and educational context that are suboptimal or even deterimental to the well-being of older adults; it might enable the design of environments that harness more of the resources that remain in old age (Baltes & Baltes, 1990). In order to learn about developmental reserve capacity, research relies on 'stress' or 'challenge' tests similar to those used in biology and medicine. The researcher manipulates the conditions that support and interfere with behavior and thereby reveals the range and limits of current and of developmental (age-indexed) plasticity. However, the 'testing-the-limits' approach (Baltes, 1987) goes beyond stress and challenge tests; in lifespan research, it also explicitly includes the engineering of conditions under which development is enhanced and optimized (Lindenberger & Baltes, 1994; Weinert, 1992).

Developmental and aging research in psychology is also guided by *interactionist* and *contextualist theories* (Lerner, 1991; Magnusson, 1988). Most interactionist and contextualist orientations in psychology regard individuals as (1) active organisms, (2) co-producers of their own development, (3) socially embedded, and (4) participants in cultural-historical change. Major parts of adult life, therefore, are outcomes of individual actions and proactions (anticipative behavior). Moreover, and this feature may set humans apart from infra-humans, individual actions include intentional subjective 'reconstructions' of the past and 'pro-constructions' of the future. The fact that individuals, as they age, construct themselves and their environments is often associated with a particular general theoretical orientation to the study of behavior which in the German tradition is called *action theory* (Brandstädter & Greve, 1994).

Contextual effects associated with *cultural conditions* and *historical change* are especially important for interactionist conceptions of psychological aging (Baltes, 1993; Lerner, 1991). As described earlier in this chapter, the facts and processes of old age are not fixed or immutable because both cultural and psychological aspects of aging are continually evolving. Comparative cross-cultural and cross-cohort (historical) research has revealed the wide range of functioning that can emerge in different cultural contexts and at different historical moments. The investigative approaches that seem particularly suited for revealing these kinds of influences are, first, cohort research or the study of individuals born at different points in historical time within a given society (Nesselroade & Baltes, 1979). A second approach involves the comparative analysis of lifespan development of different subgroups of the same population. By means of these and related methods, research has produced impressive evidence of the powerful influence of environmental and cultural factors on psychological aging.

Comparative contextural research on various aspects of psychological functioning, then, ranging from mental health to basic intelligence has yielded ample evidence that the 'nature' of human aging is inherently not only 'biological' but also 'cultural' (Baltes, 1993). The interactionist scenario of human development states that the level of psychological functioning in old age and age-associated changes in adaptive capacity are profoundly influenced by interactions and transactions with the cultural environment, by the range of opportunities and constraints provided by the cultural-environmental context, and by how individuals 'transport' (partly through their own behavior) these influences into old age.

The last items in Table 22.1 suggest that contemporary psychologists interested in the whole of life are searching for a *general theory of development* (Brent, 1978; Ford & Lerner, 1992), a theory that would consider explicitly the intricate dynamics between growth and decline as well as the systemic and transactional properties of human functioning. Not surprisingly, therefore, developmental and gerontological psychologists have begun to revisit their 'developmental' colleagues in the natural sciences and biology to explore common ground. The consequence of such interactions is that Eigen's and Prigogine's work on self-organizing systems (Brent, 1978) and chaos theory (Barton, 1994), for instance, are advanced as general frameworks worthwhile of exploration. We will turn to this topic in our concluding section.

FACTS AND FRONTIERS ABOUT PSYCHOLOGICAL AGING: A SUMMARY

This section summarizes and organizes what we regard as some of the most critical findings on the nature of psychological aging. We draw several general conclusions from the available evidence, and these seem to be shared by others in the field of aging, although the specific weighting and evaluation of different pieces of evidence is likely to vary among investigators. One serious limitation of our conclusions must be acknowledged, however. The available evidence comes primarily from the study of what Bernice Neugarten has called the 'young-old', covering the age range of approximately 60 to 75 years. Thus, the conclusions presented in this section may change, perhaps even dramatically, in the face of new findings from investigations of the very old (Baltes et al., 1993; Poon, 1992).

CONCLUSION 1: AGING REVEALS MUCH INTERINDIVIDUAL VARIABILITY (HETEROGENEITY) AND MULTIDIRECTIONALITY

Two widely (though not universally) shared assumptions that have been held since the beginning of gerontology are, first, that persons who have reached old age will be highly similar to each other, and secondly, that age-related

Table 22.2. *A meta-analysis of observed interindividual variability in 185 human aging studies*

| Variability with age | Indicators: % of studies | | | |
	Biological	Personality	Cognition	Social
Increasing	75	57	79	50
Decreasing	8	14	21	50
Uncertain	17	29	0	0

(From Nelson & Dannefer, 1992.)

changes are primarily a matter of decline. The main determinants of aging were often assumed to be sufficiently powerful and uniform, thus molding each individual in the same manner. However, the scientific evidence from long-term longitudinal studies does not corroborate this expectation (Birren & Bengtson, 1988; Lehr & Thomae, 1987; Nesselroade, 1989). Death certainly is unavoidable, but the individual pathways toward death appear highly variable. There are 80 year-olds who in some aspects of the mind and behavior appear like 40 year-olds and *vice versa*. And perhaps even more surprising, it appears that substantial interindividual variability occurs not only in behavioral but also biomedical functioning (Rowe & Kahn, 1987).

One concrete demonstration of large individual variability in old age comes from the meta-analysis of gerontological studies by Nelson & Dannefer (1992) which is summarized in Table 22.2. The findings show that interindividual variability increases with age. The increase is noteworthy because, everything else being equal, one would expect a decrease in individual variability if for no other reason than age-associated population changes due to selective mortality. Mortality is not random.

To obtain good estimates on heterogeneity in the course of aging, longitudinal and comparative research is necessary (Magnusson, 1988; Nesselroade & Baltes, 1979). Specific examples demonstrating sizeable heterogeneity are in Schaie's work (1989) on adult intellectual development and, for the period of advanced old age, in the Berlin Aging Study. The evidence from Schaie's seminal work on the aging of intelligence is most directly relevant because it was obtained in a longitudinal assessment. His findings show that persons who, for example, traverse the age range from 60 to 80 years exhibit distinct patterns of intellectual change, with many showing stability or decreases in level of performance, but others demonstrating stability or even increases.

Psychological data dealing with advanced old age come from the Berlin Aging Study (Smith & Baltes, 1993; see also Poon, 1992). Figure 22.2 illustrates the large interindividual variability present in a heterogeneous (close to representative) sample of 70 to 105 year-old West Berlin citizens in two

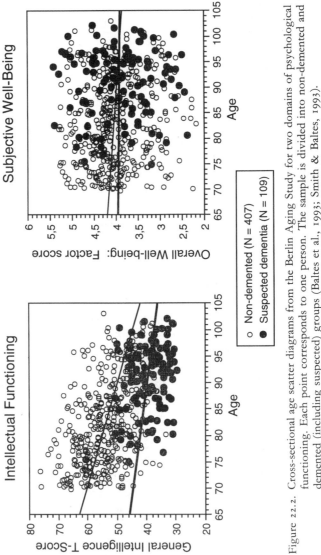

Figure 22.2. Cross-sectional age scatter diagrams from the Berlin Aging Study for two domains of psychological functioning. Each point corresponds to one person. The sample is divided into non-demented and demented (including suspected) groups (Baltes et al., 1993; Smith & Baltes, 1993).

domains of psychological functioning (intelligence, self). Note that these data are highly reliable. For the domain of intelligence, for instance, they are based on an extensive and carefully constructed battery of 14 tests of intellectual functioning.

The Berlin Aging Study offers a further window on the nature of individual variability, showing large variations in the magnitude of age correlations and in the relative independence between domains of psychological functioning (Smith & Baltes, 1993). The magnitude of the correlations for the two domains is worth noting: for the total sample, the correlation between age and intelligence is −0.57, and that between age and subjective well-being (the self) is −0.12. Moreover, the intercorrelations between these two key domains of psychological functioning turns out to be close to zero if tested by structural modeling procedures (Smith & Baltes, 1993). In other words, how well the mind functions intellectually has little or no relationship with how persons characterize their subjective state of wellness. The latter finding emphasizes the multidimensionality or independence of psychological functions within a given person.

One method used to gain insight into large interindividual differences in old age involves grouping individuals based on the relative standing on different marker variables such as intelligence, mental health, and subjective well-being. This kind of research, consistent with the notion of sizeable heterogeneity and multidimensionality, points to the existence of a relatively large number of 'change and functioning types.' In the Berlin Aging Study, for instance, 10 such clusters were found to represent 156 persons in the age range from 70 to 105 years (Smith & Baltes, 1993). These clusters exhibit clear age differences in composition, with some including primarily old-old persons, others young-old persons, and yet others were close to age-specific.

A similar conclusion is offered by Schaie (1989) who used hazard functions to categorize subjects based on the number of mental abilities in which they, over the age range from about 50 to 85, exhibited gains, stability, or decline. As illustrated in Figure 22.3, such a multivariable-change approach to clustering subjects seems to result in a more appropriate representation of the interindividual variability components of age functions than is suggested by single-group representations.

The next step in this line of inquiry is to identify the life history and concurrent conditions that regulate the commonalities and differences among the subjects. Toward this goal, one major approach has been the search for the genetic and experimental origins of the obtained individual variability. Particularly promising data come from the Swedish Adoption/Twin Study of Aging (Plomin et al., 1994) in which 112 pairs of identical and fraternal twins reared apart and 111 matched twins reared together were compared and heritability coefficients were computed to assess the extent of genetic influence on individual differences in cognitive abilities during the last half of life. Heritability coefficients for most cognitive abilities were close to or larger

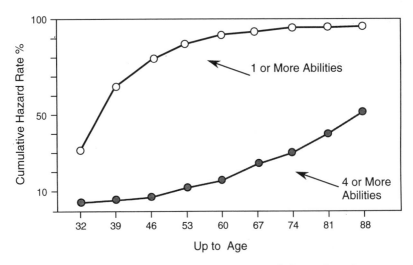

Figure 22.3. Cumulative hazard functions of intellectual decline in five primary mental abilities based on a large set of cross-cohort longitudinal studies (Schaie, 1989). Hazard rates indicate percentage of subjects at a given age who have shown significant decline in one or four or more abilities.

than 0.50; for a factor-analytically derived 'overall' measure of general cognitive ability, it was 0.80 (suggesting that under the current genetic and environmental conditions, 80% of the reliable interindividual variance in a factor of 'general' intelligence could be attributed to genetic factors). Such data show that (at least in the Swedish gene-environment context) genetic factors continue to be powerful regulators of individual differences in old age. (Note, however, that such behavior-genetics data do *not* capture the main component of experiential effects in development, namely the *level* of functioning reached as a function of cultural factors. Irrespective of level, behavior-genetics research only accounts for the source of individual differences.)

Efforts to capture the heterogeneity and multidirectionality of old age and to discover their causative sources are driven by a number of different questions. One of them concerns the possibility that the available evidence is tainted by a methodological artifact that derives from our subjective, 'forward' looking conceptions of lifetime. At present, studies of old age define age as 'distance from birth.' However, it might be more productive to plot the relevant age data backward, that is, as distance from death (Riegel & Riegel, 1972), and this kind of mapping might reveal more similarity between aging persons than is evident in age functions that originate from birth.

A further critical method-issue are the different sources and components of variability that might 'cause' heterogeneity in old age (Craik & Salthouse, 1992). Progress in understanding the multidirectionality and heterogeneity in old age might come when we attempt to distinguish more carefully between, for example, interindividual differences at one point in time, interindividual differences in age change (across time), intra-individual (within-person) variability, interbehavioral differences, as well as differences in level and rank order between individuals (Nesselroade, 1989).

Another example of an important source of age-related individual variability in cognitive aging is recent evidence showing that as people reach advanced old age, sensory systems (vision, hearing) become more and more important in the regulation of intellectual functioning. In the Berlin Aging Study, for instance, vision and hearing abilities were such powerful (correlational) predictors for 70 to 100 year-olds that they accounted for most of the age variance in a battery of 14 tests of intelligence (Lindenberger & Baltes, 1994). In earlier periods of adulthood, hearing and vision display much lower correlations with intelligence.

CONCLUSION 2: NORMAL, OPTIMAL, AND PATHOLOGICAL AGING

The difference between normal and pathological development is especially critical for aging research because pathology is not randomly distributed across age and some forms show dramatic increases in late adulthood. Perhaps the most familiar example is senile dementia of the Alzheimer's type. Up to age 70, this illness has prevalence and incidence rates of close to zero, but beyond 70, the prevalence and incidence rates increase substantially. Current estimates set prevalence rates of about 10% for the eighth, 25% for the ninth, and 40% for the tenth decade of life. One implication of these findings is that age functions revealed by investigations of older adults may be confounding the behavior/performance of adults with and without dementia.

The distinctions between normal, optimal and pathological or sick aging, however, attractive as they are, are not easily drawn (Fozard, Metter & Bryant, 1990; Fries, 1989; Gerok & Brandtstädter, 1992; Manton, 1989; Rowe & Kahn, 1987). In general, the following definitions hold. *Normal aging* refers to growing old without a manifest illness whether physical or mental. Up to age 70 or 80, this is a fairly frequent event. *Optimal aging*, the kind of aging that would be possible under 'optimal' personal and environmental conditions, refers to a kind of utopia. Understanding the conditions for optimal aging is the primary research motivation for many gerontologists. Finally, *pathological aging* refers to a process of aging where there is clear evidence for physical or mental illness. The classical example is senile dementia of the Alzheimer's type.

The juxtaposition of these differing phenotypes of aging provides another example of the multiple faces (heterogeneity) of human aging. In Figure 22.2, we had illustrated this point by computing two regression lines each for two domains of psychological functioning: intelligence and subjective well-being. The regression lines in the left part of the figure show substantial differences in cognitive efficacy for individuals with and without Alzheimer's dementia. As to subjective well-being, however, there is no differential effect. Decomposing age functions in such a manner is not only important to obtain meaningful aging statistics, it is also important for methodological and conceptual reasons (Fozard et al., 1990).

Two further research projects illustrate the same point. The first is research by Margret Baltes (Baltes, M. M., Kühl & Sowarka, 1992) aimed at exploring qualitative (discontinuous) differences in cognitive plasticity between normal aging and Alzheimer's dementia-related aging. These investigators demonstrated that older persons diagnosed as at risk for Alzheimer's dementia showed no gain from cognitive training with a standardized intervention program while all normal control subjects did show gains.

This and related work demonstrate that because of the role of age-associated pathology and age-correlated changes in the incidence of different pathologies, population-based aggregates rarely represent a good estimate of the 'typical' course of aging. Separating sources of normal and pathological aging, therefore, is a major task of gerontological research, as is the theoretical question of what constitutes normal and pathological conditions (Fozard et al., 1990; Gerok & Brandtstädter, 1992) and how subgroups formed on such a basis can be used to pinpoint the specific factors involved in processes of aging.

CONCLUSION 3: OPPOSING FACES OF PLASTICITY IN OLD AGE: BIOLOGICAL-GENETIC FACTORS AND CULTURE-BASED LEARNING

The lifespan dynamic between growth and decline, gains and losses, is highlighted most directly by the interplay between biological-genetic factors and culture-based learning. On the one hand, there is sizeable developmental reserve capacity (plasticity) in old age which can be utilized to create better states of aging – more plasticity than one would generally expect based on our negative views of aging. On the other hand, there is clear evidence for age-related losses in the extent of plasticity. In psychology, this juxtaposition can be used also to make explicit the differential role of biological-genetic versus culture-based learning in the regulation of aging as well as their interaction.

We have evidence from two areas of psychological functioning – cognition (intelligence, memory) and the self – that illustrates these two opposing faces of plasticity. For the domain of cognition and intelligence, our own studies can be used to illustrate the type of data available (Baltes, 1993). Research programs and findings by others, such as by Salthouse (1991), Schaie (1989), and Horn & Hofer (1992) can be invoked for the same purpose. For the domain of the self, we report concepts and data from work on self-regulation, the psychology of control, and subjective well-being (Brandtstädter & Greve, 1994; Cartensen, 1993; Heckhausen & Schulz, 1993; Markus & Hertzog, 1991).

Limits to plasticity in the fluid-mechanics of intelligence: working memory

In our work on cognitive aging, we explored first what we call 'developmental reserve capacity' of the aging mind and then its limits near asymptotic functioning after cognitive engineering and extensive practice (Baltes & Kliegl, 1992). Secondly, we attempted to identify bodies of cognitive skills and knowledge in which aging may harbor special strengths (such as wisdom as an instantiation of the crystallized pragmatics of intelligence) or conspicuous weaknesses (such as working memory as an instantiation of the mechanics of intelligence).

The general strategy used for this purpose involves contrasting performance on tasks (tests) that tap two main categories of intelligence that are expected to exhibit different lifespan trajectories, namely, the fluid 'mechanics' of intelligence with the crystallized and knowledge-based 'pragmatics' of intelligence (Baltes, 1993). In accord with Cattell and Horn (Horn & Hofer, 1992), our general expectation is that there is a loss with aging in the mechanics of the mind, but that pragmatic knowledge is an important modulator which can enrich the mind in important new ways including the compensation of aging losses in the cognitive mechanics.

Figure 22.4 illustrates our research method and its underlying assumptions (Baltes, 1993). The upper part of Figure 22.4 suggests that it is theoretically useful to distinguish between two main categories of intellectual functioning: the fluid mechanics and the crystallized pragmatics. In analogy to computers, these two categories can be linked to the hardware (cognitive mechanics) and the software (cognitive pragmatics) of the mind. The distinction between mechanics and pragmatics does not imply that they are completely independent of each other. Instead, they must always interact in practice, with the pragmatics building on the mechanics.

The cognitive mechanics reflect the neurophysiological architecture of the brain as it has developed during evolution, the ways and means of the 'adapted mind' (Barkow, Cosmides & Tooby, 1992). We assume that, at the operational level, the cognitive mechanics are indexed by the speed and accuracy of elementary processes of information input, visual and motor memory, and processes of discrimination, comparison and categorization and their application in working memory. Conversely, the cognitive pragmatics can be understood as the culture-based software of the mind. They reflect the kind of knowledge and information that cultures offer as 'bodies of factual and procedural knowledge about the world and human affairs and individuals

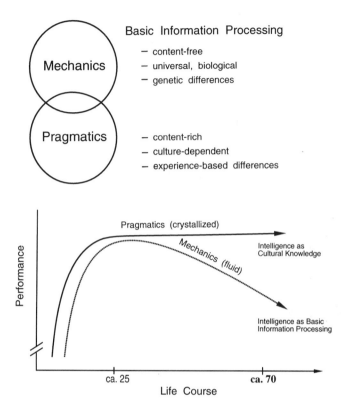

Figure 22.4. Lifespan research on two categories of human intelligence: fluid mechanics vs. crystallized pragmatics. The top section defines the categories, the bottom section illustrates the postulated lifespan trajectories. (After Baltes, 1993; Horn & Hofer, 1992.)

acquire and transform as they participate in culture-based socialization.' Examples of cognitive pragmatics are reading and writing skills, language comprehension, educational qualifications and professional skills, and also the kind of knowledge about the self and about life skills that are relevant in the planning, conduct, and interpretation of life (Baltes, 1993; Brim, 1992).

As shown in the lower part of Figure 22.4, a critical feature of the theory of fluid mechanics versus crystallized pragmatics is the form of their putative ontogenetic trajectories. It is postulated that each of these categories of intellectual functioning is regulated predominantly by a different set of determining sources: biological-genetic (including health) for the mechanics versus environmental-cultural (including learning) for the pragmatics. Because of this differential control by biological versus cultural factors, the model postulates that distinct age trajectories result.

Empirical evidence in support of this conception of cognitive aging has come from several sources. We begin by summarizing evidence relevant to the fluid mechanics of the mind. In this domain, highly consistent findings of age-related decline have come both from descriptive aging research and from experimental work (Hertzog & Schaie, 1988; Horn & Hofer, 1992; Salthouse, 1991). The findings from intervention research that explored the range of plasticity in old age seem most critical.

On the one hand, it has been repeatedly demonstrated with tasks and tests that index the fluid mechanics of the mind that most older adults (excluding those who have a brain-related disease such as Alzheimer's) are able to benefit from training and practice (Baltes, 1993; Schaie & Willis, 1986; Willis, 1991). Thus, it appears that for individuals who age without brain pathology, the basic structure and function of the mechanics of the mind (at least up to the age range from 70–80 years) remain intact. Research has revealed latent cognitive reserves that can be activated and utilized for new domains of learning. This fact is important because it lays the groundwork for the operation of the second category of intellectual functioning, that is, the pragmatics of intelligence. On the other hand, and in contrast to these positive findings, research has also shown that when difficult tasks and tests are used, or when young and old adults are studied near the limits of their performance potential, older adults display significant aging losses in speed and accuracy of information processing (Baltes, 1993; Salthouse, 1991). In fact, negative age differences become more and more pronounced as task difficulty increases and subjects' maximum performance potential is studied near its limits (Baltes & Kliegl, 1992; Mayr & Kliegl, 1993).

The latter finding was highlighted by an investigation with healthy and well-educated young and older adults who participated in 38 training sessions focused on using the method of loci, a well-known mnemonic strategy. We used the method of loci in order to assess the limits of working memory, treating it as a model case for the mechanics of intelligence (Baltes & Kliegl, 1992). It is important to emphasize at the outset that our research goal was not only the study of a specific memory technique; instead, we hoped to tap more general processes of working memory, including imagination, the ability to form new associations, to create and store mental images, and to link stimuli to specific locations. In other words, mental imagination and associative ability are seen by us not only as key components of the method of loci but also as fundamental constituents of many other cognitive activities.

Figure 22.5 summarizes results from one study of this research program. The magnitude and robustness of the aging loss obtained when using the method of loci is dramatic. Even after extensive training, older adults do not reach the same level of performance displayed by young adults after a few sessions of training. In fact, after 36 sessions of instruction and practice, none of the older adults performed at or above the average level of young adults. Not shown in Figure 22.5 is another finding dealing with speed of information processing (Salthouse, 1991). In the Kliegl, Baltes et al. studies, older subjects

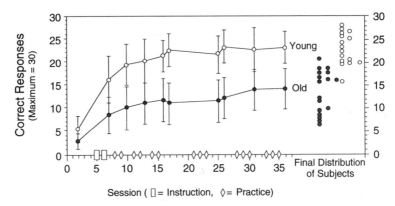

Figure 22.5. Testing the limits of working memory (an example of cognitive mechanics) in young and older adults using the Method of Loci and serial learning of word lists. (From Baltes & Kliegl, 1992.)

needed about three to four times more time to achieve the same level of performance as young adults.

Much effort in cognitive aging research is devoted to identifying more precisely the components relevant for the negative age effect in fluid tasks of information processing and problem solving (Craik & Salthouse, 1992; Kliegl, Mayr & Krampe, 1994; Salthouse, 1991). Mayr & Kliegl (1993), for instance, have investigated the separate and joint effect of components of 'cognitive complexity.' In their work, they demonstrated that the speed loss due to aging is a direct function of the degree of complexity of a given task. In 'easy' cognitive tasks, tasks that require only the repeated application of a single processing step (such as comparing stimuli along the dimension of size), older 'normal' persons took about 50% longer than young adult controls. As the tasks became more complex (such as comparing stimuli along two dimensions – size and location), the aging loss was magnified with older adults requiring about 100% more time than young adults. In other words, and this is in line with testing-the-limits methodology, the more complex or difficult the tasks the greater the age-related loss.

Taken together, these findings point to a substantial age-related loss in what we consider to be one of the two main categories of intellectual functioning – the fluid mechanics of intelligence. When it comes to the 'hardware-like' cognitive mechanics and the speedy and accurate functioning of basic mechanisms of information processing, old age takes its toll, not unlike the aging loss we observe in physical and biological functioning. Such an outcome is consistent with the two-component model of intelligence. The fluid mechanics are assumed to be primarily regulated by biological-genetic factors, and 'biology is not a friend of old age.'

Stability and advances in crystallized pragmatics: wisdom

The two-component model of intellectual development maintains that the fluid mechanics of the mind decrease with age, whereas other domains of intelligence, especially those associated with the crystallized pragmatics may show stability or even increases in old age. We expect to find the latter trends in those aspects of cognition that are primarily knowledge-dependent (Baltes, 1993; Weinert, 1992), and in psychology, supporting evidence comes from research on expert systems and on professional skills including the arts (Ericsson & Smith, 1991; Simonton, 1988). Persons with much practice and knowledge-based expertise outperform those without such expertise, even when their basic mechanics of information processing are substantially worse. We regard expert systems as prototypes of the facilitative role of culture and socialization in human development.

Cognitive pragmatics also play an important role in compensating for age-related losses in the mechanics of intelligence (Baltes & Baltes, 1990; Bäckman & Dixon, 1992). Factual and procedural knowledge can not only enrich the mind but might also compensate for deficits in cognitive mechanics. In the field of cognitive aging, research by Salthouse (1991) illustrates the significance of knowledge-based, pragmatic strategies in compensating for losses in cognitive mechanics. Salthouse investigated how older typists are able to maintain high levels of performance, even though we expect their psychomotor and reaction skills to exhibit losses. Figure 22.6 summarizes Salthouse's research while at the same time adapting his data to the distinction between mechanics and pragmatics and their interactive relationships.

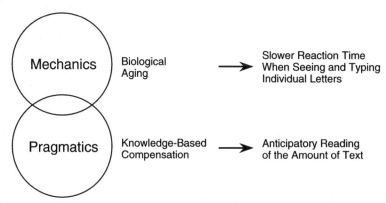

Figure 22.6. An example of compensatory interaction between mechanics and pragmatics of intelligence: older typists can maintain a high level of functioning by reading further ahead in the text to be typed, despite a loss in speed when typing individual letters. (Based on Salthouse, 1984.)

According to Salthouse (1991), effective typing is governed by two major components. The first component is the psychomotor reaction time necessary to translate the recognition of a given letter into a stroke on the keyboard. The second component is the amount of text previewed by the typist. When studying older expert typists, Salthouse was able to show that they have slower reaction times (cognitive mechanics) than comparable young adult typists with comparable typing skill, but that they can use anticipatory reading as a compensatory technique. By doing so, older typists can type as fast as young adults. In other words, older expert typists appear to use a knowledge-based pragmatic – anticipatory reading, to compensate for a deficit in the speed of psychomotor mechanics (Salthouse's work actually showed that reducing the length of text available for preview has a larger negative effect on older than younger typists).

Having demonstrated the enriching and compensatory role of knowledge, we inquire about crystallized pragmatics in old age. Are there indeed bodies of knowledge and procedural strategies of problem solving (that is, forms of pragmatic-crystallized intelligence) which exhibit stability or advances in the course of aging (Sinnott & Cavanaugh, 1991)? In our own work (Baltes & Staudinger, 1993), we are exploring this for the case of wisdom, putatively one possible prototype of a specific form of old-age intelligence (see also Sternberg, 1990).

By integrating perspectives offered by different lines of scholarship (psychological lifespan theory, psychology of expertise, and adult personality development), we first specify the content domain of wisdom and define it as an 'expertise in the fundamental pragmatics of life permitting exceptional insight and judgment involving complex and uncertain matters of the human condition' (Baltes & Staudinger, 1993). The body of knowledge associated with wisdom deals with the conduct, interpretation and meaning of life. It entails, for example, insight into the core conditions of life and the course of life, including its plasticity and limitations. Furthermore, the body of wisdom-associated knowledge contains information concerning the structure, dynamics and weighting of life goals, their likely sequencing, and the meaning of life.

Thus far, our main methodological strategy in the investigation of wisdom has been to ask persons to respond to difficult life problems by thinking aloud about the problems (after they have practiced the method of thinking aloud) and to record their answers. Subsequently, the answers are transcribed and evaluated in terms of a family of five criteria (factual knowledge, procedural knowledge, lifespan contextualism, relativism of values and priorities, recognition and management of uncertainty) which we delineated as being part of a well-developed knowledge system about the fundamental pragmatics of life, that is, the domains of expertise that we have identified as wisdom-related.

Our research on wisdom is still in its infancy. The initial results, however, are rather encouraging (Baltes & Staudinger, 1993). In several studies, for example, adults of differing ages and experiential backgrounds were asked to think aloud about various problems of life planning, life management and life review. An example would be the following vignette: 'Imagine a good friend of yours is calling you on the phone to tell you that she can't go on anymore, that she has decided to commit suicide. What should one consider and do?'

A sample of our findings is reproduced in Figure 22.7. First, unlike what is often found with traditional measures of intellectual functioning, we obtained no evidence for lower performance of older adults. On the contrary, older adults produced more than their statistical share of top responses. This was particularly true when subjects were considered who had a life history of wisdom-related training and experience such as clinical psychologists or persons nominated for being wise. These findings stand in clear contrast with evidence from work on the fluid 'mechanics' of the mind (e.g. on primary memory) where no older adults are found in the top region of the performance distribution. Of course, our findings do not show that old age guarantees wisdom; the only thing that growing old guarantees is more opportunities for growth in the domains of knowledge that underlie professional expertise and wisdom.

We do not know whether, or at what age, older adults' relative advantage on pragmatic tasks of life is limited by other negative factors that increase with age (e.g. losses in the cognitive mechanics discussed above or the increasing frequency of old age-related dysfunctions in brain structure and function). Our own interpretation of the data is that, on average, the ninth

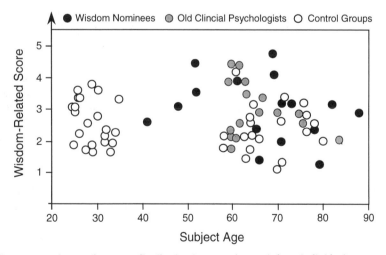

Figure 22.7. Age performance distribution in research on wisdom: individual responses from three comparison groups in two wisdom tasks. (After Baltes & Staudinger, 1993.)

decade of life represents some sort of threshold, at least under present-day conditions. Schaie's (1989) hazard functions support such a view. Similarly, in our work on wisdom, even in persons who were nominated by strict criteria as being wise, if they were older than 80 or so, their performances on wisdom-related tasks tended to decline. However, these are impressions awaiting more careful analysis. In any case, it seems reasonable to assume that culture- and expertise-based processes are delimited by a threshold of biological capacity, and that at some point we can no longer compensate for our declining biological resources. Culture-based knowledge is 'power'. However, for cultural and experiential factors to be expressed, a minimum or threshold amount of neurophysiological efficacy is necessary.

The self in old age: another example of plasticity

Another area of aging research, which can be viewed as a further instantiation of cognitive pragmatics and which speaks to psychological plasticity and multidirectionality in old age, is self-related functioning. The self system includes such components as identity, life goals, subjective well-being, and the sense of psychological control.

Because our expectations of old age are generally negative, the results obtained from investigations of how self-related indicators vary with old age are surprising. Despite the objective and subjective losses in reserve capacity and the age-associated increases in morbidity and mortality, older adults (and this includes the very old) do not show a reduction in various indicators related to the self, such as self-esteem, sense of personal control, or depressivity including psychiatric depression (Filipp & Klauer, 1986; Lachman, 1986). To illustrate this, Figure 22.2 includes information relevant to subjective well-being.

What psychological principles can account for this counterintuitive finding or paradox (Baltes, 1993)? Why should objective losses and subjective experiences of aging losses not result in a weakening of older adults' sense of self-esteem and personal control? Recently, there has been an outpouring of psychological work dealing with this topic of a resilient self in old age (e.g. Baltes & Baltes, 1990; Brandtstädter & Greve, 1994; Brim, 1992; Filipp & Klauer, 1986; Heckhausen & Schulz, 1993; Markus & Herzog, 1991; Ryff, 1991; Staudinger, Marsiske, & Baltes, 1993). At least three interrelated principles have been advanced to capture the remarkable power of the self to reorganize and readjust our identity and selfhood in response to rather differing life circumstances.

A first important avenue toward maintaining a positive sense of self is the principle of '*multiple or possible selves.*' Our self involves more than one self, it is a system of selves. Thus, most humans have rather differing expectations of who they are, who they were, who they would like to be, who else they could be, and who they would not want to be at all. Because we have a whole system of selves, it is possible that when one self is challenged by an injury (e.g. being an athlete), for example, another self (e.g. being a lover of music) is there to take its place.

A second important principle of self-management is a subjectively constructed *change in goals and levels of aspirations* (Brim, 1992; Heckhausen & Schulz, 1993). If it is not possible to achieve certain goals, one's level of aspiration and structure can be altered, or new goals can be considered. It is also possible for one to modify the time span in which these goals are to be reached, for example, by moving goals back and forth in one's lifetime perspective. In fact, Brandtstädter and his colleagues have demonstrated that during adulthood people seem to get better at using this principle. That is, older adults seem to become more flexible in accommodating their life goals to new circumstances rather than being goal-tenacious (Figure 22.8). Heckhausen & Schulz (1993) have employed the principle of primary versus secondary control to make a similar point. Primary control involves the pursuit of the same goals with established and new means. Secondary control involves adjusting goals and means to external circumstances by internal cognitive reconstruction and thereby creates a new life scenario. With age, Heckhausen and Schulz argue that people increasingly tend to select mechanisms of secondary control.

The third principle of self-management involves the *process of social comparison* and the possibility of finding new points of comparison when circumstances have changed. New reference groups are often available, thus

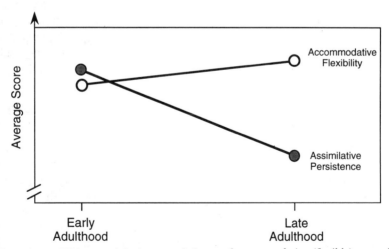

Figure 22.8. With age, adults increase their use of accommodative (flexible) strategies of adaptation and coping (simplified after Brandtstädter & Greve, 1994). Assimilative coping involves tenacious goal pursuit, accommodative coping is related to flexible goal adjustment.

permitting a reorganization of one's standards and values. For instance, if we are struck by an illness, there are usually others who have experienced the same or a worse fate. Those with a heart attack increasingly compare themselves to others who also had heart attacks. As we grow old, others also grow old. Because we can also find others in worse circumstances, they permit us to make downward comparisons (Heckhausen & Schultz, 1993). As a result, the experience of aging and old age can be seen in a new light, and a positive sense of the self can be maintained.

In sum, our selves have remarkable resiliency and adaptive capacity for reorganization and maintaining integrity. It seems possible for most older persons to continue to use this dynamic and adaptive feature of the self as a kind of protective shield against the adversities associated with becoming old. Some people are more effective in this than others, of course. *Being old, however, is not a risk factor where negative emotional states associated with the self are concerned.* On the contrary, the emerging evidence demonstrates that older individuals can acquire substantial knowledge of the factors and processes that permit effective mastery. Although analogies carry the risk of oversimplification, it is possible, as Brandstädter and Greve (1994) have suggested, to compare these processes with the concept of immunization as used in biology and medicine. In a similar way, many aging individuals may rely more extensively on high-level self-protective and immunizing strategies.

THREE INTEGRATIVE PERSPECTIVES

In this concluding section, we offer three integrative perspectives. We do this for two reasons. The first is our conviction that these perspectives serve to move us toward a more systemic view and exploration of psychological aging. The second reason concerns the intent of this book, which is to highlight interdisciplinary linkages.

The lifespan: a changing dynamic between growth (gains) and decline (losses)

At the outset of this chapter, we examined the overall dynamic of the life course which centers around biological-genetic and environmental-cultural factors, on what cultural anthropologists have called the 'hiatus' of life: growth and decline. Psychological-developmental theory of the lifespan suggests that this dynamic is not one of sequence (growth followed by decline) but rather one of a change in proportion. On the psychological level, growth is possible even in old age, and decline begins already at birth (Baltes, 1987).

Figure 22.9 summarizes our general view on the changing dynamic of growth and decline across the lifespan. The left-hand side of this figure reports data from a study that examined adults' view of the life course (Heckhausen,

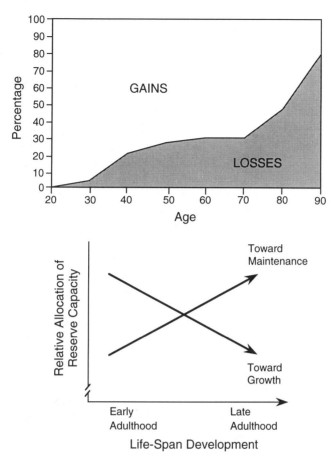

Figure 22.9. Gains and losses in attributes and functions across the lifespan. The top section of figure shows subjective expectations based on Heckhausen et al. (1989). The bottom section illustrates the interplay between age changes in plasticity and allocation of reserve capacity into two general goals of life management: maintenance vs. growth (after Staudinger et al., 1993).

Dixon & Baltes, 1989). The study used several hundred attributes (such as intelligent, energetic, helpful, healthy) and subjects were asked to use these in order to indicate what age changes they expected for each decade of adult life. Gains were defined as increases in desirable attributes (such as intelligent), and losses as increases in undesirable attributes (such as rigid). Subjects of all adult ages reported the pattern displayed in the upper part of Figure 22.9, that is, a systematic shift toward an increasingly less favorable balance. Also notable, however, is that even in advanced old age, subjects expected some positive changes, for instance, in the attribute of 'being wise'.

This shifting balance of anticipated growth and decline seems reasonably consistent with the empirical evidence that we presented earlier in this chapter. Plasticity and efficacy of functioning continue to be manifest for many into old age. However, on average two facts limit what is possible (Staudinger, Marsiske & Baltes, 1993). First, when the limits and range of plasticity in psychological functioning are tested, older adults demonstrate lower levels and an increasing need for time and accuracy control in tasks of basic information processing (cognitive mechanics). As a consequence, during a given time period (e.g. an hour, a day) fewer cognitive activities are possible. Although relevant research is not known to us, it is likely that this reduction in plasticity is not only cognitive, but that it also has an 'energetic' or motivational component (see also Carstensen, 1993). Secondly, with increasing age, there is, aside from processes of normal aging, the fact of age-related increases in physical morbidity. These are challenges to 'maintenance of function' and require attention.

The lower part of Figure 22.9 is an attempt by Staudinger, Marsiske and Baltes to highlight the interactive result of the two streams of age-related change: loss in level and range of plasticity and age-related increases in risk and morbidity factors (Staudinger et al., 1993). These authors propose that with increasing age, and more so as individuals reach advanced old age, their developmental resources (plasticity) must be allocated increasingly to maintenance and to avoidance of negative outcomes, thus leaving fewer resources that can be allocated to growth and positive change. One study which has produced results consistent with this overall dynamic is work by a research group of the Berlin Aging Study (Baltes, M. et al., 1993). When examining the relative impact of biological-medical conditions versus psychological functioning on the level and scope of everyday competence in old and very old persons, a broadly ranging everyday life style was possible only if two conditions were present: physical competence and psychological competence.

Selective optimization with compensation

The second integrative perspective reflects work on the nature of 'successful' aging. Successful aging is a concept which during the last decade has attracted much attention in gerontology, in part because the term explicitly challenges the negative stereotype of aging and forces investigators to explore the potential of old age (Baltes & Baltes, 1990; Rowe & Kahn, 1987). Moreover, the concept of successful aging forces researchers to spell out outcome criteria for aging well, outcome criteria that extend beyond longevity and consider the psychological quality of life as measured by such variables as life satisfaction, a sense of efficacy and control, or meaning of life.

We have speculated about general strategies of mastery that can describe the effective management of life in the face of age-associated losses in mental and physical reserves. One such strategy is 'selective optimization with compensation' (Baltes, 1987; Baltes & Baltes, 1990), that is, the notion that good or successful aging is based on the interplay among three components: *selection, optimization* and *compensation*. A real-life example of how this strategy is realized was provided by a television interview with the 80 year-old pianist Rubinstein. When asked how he succeeded in remaining such an admired concert pianist, Rubinstein mentioned three factors. First, he noted that he dealt with the weaknesses of old age by reducing the scope of his repertoire and by playing fewer pieces (an example of selection). Secondly, with the pieces selected he spends more time at practice than earlier in his life (an example of optimization). Thirdly, he uses special strategies such as slowing down his play before fast segments, thereby creating the impression of faster tempo than is objectively true (an example of compensation).

This selective optimization with compensation strategy is consistent with the conclusions presented earlier in this chapter (see also Baltes & Baltes, 1990). The first component of the strategy, selection, can be viewed as the correlate or outcome of an aging-associated reduction in reserve capacity (plasticity). Such a reduction objectively and subjectively mandates a reduction of certain activities (those falling below threshold levels) and in the sheer number of high performance life domains. The second component, optimization, illustrates that it is possible to maintain high levels of functioning in some areas, by practice and the acquisition of new bodies of knowledge and technology. The third component, compensation, becomes relevant when life tasks require a level of capacity beyond the current level of performance potential and alternative ways and means to reach the desired goals can be substituted (Bäckman & Dixon, 1992). We experience such needs for compensation especially in situations characteristic of high mental or physical demands, such as when having to think and memorize new material very fast, or reacting quickly when driving a car, or when climbing a mountain, or having to run fast. In addition, it is the occurrence of illness which makes the need for compensation most salient, and as described earlier, such events are more likely to happen in old age than at earlier periods of the lifespan.

We maintain that the process of optimization through selection and compensation is a general, prototypical process of effective management of old age. Its phenotypic manifestation, however, will vary widely between individuals. Thus, while all aging individuals are likely to engage in some form of selection, optimization and compensation, the specific phenotypic form (expression) of mastery will vary depending upon individuals' life histories and their patterns of interests, values, health, skills and resources (Thomae, 1979).

To prevent a possible misunderstanding, we emphasize that selective optimization with compensation is not specific to old age; we assume that it is a process that operates in all phases of life (Baltes, 1987). We assume, however, that ontogenetic selection pressure for this general strategy increases with age. Because of aging losses in plasticity and age-associated increases in morbidity, the intensity and prevalence of this strategy is likely to take on added functional significance in old age. Moreover, from a psychological perspective, as they move toward old age, individuals seem to display good pragmatic competence in understanding those core conditions that define what is possible or not possible, to apply such knowledge in personal development and adaptation, and thereby to attempt to solve the hiatus created by the challenges and reduced opportunities of an aging body.

The link between psychological models of growth and decline to general biological and physical theories of change

Our final general perspective is a first effort to relate a psychology of aging to conceptual work in physics and biology (Barton, 1994; Brent, 1978). Specifically, we explore briefly to what extent two concepts – self-organization and exchange entropy – might provide new insights and opportunities for interdisciplinary exchange and collaboration.

The notion of self-organization is familiar from Prigogine (Prigogine & Stengers, 1984), Maturana (Maturana & Varela, 1980) and others who have argued that all living systems, such as human beings and human minds, have the capacity for self-organization, thus enabling them to adapt in particular ways. A system or process is said to be self-organizing if its 'structure or pattern emerges . . . without specification from the environment' (Barton, 1994, p. 7). One commonly cited example of such a system is the biological cell. The 'transactions inside the cell are determined by the pattern of organization within that cell, and they produce the materials required for the operation of the cell itself . . . the characteristic "metabolism, growth, and replication" all take place within the bounds of the cell (and according to the pattern of organization that would distinguish an epithelial cell from a retinal cell, for example).'

Some collections of individuals (e.g. a self-help group, a music club) provide another example of self-organization and they illustrate the difference between various kinds of systems. By virtue of the particular individuals in a group, each with his/her own needs, desires, strengths and weaknesses, a certain pattern of interaction emerges among them. The group creates and defines itself, in a recursive manner, by the unique pattern of interaction among the members; it is simultaneously cause and consequence of interactions among the members. In contrast to the biological cell which is bounded by a physical barrier – the cell membrane, however, a group of individuals (like the systems implicated in psychological aging) is not delimited by a physical barrier, but only by the interaction among its constitutive components. The latter type of systems are said to be operationally closed (Varela, 1978).

Operationally closed systems can freely exchange both matter and energy with their environment, but they are closed to information. Thus, a change in its niche cannot 'instruct' such a system and cannot selectively influence its functioning; a niche change can serve only as an environmental event that perturbs the system and presents it with new constraints and opportunities.

The concept of operationally closed, self-organizing systems might give new insights into psychological aging because the mind is composed of a myriad of functions/systems that are continually changing, and thus it must always be engaged in adaptation. Like a Russian doll where one entire whole is contained inside another, or like the social fabric of a community where groups/clubs overlap to varying degrees, the human mind comprises a vast collection of systems that are embedded in (or overlap) each other (Ford & Lerner, 1992; Lerner, 1991). In this way, each system must operate in the context of, or the niche shaped by, a multitude of other systems. Systems do not 'instruct' each other, but they are intimately linked and provide both opportunities and constraints for each other. Consequently, when one or more of these systems change with age, this change alters the niche (i.e. introduces new constraints or opportunities for other systems) and thus perhaps the functioning of other systems.

A concrete example is the age-related change in working memory which in turn influences the operation of the systems involved in reading, language comprehension and problem solving. For another example, Salthouse's studies with young and older typists that we reported earlier in this chapter show how the cognitive system adapts to a reduction in motor speed. A system's precise adaptation to – compensation for – change in its niche depends on a variety of factors, however, including the specific new constraints imposed or opportunities afforded by that change, its dependence on resources that are no longer available, and its plasticity or capacity to organize itself into new patterns.

As a physical entity, the human being is also subject to the second law of thermodynamics, thus positioned on the relentless path toward an ever greater degree of entropy or disorganization. But open, living systems have the capacity to overcome (at least ward off for a time) the inevitable fate that follows from the second law by 'harvesting' or 'living off' low entropy structures in their environment or niche. As described in Brent (1978), Prigogine used the notion of exchange entropy to discuss this process, suggesting that living systems become more organized by exploiting low entropy resources in their niche and returning higher entropy structures as 'waste' products to their niche. Thus, to the extent that a system is more effective at exchanging low entropy (i.e. organized) input for higher entropy (disorganized) output than its base rate tendency toward entropy, its net organization/complexity will increase over time. Consistent with these ideas, and with our previous discussion of the dynamic interplay between gains and losses across the lifespan, we speculate that across the human lifespan, the overall entropy exchange efficiency might increase in childhood and perhaps in early adulthood, be maintained through adulthood, but then undergo a gradual decline in old age.

In the field of developmental psychology and considering the 'mindfulness' of human behavior, Brent (1978) has taken the notion of exchange entropy one step further by exploring the fact that human beings are comprised of both biological and symbolic (knowledge) systems. These systems occupy and exploit their own pool of low entropy structures, and their combination enables the unique adaptation exhibited by human beings. The difference between symbolic and biological systems can be mapped onto our distinction between the pragmatics and mechanics of mind, thus enabling speculations about two distinct lifespan functions in entropy exchange efficiency similar to the two lifespan trajectories displayed by the fluid mechanics and crystallized pragmatics of intelligence (see Figure 22.4). The entropy exchange efficiency of the biological-mechanics of mind is likely to show a rapid increase in childhood, peak in young adulthood, and then decline toward old age. By contrast, the entropy exchange efficiency of the symbolic pragmatics of mind is likely to grow more slowly at the onset of life, increase and grow well into adulthood, and maintain itself well into old age, at least as long as no major brain-related dysfunctions occur.

OUTLOOK

Neither the biological matrix of the human species nor the current state of the cultural world ought to be viewed as natural, fixed representations of 'the' nature of human aging. Rather, like many other facets of the human condition, aging is to a significant degree the product of individual and societal conditions. The nature of aging itself is subject to continuous evolution, and because of the historical infancy of our aging society, we need to extend our vision beyond the conditions of our current reality.

The many faces of aging reflect the fact that it is an evolutionary and modifiable process. The family of conclusions and perspectives offered in this chapter constitutes a blueprint or chart for specific future research directions. We remain guided by the fact that biology sets unavoidable limits to the spectrum of possibilities in old age, that the deficient state of biological structure and function becomes more and more conspicuous in old age. Importantly, however, we regard this very fact as a challenge for cultural evolution and psychological optimization. States of deficit and limitations are powerful catalysts for cultural progress and new forms of mastery or cultural innovation. By accepting this challenge, it may be possible not only to learn more and more about the reserve capacities of old age, but also about the conditions of a 'culture of old age' whose primary commitment is the conquest of the deficits of biological aging and the creating of conditions facilitative of high levels of subjective well-being, agency, and a sense of personal control.

We began this chapter with the observation that gerontology and old age in an interesting way are 'young'. Indeed, psychological research on human aging is in its infancy. The scope, precision and applicability of relevant theories leave much to be desired. Interdisciplinary linkages, for instance between the biological, psychological and social aspects of human aging, are largely unexplored, and neurobiological substrates and correlates of the phenomena await specification. However, in our view some progress has been made. Simple decline and deterioration models of human aging should no longer be part of gerontology. Both potential and limits, gains and losses, are part of the psychology of aging, and the analysis of their interaction is the challenge of future scholarship.

REFERENCES

Bäckman, L. & Dixon, R. (1992) Psychological compensation: a theoretical framework. *Psychological Bulletin*, **112**, 259–83.

Baltes, M. M., Kühl, K.-P. & Sowarka, D. (1992) Testing for limits of cognitive reserve capacity: a promising strategy for early diagnosis of dementia? *Journal of Gerontology: Psychological Sciences*, **47**, 165–7.

Baltes, M. M., Mayr, U., Borchelt, M., Maas, I. & Wilms, H.-U. (1993) Everyday competence in old and very old age: an interdisciplinary perspective. *Ageing and Society*, **13**, 657–80.

Baltes, P. B. (1987) Theoretical propositions of life-span developmental psychology: on the dynamics between growth and decline. *Developmental Psychology*, **23**, 611–26.

Baltes, P. B. (1993) The aging mind: potential and limits. *Gerontologist*, **33**, 580–94.

Baltes, P. B. & Baltes, M. M. (eds.) (1990) *Successful Aging: Perspectives from the Behavioral Sciences*. New York: Cambridge University Press.

Baltes, P. B. & Kliegl, R. (1992) Further testing of limits of cognitive plasticity: Negative age differences in a mnemonic skill are robust. *Developmental Psychology*, **28**, 121–5.

Baltes, P. B., Mayer, K. U., Helmchen, H. & Steinhagen-Thiessen, E. (1993) The Berlin Aging Study (BASE): overview and design. *Ageing and Society*, **13**, 483–515.

Baltes, P. B. & Mittelstrass, J. (eds.) (1992) *Zukunft des Alterns und gesellschaftliche Entwicklung*. Berlin: De Gruyter.

Baltes, P. B. & Staudinger, U. M. (1993) The search for a psychology of wisdom. *Current Directions in Psychological Science*, **2**, 75–80.

Barkow, J. H., Cosmides, L. & Tooby, J. (eds.) (1992) *The Adapted Mind: Evolutionary Psychology and the Generation of Culture*. New York: Oxford University Press.

Barton, S. (1994) Chaos, self-organization, and psychology. *American Psychologist*, **49**, 5–14.

Birren, J. E. (ed.) (1959) *Handbook for Aging and the Individual: Psychological and Biological Aspects*. Chicago, Ill.: University of Chicago Press.

Birren, J. E. & Bengtson, V. L. (eds.) (1988) *Emergent Theories of Aging*. New York: Springer.

Brandtstädter, J. & Greve, W. (1994) The aging self: stabilizing and protective processes. *Developmental Review*, **14**, 52–80.

Brent, S. B. (1978) Prigogine's model for self-organization in nonequilibrium systems: its relevance for developmental psychology. *Human Development*, **21**, 374–87.

Brim, G. (1992) *Ambition: Losing and Winning in Everyday Life*. New York: Basic Books.

Brock, D. B., Guralnik, J. M. & Brody, J. A. (1990) Demography and epidemiology of aging in the United States. In Schneider, E. L. & Rowe, J. W. (eds.) *Handbook of the Biology of Aging*. San Diego, Calif.: Academic Press, pp. 3–23.

Carstensen, L. L. (1993) Motivation for social contact across the life-span: A theory of socioemotional selectivity. In Jacobs, J. (ed.) *Nebraska symposium on motivation* (Vol. 40). Lincoln, Nebr.: University of Nebraska Press, pp. 205–54.

Craik, F. I. M. & Salthouse, T. A. (eds.) (1992) *The Handbook of Aging and Cognition*. Hillsdale, NJ: Erlbaum.

Durham, W. H. (1990) Advances in evolutionary culture theory. *Annual Review of Anthropology*, **19**, 187–210.

Edelman, G. M. (1987) *Neural Darwinism: the Theory of Neuronal Group Selection*. New York: Basic Books.

Ericsson, K. A. & Smith, J. (eds.) (1991) *Towards a General Theory of Expertise: Prospects and Limits*. New York: Cambridge University Press.

Filipp, S.-H. & Klauer, T. (1986) Conceptions of self over the life span: reflections on the dialectics of change. In Baltes, M. M. & Baltes, P. B. (eds.) *The Psychology of Control and Aging*. Hillsdale, NJ: Erlbaum, pp. 167–205.

Ford, D. H. & Lerner, R. M. (1992) *Developmental Systems Theory: An Integrative Approach*. London: Sage.

Fozard, J. L., Metter, E. J. & Bryant, L. J. (1990) Next steps in describing aging and disease in longitudinal studies. *Journal of Gerontology: Psychological Sciences*, **45**, 116–27.

Fries, J. F. (1989) The compression of morbidity: near or far? *Milbank Memorial Fund Quarterly*, **67**, 208–32.

Gerok, W. & Brandtstädter, J. (1992) Normales, krankhaftes und optimales Altern: Variationen und Modifikation. In Baltes, P. B. & Mittelstrass, J. (eds.) *Zukunft des Alterns und gesellschaftliche Entwicklung*. Berlin: de Gruyter, pp. 356–85.

Gruman, G. J. (ed.) (1979) *Roots of Modern Gerontology and Geriatrics*. New York: Arno Press.

Heckhausen, J., Dixon, R. A. & Baltes, P. B. (1989) Gains and losses in development throughout adulthood as perceived by different adult age groups. *Developmental Psychology*, **25**, 109–21.

Heckhausen, J. & Schulz, R. (1993) Optimization by selection and compensation: Balancing primary and secondary control in life-span development. *International Journal of Behavioral Development*, **16**, 287–303.

Hertzog, C. & Schaie, K. W. (1988) Stability and change in adult intelligence: 2. Simultaneous analysis of longtitudinal means and covariance structures. *Psychology and Aging*, **3**, 122–30.

Horn, J. L. & Hofer, S. M. (1992) Major abilities and development in the adult period. In Sternberg, R. J. & Berg, C. A. (eds.) *Intellectual development*. New York: Cambridge University Press, pp. 44–99.

Kliegl, R., Mayr, U. & Krampe, R. Th. (1994) Time-accuracy functions for determining process and person differences: an application to cognitive aging. *Cognitive Psychology*, **26**, 134–64.

Lachman, M. E. (1986) Personal control in later life: stability, change, and cognitive correlates. In Baltes, M. M. & Baltes, P. B. (eds.) *The Psychology of Control and Aging*. Hillsdale, NJ: Erlbaum, pp. 207–36.

Lehr, U. & Thomae, H. (Hrsg.) (1987) *Formen seelischen Alterns: Ergebnisse der Bonner Gerontologischen Längsschnittstudie (BOLSA)*. Stuttgart: Enke.

Lerner, R. M. (1991) Changing organism-context relations as the basic process of development: a developmental contextual perspective. *Developmental Psychology*, **27**, 27–32.

Lindenberger, U. & Baltes, P. B. (1994) Sensory functioning and intelligence in old age: A powerful connection. *Psychology and Aging*, **9**, 339–55.

Lindenberger, U. & Baltes, P. B. (1994) Intellectual aging. In Sternberg, R. J. et al. (eds.) *Encyclopedia of Intelligence*. New York: Macmillan, pp. 52–66.

Magnusson, D. (1988) *Individual Development from an Interactional Perspective: A Longitudinal Study*. Hillsdale, NJ: Erlbaum.

Manton, K. G. (1989) Life-style risk factors. *Annals of the Academy of Political and Social Sciences*, **503**, 72–88.

Markus, H. R. & Herzog, A. R. (1991) The role of the self-concept in aging. *Annual Review of Gerontology and Geriatrics*, **11**, 110–43.

Marsiske, M., Lang, F., Baltes, M. M. & Baltes, P. B. (1995) Selective optimization with compensation: life-span perspectives on successful human development. In Dixon, R. A. & Bäckman, L. (eds.) *Compensation for Psychological Defects and Declines: Managing Losses and Promoting Gains*. Hillsdale, NJ: Erlbaum, pp. 35–79.

Maturana, H. & Varela, F. (1980) *Autopoiesis and Cognition: The Realization of the Living*. Boston: D. Riedel.

Mayr, U. & Kliegl, R. (1993) Sequential and coordinative complexity: age-based processing limitations in figural transformations. *Journal of Experimental Psychology: Learning, Memory and Cognition*, **19**, 1297–320.

Nelson, A. E. & Dannefer, D. (1992) Aged heterogeneity: fact or fiction? The fate of diversity in gerontological research. *Gerontologist*, **32**, 17–23.

Nesselroade, J. R. (1989) Adult personality development: Issues in addressing constancy and change. In Rabin, A. I., Zucker R. A., Emmons, R. A. & Frank, S. (eds.) *Studying Persons and Lives*. New York: Springer, pp. 41–85.

Nesselroade, J. R. & Baltes, P. B. (eds.) (1979) *Longitudinal Research in the Study of Behavior and Development*. New York: Academic Press.

Plomin, R., Pedersen, N. L., Lichtenstein, P. & McClearn, G. E. (1994) Variability and stability in cognitive abilities are largely genetic later in life. *Behavior Genetics*, **24**, 207–15.

Poon, L. W. (ed.) (1992) *The Georgia Centenarian Study*. Amityville, NY: Baywood.

Prigogine, I. & Stengers, I. (1984) *Order out of Chaos*. New York: Bantam.

Riegel, K. F. & Riegel, R. M. (1972) Development, drop, and death. *Developmental Psychology*, **6**, 306–19.

Rowe, J. W. & Kahn, R. L. (1987) Human aging: usual and successful. *Science*, **237**, 143–9.

Ryff, C. D. (1991) Possible selves in adulthood and old age: a tale of shifting horizons. *Psychology and Aging*, **6**, 286–95.

Salthouse, T. A. (1984) The skill of typing. *Scientific American*, **250**, 128–35.

Salthouse, T. A. (1991) *Theoretical Perspectives on Cognitive Aging*. Hillsdale, NJ: Erlbaum.

Schaie, K. W. (1989) The hazards of cognitive aging. *The Gerontologist*, **29**, 484–93.

Schaie, K. W. & Willis, S. L. (1986) Can adult intellectual decline be reversed? *Developmental Psychology*, **22**, 223–32.

Shock, N. W. (1977) System integration. In Finch, C. E. & Hayflick, L. (eds.) *Handbook of the Biology of Aging*. New York: Van Nostrand Reinhold, pp. 639–65.

Simonton, D. K. (1988) Age and outstanding achievement: what do we know after a century of research? *Psychological Bulletin*, **104**, 251–67.

Sinnott, J. D. & Cavanaugh, J. C. (eds.) (1991) *Bridging Paradigms: Positive Development in Adulthood and Cognitive Aging*. New York: Praeger.

Smith, J. & Baltes, P. B. (1993) Differential psychological aging: profiles of the old and very old. *Ageing and Society*, **13**, 551–87.

Staudinger, U. M., Marsiske, M. & Baltes, P. B. (1993) Resilience and levels of reserve capacity in later adulthood: perspectives from life-span theory. *Development and Psychopathology*, **5**, 541–66.

Sternberg, R. J. (ed.) (1990) *Wisdom: Its Nature, Origins and Development*. New York: Cambridge University Press.

Thomae, H. (1979) The concept of development and life-span developmental psychology. In Baltes, P. B. & Brim, O. G., Jr. (eds.) *Life-span Development and Behavior, Vol. 2*. New York: Academic Press, pp. 282–312.

Varela, F. J. (1978) The lessons of natural history for systems theory. In Klir, G. J. (ed.) *Applied General Systems Research*. New York: Plenum Press, pp. 77–84.

Weinert, F. E. (1992) Altern in psychologischer Perspektive. In Baltes, P. B. & Mittelstrass, J. (Hrsg.) *Zukunft des Alterns und gesellschaftliche Entwicklung*. Berlin: DeGruyter, pp. 180–203.

Willis, S. L. (1991) Cognition and everyday competence. In Schaie, K. W. (ed.) *Annual Review of Gerontology and Geriatrics, Vol. 11*. New York: Springer, pp. 80–109.

23 Genetics of aging and Alzheimer's disease

JOHN HARDY

PREAMBLE

Much of what happens to us may seem chance happenstance. However, each of us is born into specific circumstances and with specific alleles at the many variable genetic loci. Historically, these two influences on our behavior – the environment and our genetic load – have been cast as opposing pillars in largely sterile 'nature' versus 'nurture' debates which have dominated much of psychology and psychiatry. Gradually, these unresolved debates are being put aside as more and more come to appreciate that individuals' behaviors are determined by the interaction of their genetic make up with their environment and their experience of their previous environments.

Until recently, it was not possible to quantify rigorously either genetic make up or individual's environments and behaviors. However, the recent explosive advances in molecular biology and computing are changing this situation rapidly. In particular, the many overlapping human genome projects are not only sequencing and storing large sections of the human genome, but also, they are beginning to allow the variability of this sequence information to be determined. It is my suspicion that this enterprise will reveal that the human genome is much more variable than is presently expected: at present, typically, a gene is cloned, sequenced once, and the information stored. Almost no genes have been systematically checked for variability between individuals.

Potentially, the occurrence of any observed sequence variation can be correlated with various traits and behaviors. This operation is laden with opportunities, but also fraught with potential problems related to the ethical use of this information. My intention in raising the point in this preamble to the main text of this chapter is to alert the reader, both to opportunities and hazards of molecular biology in general, and human molecular genetics in particular offer. These disciplines and this new information will have an enormous impact on society, on medicine and on the fields of psychology, sociology and psychiatry in particular. In this chapter, I shall discuss how molecular genetics has helped us to (partially) understand the riddles of the causes of dementia and also to discuss how understanding the genetics of common diseases helps us in understanding the genetics of longevity.

THE GENETICS OF ALZHEIMER'S DISEASE

The four major causes of death in the Western world are cancer, heart disease, stroke and dementing illnesses. Among the dementias, Alzheimer's disease (AD) is by far the most prevalent and probably accounts for about 75% of all the dementias.

It is clear that AD clusters in families and that a family history is a potent risk factor for the disease (Van Duijn et al., 1991). However, while many families in the literature display straightforward autosomal dominant inheritance of early onset disease (St George Hyslop et al., 1989), the mode of inheritance of the disease in an epidemiological context has not been clear. However, over the last three years, molecular genetic analyses of families multiply-affected by disease have started to allow an unraveling of the genes involved in the disease process as well as their mode of action.

Three genes have been shown to be involved in the etiology of the disease: these are the amyloid precursor protein (APP) gene on chromosome 21 (Goate et al., 1991), an, as yet unidentified gene on chromosome 14 (Schellenberg et al., 1992b) and the apolipoprotein E (ApoE) gene on chromosome 19 (Strittmatter et al., 1993).

APP genetics

The ages at which these genetic loci act are distinct. Thus, mutations in the APP gene, although very rare, are a major cause of fully penetrant, autosomal dominant AD with an onset range from 50–60 years (Goate et al., 1991, Chartier Harlin et al., 1991, Mullan et al., 1992, Hendricks et al., 1992). Very few families with APP mutations have an age of onset below this range (e.g. Murrell et al., 1991), and none, so far, above this age (while, conventionally, we speak of the APP mutations as giving rise to an autosomal dominant disorder, in fact, no mutation homozygotes have been identified). The effects of these mutations is to cause a greater proportion of APP to be metabolized to insoluble beta-amyloid (see Hardy and Duff, 1993 for review).

Chromosome 14 genetics

The chromosome 14 locus appears to cause fully penetrant, autosomal dominant disease with an onset age from 30–50 years (Schellenberg et al., 1992b). Within this age range it is the major (possibly the only) locus, apart from those few families with APP mutations in this age range. Very few families with the chromosome 14 locus form of the disease have an onset age above 50 years (e.g. FAD3) (St George Hyslop et al., 1992) (again, while this form of the disorder is conventionally described as a fully penetrant, autosomal dominant, there have been no documented mutant locus homozygotes).

ApoE genetics

The ApoE is variable locus on chromosome 19 with three common variants: E2 (ca. 10%), E3 (ca. 75%) and E4 (ca. 15%). These isoforms differ at amino acids 112 and 158. E2 has cysteine at both sites, E3 has cysteine at 112 and arginine at 158 and E4 has arginine at both sites. The three haplotypes give rise to six genotypes: E2E2 (ca. 1%); E2E3 (ca. 15%); E2E4 (ca. 3%); E3E3 (ca. 55%); E3E4 (ca. 23%); E4E4 (ca. 3%) (Davignon, Gregg & Sing, 1990). An association between markers on chromosome 19 and late onset AD had previously been reported and confirmed (Schellenberg et al., 1987; Pericak-Vance et al., 1991; Schellenberg et al., 1992a). Strittmatter and colleagues (1993) reported a very strong association between late onset AD and the E4 allele of ApoE in familial AD, a result they later extended to apparently sporadic disease (Saunders et al., 1993) and which has been multiply confirmed (e.g. Houlden et al., 1993b). However, it is clear that while the association between the E4 allele and AD is very strong in late onset AD, it is also important in early onset disease (Van Duijn et al., 1994). Indeed, the association between the E4 allele and disease starts to rise at around 45 years. Unlike the case with APP mutations and the chromosome 14 locus, it is clear that E4 homozygotes have a greatly increased risk for the development of disease (Corder et al., 1993). Thus, E3E4 heterozygotes have an increased risk for disease development of about threefold by the age of 75 years and that E4E4 homozygotes have an eightfold increase in risk for disease development by this age (Corder et al., 1993; data not based on epidemiological assessment). Furthermore, it is also clear that the E2 allele is associated with decreased risk of developing the disease and E2 homozygotes with a greatly decreased risk (Talbot et al., 1994; Corder et al., 1994).

Related to this ApoE genotype data in AD cases from the general population, it is clear that ApoE genotype influences the expression of the disease in cases where the primary lesion is at the amyloid locus. Thus, the E2 allele leads to a later onset of disease in cases with amyloid mutations (Houlden et al., 1993a) and in Down syndrome (Hardy et al., 1994) whereas, the E4 allele is associated with an earlier onset age of dementia in these cases. Indeed, the whole effect of the ApoE genotype appears to be simply summarized thus: relative to the common E3E3 genotype, E3E4 increases the risk of disease by an amount equivalent to five years of age, E4E4 by an amount equivalent to 10 years of age, E2E3 decreases the risk of disease by an amount equivalent to five years of age, E2E2 by an amount equivalent to 10 years of age. The one known exception to this general rule is chromosome

14 encoded disease which is not modulated by ApoE genotype (Van Broeckhoven et al., 1994b).

Calculations determining the proportion of risk of developing AD encoded by the ApoE locus are, as yet, imprecise because of the lack of good epidemiological data. However, a recent calculation (Corder et al., 1994) suggested that 80% of the risk of developing AD (relative to the low risk, E2E3 genotype) was encoded at the ApoE locus. This calculation, while crude, suggests that if everyone was E2E3, the prevalence of AD would be reduced by 80%. Since AD is a major cause of death in the age range 65–80 years, it is perhaps unsurprising that certain ApoE genotypes are associated with longevity (*vide infra*).

APoE AND HEART DISEASE

The findings relating ApoE to the pathophysiology of AD came as a surprise, since the only well-defined role of ApoE is in cholesterol and lipid transport (Mahley, 1988). The E4 allele is associated with higher blood cholesterol levels and with a higher incidence of coronary artery disease (Davignon et al., 1988). Thus, ApoE4 (which is probably the ancestral allele since other species have arginine at the equivalent sites) is a risk factor for the development of two of the four leading causes of death in the Western world and the ApoE2 allele is associated with protection against these two causes of death.

THE GENETICS OF LONGEVITY

With this background, it is not surprising that the frequency of the ApoE4 allele decreases with age and that of the ApoE2 allele increases with age (Louhija et al., 1994 and references therein). Indeed, studies of centenarians indicate that individuals with an E2 allele were twice as likely and individuals with an E4 allele half as likely at ApoE3 homozygotes to live to 100 years (Schachter et al., 1994). These effects are more pronounced in homozygotes. It would seem that ApoE2 homozygotes have a fourfold increase in their chances of reaching 100 years and that ApoE4 homozygotes almost never reach this age (Schachter et al., 1994).

DISCUSSION

These findings relating simply assessed genotypes to the risks of major causes of mortality and morbidity and to the chances of achieving longevity are likely to have a profound impact on the practice of health care. So far, widespread genetic analysis occur in only two circumstances: in families with life-threatening illnesses such as cystic fibrosis or Huntington's disease, and population screening for relatively common, manageable diseases such as phenylketonuria. Predictive testing for common, late onset causes of mortality and morbidity has more complex and wide-ranging effects, especially if these diseases are untreatable. Among the questions which have to be answered are:

(1) *Does the individual have the right to know his own genome?* My prejudice is that individuals should have this right, not least for the pragmatic reason that the tests are so simple that schoolchildren could carry them out using increasingly available simple laboratory equipment. Thus, I think it is likely to be impractical to prevent this information being gained. Furthermore, some of the information is likely to have immediate heath care benefits. For example, ApoE4 homozygotes could be cautioned (in a focused way) to have low cholesterol diets.

(2) *Do insurers have the right to know their client's genome?* The simple answer to this would seem to be 'no'. But if this is the case, clearly, for example, ApoE4 homozygotes could insure themselves for long-term care when they were in their fifties in the almost certain knowledge they would need such care when they got AD. In contrast, E_3E_2 heterozygotes could forego such coverage since they would be fairly confident that they would not need it.

(3) *Should employers have the right to know their employee's genome?* With regard to AD and heart disease, there is little reason why employers would find this information useful. However, as genetic associations for other, more 'personality-related' traits are identified this issue is likely to become of greater importance and difficulty.

These are just three of many questions which the progress in human molecular genetics pose: there are many other variants (should prospective spouses know each other's genome; should parents be able to choose their offspring's genetic characteristics; etc?). There are no correct answers to these questions: rather, societies will have to choose the answers which fit best with their plans for their futures. For such decisions to be made, it is vital that there is informed debate about the issues involved. For there to be informed debate, we desperately need better public education about genetics. An understanding of biology, based upon genetics, is as central and important to our future as are math and language. The present situation, where even specialists in other areas of the biology-based sciences from biochemistry to sociology are woefully ignorant of the fundamentals of genetics, does not bode well for the intelligence of the debate.

REFERENCES

Chartier Harlin, M. C., Crawford, F., Houlden, H., et al. (1991) Early onset Alzheimer's disease caused by mutations at codon 717 of the β-amyloid precursor protein gene. *Nature*, **353**, 844–6.

Corder, E. H., Saunders, A. M., Strittmatter, W. J., et al. (1993) Gene dose of Apolipoprotein E type 4 allele and the risk of Alzheimer's disease in late onset families. *Science*, **261**, 921–3.

Corder, E. H., Saunders, A. M., Risch, N. J., et al. (1994) Protective effect of apolipoprotein E type 2 allele for late onset Alzheimer's disease. *Nature Genetics*, **7**, 180–4.

Davignon, J., Gregg, R. E. & Sing, C. F. (1988) Apolipoprotein E polymorphism and atherosclerosis. *Arteriosclerosis*, **8**, 1–21.

Goate, A., Chartier Harlin, M. C., Mullan, M., et al. (1991) Segregation of a missense mutation in the amyloid precursor protein gene with familial Alzheimer's disease. *Nature*, **349**, 704–6.

Hardy, J., Crook, R., Perry, R., Raghavan, R. & Roberts, G. (1994) ApoE genotype and Down syndrome. *Lancet*, **343**, 979–80.

Hardy, J. & Duff, K. (1993) Heterogeneity in Alzheimer's disease. *Annals of Medicine*, **25**, 437–40.

Houlden, H., Collinge, J., Kennedy, A., et al. (1993a) ApoE genotype and Alzheimer's disease. *Lancet*, **342**, 737–8.

Houlden, H., Crook, R., Duff, K., Collinge, J., Rossor, M. & Hardy, J. (1993b) Confirmation that the Apolipoprotein E, E4 allele is associated with late onset, familial Alzheimer's disease. *Neurodegeration*, **2**, 283–6.

Hendricks, L., Van Duijn, C. M., Cras, P., et al. (1992) Presenile dementia and cerebral haemorrhage caused by a mutation at codon 692 of the beta-amyloid precursor protein gene. *Nature Genetics*, **1**, 218–21.

Louhija, J., Miettinen, H. E., Kontula, K., et al. (1994) Aging and genetic variation of plasma apolipoproteins: relative loss of apolipoprotein E4 phenotype in centenarians. *Arteriosclerosis and Thrombosis*, **14**, 1084–9.

Mahley, R. W. (1988) Apolipoprotein E: cholesterol transport protein with an expanding role in cell biology. *Science*, **240**, 622–30.

Mullan, M., Crawford, F., Axelman, K., et al. (1992) A new mutation in APP demonstrates that pathogenic mutations for probable Alzheimer's disease frame the beta-amyloid sequence. *Nature Genetics*, **1**, 345–7.

Murrell, J., Farlow, M., Ghetti, B. & Benson, M. (1991) A mutation in the amyloid precursor protein associated with hereditary Alzheimer's disease. *Science*, **254**, 97–9.

Pericak-Vance, M. A., Bebout, J. L., Gaskell, P. C., et al. (1991) Linkage studies in familial Alzheimer's disease: evidence for chromosome 19 linkage. *American Journal of Human Genetics*, **48**, 1034–50.

Saunders, A. M., Strittmatter, W. J., Schemechel, D., et al. (1993) Association of apolipoprotein E allele (e4) with late onset familial and sporadic Alzheimer's disease. *Neurology*, **43**, 1467–72.

Schachter, F., Faure-Delanef, L., Guenot, F., et al. (1994) Genetic associations with human longevity at the APOE and ACE loci. *Nature Genetics*, **6**, 29–32.

Schellenberg, G. D., Bird, T., Wijsman, E., et al. (1992a) Genetic association and linkage analysis of the apolipoprotein CII locus and familial Alzheimer's disease. *Ann. Neurol.*, **31**, 223–7.

Schellenberg, G. D., Bird, T., Wijsman, E., et al. (1992b) Genetic linkage evidence for a familial Alzheimer's disease locus on chromosome 14. *Science*, **258**, 668–71.

Schellenberg, G. D., Deeb, S. S., Boehnke, M., et al. (1987) Association of an apolipoprotein CII allele with familial dementia of the Alzheimer type. *Journal of Neurogenetics*, **4**, 97–108.

St George Hyslop, P. H., Haines, J. L., Rogaev, E., et al. (1992) Genetic evidence for a novel familial Alzheimer's disease locus on chromosome 14. *Nature Genetics*, **2**, 330–4.

St George Hyslop, P. H., Myers, R. H., Haines, J. L., et al. (1989) Familial Alzheimer's disease: progress and problems. *Neurobiological Aging*, **10**, 417–297.

Strittmatter, W. J., Saunders, A. M., Schmechel, D., et al. (1993) Apolipoprotein E: high avidity binding to beta-amyloid and increased frequency of type-4 allele in late onset familial Alzheimer's disease. *Proceedings of the National Academy of Science of the USA*, **90**, 1977–81.

Talbot, C., Lender, C., Craddock, N., et al. (1994) Protection against Alzheimer's disease with ApoE E2. *Lancet*, **343**, 1432–3.

Van Duijn, C. M., de Knijff, P., Cruts, M., et al. (1994) Apolipoprotein E4 allele in a population based study of early onset Alzheimer's disease. *Nature Genetics*, **7**, 74–8.

Van Duijn, C., Stijnen, T., Hofman, A. (1991) Overview of the EURODEM case control studies. *International Journal of Epidemology*, **20** Suppl. 2.

Van Broeckhoven, C., Backhovens, H., Cruts, M., et al. (1994) ApoE genotype does not modulate age of onset in families with chromosome 14 encoded Alzheimer's disease. *Neuroscience Letters*, **169**, 179–80.

24 Aging and molecular biology

DAVID G. MORGAN AND MARCIA N. GORDON

INTRODUCTION

Changes at the molecular level underlie a number of critical steps in embryogenesis and maturation of organisms into reproductively competent adults (Davidson, 1986). A fundamental question in the field of biogerontology is the degree to which changes associated with adult development and senescence might also cause similar changes at the molecular level. The view of some biogerontologists that adult development and aging is a continuation of the genetic program guiding the maturation of the organism, supports a primary role for molecular changes in driving aging processes. However, importantly, this perspective is not necessary for molecular alterations to be considered primary in the aging process. While 'molecular biology' has recently become associated with the study of nucleic acid polymers, this chapter will encompass a broader definition of the term molecules.

The chapter will be organized into three major sections. The first will briefly describe several theories that have attempted to explain age-related phenomena at the molecular level, identify specific predictions of these theories, and briefly summarize the evidence supporting (or refuting) these theories. The second section will summarize the regulations of genes by specific challenges, and changes in macromolecular regulation associated with aging. In the third section, recent data from the authors' laboratory relevant to these issues will be presented.

A significant question regarding adult development and senescence concerns the degree to which molecular changes found in aged organisms are the cause of organismic aging, rather than a result of primary changes occurring at other loci. Although sizeable in number, attempts at gerontological Thomism have been futile; there has yet to be a prime mover identified for the phenomena of aging. Increasingly, this frustration has led many biogerontologists to a conversion that aging, by analogy with complex disease processes such as heart disease or cancer, has multiple etiologies, and that attempts to single out specific causative agents will not be successful. Such a perspective is consistent with the population geneticists notion that aging arises within species because of the reduction in selective pressure on organisms as they grow older, thus favoring potentially pleiotropic genes, which enhance survival during early development, but have neutral or deleterious consequences once reproductive and progeny support events have been completed. This argument might also predict that the 'causes' of aging in different organisms and different tissues within an organism need not be mechanistically related, to the extent that different selective pressures operate independently on these tissues or organisms during early development. In the absence of compelling support for specific hypotheses, it is hard to determine whether this shift represents cyclic pendulum-like movements or a permanent realignment of paradigmatic emphasis.

The breadth of information on this topic is considerable, covering a number of organisms and *in vitro* systems. To retain a manageable scope, this review will focus upon *in vivo* aging in mammals, with only occasional reference to other organisms and in vitro aging. For a more inclusive review the reader is referred to Finch (1990).

MOLECULAR THEORIES RELATED TO ADULT DEVELOPMENT AND AGING

The theories described in this section are not intended to be exhaustive, but represent several of the hypotheses that have been carefully elaborated by several different investigators. Often, these theories lead to testable predictions. One theory (error castrophe) has not been fully supported by experimentation, but the remaining theories have some modicum of support from the experimental literature. Importantly, given the potential that aging is a multifactorial process, many of these theories may be partially correct and contribute in synergistic manners to produce the phenomena of aging.

Error catastrophe theory

Built upon the engineering concept of catastrophe theory, which explains phenomena such as the sudden failure of a bridge after years of accumulated damage, Orgel (1963) proposed that aging resulted from an accumulation of cells with damaged synthetic machinery. The concept is that damage occurs at a gradual rate to all molecules within a cell, but that turnover or repair activities prevent this damage from dramatically modifying cell function. However, at some point damage occurs to some molecule(s) involved in the generation of other macromolecules, either as a mutation or misincorporation of an amino acid into a protein. Damage is then propagated by generation of other aberrant molecules, for example, by misincorporation of amino acids into proteins, which leads to a vicious cycle of further damage to the synthetic apparatus. Rapidly, many of the molecules in the cell become dysfunctional, leading to tissue and organ impairments representative of physiological changes over the lifespan.

The error catastrophe theory predicts that in aged, senescent organisms, there should be the accumulation of aberrant molecules; proteins with misincorporated amino acids, or abnormal lipid structures. In addition, the protein synthetic machinery of at least some cells should lack the fidelity found in younger cells when tested *in vitro*, because of 'damaged' components of the synthetic machinery. In general, both predictions have been demonstrated *not* to occur with aging. An additional consideration is that the error catastrophe theory predicts that aging should occur suddenly (like a bridge collapse) rather than progressively following the attainment of reproductive competence. Unfortunately for error catastrophe theory, it has led to testable predictions that have been found not to be true.

Orgel's hypothesis led to a number of attempts to identify dysfunctional proteins in aged organisms. One common method to identify the presence of enzymes that might be dysfunctional was to compare the ratio of enzyme activity to immunoreactivity (specific activity) of an enzyme. Many of these data were reviewed by Reff (1985). Some, but by no means all, of the examined enzymes displayed a decreased specific activity with age, superficially supporting a prediction of Orgel's hypothesis (but also consistent with the cumulative damage hypothesis and several others). Importantly, for some of these enzymes, a cycle of denaturation followed by renaturation reversed the age-related reduction in specific activity (Yuh & Gafni, 1987). This indicated that, at least for these examples, the changes responsible for the decline in specific activity with age were post-translational and reversible. This is not consistent with Orgel's hypothesis, which would have predicted misincorporation of amino acids that could not be reversed by denaturation/renaturation.

Mori, Mizuno & Gato (1979) examined the accuracy of protein synthesis in a cell free system. No differences were found in the capacity of ribosomes from young and old donors to synthesize proteins faithfully. Another study (Popp et al., 1976) looked for the misincorporation of isoleucine into globin (normally lacking of isoleucine). No differences in the error rate was found with age in human globin. There is also no correlation of isoleucine misincorporation into globin with maximum lifespan in different animals (Hirsch et al., 1980). These results have led to the dismissal of the error catastrophe hypothesis as a meaningful explanation for molecular changes with aging.

Cumulative damage theories (oxidation, glycation, cross-linking)

Cumulative damage theories start with the same premise as error castrophe theory; that molecules are continuously suffering hits during routine cell activity which damage their function. With aging, there is an accumulation of damaged molecules which impairs cell (and thus tissue/organ) function. A catastrophe component might enter this scenario if the mechanisms by which molecules are replaced or repaired were to become defective, leading to exponential increases in the fraction of dysfunctional molecules.

One difference between these theories concerns the type of agent causing damage. In oxidative damage theories, oxygen radicals are the culprits. Free radicals are formed as intermediates during the reduction of molecular oxygen in mitochondrial electron transport, a number of enzymatic reactions, and may also be formed by the interactions of other agents with water, such as ionizing radiation, unchelated iron, or nitrites. The oxygen radicals extract electrons from other molecules, most often converting them into radicals which propagate the molecular damage by chain reaction. A variety of antioxidant defenses are found within cells which inactivate free radicals. Additionally, cells have repair/replacement mechanisms for most molecules which diminish the long-term consequences of oxygen radical damage. Oxidative damage has also been proposed as a causative factor in cancer, atherosclerosis and neurodegeneration as well as aging (Ames et al., 1993).

In glycation theory, glucose is the damaging agent (Cerami, 1985). Specifically, glucose is proposed to attach to molecules in a nonenzymatic covalent manner via Schiff base formation and condensation into Amadori products. In the presence of metal ions, the Amadori products proceed via Maillard reactions to form stable advanced glycosylation end products, resulting in inter- and intra-molecular crosslinkages (Monnier et al., 1991). The cross-linking is believed to decrease the functions of the affected molecules and lead to aging. This theory developed from the recognition that many symptoms of diabetes resembled advanced aging. Diabetes is proposed to be a segmental progeroid syndrome.

Bjorksten also proposed a cross-linking theory of aging in the 1940s. This theory focused on a special role for collagen cross-linking, but mechanistically predicts the same consequences as the oxidative and glycation theories, if expanded to include other molecules. It is also important to consider that these agents causing molecular damage may interact in a synergistic manner. Kristal & Yu (1992) have elegantly argued that oxidative damage predicts greater degrees of glycation, and that glycation products are expected to promote free radical formation.

These cumulative damage theories predict that damaged proteins and lipids will accumulate with age. In addition, these damaged molecules should bear the atomic scars of oxidative or glycative damage. One might predict that for aging to assume its progressive nature, the amount of oxidation and/or glycation of molecules should increase in parallel with organismic aging, owing to either increased concentrations of oxygen radicals and glucose, or declines in the defenses against such damage. Kristal & Yu propose that damage does occur to the cellular repair, removal and/or replacement systems over the lifespan, and this leads to a self-perpetuating cycle of gradual accumulation of damaged molecules, further reducing repair/replacement functions, and so on.

There is increasing evidence to support a role for cumulative damage to macromolecules during aging. There is some evidence that the antioxidant mechanisms which normally regulate oxidative damage are diminished with age. The redox state of glutathione shifts towards the oxidized form in aged rats (Noy, Schwartz & Gafni, 1985), and the activities of catalase and superoxide dismutase decline in some (but not all) tissues (Semsei, Rao & Richardson, 1989). Dietary restriction, a well-characterized lifespan extending treatment in rodents, slows the changes in catalase and superoxide dismutase, and reduces the age-related increase in oxidative damage to lipids found in liver (Rao et al., 1990). Over-expression of these antioxidant enzymes in transgenic flies increases median and maximum lifespan (Orr & Sohal, 1994). Recently, support has emerged for a role of free radicals in causing neurodegeneration, specifically a familial form of amyotrophic lateral sclerosis. Deng et al. (1993) have demonstrated reduced Cu/Zn superoxide dismutase activity in ALS families carrying a mutation in this gene. Linkage indicates that this defect causes the disease in an autosomal dominant fashion. Although these data support the capacity of oxygen radicals to damage tissues, this finding questions the universality of the free radical hypothesis of aging. Why is the disorder in these individuals ALS and not a form of progeria? Why is the primary degeneration in lower motor neurons (not a typical finding during human aging), and not other regions more commonly affected by age (e.g. hippocampus; substantia nigra)? Resolving these and similar questions should identify more precisely the roles of oxidative damage in aging processes.

Advanced glycosylation end-products accumulate in a variety of long-lived proteins over the lifespan. Tissues accumulating such products include skin (Monnier et al., 1991), the eye lens crystallins, collagen, myelin and hemoglobin (Lee & Cerami, 1990). Furthermore, in some instances, artificially induced oxidative damage can produce alterations in enzymes which behave the same as those found in aged tissues (Cook & Gafni, 1988).

However, it is important to recognize that damage to macromolecules occurs at all ages. Certainly, for long-lived proteins, cumulative damage may impair function on a timescale approximating the lifespan of the organism, but the bulk of proteins turn over with half lives that are very small fractions of the organismic lifespan. Hence, given generally accepted half lives, damage to these proteins should not induce the progressive changes associated with physiological aging because new proteins replace those that are damaged. One potential explanation is that, at least for some rodent tissues, there is a reduction in the rate of protein synthesis with aging (reviewed in Reff, 1985; Danner & Holbrook, 1990; Finch, 1990: ch. 7). It should be recognized that this literature is not without contradictions, and there are significant technical difficulties in performing turnover studies which involve correcting for precursor pool activities and reutilization of label. The majority of studies support the conclusion that the rate of protein elongation, but not initiation, is diminished over the rodent lifespan. Corresponding declines in protein degradation maintain steady state protein levels, but with extended half lives. Thus far, the small number of studies in humans have not found reductions in protein synthesis. Nonetheless, an extended residence time of proteins and other macromolecules in older organisms may allow molecular damage to have a progressive impact over the lifespan.

Somatic mutation theory

This is a DNA variant of the cumulative damage theories. The basis for the hypothesis is a gradual accumulation of mutations in the DNA of somatic cells. These mutations would modify protein function by specifying aberrant amino acid sequences and lead to cell, tissue and organ dysfunction. While there is some evidence for an increase in chromosomal abnormalities in somatic cells over the lifespan, Slagboom & Vijg (1992), in reviewing this literature, conclude that 'accumulation of mutations does not necessarily occur with aging'. However, two genomic changes which future research may emphasize in this regard are the age-related increase in mitochondrial DNA deletions in nondividing cells (Cortopassi & Arnheim, 1990), and the loss of chromosomal telomere repeats with aging both *in vitro* and *in vivo* (Hastie et al., 1990).

Gene derepression theory

Cytosine methylation is believed in some instances to be linked with gene repression, and to be one mechanism involved in differentiation. Evidence suggests that aging is associated with a loss of methylation, and this leads to inappropriate gene expression (Holliday, 1987; Mays-Hoopes, 1989). One example is reactivation of genes on the inactivated X chromosome in aged organisms (Wareham et al., 1987). However, further work indicated that much of this reactivation occurs early in the lifespan and should be considered a maturational rather that age-related change (Migeon, Axelman & Beggs, 1988).

Cutler (1982) elaborated a version of this theory called the dysdifferentiation theory of aging in which he predicted that a number of genes would be increasingly expressed in inappropriate tissues during aging. This inappropriate gene expression, again, might disrupt normal cell function leading to aging and senescence. Although there are a few cases of inappropriate tissue expression of some genes with aging, these appear to be exceptions, not examples. Sato et al. (1990) examined a number of tissue specific genes for inappropriate expression using sensitive methodology and failed to detect such changes in aged organisms. In addition, a substantial anatomical literature does not reveal gross changes in the differentiated characteristics of most organs with aging. Thus, while a potential explanation for isolated phenomena, the generality of the dysdifferentiation hypothesis appears limited.

A corollary of this hypothesis might include gene rearrangements to confer inappropriate expression. Evidence for rearrangements derives from the spontaneous age-related increase in vasopressin immunopositive neurons in the Brattleboro rat (homozygous for a deletion in the vasopressin gene; van Leeuwen et al., 1989), and the age-related increase in the number of hepatocytes immunopositive for albumin in the analbuminemic rat (Esumi et al., 1985). While intriguing as a potential mechanism for not only aging, but possibly carcinogenesis, these isolated findings have yet to be confirmed in other loci.

Endocrine theories of aging

The basic premise of the endocrine theories is that aging results in changes in (a) the steady-state levels of hormones, (b) dynamic responses of hormones to environmental challenges, and/or (c) changes in the sensitivity of tissues to these hormones. There are a number of variations on this theory, depending upon which hormone is being discussed. These endocrine changes cause inappropriate regulation of the expression of hormone-sensitive gene products with aging, resulting in altered cell growth, tissue physiology and organ function, ultimately leading to aging and senescence. These theories predict that changes in hormone levels are the events driving the changes in gene expression that occur with aging. There are ample examples of changes in gene expression which are secondary to hormonal changes. For example, the diminished induction of liver tyrosine amino transferase by cold stress is secondary to the diminished corticosterone response to the stress (Finch, Foster & Mirsky, 1969; Wellinger & Guigoz, 1986). The age-related decline of the male specific urinary protein $\alpha 2u$-globulin is secondary to the age-related decline in liver androgen receptor density, and thus diminished tissue responsiveness to testosterone; reduced testosterone levels with age magnify this decline (Roy et al., 1983). These age-related changes in $\alpha 2u$-globulin synthesis and transcription are attenuated in rats treated with dietary restriction (reviewed in Heydari & Richardson, 1992). These theories have some difficulty explaining age-associated changes in the expression of genes which are not regulated by hormones, although complex cascading interactions can be envisioned.

Anatomical theories

These theories claim that aging causes changes in the types and quantities of cells comprising specific organs (e.g. brain). Thus changes in the relative portions of different cell types would lead to differences in the tissue expression of certain genes consistent with the transition in cell types. As one example, during brain aging there are reports of neuron loss, and associated glial proliferation (reviewed in Finch & Morgan, 1990). Thus, changes in gene expression could be observed which are secondary to the shifts in cell types.

GENE REGULATION DURING AGING

A large number of studies have documented changes in chemical markers of aging in most tissues of the body. This author has shared in reviews of the literature concerning chemical markers of brain aging, with an emphasis on synaptic markers (Morgan & Finch, 1988; Morgan & May, 1990; Morgan, 1992). In general, it is difficult to synthesize definitive conclusions about the neurochemical markers of aging because the results reported are usually inconsistent. For virtually every report identifying a change with age, there is at least one contradictory report. It should also be recognized that many 'negative' findings (i.e. those for which no significant age-related change is detected) remain unpublished unless they are used to contrast with a marker that does change with age. Thus the number of reports failing to detect age-related changes underestimate the actual number of such findings.

In addition to the biochemical literature, there is an emerging parallel literature describing the use of molecular tools to identify changes in RNA levels and transcription with aging. Two recent reviews summarize the scattered reports that have appeared thus far (Danner & Holbrook, 1990; Thakur et al., 1993), and this chapter will not duplicate these compendia. As consensus emerges from these descriptive studies, they may lead to the development of more hypotheses concerning select aspects of aging. Increasingly, these molecular studies measure not only steady state levels of RNA, but changes in transcription, RNA stability and correlations with cognate protein levels and activities.

However, it is anticipated that as for the biochemical markers, the molecular marker literature will also be fraught with contradictory reports. To minimize the inconsistency, there are several considerations which must increasingly be satisfied before descriptive studies of this type are accepted for publication. Adherence to rigorous experimental design should aid in reducing the inconsistency. The considerations include:

(1) *Inclusion of more than two age groups.* The phenomena of aging are progressive after reproductive competence (at least in mammals). True markers of aging (what Finch, 1990, terms 'eugeric' changes) should also develop progressively, although not necessarily linearly, with age. Importantly, at least three of these age groups should be at ages beyond the period of biological maturation for that species (roughly 3 months in rodents; 18 years in humans). Additionally, including ages beyond the 50% survival point for the oldest age groups should be done cautiously. Together, these precautions will avoid erroneously attributing as 'aging-related' effects that are either late maturational changes, or secondary to pathology in other organs (pathogeric changes). Gene induction/repression studies should include multiple time points to distinguish changes in magnitude from changes in latency (*vide infra*).

(2) *Careful necropsy should be performed on all subjects.* While detailed pathology of aged rodents is a limitless realm of investigation, the investigator should at least examine for gross pathologic abnormalities. Body weights should be collected for several months before the animal is killed as an index of general health. We (and others) have found that body weights typically decline 10–25% in the months and weeks before natural death in rodents (Goss, Finch & Morgan, 1990). At the minimum the viscera should be examined for tumors, enlarged spleens, presence of food boli, abnormal appearance of lungs, heart, liver, reproductive organs. Kidneys should be incised and examined for stones or enlarged cisterns. If F344 rats are used, renal sections may be taken to score for renal pathology, an invariant age-related pathology in these rodents and the most common cause of natural death. The *n* for the older age groups should be increased so that animals with significant pathology can be culled from the study without compromising the statistical power of the experiment.

(3) *Several markers should be measured in the same sample preparation, including some which are not expected to change to control for general changes in sample properties affecting measurements.* When negative results are obtained, the power of the experiment should be evaluated, and the size of the difference which would have resulted in a significant change should be reported. Many age-related changes are small by molecular standards (30% is not uncommon). If no change is detected, but the *n* and variance are such that 50% differences would have been required to observe statistically reliable differences, the study can hardly be considered a 'negative' finding. It should be remembered that failing to reject the null hypothesis in inferential statistics does not mean there is no change, but simply that the experiment was unable to detect a change. This lesson is frequently forgotten in biological aging research (and in most of biology). It should also be recognized that most cross-sectional studies of aging violate a critical assumption of statistical analysis; age cannot be assigned randomly as an independent variable. Cohort effects must be considered, even for inbred or hybrid strains.

Rigid adherence to these experimental design considerations may avoid some of the inconsistencies that have muddied the waters in past aging studies.

While the descriptive studies of changes in steady-state levels of specific RNAs and proteins are valuable in aging research, increasingly, experiments which examine the dynamics of gene regulation and interventions which modify gene regulation are important in dissecting the causes of age-related changes. The induction of genes during the lifespan has been studied for the last 25 years, and some patterns of changes in gene induction have emerged, although they do not apply uniformly. The activation or inactivation of genes in response to environmental challenges may be the most critical molecular changes during aging. Perhaps the best characterization of aging processes at the physiological level is the loss of homeostatic capacity. Environmental challenges, which in young organisms were easily compensated for physiologically, often become life-threatening in aged organisms. Identifying the basis for this loss of homeostatic capacity is fundamental to aging research at the biological level. One intriguing possibility is that with age there is diminished capacity to alter gene expression in response to environmental challenges. This would dampen the ability of cells and tissues to respond sufficiently to the challenge and return to the homeostatic set point. If the diminution in gene induction arises because of changes in the nucleus which are generalizable, then a primary cause of many age-related phenomena may be identified. The molecular tools to begin addressing this question are now available.

Gene induction by environmental regulators in aging research has led to four general classes of results, summarized in the textbook by Timiras (1988). One outcome of gene induction studies is stability across the lifespan. A second potential outcome is a decreased magnitude of the peak level of induction with aging. A third alternative is that the same magnitude of induction is achieved, but the latency to the peak response is delayed relative to the response in young organisms. The fourth outcome is that both magnitude and latency are modified. The literature on decreased protein turnover with aging (discussed above) is consistent with the hypothesis that impaired gene regulation is responsible for aging; RNA synthesis is similarly reported to decline with age (reviewed in Reff, 1985 and Danner & Holbrook, 1990). Theoretically, a slower rate of RNA synthesis, if uniform, would slow the rate of mRNA increase in response to an environmental challenge, delaying induction. Delayed rates of induction might also diminish magnitude if the immediate signal invoking increased RNA polymerase activity wanes rapidly, before maximal levels of transcripts are achieved. Conversely, decreased rates of protein (and potentially RNA) degradation may further hinder the capacity of cells to rapidly respond if decreased activity of a protein is the response required to maintain homeostasis; it will take longer for a shut off of transcription/translation to result in lower levels of gene product.

While the scenario described above is enticing, the available evidence suggests that extranuclear factors are usually responsible for changes in gene regulation following environmental challenge. A few examples serve to illustrate this point. In the section on endocrine theories of aging above, two examples of altered gene regulation that are secondary to endocrine system changes are described. The age-related decline in $\alpha 2$U-globulin in male rat liver is secondary to declines in testosterone and declines in liver androgen receptors during aging. Similarly, the induction of tyrosine aminotransferase by cold exposure is diminished with age, but this is secondary to diminished elevations of corticosterone caused by the cold exposure in old mice. Importantly, direct injections of glucocorticoid causes similar inductions at all ages, indicating the nuclear machinery for up-regulating this gene is intact (Finch, Foster & Mirsky, 1969).

Blake et al. (1991) confirmed that increased ambient temperature up-regulated the HSP70 heat shock RNA family to a lesser extent in old rats. However, these researchers carefully monitored the colonic temperature of the young and aged rats, and found that aged rats increased colonic temperature less than young rats when challenged with the same elevation of ambient temperature. When the data were corrected for the amount of change in colonic temperature, there was no age-related difference in the heat shock response with age. Thus, here the alteration in gene induction was secondary to an increased capacity to maintain thermostasis in the older rats when challenged with increased ambient temperatures. Potentially, this resides in the lower volume to surface area ratio of the older, heavier rats.

Hobbs et al. (1993) examined the induction in cytokine gene expression after activation of CD4+ T cells. CD4+ spleen cells were isolated from young and old mice and activated in vitro with antibodies directed against CD3. The induction of RNA for IL-2, TNFα and TNF-β were not different in cells from young and old mice, nor were there changes in the secretion of these lymphokines. However, the induction of RNA for IL-3, IL-4, IL-5 and IFN-gamma, and the secretion of these lymphokines was diminished in cells from old mice. Critically, these authors also examined the subtypes of CD4+ cells in the different age groups. T cells from old mice had a higher proportion of cells expressing large quantities of the CD44 antigen. The expression of this marker is thought to identify memory T cells rather than CD44-negative naive or virgin cells. When CD4+ T cells were separated into CD44 high and CD44 low subpopulations, the CD44 high population was found to have diminished induction of IL-3, IL-5 and IFN-gamma, even when obtained from young rats. Thus, rather than representing an age-related change in gene regulation, the age-related changes in lymphokine induction in activated T cells are secondary to a gradual shift in the subpopulations present within the CD4+ population of cells over the lifespan.

These examples represent three mechanistically distinct cases where diminished gene induction with aging is secondary to age-related changes other than the transcriptional apparatus. These data dictate that future studies documenting changes in gene regulation with aging carefully dissect the phenomenon to determine whether the transcriptional response to the immediate stimulus (steroid hormone levels; intracellular second messengers) are similarly modified, or whether the age-related defect is upstream in the information pathway.

ENHANCED INDUCTION OF GLIAL MARKERS
IN RESPONSE TO MODEST SYNAPTIC
DEAFFERENTATION IN AGED RODENT BRAIN

The author's laboratory has an enduring interest in the regulation of brain function with aging. Some of this effort has focused on nonneuronal cells, specifically astrocytes and microglia. With aging, there is increased steady state expression of glial fibrillary acidic protein (GFAP) in astrocytes, and the MHC class II antigen (recognized by the antibody OX6) in microglia. Conversely, several other astrocyte marker proteins and the microglial complement receptor 3 do not change with age (Goss, Finch & Morgan, 1991; Gordon & Morgan, 1991; 1992).

Some of these glial markers react to brain injury; O'Callaghan & Jensen (1992) have proposed that GFAP is a universal marker of neuronal damage, and one of the most sensitive available. The reactions of nonneuronal cells have been frequently suggested to play a role in the functional reorganization that occurs after brain injury. Hence, we investigated the induction of these markers after brain injury during aging.

Our first studies examined the hippocampus in mice with knife cuts of the fornix. This experimental preparation was chosen because the transection would produce a modest deafferentation of the target structure (loss of 10–15% of synapses; analogous to usual aging changes) that should be of the same magnitude in animals of all ages (neurotoxins, for example, are notorious for producing greater damage in old animals). Preliminary studies confirmed that knife cuts produced unilateral loss of 90% of the acetylcholinesterase staining in hippocampus, and established that peak induction of GFAP RNA in 7 month-old mice occurred between two and four days, and returned to baseline between eight and 16 days (Goss & Morgan, 1993). The increase in GFAP RNA in the hippocampus was bilateral, even though the cholinesterase staining demonstrated unilateral deafferentation. In the striatum, near the transection site, the GFAP RNA increase was confined to the lesioned side of the brain.

We next performed a time course study in mice of 3, 14 and 23 months of age. The time points were 0 (unlesioned controls), two, five, and 10 days (because of mortality in quarantine, the 10 day point was not examined for the 23 month-old group). The RNA for GFAP, S-100 protein, glutamine synthetase, apolipoprotein E, clusterin and amyloid precursor protein were measured by in situ hybridization. In hippocampus, young mice exhibited a slight increase in GFAP RNA at two days after transection which returned to baseline at days 5 and 10. In 14 month-old mice, the elevations were present at both two and five days, before returning to baseline at 10 days. The oldest mice showed the greatest elevations in GFAP RNA, and this was present at five days after the transection. Only a slight increase was observed at two days. A similar pattern of GFAP induction, with the greatest elevations found in old mice and intermediate inductions in middle aged mice, was also observed in the striatum, although this elevation was strictly unilateral. Another important difference between the striatum and hippocampus was that the striatal induction in the old mice was apparent two days after the transection, much like the young mice, while the hippocampal increase was delayed relative to the young animals (Goss & Morgan, 1995). Thus, the aged mice appeared to generate an exaggerated response to the stimulus of modest deafferentation (roughly 10% of synapses) regarding GFAP RNA induction. Clusterin RNA and apolipoprotein E RNA were induced at the site of the transection. These RNAs continued to increase up to 10 days after transection, and were induced to the same extent in mice of different ages. S-100, glutamine synthase and amyloid precursor protein RNAs were not modified by the transection.

A second deafferentation study was initiated to generalize these findings. In this experiment, F344 rats of 6, 15 and 24 months were lesioned unilaterally with 6-hydroxydopamine in the nigrostriatal pathway. Rats were killed at 0 (unlesioned controls), 2, 4, 7 and 14 days. Similar to the fornix transection, this lesion also produces a modest (10%) deafferentation of the ipsilateral striatum. The completeness of the lesions was determined by tyrosine hydroxylase (TH) immunostaining of the striatum and nigra. These stains revealed virtually complete loss of striatal immunostaining for this marker of dopaminergic synapses in rats of all ages. Cell counts in the nigra confirmed the uniformity of dopaminergic neuron loss at all ages.

Striatal sections were next immunostained for GFAP, S-100, complement receptor 3 and MHC class II antigen. The GFAP data confirmed the results in the mouse study using fornix transections (Figure 24.1). In the young rats, GFAP immunostaining (quantified by densitometric image analysis) increased slightly at four and seven days, but returned to baseline values at 14 days. In the oldest rats, GFAP immunostaining was elevated slightly at two days, substantially at four and seven days, and continued to increase at 14 days. The middle-aged rats were again intermediate, with elevations peaking between four and seven days, and returning near baseline by 14 days. No effects of the lesion were observed in the contralateral striatum. As in the mouse study, S-100 protein, another astrocyte marker, was unaffected by the lesion or aging.

Microglial activation, monitored with an antibody directed against the MHC class II antigen (OX-6), was absent in young rats, and only slightly elevated above baseline at seven days in middle aged rats. However, in the old rats, the immunostaining for MHC-II increased dramatically up to 14 days (Figure 24.2). Conversely, the immunostain signal for the complement receptor 3 stained with antibody OX-42 was not induced at any age by this modest deafferentation signal. Similar to the astrocyte results, no changes in microglial staining characteristics were observed contralateral to the lesion.

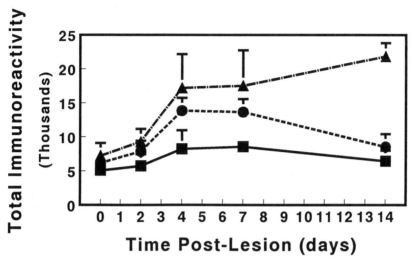

Figure 24.1. Striatal GFAP immunoreactivity ipsilateral to nigrostriatal bundle lesions. Rats of 6, 15 or 24 months were injected with 8 μg 6-hydroxydopamine into the nigrostriatal bundle slightly anterior to the ventral tegmental area (A10). Rats were perfused under pentobarbital anesthesia with freshly prepared 3.7% paraformaldehyde (in phosphate buffer, pH 7.4) and post-fixed for 24 hours. Twenty micron frozen sections were stored at 4°C in PBS until used for immunocytochemistry. Sections were incubated in primary antibody overnight and with peroxidase conjugated secondary antibody for 30 minutes. Reaction with diaminobenzidine was for 5 minutes. Immunoreaction product was quantified by micro-densitometry using a true color image analysis system. Hue, saturation and intensity (HSI) thresholds for positive identification of reaction product were established at the beginning of each analysis session using four calibration slides which spanned the range of reaction product intensities found in the experimental sections. The identification thresholds were then held constant throughout the analysis session. Both the area of positive reaction product and the density of the reaction product were measured and summed to produce a measure of total immunoreactivity for each field (integrated optical density is the summed optical density of all pixels within the HSI segment representing positive immunoreactivity). Four striatal fields from 4 sections from each rat (16 measurements) were averaged to produce the datum for that brain region. Total n in each group is equal to the number of rats (5–6) not the number of measurements. The value for aged rats significantly exceeded the value for young rats at 4, 7 and 14 days; and the value for middle aged rats at 14 days (P < 0.05 or 0.01).

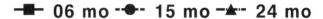

MHC Class II Antigen Immunoreactivity (Ipsilateral)

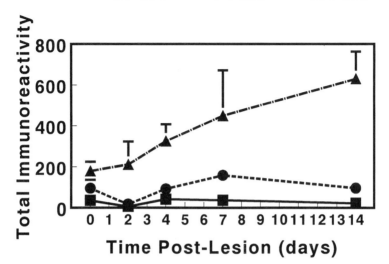

Figure 24.2. MHC Class-II antigen immunoreactivity ipsilateral to nigrostriatal bundle lesions. Sections from the experiment described in Figure 24.1 were similarly reacted with antibody OX-6. Total immunoreactivity (integrated optical density) in the aged rats exceeded the young rats at 2, 4, 7 and 14 days. The values for the aged rats exceeded the values for the middle aged rats at 2, 4, and 14 days.

Together, these studies develop a picture of an altered reactivity of aged brain to modest deafferentation of the type which might occur gradually with usual aging, occasionally at sites deafferented by stroke or other trauma, or progressively in degenerative diseases such as Alzheimer's or Parkinson's diseases. Under these circumstances, the aged brain appears to generate an exaggerated response, compared to young rodents, with middle-aged animals producing an intermediate response. Specifically, the reponse involves up-regulation of markers of reactivity (GFAP, MHC class II antigen) without substantial proliferation of cells, as evidenced by the failure of constitutive markers for astrocytes and microglia to changes in these studies. While it is impossible to make direct comparisons, the mouse transection model examining hippocampal RNA gave qualitatively similar results as the rat 6-hydroxy-dopamine lesion model examining striatal immunostaining. The common features of these models involve modest deafferentation (10% loss of synapses) using lesions located distal from the site being examined. The common result is that glia in aged animals exhibit larger reactions (not involving proliferation) to the deafferentation. It is tempting to speculate that these exaggerated reactions may relate to the diminished functional recovery observed after brain injury in aged organisms, but this issue still needs to be addressed in subsequent experimentation.

From the perspective of the present review, these data indicate that induction of RNA and protein is not necessarily diminished with age. Clearly, examples are available that not only similar, but even larger inductions of protein and RNA can be observed in aged rats relative to young rats. The progressive nature of the change in induction, with middle-aged rats displaying intermediate responses enhances the probability that this is a eugeric age-related phenomenon and not secondary to late life disease. In addition to changes in latency and/or magnitude of induction, these data introduce duration as another parameter of induction which might be modified with age. In the rat study described above, the duration of increase in the GFAP and MHC markers far outlasted any elevations observed in younger rats. In fact, the greatest values were observed at the longest time points. A similar increased duration of a response in aged rats was reported for blood corticosterone elevation produced by immobilization stress in aged rats (Sapolsky, Krey & McEwen, 1986). It is unlikely that a similar corticosterone response underlies these data, as corticosterone down-regulates GFAP immunoreactivity in rats (O'Callaghan, Brinton & McEwen, 1989, but it should be recognized that failure to turn off a response may be just as debilitating as failure to initiate a response. The examination of lymphokines in this or similar models may identify other regulators of GFAP which might mediate the exaggerated reaction to deafferentation in aged rodents.

CONCLUSIONS

Molecular changes that are observed in aged organisms may arise for a number of reasons. One impetus for pursuing such studies is to identify causal mechanisms responsible for the phenomena of aging, the manipulation of which might modify the aging process. A number of candidate mechanisms for the 'prime mover' of aging have been proposed, but none have fulfilled all the criteria necessary for this role. Increasingly, it is unlikely that any single mechanism will fulfill this putative function.

General changes in protein and RNA synthesis are intriguing potential mediators of the phenomena of aging. The scenario of increased residence time (half life) of proteins and cognate mRNAs during aging, allowing damaging agents (oxygen radical, glucose, etc.) greater impact on the functional status of these molecular populations could explain most changes observed with mammalian aging at even a physiological and organismic level. General changes in macromolecular synthetic and degradation rates might also explain diminished and delayed regulation of gene expression with aging, further contributing to reduced homeostatic capacity. Unfortunately, consistent, generalized changes in macromolecular biosynthesis have been difficult to document. In the absence of universally accepted methodology for the measurement of macromolecular synthesis rates, it is difficult to embrace this hypothesis fully. Nevertheless, this issue deserves continuing scrutiny as more sophisticated methodologies are developed.

Changes in the regulation of specific genes observed with aging have in many instances been found to involve extranuclear factors rather than modified transcription or translation capacity. Changes in cell populations or sensitivity to hormones with aging often underlie changes in gene regulation, and the identification of increased inducibility of some genes (GFAP) indicates that reduced synthetic rates are not universal concomitants of aging.

There are a number of well-described changes in physiological systems with aging, and generalized declines in homeostatic capacity. In addition, there are generally accepted changes in hormonal status which have been identified. Changes in cell function are believed to underlie these organismic level changes, and, following reductionist logic, molecular changes should be found which are responsible for the changes in cells, tissues and systems. However, as of this time, the molecular changes which are observed appear secondary to the physiologic and hormonal changes, rather than vice-versa. The search continues for a fundamental molecular change which directs the subsequent phenomena. Importantly, this form of Thomist reductionism need not apply. Aging may indeed be a hodgepodge of accumulated evolutionary pleiotrophisms, lacking common molecular determinants, but resulting in similar physiological changes in many organisms, primarily because of similar advantages conferred during development, maturation and reproduction. The frustrations, thus far, in identifying a unitary cause of aging, either molecular, hormonal or physiological, lead to this conclusion in an apologetic manner. Nevertheless, the quest will continue by describing even more age-related phenomena and attempting to intervene in the aging process with agents testing specific hypotheses of aging.

REFERENCES

Ames, B. N., Shigenaga, M. K. & Hagen, T. M. (1993) Oxidants, antioxidants and the degenerative diseases of aging. *Proceedings of the National Academy of Science of the USA*, **90**, 7915–22.

Blake, M. J., Fargnoli, J., Gershon, D. & Holbrook, N. J. (1991) Concomitant decline in heat-induced hyperthermia and HSP70 mRNA expression in aged rats. *American Journal of Physiology*, **260**, R663–R667.

Cerami, A. (1985) Hypothesis: glucose as a mediator of aging. *Journal of the American Geriatrics Society*, **33**, 626–34.

Cook, L. L. & Gafni, A. (1988) Protection of phosphoglycerate kinase against in vitro aging by selective cysteine methylation. *Journal of Biological Chemistry*, **263**, 13991–3.

Cortopassi, G. A. & Arnheim, N. (1990) Deletion of a specific mitochondrial DNA in tissues of older humans. *Nucleic Acids Research*, **18**, 6927–33.

Cutler, R. G. (1982) The dysdifferentiation hypothesis of mammalian aging and longevity. In Giacobini, E. (ed.) *The Aging Brain: Cellular and Molecular Mechanisms of Aging in the Nervous System.* New York: Raven Press, pp. 1–19.

Danner, D. B. & Holbrook, N. J. (1990) Alterations in gene expression with aging. In Schneider, E. L. & Rowe, J. (eds.) *Handbook of the Biology of Aging.* San Diego: Academic Press, pp. 97–115.

Davidson, E. H. (1986) *Gene Activity in Early Development.* 3rd Edition. New York: Academic Press.

Deng, H. X., Hentani, A., Tainer, J., Iqbal, Z., Cayabyab, A., Hung, W.-Y., Getzoff, E. D., Hu, P., Herzfeldt, B., Roos, R. P., Warner, C., Deng, G., Sorianao, E., Smyth, C., Parge, H. E., Ahmed, A., Roses, A. D., Hallewell, R. A., Pericak-Vance, M. A. & Siddique, T. (1993) Amyotrophic lateral sclerosis and structural defects in Cu, Zn superoxide dismutase. *Science*, **261**, 1047–51.

Esumi, H., Takahashi, Y., Makino, R., Sato, S. & Sugimura, T. (1985) Appearance of albumin producing cells in the liver of analbuminemic rats on aging and administration of carcinogens. *Advances in Experimental Biology and Medicine*, **190**, 637–50.

Finch, C. E. (1990) *Longevity, Senescence and the Genome.* Chicago: University of Chicago Press.

Finch, C. E., Foster, J. R. & Mirsky, A. E. (1969) Aging and the regulation of cell activities during exposure to cold. *Journal of General Physiology*, **54**, 690–712.

Finch, C. E. & Morgan, D. G. (1990) RNA and protein metabolism in the aging brain. *Annual Review of Neuroscience*, **13**, 75–87.

Gordon, M. N., Berg, D. G., Flores, C. M. & Morgan, D. G. (1990) Increased GFAP expression in aged rat brain revealed by quantitative immunohistochemistry. *Society for Neuroscience Abstracts*, **16**, 347.

Gordon, M. N. & Morgan, D. G. (1991) Increased GFAP expression in the aged rat brain does not result from increased astrocyte density. *Society for Neuroscience Abstracts*, **17**, 53.

Gordon, M. N., Myers, M. A., Perlmutter, L. S. & Morgan, D. G. (1992) Microglia of the aged rat brain. *Society for Neuroscience Abstracts*, **18**, 1488.

Goss, J. R., Finch, C. E. & Morgan, D. G. (1990) GFAP RNA increases during a wasting state in old mice. *Experimental Neurology*, **108**, 266–8.

Goss, J. R., Finch, C. E. & Morgan, D. G. (1991) Age-related changes in glial fibrillary acidic protein RNA in the mouse brain. *Neurobiology of Aging*, **12**, 165–70.

Goss, J. R. & Morgan, D. G. (1993) The effects of age on glial fibrillary acidic protein RNA induction by fimbria/fornix transection in mouse brain. *AGE*, **16**, 15–22.

Goss, J. R. & Morgan, D. G. (1995) Enhanced glial fibrillary acidic protein RNA response to fornix transection in aged mice. *Journal of Neurochemistry*, **64**, 1351–60.

Hastie, N. D., Dempster, M., Dunlop, M. G., Thompson, A. M., Green, D. K. & Allshire, R. C. (1990) Telomere reduction in human colorectal carcinoma and with aging. *Nature*, **346**, 866–8.

Heydari, A. R. & Richardson, A. (1992) Does gene expression play any role in the mechanism of the antiaging effect of dietary restriction? *Annals of the New York Academy of Science*, **663**, 384–95.

Hirsh, G. P., Popp, R. A., Francis, M. C., Bradshaw, B. S. & Bailiff, E. G. (1980) Species comparisons of protein synthesis activity. *Advances in Pathobiology*, **7**, 142–59.

Hobbs, M. V., Weigle, W. O., Noonan, D. J., Torbett, B. E., McEvilly, R. J., Koch, R. J., Cardenas, G. J. & Ernst, D. N. (1993) Patterns of cytokine gene expression by CD4+ T cells from young and old mice. *Journal of Immunology*, **150**, 3602–14.

Holliday, R. (1987) The inheritance of epigenetic defects. *Science*, **238**, 163–70.

Kristal, B. S. & Yu, B. P. (1992) An emerging hypothesis: Synergistic induction of aging by free radicals and Maillard reactions. *Journal of Gerontology*, **47**, B107–B114.

Lee, A. T. & Cerami, A. (1990) Modifications of proteins and nucleic acids by reducing sugars: Possible role in aging. In Schneider, E. L. & Rowe, J. (eds.) *Handbook of the Biology of Aging*. 3rd Edition. San Diego: Academic Press, pp. 116–30.

Mays-Hoopes, L. (1989) Development, aging and DNA methylation. *International Review of Cytology*, **114**, 118–20.

Migeon, B. R., Axelman, J. & Beggs, A. H. (1988) Effects of aging on reactivation of the human X-linked HPRT locus. *Nature*, **355**, 93–6.

Monnier, V. M., Sell, D. R., Nagaraj, R. H. & Miyata, S. (1991) Mechanisms of protection against damage mediated by the Maillard reaction in aging. *Gerontology*, **37**, 152–65.

Morgan, D. G. (1992) Neurochemical changes with aging: predisposition towards age-related mental disorders. In Birren, J. E., Sloane, R. B. & Cohen, G. D. (eds.) *Handbook of Mental Health and Aging*. 2nd Edition. San Diego: Academic Press, pp. 175–200.

Morgan, D. G. & Finch, C. E. (1988) Dopaminergic changes in the basal ganglia. *Annals of the New York Academy of Science*, **515**, 145–60.

Morgan, D. G. & May, P. C. (1990) Age-related changes in synaptic neurochemistry. In Schneider, E. L. & Rowe, J. W. (eds.) *Handbook of the Biology of Aging*. 3rd Edition. New York: Academic Press, pp. 219–54.

Mori, N., Mizuno, D. & Gato, S. (1979) Conservation of ribosomal fidelity during aging. *Mechanisms of Ageing and Development*, **10**, 379–98.

Nichols, N. R., Osterburg, H. H., Masters, J. N., Millar, S. L. & Finch, C. E. (1990) Messenger RNA for glial fibrillary acidic protein is decreased in rat brain following acute and chronic corticosterone treatment. *Molecular Brain Research*, **7**, 1–7.

Noy, N., Schwartz, H. & Gafni, A. (1985) Age-related changes in the redox status of rat muscle cells and their role in enzyme aging. *Mechanisms of Ageing and Development*, **296**, 63–9.

O'Callaghan, J. P., Brinton, R. E. & McEwen, B. S. (1989) Glucocorticoids regulate the concentration of glial fibrillary acidic protein throughout the brain. *Brain Research*, **494**, 159–61.

O'Callaghan, J. P. & Jensen, K. F. (1992) Enhanced expression of glial fibrillary acidic protein and the cupric silver degeneration reaction can be used as sensitive and early indicators of neurotoxicity. *Neurotoxicology*, **13**, 113–22.

Orgel, L. E. (1963) The maintenance of the accuracy of protein synthesis and its relevance to aging. *Proceedings of the National Academy of Science of the USA*, **49**, 512–17.

Orr, W. C. & Sohal, R. S. (1994) Extension of lifespan by overexpression of superoxide dismutase and catalase in Drosophila Melanogaster. *Science*, **263**, 1128–30.

Popp, R. A., Bailiff, E. G., Hirsch, G. P. & Conrad, R. A. (1976) Errors in human hemoglobin as a function of age. *Interdisciplinary Topics in Gerontology*, **9**, 209–18.

Rao, G., Xia, E., Nadakavukaren, M. J. & Richardson, A. (1990) Effects of dietary restriction on the age-dependent changes in the expression of anti-oxidant enzymes in rat liver. *Journal of Nutrition,* **120**, 602–9.

Reff, M. E. (1985) RNA and protein metabolism. In Finch, C. E. & Schneider, E. L. (eds.) *Handbook of the Biology of Aging.* 2nd Edition. New York: Van Nostrand, pp. 225–54.

Roy, A. K., Nath, S. T., Motwanee, N. M. & Chattergee, B. (1983) Age-dependent regulation of the polymorphic forms of alpha-2-u globulin. *Journal of Biological Chemistry,* **258**, 10123–7.

Sapolsky, R. M., Krey, L. & McEwen, B. (1986) The neuroendocrinology of stress and aging: The glucocorticoid cascade hypothesis. *Endocrine Reviews,* **7**, 284–301.

Sato, A. I., Schneider, E. L. & Danner, D. B. (1990) Aberrant gene expression and aging: examination of tissue-specific mRNAs in young and old rats. *Mechanisms of Ageing and Development,* **54**, 1–12.

Semsie, I., Rao, G. & Richardson, A. (1989) Changes in the expression of superoxide dismutase and catalase as a function of age and dietary restriction. *Biochemical and Biophysical Research Communications,* **164**, 620–5.

Slagboom, P. E. & Vijg, J. (1992) The dynamics of genome organization and expression during the aging process. *Annals of the New York Academy of Science,* **673**, 58–69.

Thakur, M. K., Oka, T. & Natori, Y. (1993) Gene expression and aging. *Mechanisms of Ageing and Development,* **66**, 283–98.

Timiras, P. S. (1988) *Physiological Basis of Geriatrics.* New York: Macmillan.

van Leeuwen, F., van der Beek, E., Seger, M., Burbach, P. & Ivell, R. (1989) Age-related development of a heterozygous phenotype in solitary neurons of the homozygous Brattleboro rat. *Proceedings of the National Academy of Science of the USA,* **86**, 6417–20.

Wareham, K. A., Lyon, M. F., Glemister, P. H. & Williams, E. D. (1987) Age-related reactivation of an X-linked gene. *Nature,* **327**, 725–7.

Wellinger, R. & Guigoz, Y. (1986) The effect of age on the induction of tyrosine amino transferase and tryptophan oxygenase genes by physiological stress. *Mechanisms of Ageing and Development,* **34**, 203–17.

Yuh, K. C. & Gafni, A. (1987) Reversal of age-related effects in rat muscle phosphoglycerate kinase. *Proceedings of the National Academy of Science of the USA,* **84**, 7458–62.

25 Commentary **Biological bases for plasticity during aging of individual life histories**

CALEB E. FINCH

INTRODUCTION

This chapter considers issues raised in the three chapters that addressed mechanisms in brain aging, but also draws from the other presentations. A major theme of this book is the mechanisms or pacemakers that govern the timing of life history stages and that may set limits on the range of phenotypic variations, including the duration of a particular stage. Collectively, these variations represent plasticity.

To introduce the following discussion of plasticity in mammalian life histories, I give two examples that indicate the breadth of plasticity (Bateson, Chapter 1; Finch, 1990). The Atlantic and Pacific salmon have subpopulations of males ('jacks') that mature a year early and, despite their small size, are effective in mating by being able to sneak around the larger males. In the case of social insects, even more diverse life histories arise from the same genotype and batch of eggs. Honeybee castes include very long-lived queens that can live at least five years; short-lived workers that can live two months, if born in the Spring; and workers that survive to the next Spring, if born later in the summer. These and many other examples support the concept that plasticity in life history recurs throughout the animal and plant kingdoms, to which human life history is no exception. In many species, the nervous and endocrine systems have fundamental roles in determining behaviors that expose individuals to various opportunities and risks (Finch & Rose, 1995; Mobbs & Finch, in press).

However, *some* boundary values on plasticity must derive from constitutional features of the body plan, but also the particular genes that an individual carries. Constitutional constraints on life history trajectories represent biology in a general sense, such as the limited capacity for regeneration of appendages and nondividing neurons, as found in all adult birds and mammals. Constitutional constraints also include the characteristics of individuals that are determined by how the environment interacts with genes. Ultimately, the upper limit to the human lifespan is determined by the accelerations of mortality that seem to be remarkably similar in populations that, nevertheless, differ widely in the incidence of specific diseases (Finch et al., 1990; Finch, Pike & Witten, 1990, pp. 16 & 161), for example, breast cancer (Henderson, Tomlinson & Gibson, 1984). Inquiry into these questions is helped by examining life history from a broad perspective that includes population biology concepts on how natural selection interacts with aging.

DOMAINS IN HUMAN LIFE HISTORY

The major functionally distinct phases of the human life history can be considered as two major domains: development and adult, each of which has four discrete phases (Figure 25.1, 25.2). *Development* includes two prefertilization phases of the oocyte in the grandmother and mother, respectively (Figure 25.2); the fetal and postnatal phases (Figure 25.1). *Adult* includes the young adult, parental, midlife, and frail phases. Each of these phases has a range of values that endows the individual life history with considerable, but not absolute plasticity (Figure 25.1). While it may seem trivial to recall that allelic differences may influence the duration or functions of any of these stages, even in genetically identical organisms like the inbred flies, worms, and mice of developmental biologists, individuals display variations in the timing of major events during postnatal development and aging, for example, the maximum individual adult lifespan in the worm *Caenorhabditis* is typically more than twice the mean (Johnson, 1987). Sources of these and other non-genetic variations will be considered later. The following discussion is not comprehensive, but aims to give examples that trace influences between

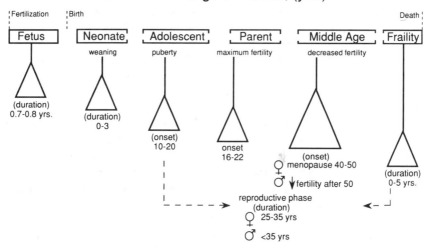

Post Fertilization Domains of Life History
Normative Range of Values, (yrs.)

Figure 25.1. The major temporal domains of the human lifespan, beginning with the prefertilization phases of the oocyte. (Original figure by author.)

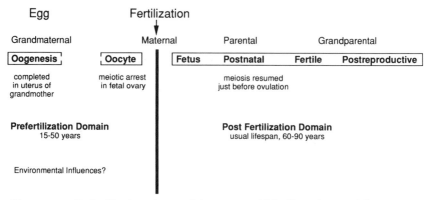

Figure 25.2. Prefertilization phases of the oocyte which allow the possibility, so far unproven, of environmental influences on an individual before fertilization in either the grandmother's uterus or in the maternal ovary. (Original figure by author.)

the different mammalian life phases that influence the range of outcomes during aging.

Prefertilization phases

Virtually all mammals lack *de novo* oogenesis after birth, that is, no new eggs are differentiated as cells after birth, with a few possible exceptions in prosimians (Finch, 1990: 154–5, 165). This important biological feature of mammalian reproduction appears to have existed for at least 85 million years and may be an evolutionarily primitive trait that was already established in the early ancestors of mammals (Figure 25.3). Oocytes remain in an arrested state of meiosis in the ovary, from before birth until the oocyte and its surrounding follicle are stimulated during reproductive cycles to complete cell maturation.

The standard concept of mammalian life history neglects the potential for environmental influences before fertilization. In fact, the human egg or oocyte has already existed for at least 15 years in most individuals (the earliest usual first pregnancy), because oocytes are formed before birth. Thus, the egg that gave rise to each of us was formed in our mother while she existed as a fetus in our *grandmother* (Figure 25.2).

The extended prefertilization life of the oocyte may be subject to distinct environmental influences during the pregnancy of the grandmother and then during the postnatal life of the mother before the egg is finally fertilized (Figure 25.2). This means that for a typical maternal age of 25 years, the

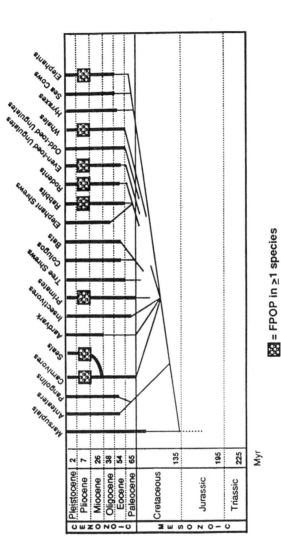

Myr

= FPOP in ≥1 species

Figure 25.3. The taxonomic distribution of fixed oocyte pools in placental mammals. The lines with boxes represent mammalian orders in which at least one species has shown the absence of de novo oogenesis as adults and has shown evidence of menopause or its equivalent through the age-related depletion of oocytes. From Finch (in press), originally published in vom Saal et al., 1994. The occurrence of fixed oocyte pools in orders that phylogenetically separated more than 80 million years ago suggests that this developmental trait is evolutionarily primitive in mammals.

oocyte existed about five months in the grandmother and then 24 years in the mother. The primary oocyte of mammals is a small cell (diameter of 20 μ in humans and 10 μ in mice). Studies on mice show that protein synthesis occurs at a very low, but definite level (Wasserman & Albertini, 1994). DNA synthesis is arrested in the chromosomes, but probably not in the few self-replicating mitochondria that are present. One may suppose that the primary oocyte has an inventory of enzymes that repair damage from ever-present free radicals that inevitably arise from oxidative metabolism. There may be limits, however, on the capacity for repair. For example, maternal smoking induces chemical changes in placental DNA, that is, in cells which are derived from embryonic membranes (Everson et al., 1986); there is no information on whether smoking alters the DNA of the ovary within the fetus, however.

The first examination of this extended maternal prefertilization phase for environmental effects resulted from this symposium. Conversations between this author and John Loehlin stimulated an examination of maternal age effects on within-pair variance in several behavioral traits in MZ versus DZ twins. While no age effects were found that might reflect maternal environmental influences on the oocyte, further inquiry is warranted. The strong maternal age effect on the increased risk of Down syndrome and other chromosomal anomalies may turn out not to be due to oocyte age *per se* (pp. 496–7, below).

Prematurational phases

The fetus

The duration of gestation is relatively fixed in humans, with less variation than observed in some other mammals that can delay implantation of the fertilized egg for extended times. For example, mice can delay implantation (preimplantation diapause) during nursing for longer than the gestational period itself, about three weeks. The record for diapause is held by the long-nosed armadillo, in which it lasts at least four years (Storrs, Burchfield & Rees, 1989). Humans do not appear to have the capacity for delayed implantation and the normative gestation length is 280 days with a range of ± 12 days.

Fertilization of the egg initiates the life history of the individual as genetically defined. Environmental factors can influence the conceptus even before implantation and organogenesis, including with regards to infections. The best characterized effects of the maternal environment have been shown later in gestation, when maternally derived hormones, nutrients, and toxins can cause major perturbations in the health of the fetus. Familiar examples are syndromes caused by exposure to diabetes during pregnancy, which can predispose to childhood obesity (Silverman, Landsberg & Metzer, 1994) and may dispose to later onset diabetes and numerous sequelae that increase morbidity and mortality, for example hypertension, stroke and arthritis. The converse, inadequate nutrition during pregnancy causes neonates to have subnormal birth weights. To resolve maternal and fetal effects of malnutrition, Zamenhof, Von Marthens & Grauel (1972) cross-fostered rats that were born from malnourished dams and observed that the brain cell number (DNA content) remained below normal up to two generations later. It was hypothesized that the pups had deficient nursing behavior, which stunted their development, with consequences for the next generation.

The gender of the neighboring fetus ('fetal position effects') has quantitative effects on adult reproductive behavior in gerbils, mice, and rats (vom Saal et al., 1994). Females flanked by males (2M females) have longer intervals between ovulation as young adults than do females flanked by females (0M females). Moreover, 0M females show an earlier loss of fertility during aging and more masculine behaviors (vom Saal & Moyer, 1985). These striking alternate reproductive phenotypes are the result of different exposures to sex steroids *in utero* and are also found in males. Furthermore, vom Saal, Finch & Nelson (1994) describe fetal position effects on prostate development that might be factors in outcomes of hypertrophy and hyperplasia during prostate aging, by their influence on the sensitivity of the prostate to sex steroids. These examples from rodents demonstrate how subtle differences in sex steroid levels during development can influence outcomes of aging.

Human twins may show an analogous phenomenon, a subtle sex difference of auditory function in which the cochlea emits weak 20 decibel tones that are more common in females than males. McFadden (1993) found that female twins with a female co-twin emitted more 20 decibel tones than when the co-twin was male. Fetal testosterone may be involved, since it is much higher in males than females towards the end of the first trimester when the cochlea had developed.

The role of fetal testosterone in other features of human brain development is unknown, although there is ample evidence for the importance of fetal androgens in the sexual differentiation of the hypothalamus in rodents (Gorski Chapter 16). As described by Goy (Chapter 15), primates are also subject to influences on behavior from prenatal exposure to sex steroids. The relatively rare sexual differentiation syndromes caused by maternal androgens, for example, the adrenogenital syndromes, cause abnormal morphogenesis of the genitalia that can be corrected, but effects on neuroanatomy or behavior are not known.

Postnatal phases

As an example of postnatal experience that influences outcomes in aging, handling of infant rats has effects on the regulation of glucocorticoids in adults that in turn appear to cascade into hippocampal damage during aging. In a thyroid-dependent mechanism, neonatally handled rats show briefer elevations of corticosterone in response to restraint stress as young adults (Meany et al., 1988; Sapolsky, 1992). The implied greater lifetime exposure to corticosterone was associated with greater hippocampal neuron loss in old age. This important study complements observations that astrocytic hyperactivity is correlated with elevations of corticosterone and that hippocampal neuron loss and astrocytic hyperactivity can be reduced in old rats that are adrenalectomized and allowed to age with little exposure to corticosterone (Landfield, 1994).

Differences in reactivity of human infants that predict later childhood behavior (Kagan, Chapter 19) may be influenced by genetic factors. The putative association or reactivity with particular cranio-facial features with different neural connectivity would be consistent with hereditary influences on neural crest cell migration, since many cranio-facial anatomical components are of neural crest origin.

Adult domains

Puberty

In all mammals, sexual maturation can occur over a wide range of times. By the time of birth, the external genitalia are formed and can respond to elevations of sex steroids that induce genital enlargement, hair, and so on. In rare cases, menarche can occur as early as the first month after birth. The physiological capacity for reproduction is also present far earlier than the usual age of puberty. In Escomel's famous case, a 5 year-old girl became pregnant and was delivered of a normal baby by Cesarean section (Wilkins, 1965). Precocious puberty can result from brain injuries, e.g. tumors that impinge on the pineal (Kitay & Altschule, 1964). The early postnatal competence of sex steroid target organs to respond to hormones gives an enormous plasticity in the timing of puberty. Evolutionary considerations suggest that the timing of sexual maturation must be coordinated with the environment, in order to optimize reproduction with respect to nutrition, social circumstances, and so on. If puberty were timed by a rigidly programmed pacemaker, this would be maladaptive in evolutionary terms if nutrition or social conditions were unfavorable. In most animals, neural and hormonal processes coordinate developmental and adult life history transitions with the environment (Finch & Rose, 1995).

The historical trend for faster growth of children and earlier puberty by several years during the last 200 years in Europe as publicized by Tanner (1962) may nevertheless have varied widely depending on local conditions (Bullough, 1981). Earlier puberty most likely represents the response to improved environment through the reductions of childhood disease and better diet, rather than a genetic change. The normative range of menarche over the past 200 years spans at least 10 years (Figure 25.1). According to a current view, the puberty is sensitive to some metabolic or hormonal correlate of growth through a hypothetical regulator, the 'sommatometer' (Plant, 1994). Neural loci by whatever name are located in the brain, in regions of the hypothalamus and limbic system that regulate the pulsatile secretion of GnRH. Increases of frequency and amplitude during puberty drive the pituitary production of gonadotropins, and that, in turn, increase sex steroid production by the ovary or testis.

The timing of puberty has important influences on the outcomes of adolescence. Magnusson (1988) has shown that girls with relatively early menarche tend to seek peers on the basis of their biological stage rather than chronological age, thereby curtailing a phase of childhood. The earlier maturing girls tend to marry earlier, start families and are less apt to continue their education, at least during the child-rearing phase of their lives. In view of the inverse association of the extent of education with later risks of Alzheimer's disease, as found in populations from Asia, Europe and North America (Katzman, 1993; Stern et al., 1994), a prediction is that early puberty, by truncating education, will prove to be a risk factor for cognitive dysfunctions later in life. Another delayed outcome of the age of puberty is the greater risk of breast cancer in women with earlier menarche (Pike et al., 1983).

Midlife

Females. As described above, the ovary has a fixed number of primary oocytes by birth in humans and most other mammals. By the time of puberty, more than 50% are already lost through a poorly understood process of follicular atresia. The rate of loss resembles radioactive decay, with a fixed proportion of primary oocytes disappearing each year. As the ovary approaches depletion during maternal aging, menstrual cycles lengthen and eventually cease at menopause. Menopause occurs naturally between 40 to 55 years, which spans an even wider range than does puberty (Gosden, 1985; vom Saal et al., 1994). Complete exhaustion of the oocytes is not accepted as the main factor in the timing of menopause (Richardson, Senikas & Nelson, 1987). Strains of mice with different numbers of oocytes at birth show corresponding differences in the age when oocytes are depleted (Faddy, Gosden & Edwards, 1983).

The ovary provides a pacemaker for the duration of the fertile period in women that depends on the rate of oocyte loss and that leads to menopause. The numbers of oocytes present at birth may be the main determinant of the age of menopause. In neonatal girls, the number of oocytes varies twofold between individuals (Figure 25.4). Because inbred mice with negligible residual heterozygosity show a similar range in the numbers of oocytes between individuals (Gosden et al., 1983; Faddy et al., 1983), it is not likely that genetic polymorphisms cause these variations. Nevertheless, genetic influences are clearly shown in inbred mice that differ between strains in the numbers of oocytes at birth (Faddy et al., 1983) and in the rate of loss during aging (Jones and Krohn, 1961).

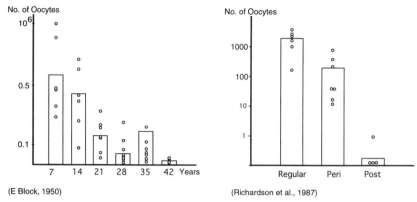

Figure 25.4. Variations in the numbers of primordial follicles (oocytes). Left panel, across the reproductive lifespan, redrawn from Block (1950). Right panel, surgical specimens from women aged 45–55 years, showing that follicles are depleted when cycles cease. (Redrawn from Richardson et al., 1987.)

However, the rate of oocyte loss is also subject to influences from the internal (hormonal) and external environment (nutrition). In rodents, removal of the pituitary (hypophysectomy) greatly shows the rate of oocyte loss (reviewed in Finch, 1990). Diet can also be a factor in outcomes of reproductive aging. Mice maintained on calorically restricted diets that extend the lifespan also have slowed loss of oocytes (Nelson, Gosden & Felicio, 1985). While calorically restricted diets generally improve the health of aging rodents and reduce the incidence of glycated and oxidized proteins (see Morgan and Gordon, Chapter 24), fertility is greatly reduced. When calorically restricted rodents are returned to *ad libitum* diets, fertility is regained at ages (18–23 months) that are far later than the usual age of the last litter (Nelson et al., 1985). These findings show a great plasticity in the aging of the reproductive system. Recent success in achieving fertility beyond 60 years (10 years after the usual age of menopause) shows that the uterus and the neuroendocrine support system for pregnancy and parturition are not on the same clock as the ovary.

The increase of the Down syndrome and other chromosomal anomalies with maternal age may also be a direct consequence of oocyte depletion that may also be open to intervention. Simulation of oocyte loss during aging by removing one ovary in young mice prematurely increased fetal chromosomal anomalies, as well as the loss of fertility (Brook et al., 1984). Conversely, it may be possible to reduce the risk of birth defects by hormonal interventions.

Another consequence of ovarian aging is the loss of estrogens after menopause. A benign outcome is that breast cancer risks tend to slow, because many abnormal growths in the breast and other reproductive tract loci are commonly estrogen-dependent (Henderson et al., 1994). On the other hand, there are adverse effects of menopause that can greatly restrict health in later years. Estrogen loss also accelerates the general trend for loss of bone mineral (Riggs & Melton, 1986), leading to osteoporosis and frequent spontaneous fractures that are a particular curse of aging in older Caucasian women (Cummings et al., 1985). Estrogen replacements are being used increasingly as an intervention to slow the loss of bone mineral. The combination of estrogen with progesterone, as used in combined oral contraceptives, may not only slow bone loss, but may reduce on an absolute basis the risk of reproductive tract tumors at later ages (Pike et al., 1983). There are also hints that estrogen may reduce the risk of Alzheimer's disease (Buckwalter et al., 1993; Henderson & Paganini-Hill, 1994), which would be consistent with the presence of estrogen receptors in the cholinergic projection neurons that supply most of the frontal cortex (Torran-Allerand et al., 1992). In summary, the fixed ovarian stock of oocytes and hormone producing follicles can be viewed as a pacemaker for health in women during later years. The vast clinical experience acquired during the last 30 years in sex steroid usage gives a major basis for future interventions.

Midlife in males. While men do not show an exact equivalent of menopause, there is a gradual decline in fecundity that has diverse causes (Finch, 1990, pp. 167–8). The prostate tends to become enlarged in almost all men by 65, which can directly and indirectly alter reproductive functions. While the risk of partial or complete impotence increases with age (Feldman et al., 1994), a sizable subgroup of older men maintain full sexual capacity. Paternity is documented into the nineties, at least 35 years after the oldest natural childbirth in women (Seymour, Duffy & Koerner, 1935). Testosterone tends to decline, as measured by average values as well as the frequency and amplitude of the ultradien pulses (Deslypere et al., 1987). The possible role of sex steroids in cognitive dysfunctions of men is unknown.

Midlife in general. Ongoing longitudinal studies of ages 30–64 show a remarkable diversity of social changes in men as well as women, for example, whether children are still living at home, the marital status, employment, and so on (the MacArthur Foundation Network in Successful Midlife Development, or MIDMAC). Except for the loss of fertility at menopause, there is no indication that any biological clock drives social transitions in the transition from young adult into later ages (Bumpass & Aquilino, 1995). A very positive change during midlife is the sharp decline of antisocial behavior (Rutter, Chapter 20). Among physiological changes that might be considered are decreased secretions of sex steroids by the gonads or the weak adrenal androgen DHEA (Finch, 1990: 187–8) or to the subtle declines of receptors for monoaminergic neurotransmitters that can be detected during middle age, as shown in collaborative studies with Bengt Winblad (Morgan, May & Finch, 1987).

Frailty

Midlife is also marked by increased the risk of numerous diseases (cancer, angina, hypertension, etc.) that underlie the exponential acceleration of mortality during midlife that is observed in all human populations (Jones, 1956; Finch et al., 1990). By the average lifespan and at later ages, it is common to have a phase of increasing frailty and dependence, due to diverse causes that include osteoporotic fractures, vascular impairments, and Alzheimer's disease. The epidemiology of frailty is incompletely documented. One survey indicates that more than 50 percent of one population aged 65 and older were in good health the year before their death (Brook, Gosden & Chandley, 1992). Thus, the existence of a senium or defined phase or morbidity before death at later ages may not be as clear as traditionally believed. Most people appear to age successfully, unless Alzheimer changes become prominent (Berkman et al., 1993). Observations that glial responses to experimental lesions are greater in older rodents (Morgan & Gordon, Chapter 24) may be a clue to the accelerating prevalence of Alzheimer changes after 60 years, since some glial activities are neurotoxic.

Maximum lifespan

The present lifespans for humans certainly exceed 110 years. According to the *Guinness Book of World Records* (Russell, 1987) Shigichio Izumi lived 120 years. The accelerations of mortality that occur throughout all populations during midlife at least into the eighth decade (Jones, 1956; Finch et al., 1990) *require* a statistical maximum lifespan in finite populations (Finch & Pike, in press). However, evidence that the acceleration slows at later ages beyond the average lifespan (Kannisto, 1994) could allow survival to even greater years. The remarkable demographic growth of age groups over 80 years throughout the world (Kannisto, 1994), if they prove to continue beyond 110 years, may challenge the lifespan records for humans. We will know within a human generation from now if the upper limit to lifespan was altered by technological progress as much as the life expectancy. As a biologist, I can not resist observing that the average and record lifespans for laboratory rodents have increased more than 50 percent in the last 30 years, due to better husbandry and optimized diet.

LIMITS OF GENETICS

The wide variability between individuals in the numbers of oocytes even at birth is at first sight contrary to expectations that variations between genetically similar individuals should be modest. The role of fluctuations in cell numbers is implicit. The phenomenon of developmental noise is well recognized by developmental biologists fluctuations in asymmetry, for instance, in the numbers of veins on the wings of flies on each side of the body, or the numbers of teeth on each side of the mouth in mice (Phelan & Austad, 1994). Inbreeding appears to generally increase developmental noise. An explanation of variable numbers of oocytes can be found in developmental mechanisms that determine cell lineages and cell type.

In mammals, like other vertebrates examined, embryogenesis is characterized by the lack of a rigid determination of cell type or cell fate. Cells migrate within the embryo over relatively large distances, as shown for the primordial germ cells that collect to form the gonads. Not all of these cells reach their destination and stragglers can be identified as ectopic germ cells that mostly disappear before puberty (Upadhyay & Zamboni, 1982). O'Leary (Chapter 2) describes the dispersal of clonally related cells by migration during brain development within a generalized protocortical map that does not precisely specify where each neuron will reside or what its connections will be. Beside some degree of imprecision in migration, the fate of cells also depends on its neighbors. In vertebrates, it is well established that many more neurons are produced for example, than survive – see chapters by O'Leary, Purves and Edelman & Tonini (Chapters 2, 8 and 9 respectively). The prominence of cell death on a large scale throughout development of vertebrates implies the necessity of trimming back excess cells and the 'exuberance' of excess connections (Changeaux, Chapter 6). For most other parts of nervous systems, there is no information on how much of this variation survives development, but some degree of variability, however, persists. Furthermore in the brain, there is a mystery about how different neurotransmitter receptor subunits become distributed and localized at their terminals (Changeaux, Chapter 6).

Some parts of the nervous system show a fixed probability at each division that one of the daughter cells will survive as a neuron. The distribution of numbers of neurons in a specialized neural organ of frogs, the lateral line system varies between locations in the same individual over a tenfold range (Winklbauer & Hausen, 1983) (Figure 25.5). Apparently in this organ, the survival of neurons is determined by a series of binary choices with a fixed probability, like a string of coin tosses (heads, the cell wins and survives; tails, the cell dies). The resulting distribution of neurons in the lateral line fits the binomial distribution. This situation contrasts with that in many invertebrates, like the worm *Caenorhabditis*, in which the lineage of every cell in the embryo and adult can be traced with great precision, a rigid process of cell determination that predestines which cells become neurons, for example, and which cells die. In this species, the total number of cells in the nervous system and other organs is almost invariant between individuals.

Surprisingly, there are very few studies to evaluate the extent of variations between individuals of neuron number in mammals. Two computer-based analyses of brains from neurologically healthy humans displayed the same

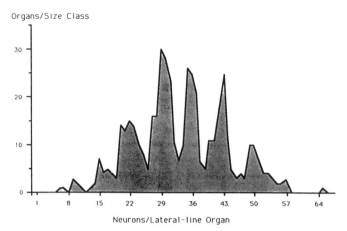

Figure 25.5. The distribution of numbers of neurons in a specialized neural organ of frogs, the lateral line system, in which there are tenfold differences in neuron number within the same individual. (Redrawn from Winklbauer and Hausen, 1983.)

range of variations, which were a remarkable $\pm 50\%$ range about the mean *between* individual adults (Henderson et al., 1980; West, 1993). In particular, highly accurate stereological methods showed that the numbers of neurons in the hippocampal formation did not change between 13 and 85 years in the granule neuron-, CA1-, or CA3-neuron layers. This range is consistent with the 10–20% coefficients of variation that may be calculated from almost any study on neuron density in vertebrates.

For neuron populations that are at risk for loss or irreversible damage during aging and diseases like Alzheimer's and stroke, the numbers of neurons in the hippocampus, for example, might set the threshold age of dysfunction. Similar arguments can be made for the neurons that regulate blood pressure in the brain stem, in which blood pressure fluctuations increased in proportion to the size of experimental lesions of the A2 neuron group (Talman, Snyder & Reis, 1980) (Figure 25.6). In contrast, the substantia nigra shows a much higher threshold for neuron loss before functions are compromised, as observed in Parkinsonism (Bernheimer et al., 1973).

Variations in neuron number are hypothesized by Edelman (1987: 58) as one of the sources of cytoarchitectonic variations that are a substrate for variations between individuals in neural circuitry, including cortical maps. In Chapter 16, Gorski comments on hypothalamic nuclei that show sex differences in numbers of neurons that are statistical trends and not absolute differences, which again implies some stochastic variations in neuron number. I wonder whether nonprogrammed variations in neuron number that influence neural circuit development could be a basis for deviant behavior during childhood or later.

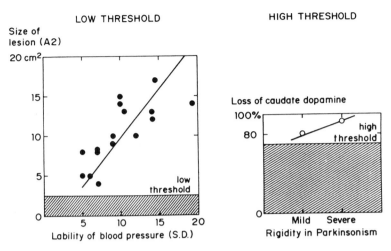

Figure 25.6. Brain regions differ in the extent of neuron loss that can be tolerated
before dysfunctions are manifest. One region with a low threshold for
loss is the brain stem A2 dopaminergic locus, in which even small lesions
cause fluctuations in blood pressure (Talman et al., 1980). In contrast,
the substantia nigra can withstand much greater loss of neurons
before major abnormalities are manifested (Bernheimer et al., 1973).
(Redrawn from Finch, 1990.)

Other insights are given by variations in oocyte numbers which are
available from inbred mice. Although allelic variations in genes clearly
influence the numbers of cells in adult vertebrates, the genetic determinants
appear to set the range of cell numbers for any type of cell, rather than an
absolute number. These variations could be a major substrate in the individual
variations of life history. At least for oocytes, there is a correspondence
between the numbers in the neonate and the age of ovarian depletion. Thus,
one of the most vital parameters of life, the age when fertility is lost at
menopause, appears subject to considerable non-genetic variability. It would
be valuable to know the degree of concordance shown by identical twins in
the age of menopause. An obvious hypothesis is that variations in the age of
puberty of identical twins in the same environment represents developmental
variations in the number of neurons, whereas variations in the age of menopause represents developmental variations in the numbers of ovarian oocytes.

This evidence suggests the need for another term to the standard equation
for sources of phenotypic variance that represents stochastic (unprogrammed)
variations in cell number V_{SVCN}. Stochastic variations in cell number are
themselves subject to genotypic (G) and environmental (E) factors, but should
be distinguished from G × E interactions that more typically represent
external environmental effects on gene expression.

$$V_{phenotype} = V_G + V_E + V_{G \times E} + V_{SVCN}$$

EVOLUTION AND AGING

The delay of many age-related dysfunctions until midlife or later can be rationalized by theory from population biology. A line of reasoning founded by Fisher, Haldane, Medawar, and Williams posited that the force of natural selection declines during aging for a simple reason (Rose & Finch, 1993; Bateson, Chapter 1). In the world of natural populations of animals and plants, attrition is always high because of dangers from predation, starvation, accidents and infections (Austad, 1994; Rose, 1991). Consequently, adult mortality rates are typically 5–25% per year for large animals and may be even greater for smaller ones. This high degree of attrition causes an exponential decline of survivors to later ages in natural populations. Consequently, most of the reproduction in natural populations is accomplished by young adults, with older individuals contributing proportionately less to the gene pool. In terms of population genetics, this high attrition of mature adults is considered equivalent to the statement that the 'force of natural selection declines during aging' (Rose, 1991). The argument is then made that the weaker force of natural selection on older individuals is permissive for the accumulation of genes in the population through spontaneous mutation that have delayed adverse effects. In general, a hereditary disease or dysfunction that emerges in later years will have little effect on the fitness of the individual because the main reproductive period has already occurred. This inductive argument has been developed in detail for various cases from the Euler–Lotka model of population growth:

$$\sum_{t=1}^{\infty} e^{-rt}s(t)f(t)\,\mathrm{d}t = 1,$$

where r is the Malthusian parameter of population growth for which the equation may be solved, given either the function or a range of values for $s(t)$ and $m(t)$; $s(t)$ is the proportion of the population surviving from birth to age t; $f(t)$ is the fecundity per individual at age t. The Euler–Lotka equation serves the role in population genetics of physicists' equations of state.

The lifespan *per se* is not viewed as contrained by evolutionary biologists, who point to the enormous range of lifespans in species of plants and animals, that vary over nearly a millionfold range (Finch & Rose, 1995). The reproductive schedule that is the foundation for the potential lifespan is considered to be a major focus of selection in life history evolution and is subject to quantitative variations in the onset of fertility, in the numbers born per mating, and in the intervals between mating. Each of these parameters are balanced against sources of mortality, such as the increased mortality that comes from reproduction *per se*. A well-studied example is the increased mortality observed in red deer that are nursing, where nutrient drain is considerable (Clutton-Brock, Albon & Guinness, 1988).

Predictions from the argument that the force of natural selection decline during aging are that adverse features of aging will tend to be caused by a variety of mutations. As Hardy describes (Chapter 23), at least three different chromosomes contain alleles that cause Alzheimer's disease. The loss of fertility at midlife due to ovarian oocyte depletion likewise would not have been selected against because so few individuals would be able to survive to that age range were it not for the many amenities of civilization. However, one should not ignore observations that some individuals survive to the grandparental generation in many wild populations, for example, elephants, chimpanzees and whales (Finch, 1990: 166).

Besides the specific genes like those that cause Alzheimer's disease, there is no clear basis for selection against certain age-related diseases that are associated with physiological regulators. Sex steroid-dependent abnormal growths in the reproductive tract are a major class of delayed effects. A different example is the glycated proteins that can represent the nonenzymatic addition of endogenous glucose to long-lived proteins like collagen and elastin. The slow glycation processes may be pacemakers for certain age-related conditions that also appear more precipitant in type II diabetes, such as vascular disease and peripheral neuropathy (Vlassara, Bucala & Striker, 1994; Monnier et al., 1986; Kristal & Yu, 1992). The accumulation of glycated adducts is accelerated by diabetes and, in calorically restricted rodents, is slowed in association with lowered glucose (Reiser, 1994). For these delayed effects of sex steroids and glucose, there may be genotypic variations. Interventions are being tested that may reduce the impact of nonenzymatic glycation and of sex steroids.

Sex differences in gonadal changes during aging may be reconsidered here. In contrast to females, males of virtually all mammals maintain some degree of fertility throughout their lifespans. Several general features of the reproductive schedule fit with this trend. First, puberty in males tends to lag behind that of females in humans, as well as in many other mammals. Moreover, throughout the world, both men and women show clear preferences on the average for the age of the partner that favors slightly older males (Buss & Schmitt, 1993). A lively argument is underway on how this choice of partner age may be an evolutionary strategy, on the basis of the greater resources and mating efficacy of older and more experienced males. Such concepts are familiar to field biologists and imply genes that influence these behavioral outcomes, a very controversial topic. It seems plausible to recognize the importance of the reproductive schedule as a major target of evolution that also influences life expectancy and that, in the case of humans, may have led to a statistically earlier age of infertility in women than men.

DETERMINANTS OF NEURAL PLASTICITY DURING AGING

The capacity for learning in adults becomes reduced during aging even in individuals who are generally healthy, as Baltes (Chapter 22) has shown so convincingly in testing the limits of memory. This lowered ceiling for learning implies a reduction in neural plasticity, through mechanisms that may include synaptic remodelling. The brain even in Alzheimer's disease retains some capacity for synaptic remodelling, as shown by the compensatory sprouting of fibers in the hippocampal afferents that is apparently triggered by degeneration of afferents from the perforant path (Geddes et al., 1985). These local homeostatic attempts to compensate for massive neurodegeneration during Alzheimer's disease, however, do not prevent the progression of cognitive impairments. While the prevalence of familial forms of Alzheimer's disease is high (Hardy, Chapter 23), sporadic forms may be almost as common (Farrer, 1993). It may be said that a major cause of the loss of neural plasticity during aging is predestined by genes that cause neurodegeneration directly through familial Alzheimer's disease or through vascular syndromes that may also be genetic risk factors. Because the apolipoprotein E4 (apoE4) allele is associated with heart attacks as well as cerebrovascular disease (Hardy, Chapter 23), it is currently unclear as to whether apoE4 also promotes primary neurogeneration. Testing the limits of memory by training, as in the Baltes' paradigm, may prove to be a probe for incipient Alzheimer's disease or neurovascular impairments. The protective role of higher education against cognitive dysfunctions at later ages that was discussed above (p. 495) suggests that plasticity at later ages may be improved by training in the earlier years.

Besides the extreme but selective neurodegeneration observed during Alzheimer's disease, during more usual aging there is also a general trend in neurologically normal individuals for atrophy of large neurons in the hippocampus and frontal cortex (reviewed in Finch & Morgan, 1990; Finch, 1993). Neuron atrophy has often been mistaken in the past for neuron loss. However, the atrophy of some neurons in aging rats can be reversed by treatment with nerve growth factor (NGF) (Fischer et al., 1991; reviewed in Finch, 1993). Together with the evidence for compensatory sprouting in Alzheimer's disease (Geddes et al., 1985), these responses to NGF imply a considerable preservation of nerve cell functions throughout the lifespan.

In contrast to the trends for neuronal atrophy, other brain cells, the glia, show increased activity. Astrocytes are the best studied and were long-recognized to become hyperactive during normal aging in rats and humans, in the absence of obvious neurodegeneration (Nichols et al., 1993; Morgan & Gordon, Chapter 24). The age-related hyperactivity of astrocytes can be modified by manipulating glucocorticoids, as described above. Caloric restriction also blunts the age-related astrocytic activity, as measured by the cytoskeletal protein, glial fibrillary acidic protein (Nichols et al., 1995; Major et al., 1994). Some of the possible genetic controls on the promotor of this gene (Figure 25.7) indicate the integration of multiple hormonal and inflammatory axes (Laping et al., 1994a,b). We are studying the production of

A. Putative Response Elements in GFAP Genes

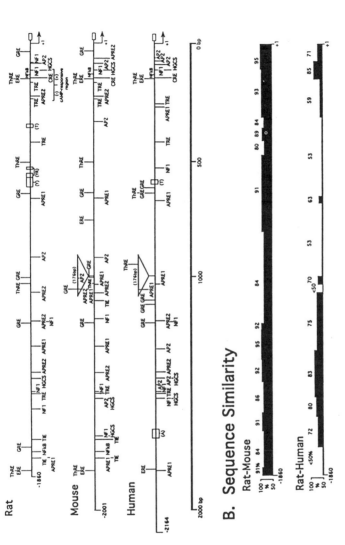

B. Sequence Similarity

Figure 25.7. Comparison of the 5′-upstream sequences of the gene for glial fibrillary acidic protein (GFAP) in humans, mice, and rats to show the organization of putative hormone response elements (redrawn from Laping et al., 1994a). We suspect that the similar clusters of response elements in these species represent integrated control regions that are sensitive to multiple hormone and inflammatory mediators, e.g. the cluster at 1200 nt in human, rat, and mouse, that contains one or more GRE (glucocorticoid response element), ThRE (thyroid hormone response element), and APRE1/2 (acute phase response element-2). This non-coding region is also highly conserved in these species that diverged more than 80 million years ago. It can be ruled out from such comparisons that these similarities resulted from convergent evolution.

complement proteins that are found in senile plaques during Alzheimer's disease (Johnson et al., 1992; Pasinetti et al., 1992), but are also expressed during normal brain development (Johnson et al., 1994). Here again, normal mechanisms in the repair of injury and tissue homeostasis may have delayed adverse effects during aging.

One basis for the profound effects of caloric restriction may be the reduced blood glucose and slower accumulation of glycation adducts observed in rats. My lab is investigating the hypothesis that glycated adducts of long-lived brain proteins stimulate microglia and astrocytes to release various cytokines. Glycated adducts occur in the senile plaques and neurofibrilliary tangles of Alzheimer brains (Smith et al., 1994; Vitek et al., 1994; Yan et al., 1994) and could be a general substrate for macrophage-mediated inflammatory mechanisms during aging as well as Alzheimer's disease. The progressive age-related accumulation of glycated proteins in the brain and elsewhere may set some upper limit on plasticity.

CONCLUSIONS

I have argued that there is enormous plasticity in outcomes of aging and that aging is not at all rigidly programmed. More than one mechanism may serve as the rate pacemaker for aging changes in any tissue, from the ovary, to the blood vessels, to the brain. Profound influences from development can be traced in rodents to the outcomes of aging. Stochastic fluctuations in cell number are a major determinant in the age when fertility is lost and could be of great significance to the threshold for dysfunction in the brain. Other hormonal influences during pregnancy have influences on adult rodents and humans, of which diabetes is a strong example. The ultimate source of plasticity is the maintenance of the inventory of genes, or the genomic totipotency which is thought not to vary between most somatic cells of young adults. The progressive age-related accumulation of glycated proteins in the brain and other tissues may, nevertheless, set some upper limit on plasticity. Meanwhile, the extensive manipulation of aging changes and risks of age-related diseases through hormones and nutrition give many targets for intervention.

REFERENCES

Austad, S. N. (1994) Menopause: an evolutionary perspective. *Experimental Gerontology*, **29**, 255–63.

Berkman, L. F., Seeman, T. E., Albert, M., Blazer, D., Kahn, R., Mohs, R., Finch, C., Schneider, E., Cotman, C., McClearn, G., Nesselroade, J., Featherman, D., Garmezy, N., McKhann, G., Brim, O., Prager, D. & Rowe, J. (1993) High, usual, and impaired functioning in community-dwelling older men and women: findings from The MacArthur Foundation Research Network on Successful Aging. *Journal of Clinical Epidemiology*, **46**, 1129–40.

Bernheimer, H., Birkmayer, W., Hornykiewicz, O., Jellinger, K. & Seitelberger, F. (1973) Brain dopamine and the syndromes of Parkinson and Huntington: clinical, morphological, and neurochemical correlations. *Journal of the Neurological Sciences*, **20**, 415–55.

Block, E. (1950) Quantitative morphological investigations of the follicular system in women. *Acta Anatomica*, **14**, 108–23.

Brock, D. B., Holmes, M. B., Foley, D. J. & Holmes, D. (1992) Methodological issues in a survey of the last days of life. In Wallace, R. B. & Woolson, B. F. (eds.) *The Epidemiologic Study of Aging*. New York: Oxford University Press, pp. 315–32.

Brook, J. D., Gosden, R. G. & Chandley, A. C. (1984) Maternal aging and aneuploid embryos: evidence from the mouse that biological and not chronological age are the important influence. *Human Genetics*, **66**, 41–5.

Buckwalter, J. G., Sobel, E., Dunn, M. E., Diz, M. E. & Henderson, V. W. (1993) Gender differences on a brief measure of cognitive functioning in Alzheimer's disease. *Archives of Neurology*, **50**, 757–60.

Bullough, V. L. (1981) Age at menarche: a misunderstanding. *Science*, **213**, 365–6.

Bumpass, L. & Acquilino, W. S. (1995) A social map of midlife: family and work over the middle life course. The John D. and Catherine T. MacArthur Foundation Research Network on Successful Midlife Development. Gilbert Brim Director. 1625 Tenth Avenue, Vero Beach, Fl 32960.

Buss, D. M. & Schmidt, D. P. (1993) Sexual strategies theory: an evolutionary perspective on human mating. *Psychol. Rev.*, **100**, 204–32.

Clutton-Brock, T. H., Albon, S. D. & Guinness, F. E. (1988) *Reproductive Success: Studies of Individual Variation in Contrasting Breeding Systems*. Chicago: University of Chicago Press.

Cummings, S. R., Kelsey, J. L., Nevitt, N. C. & O'Dowd, K. H. (1985) Epidemiology and osteoporosis and osteoporotic fractures. *Epidemiologic Reviews*, **7**, 178–208.

Deslypere, J. P., Kaufman, J. M., Vermeulen, T., Vogelaers, D., Vandalem, J. L. & Vermeulen, A. (1987) Influence of age on pulsatile luteinizing hormone release and responsiveness of the gonadotrophs to sex hormone feedback in men. *Journal of Clinical Endocrinology and Metabolism*, **64**, 68–73.

Edelman, G. M. (1987) *Neural Darwinism*. New York: Basic Books.

Everson, R. B., Randerath, E., Santella, R. M., Cefalo, R. C., Avitts, T. A. & Randerath, K. (1986) Detection of smoking-related covalent DNA adducts in human placenta. *Science*, **231**, 54–7.

Faddy, M. J., Gosden, R. J. & Edwards, R. G. (1983) Ovarian follicle dynamics in mice: a comparative study of three inbred strains and in F1 hybrid. *Journal of Endocrinology*, **96**, 23–33.

Farrier, L. (1993) Neurogenetics of aging. In *Clinical Neurology of Aging,* 2nd edn. New York: Oxford University Press, pp. 136–58.

Feldman, H. A., Goldstein, I., Hatzichristou, D. G., Krane, R. J. & McKinlay, J. B. (1994) Impotence and its medical and psychosocial correlates: results of the Massachusetts male aging study. *Journal of Urology*, **151**, 54–61.

Finch, C. E. (1990) *Longevity, Senescence and the Genome,* 2nd edn. Chicago, Ill.: University of Chicago Press.

Finch, C. E. (1993) Neuron atrophy during aging: programmed or sporadic? *Trends in Neurosciences*, **16**, 104–10. Corrigenda: aged dogs, space, and scissors. *Trends in Neurosciences*, **16**, 352.

Finch, C. E. & Morgan, D. G. (1990) RNA and protein metabolism in the aging brain. *Ann. Rev. Neurosci.*, **13**, 75–87.

Finch, C. E., Pike, M. C. & Witten, M. (1990) Slow mortality rate accelerations during aging in animals approximate that of humans. *Science*, **249**, 902–5.

Finch, C. E., Laping, N. J., Morgan, N. E., Nichols, N. R. & Pasinetti, G. M. (1993) Hypothesis: Transforming growth factor β1 is an organizer of responses to neurodegeneration. *Journal of Cell Biochemistry*, **53**, 314–22.

Finch, C. E. & Rose, M. R. (1995) Hormones and the physiological architecture of life history evolution. *Quarterly Review of Biology*, **70**, 1–52.

Finch, C. E. & Pike, M. C. (in press) Maximum life-span predictions from Gompertz mortality model. *Journal of Gerontology*.

Fischer, W., Björklund, Chen, K. & Gage, F. H. (1991) NGF improves spatial memory in aged rodents as a function of age. *Journal of Neuroscience*, **11**, 1889–906.

Geddes, J. W., Monaghan, D. T., Cotman, C. W., Lott, I. T., Kim, R. C. & Chui, H. C. (1985) Plasticity of hippocampal circuitry in Alzheimer's disease. *Science*, **230**, 1179–81.

Gosden, R. G. (1985) *The Biology of Menopause*. San Diego, Calif.: Academic Press.

Gosden, R. G., Laing, S. C., Felicio, L. S., Nelson, J. F. & Finch, C. E. (1983) Imminent oocyte exhaustion and reduced follicular recruitment mark the transition to acyclicity in aging C57BL/6J mice. *Biology of Reproduction*, **28**, 255–60.

Henderson, B. E., Pike, M. C. & Ross, R. K. (1984) Epidemiology and risk factors In Bonadonna, G. (ed.) *Breast Cancer, Breast Cancer: Diagnosis and Management*. New York: John Wiley, p. 15–33.

Henderson, G., Tomlinson, B. E. & Gibson, P. H. (1980) Cell counts in human cerebral cortex in normal adults throughout the life-span using an image analyzing computer. *Journal of Neurological Sciences*, **46**, 113–36.

Henderson, V. W. & Paganini-Hill, A. (1994) Oestrogens and Alzheimer's disease. in Asch, R. & Studd, J. (eds.) *Annual Progress in Reproductive Medicine, Vol. 2*. Lancashire: Parthenon.

Johnson, S. A., Lampert-Etchells, M., Rozovsky, I., Passinetti, G. & Finch, C. E. (1992) Complement mRNA in the mammalian brain: responses to Alzhemier's disease and experimental lesions. *Neurobiology of Aging*, **13**, 641–648.

Johnson, S. A., Pasinetti, G. M. & Finch, C. E. (1994) Expression of complement C1qB and C4 mRNAs during rat brain development. *Developmental Brain Research*, **80**, 163–74.

Johnson, T. E. (1987) Aging can be genetically dissected into component processes using long-lived lines of Caenorhabdtis elegans. *Proceedings of the National Academy of Science of the USA*, **84**, 3777–81.

Jones, H. B. (1956) A special consideration of the aging process, disease and life expectancy. *Advances in Biological and Medical Physics*, **4**, 281–337.

Jones, E. C. & Krohn, P. L. (1961) The relationships between age, numbers of oocytes, and fertility in virgin and multiparous mice. *Journal of Endocrinology*, **21**, 469–96.

Jones, H. B. (1956) A special consideration of the aging process, disease, and life expectancy. *Advances in Biological and Medical Physics*, **4**, 281–337.

Kannisto, V. (1994) *Development of Oldest-Old Mortality, 1950–1990: Evidence from 28 Developed Countries*. Odense University Press, Denmark.

Katzman, R. (1993) Education and the prevalence of dementia and Alzheimer's disease. *Neurology*, **48**, 13–20.

Kitay, J. I. & Altschule, M. D. (1964) *The Pineal Glans: A Review of the Physiological Literature*. Cambridge, Mass.: Harvard University Press.

Kristal, B. S. & Yu, B. P. (1992) An emerging hypothesis: synergistic induction of aging by free radicals and Maillard reactions. *Journal of Gerontology*, **47**, B107–B114.

Landfield, P. W. (1994) The role of glucocorticoids in brain aging and Alzheimer's disease: an integrative physiological hypothesis. *Experimental Gerontology*, **29**, 3–11.

Laping, N. J., Teter, B., Nichols, N. R., Rozovsky, I. & Finch, C. E. (1994a) Glial fibrillary acidic protein: regulation of expression by hormones, cytokines, and growth factors. *Brain Pathology*, **4**, 259–75.

Laping, N. J., Morgan, T. E., Nichols, N. R., Rozovsky, I., Young-Chan, C., Zarow, C. & Finch, C. E. (1994b) Transforming growth factor-β1 induces neuronal and astrocyte genes: Tubulin α1, glial fibrillary acidic protein, and clusterin. *Neuroscience*, **58**, 563–72.

Magnusson, D. (1988) *Individual Development from an Interactional Perspective: a Longitudinal Study*. Hillsdale, NJ.: Erlbaum.

Major, D. E., Kesslak, J. P., Cotman, C. W., Finch, C. E. & Day, J. R. (1994) Life-long dietary restriction attentuates age-related increases in glial fibrillary acidic protein (GFAP) mRNA in the rat hippocampus. *Society Neuroscience Abstract*, **20**, 50.

McFadden, D. (1993) A masculinizing effect on the auditory systems of human females have male co-twins. *Proceedings of the National Academy of Science of the USA*, **90**, 11900–904.

Meaney, M. J., Aiken, D. H. & Bhatnagar, S., Van Berkel, C. & Sapolsky, R. M. (1988) Postnatal handling attenuates neuroendocrine, anatomical and cognitive impairments related to the aged hippocampus. *Science*, **238**, 766–8.

Mobbs, C. V. & Finch, C. E. (in press) Cumulative costs of reproduction as a mechanism in neuroendocrine aging in vertebrates. *Frontiers in Neuroendocrinology*.

Money, J. & Ehrhardt, A. (1921) *Man and Woman, Boy and Girl*. Baltimore, Md.: Johns Hopkins University Press.

Morgan, D. G., May, P. C. & Finch, C. E. (1987) Dopamine and serotonin systems in human and rodent brain: effects of age and degenerative disease. *Journal of the American Geriatric Society*, **35**, 334–45.

Monnier, V. M., Vishwanat, V., Frank, K. E., Elmets, C. A., Dauchot, P. & Kohn, R. R. (1986) Relation between complications of type I diabetes mellitus and collagen-linked fluorescence. *New England Journal of Medicine*, **314**, 403–8.

Nelson, J. F., Gosden, R. G. & Felicio, L. S. (1985) Effect of dietary restriction on estrous cyclicity and follicular reserves in aging C57BL/6J mice. *Biology of Reproduction*, **32**, 512–22.

Nichols, N. R., Day, J. R., Laping, N. J., Johnson, S. A. & Finch, C. E. (1993) GFAP mRNA increases with age in rat and human brain. *Neurobiological Aging*, **14**, 421–9.

Nichols, N. R., Finch, C. R. & Nelson, J. F. (1995) Food restriction delays the age-related increases of GFAP mRNA in rat hypothalamus. *Neurobiology of Aging*, **16**, 105–10.

Pasinetti, G. M., Johnson, S. A., Rozovsky, I., Lampert-Etchells, M., Morgan, D. G., Gordon, M. N., Morgan, T. E., Willoughby, D. A. & Finch, C. E. (1992) Complement mRNA responses to lesioning in rat brain. *Experimental Neurology*, **118**, 117–25.

Phelan, J. P. & Austad, S. N. (1994) Selecting animal models of human aging: inbred stains often exhibit less biological uniformity than F1 hybrids. *Journal of Gerontology*, **49**, B1–B11.

Pike, M. C., Krailo, M. D., Henderson, B. E., Casagrande, J. T. & Hoel, D. G. (1983) 'Hormonal' risk factors, 'breast tissue age', and the age-incidence of breast cancer. *Nature*, **303**, 767–70.

Plant, T. M. (1994) Puberty in primates. In Knobil, E. & Neill, J. D. (eds.) *The Physiology of Reproduction, Vol. 2*, 2nd edn. New York: Raven Press, pp. 453–85.

Reiser, K. M. (1994) Influence of age and long-term dietary restriction on enzymatically mediated crosslinks and nonenzymatic glycation of collagen in mice. *Journal of Gerontology*, **49**, B71–B79.

Richardson, S. J., Senikas, V. & Nelson, J. F. (1987) Follicular depletion during the menopausal transition: Evidence for accelerated loss and ultimate exhaustion. *Journal of Clinical Endocrinology and Metabolism*, **65**, 1231–7.

Riggs, B. L. & Melton, J. L. III (1986) Involutional osteoporosis. *New England Journal of Medicine*, **314**, 1676–85.

Rose, M. R. (1991) *The Evolutionary Biology of Aging*. Oxford: Oxford University Press.

Rose, M. R. & Finch, C. E. (1993) *Genetics of Aging, Genetica (Special Issue)*, *Vol. 91*.

Russell, A. (ed.) (1987) *Guinness Book of World Records*. New York: Sterling Publishing Co.

Sapolsky, R. M. (1992) *Stress, the Aging Brain, and Mechanics of Neuron Death*. Cambridge, Mass.: MIT Press.

Seymour, F. I., Duffy, C. & Koerner, A. (1935) A case of authenticated fertility in a man of 94. *Journal of American Medical Association*, **105**, 1423–4.

Silverman, B. L., Landsberg, L. & Metzger, B. E. (1994) Fetal hyperinsulinism in offspring of diabetic mothers. Association with the subsequent development of diabetes. In Williams, C. L. & Sue, Y.-S. Kim (eds.) Prevention and Treatment of Childhood Obesity. *Annals of New York Academy of Sciences*, **699**, 36–45.

Smith, M. A., Taneda, S., Richey, P. L., Miyata, S., Sayre, L. M., Monnier, V. M. & Perry, G. (1994) Advanced Maillard reaction end products are associated with Alzheimer disease pathology. *Proceedings of the National Academy of Science of the USA*, **91**, 5710–14.

Stern, Y., Gurland, B., Tatemichi, T. K., Tang, M. X., Wilder, D. & Mayeaux, R. (1994) Influence of education and occupation on the incidence of Alzheimer's disease. *Journal of American Medical Association*, **271**, 1004.

Storrs, E. E., Burchfield, H. P. & Rees, R. J. W. (1989) Reproduction delay in the common long-nosed armadillo, Dasypus novemcintus L. In Redford, H. & Eisenberg, J. F. (eds.) *Advances in Neotropical Mammalogy*. Gainesville, Fla.: Sandhill Crane, pp. 535–48.

Talman, W. T., Snyder, D. & Reis, D. J. (1980) Chronic lability of arterial pressure produced by destruction of A2 catecholamine neurons in rat brain stem. *Circulation Research*, **46**, 842–53.

Tanner, J. M. (1962) *Growth at Adolescence*, 2nd edn. Oxford: Blackwell.

Torran-Allerand, C. D., Miranda, R. C., Bentham, W. D., Sohrabji, F., Brown, T. J., Hochberg, R. B. & MacLusky, N. J. (1992) Estrogen receptors colocalize with low-affinity nerve growth factor receptors in cholinergic neurons of the basal forebrain. *Proceedings of the National Academy of Science of the USA*, **89**, 4668–72.

Upadhyay, S. & Zamboni, L. (1982) Extopic germ cells: natural model for the study of germ cell differentiation. *Proceedings of the National Academy of Science of the USA*, **79**, 6584–88.

Vitek, M. P., Bhattacharya, K., Glendening, M. J., Stopa, E., Vlassara, H., Bucala, R., Manogue, K. & Cerami, A. (1994) Advanced glycation end products contribute to amyloidosis in Alzheimer's disease. *Proceedings of the National Academy of Science for the USA*, **91**, 4766–70.

Vlassara, H., Bucala, R. & Striker, L. (1994) Biology of disease: Pathogenic effects of advanced glycosylation: biochemical, biological and clinical implications for diabetes and aging. *Laboratory Investigation*, **70**, 138–54.

vom Saal, F. S., Finch, C. E. & Nelson, J. F. (1994) The natural history of reproductive aging in humans, laboratory rodents, and selected other vertebrates. In Knobil, E. (ed.) *Physiology of Reproduction, Vol. 2*, 2nd edn. New York: Raven Press, pp. 1213–314.

vom Saal, F. S. & Moyer, C. L. (1985) Prenatal effects on reproductive capacity during aging in female mice. *Biology of Reproduction*, **32**, 1111–26.

Wasserman, P. M. & Albertini, D. F. (1994) The mammalian ovum. In Knobil, E. & Neill, J. D. (eds.) *The Physiology of Reproduction, Vol. 1,* 2nd edn. New York: Raven Press, pp. 79–122.

West. M. J. (1993) Regionally specific loss of neurons in the aging human hippocampus. *Neurobiology Aging*, **14**, 287–93.

Wilkins, L. (1965) *The Diagnosis and Treatment of Endocrine Disorders of Childhood and Adolescence*, 3rd edn. Springfield, Ill.: C. C. Thomas.

Winklbauer, R. & Hausen, P. (1983) Development of the lateral line system in *Xenopus laevis*. II. Cell mutiplication and organ formation in the supraorbital system. *Journal of Embryology and Experimental Morphology*, **76**, 283–96.

Yan, S. D., Chen, X., Schmidt, A.-M., Brett, J., Godman, G., Zou, Y.-S., Scott, C. W., Caputo, C., Frappier, T., Smith, M. A., Perry, G., Yen, S.-H. & Stern, D. (1994) Glycated tau protein in Alzeimer's disease: A mechanism for induction to oxident stress. *Proceedings of the National Academy of Sciences*, **91**, 7787–95.

Zamenhof, S., Von Marthens, E. & Grauel, L. (1972) DNA cell number and protein in rat brain. Second generation (F2) alteration by maternal (Fo) dietary restriction. *Nutrition and Metabolism*, **14**, 262–70.

Index